DIAGNOSTIC RADIOLOGY IN SMALL ANIMAL PRACTICE

2nd Edition

5m Books

DIAGNOSTIC RADIOLOGY IN SMALL ANIMAL PRACTICE

2nd Edition

Edited and translated by

Silke Hecht

5m Books

First published 2008

This edition published by 5m Books Ltd 2020

Authorized translation of the second German language edition of Silke Hecht, Röntgendiagnostik in der Kleintierpraxis © 2008 by Schattauer GmbH, Stuttgart, Germany

Published by

5m Books Ltd,
Lings, Great Easton,
Essex, CM6 2HH, UK
www.5mbooks.com

A catalogue record for this book is available from the British Library.

ISBN 9781789180930
Book layout by Toynbee Editorial Services Ltd, Great Easton, UK
Printed by Replika Press Pvt Ltd, India
Photos and illustrations by Schattauer

Important note:
Medicine is an ever-changing science, so the contents of this publication, especially recommendations concerning diagnostic and therapeutic procedures, can only give an account of the knowledge at the time of publication. While utmost care has been taken to ensure that all specifications regarding drug selection and dosage and treatment options are accurate, readers are urged to review the product information sheet and any relevant material supplied by the manufacturer, and, in case of doubt, to consult a specialist. From both an editorial and public interest perspective, the publisher welcomes notification of possible inconsistencies. The ultimate responsibility for any diagnostic or therapeutic application lies with the reader.

No special reference is made to registered names, proprietary names, trademarks, etc. in this publication. The appearance of a name without designation as proprietary does not imply that it is exempt from the relevant protective laws and regulations and therefore free for general use.

Contents

Preface

It is hard to believe that more than 10 years have passed since the publication of the first German language edition of this diagnostic radiology textbook. This English version represents a translation of the second, extensively revised edition. Even though advanced imaging modalities (ultrasound, CT and MRI) continue to gain importance in veterinary medicine, the radiographic examination remains a mainstay in the diagnostic workup of small animal patients. Veterinarians in small animal practice, specialty hospitals and academia alike are routinely asked to interpret radiographs, and competence in radiographic diagnosis is expected from non-radiologist specialists in their area of expertise (surgeon, internist, neurologist, etc.). The primary goal of this book is to provide veterinary students, practitioners and specialists with a comprehensive overview of radiographic findings in diseases of small animal and exotic patients, including both common and more unusual conditions. In addition, information is provided on basic radiology principles and physics, artefacts, practical radiation safety, radiographic contrast procedures, and basic principles and applications of advanced imaging technologies. Hopefully, readers will find this book to be an interesting, educational and helpful resource for clinical practice and teaching.

I would like to thank my co-authors for their contributions, the staff members of Schattauer (now Thieme) for their support with the two prior German editions, and Sarah Hulbert and Alessandro Pasini from 5m Publishing for their help in seeing this project through. Special thanks go to Marcy Souza for her assistance with editing the exotic animal chapters. I would also like to extend my deepest gratitude to Jenny Cattermole for her superb copyediting skills. Last but not least, I would like to thank my husband Bill for his encouragement and patience.

And now – enjoy the book!

Knoxville, September 2019

Silke Hecht

Contributors

Editor

Silke Hecht, Dr. med. vet., DACVR, DECVDI
Department of Small Animal Clinical Sciences
University of Tennessee College of Veterinary Medicine
2407 River Drive
Knoxville, TN 37996, USA
shecht@utk.edu

Authors

William H. Adams, DVM, DACVR (R, RO)
Department of Small Animal Clinical Sciences
University of Tennessee College of Veterinary Medicine
2407 River Drive
Knoxville, TN 37996, USA
wha@utk.edu

Alexandra Böhler, Dr. med. vet.
University of Veterinary Medicine
Diagnostic Imaging
Veterinärplatz 1
1210 Vienna, Austria
alexandra.boehler@vetmeduni.ac.at

Gregory B. Daniel, DVM, MS, DACVR
Virginia–Maryland Regional College of Veterinary Medicine
205 Duck Pond Drive, Phase II (0442)
Blacksburg, VA 24061, USA
gdaniel@vt.edu

Randi Drees, Dr. med. vet., PhD, DACVR (R, RO), DECVDI add RadOncol, PGCertAP, MRCVS
Royal Veterinary College
Hawkshead Lane
Hatfield, Hertfordshire
AL9 7TA, United Kingdom
rdrees@rvcac.uk

Michaela Gumpenberger, Dr. med. vet.
University of Veterinary Medicine
Diagnostic Imaging
Veterinärplatz 1
1210 Vienna, Austria
Michaela.Gumpenberger@vetmeduni.ac.at

Jasmin Hassan, Dr. med. vet.
Rustenschacherallee
1020 Vienna, Austria
jasmin.hassan@gmx.net

George A. Henry, DVM, DACVR
Department of Small Animal Clinical Sciences
University of Tennessee College of Veterinary Medicine
2407 River Drive
Knoxville, TN 37996, USA
gahenry@mac.com

Eberhard Ludewig, Prof. Dr. med. vet., DECVDI
University of Veterinary Medicine
Diagnostic Imaging
Veterinärplatz 1
1210 Vienna, Austria
ludewig@vetmed.uni-leipzig.de

Federica Morandi, DVM, MS, DECVDI, DACVR
Department of Small Animal Clinical Sciences
University of Tennessee College of Veterinary Medicine
2407 River Drive
Knoxville, TN 37996, USA
fmorandi@utk.edu

Dagmar Nitzl, Dr. med. vet., DECVDI
Hönggerstr. 27
8037 Zurich, Switzerland
dnitzl@gmx.net

Stefanie Ohlerth, Prof. Dr. med. vet., DECVDI
Clinic for Diagnostic Imaging
Vetsuisse Faculty, University of Zurich
Winterthurerstraße 260
8057 Zurich, Switzerland
sohlerth@vetclinics.uzh.ch

Jürgen Schumacher, Dr. med. vet., DACZM, DECZM
Department of Small Animal Clinical Sciences
University of Tennessee College of Veterinary Medicine
2407 River Drive
Knoxville, TN 37996, USA
jschumacher@utk.edu

Tobias Schwarz, Dr. med. vet., MA, DVR, DECVDI, DACVR, MRCVS
Department of Veterinary Clinical Studies
Royal (Dick) School of Veterinary Studies
The University of Edinburgh
Roslin, EH25 9RG, UK
tobias.schwarz@ed.ac.uk

Marcy Souza, DVM, MPH, DABVP (Avian), DACVPM
Department of Biomedical & Diagnostic Sciences
University of Tennessee College of Veterinary Medicine
2407 River Drive
Knoxville, TN 37996, USA
msouza@utk.edu

1

Basic radiology principles and interpretation

Silke Hecht and Eberhard Ludewig

1.1 Introduction

When inspecting and interpreting a radiograph two basic principles have to be considered.

- A radiograph produced either by exposing an X-ray film or a digital detector is an image of the patient resulting from partial transmission of the X-ray beam through the body with variable attenuation in different tissues. Generation of a useful radiograph requires the presence of structures and organs within the body which **attenuate X-rays** differently. If this was not the case, the outer margins of an object would still be visible as they contrast with the (more radiolucent) surrounding air, but an inner structure would not be recognizable (Fig. 1.1).
- A radiograph is a two-dimensional representation of a three-dimensional object. This results in artefacts and particularities the veterinarian has to be familiar with to be able to produce useful radiographs and interpret them correctly.

1.2 Nomenclature and image orientation

The correct description of a radiograph is based on the path of the X-ray beam through the patient from point of entrance to point of exit. For example, on a **ventrodorsal** radiograph the cassette or plate is located at the back of the patient, and the X-ray beam traverses the patient from ventral to dorsal. On a **dorsoventral** radiograph the beam path is reversed. On a **laterolateral** radiograph the X-ray beam traverses the patient either from left to right or from right to left. When obtaining a **mediolateral** view the X-ray beam enters the medial aspect of a body part and exits laterally (radiographs of extremities). As the terms 'laterolateral' and 'mediolateral' are cumbersome they are usually replaced with the simple term **lateral**. On a **right lateral** view the right side of the patient, and on a **left lateral** view the left side of the patient, is positioned adjacent to the X-ray plate.

A few special nomenclature rules apply to radiographs of the extremities and the head. While radiographic views proximal to the carpus and tarsus are termed **craniocaudal** or **caudocranial**, respectively, the terminology changes to **dorsopalmar** or **dorsoplantar** and **palmarodorsal** or **plantarodorsal**, respectively, from the carpus and tarsus distally. For radiographs of the head, **cranial** is replaced with **rostral**.

Most radiographs in small animals are acquired with the patient positioned on an X-ray table and using a vertical X-ray beam. If under certain circumstances radiographs with a horizontal beam technique are necessary (e.g. for a diagnosis of pneumoperitoneum), or if special techniques are used for radiographic evaluation of the head (e.g. intraoral radiographs), this should be noted in the radiographic report.

The **evaluation of a radiograph** is principally a form of pattern recognition, similar to techniques employed

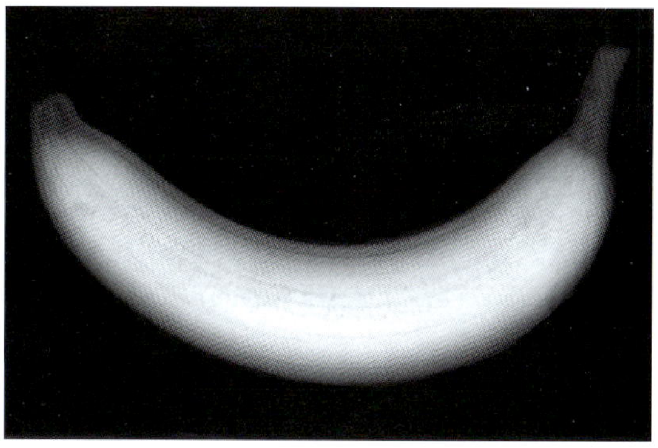

Fig. 1.1 Radiograph of a banana, which in contrast to the human or animal body lacks interior organs and appears homogeneous on a radiograph.

in machine learning. To train the investigator's eye in the recognition of normal anatomy, radiographs should always be positioned in the same orientation (i.e. following the same pattern). Following international standards, lateral views (including radiographs of extremities) should always be positioned with the cranial/rostral part of the patient towards the left and the caudal part to the right. Dorsoventral/ventrodorsal radiographs are positioned with the cranial part of the patient towards the top, the right side to the left and the left to the right of the observer. Radiographs of the extremities are oriented with the distal part at the bottom of the image.

1.3 Radiographic opacity

The X-ray permeability of a structure depends on the atomic number, the physical density and its thickness. Materials of a higher density (bone or mineral calculi) absorb more X-rays than less dense materials (gas or fat) and will appear brighter on a resultant radiograph. Similarly, thick layers of a given material will absorb more X-rays than thin layers. The most commonly used term for differences in radiographic appearance of tissues based on degree of X-ray attenuation is **opacity**. Other terms occasionally found in the literature include **radiolucency** (decreased opacity) and **radiopacity**.

There are five different **radiographic opacities** (Fig. 1.2):

- air
- fat
- soft tissue and fluid
- bone
- metal.

Several and sometimes all of these opacities may be concurrently noted on a radiograph. In Figure 1.3 the following opacities are represented:

- gas (intestinal loops and caudal lung fields)
- fat (retroperitoneal and peritoneal space)
- soft tissue and fluid (liver, kidneys, urinary bladder, etc.)
- bone (vertebrae, ribs, etc.).

The differential absorption of X-rays is useful for the interpretation of regular radiographs and is the basic concept of radiographic contrast studies. Although often

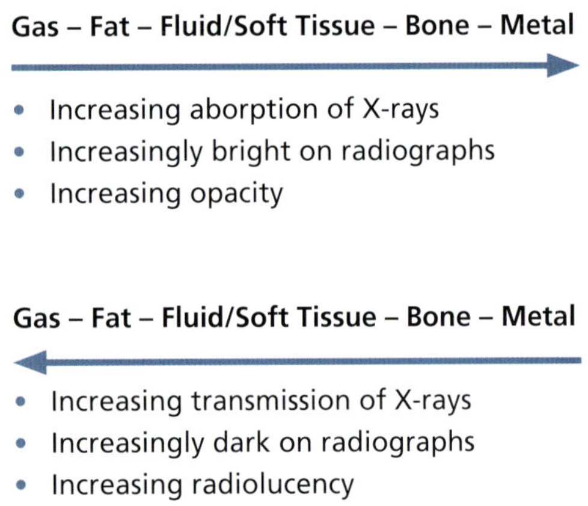

Fig. 1.2 Comparison of different radiographic opacities.

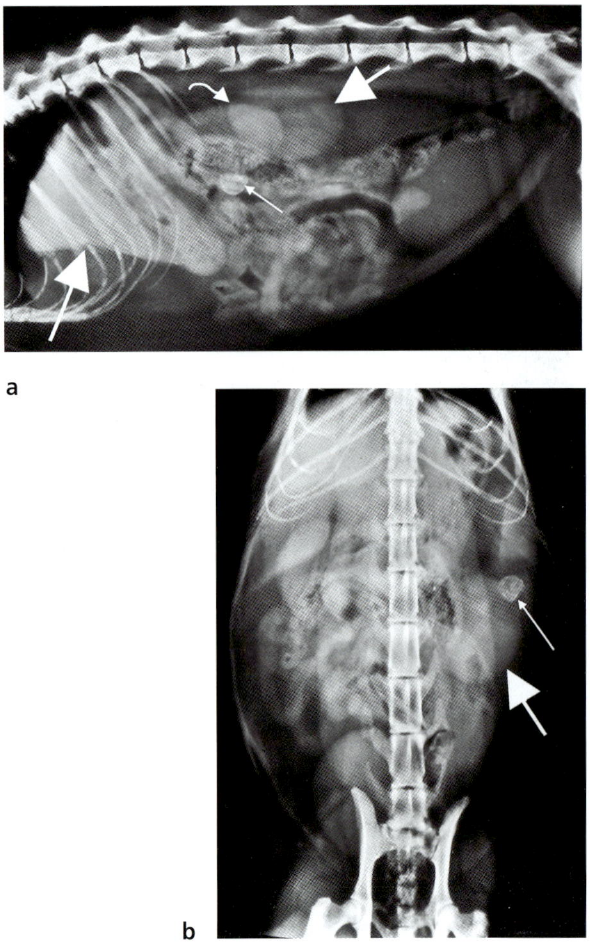

a

b

Fig. 1.3 Lateral **a** and ventrodorsal **b** abdominal radiographs of a well-nourished cat. The excellent abdominal detail is attributed to fat deposits. The margins between the caudal pole of the left kidney and adjacent retroperitoneal fat as well as the ventral liver margin and adjacent peritoneal/falciform fat are marked by large arrows. An incidental well-defined round mineral opaque structure is associated with the left mid abdominal fat (fat necrosis, 'Bates body') (*small straight arrow*). The small bent arrow indicates overlap of the caudal pole of the right kidney with the cranial pole of the left kidney, resulting in additive X-ray absorption and resultant increased opacity compared to individual kidneys (summation).

forgotten, fat is tremendously important in radiographic interpretation as it has a lower opacity than soft tissue and thus allows delineation of abdominal organs. Similarly, air (e.g. intraluminal gas in intestinal segments or air in body cavities as seen with pneumothorax) may serve as a natural contrast medium and can help delineate neighbouring structures of similar opacity.

1.4 Silhouetting and summation

The presence of different opacities within the patient results in two radiographic phenomena: silhouetting and summation. A radiographic report will often comment on structures silhouetting or summating, respectively.

1.4.1 Silhouetting

When two structures of the same or similar opacity are in physical contact with each other, their margins cannot be distinguished radiographically. Conversely, structures that are separated by material of a different opacity are easily identified. This phenomenon explains the poor serosal detail observed on abdominal radiographs in any of the following circumstances:

- very young animals with little to no abdominal fat deposits
- very thin/cachectic patients
- patients with ascites in which abdominal effusion obscures the margins of soft-tissue opaque abdominal organs (Fig. 1.4; see also section 11.3).

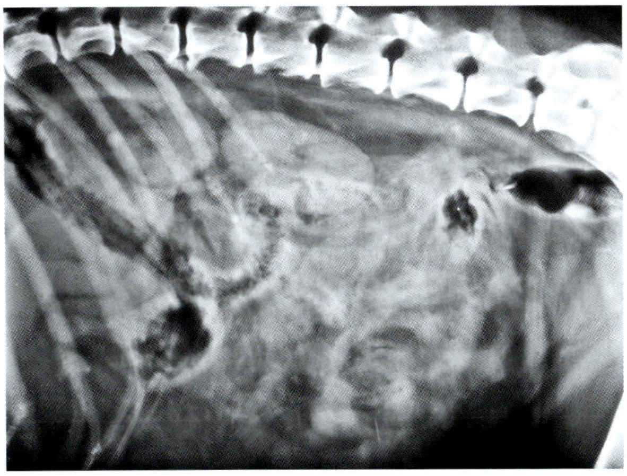

Fig. 1.4 Lateral abdominal radiograph in an 11-year-old German Shepherd Dog. There is poor serosal detail indicated by lack of visibility of abdominal organ margins due to a large volume of abdominal effusion (ascites). The kidneys are clearly delineated due to the presence of retroperitoneal fat and the absence of retroperitoneal effusion. The ultimate diagnosis in this patient was haemoabdomen due to a ruptured splenic mass.

On the other hand, there is nothing more appealing to a radiologist than abdominal radiographs of a well-nourished (fat) cat which are characterized by excellent serosal margin detail (Fig. 1.3).

Other examples of silhouetting on radiographs include:

- inability to distinguish the wall of a cardiac chamber from intraluminal blood
- obscured cardiac and diaphragmatic margins in patients with pleural effusion
- inability to diagnose tumours of the bladder wall as they are obscured by adjacent urine.

1.4.2 Summation

When two separate structures are superimposed on a radiograph their individual X-ray absorption and thus opacity are additive. A typical example is the region of increased opacity observed at the overlap of the cranial pole of the left kidney with the caudal pole of the right kidney on a lateral abdominal radiograph (see Fig. 1.3a). When summation of two soft-tissue opaque structures is observed it indicates that these are not in direct physical contact.

1.5 Radiographic perception

Our patients are three-dimensional objects (subjects) which are converted into a two-dimensional format when obtaining a radiograph. This process and the associated loss of depth perception results in an unusual appearance and potentially the inability to identify otherwise familiar structures depending on the direction of the beam in respect to the area of interest (Fig. 1.5). Full evaluation of (disease) processes occurring in a patient's body therefore requires at least two radiographs obtained with orthogonal beam orientation in most situations.

The following phenomena come into play when a radiograph is evaluated in a single projection.

- **Distortion/magnification**: Variations in distance of parts of the patient from the X-ray tube ('focus') on the one hand and the receptor (film/plate) on the other hand result in changes in apparent size of a structure (Fig. 1.6) and distortion (Fig. 1.7).
- **Superimposition of structures**: Unless aided by magnification, it is usually impossible to separately evaluate symmetric anatomic structures (e.g. vertebral transverse processes, ribs, coxofemoral joints or bones of the skull) or determine laterality of a disease process (e.g. pleural effusion or fracture) on a lateral view only. In addition to the inability to distinguish the left and right sides of the patient on a lateral view, superimposition of surrounding structures may result in complete inability to evaluate a lesion on a single projection (Fig. 1.8).

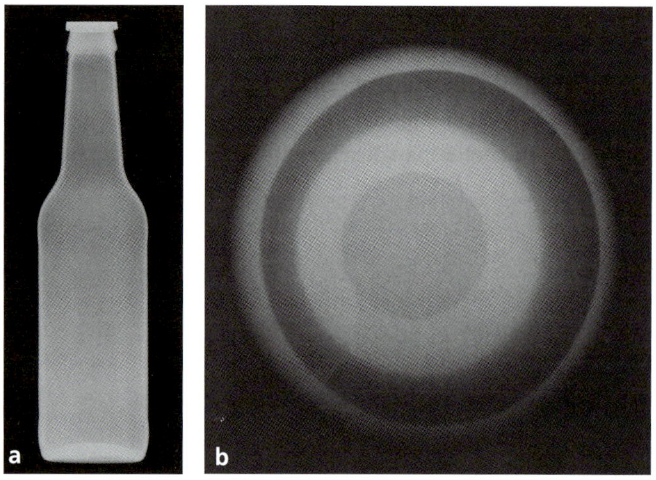

Fig. 1.5 Radiograph of a bottle.
a The object is easily recognized on this 'lateral' view.
b The orthogonal ('rostrocaudal') view makes identification of the object impossible even for experienced radiologists.

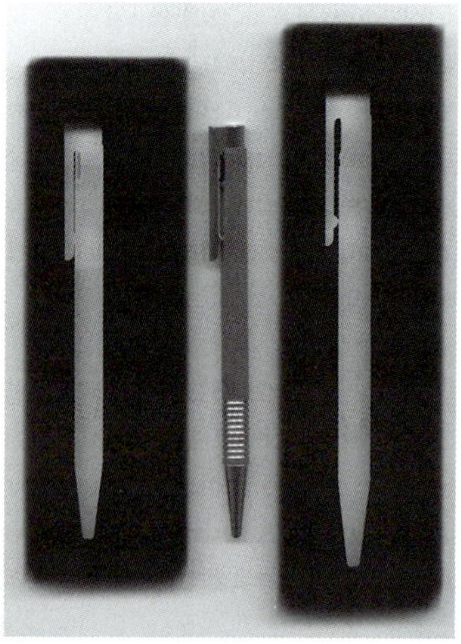

Fig. 1.6 Two radiographs of the same pen (middle picture) positioned directly on the cassette (left) and on a 13 cm foam block (right), respectively. There is notable magnification of the object on the second radiograph resulting from an increased object–film distance. Considering that certain body parts (thorax, abdomen) are often thicker than 13 cm even in small animals, the investigator has to take into account that anatomic structures distant from the plate will be magnified, possibly to a significant degree.

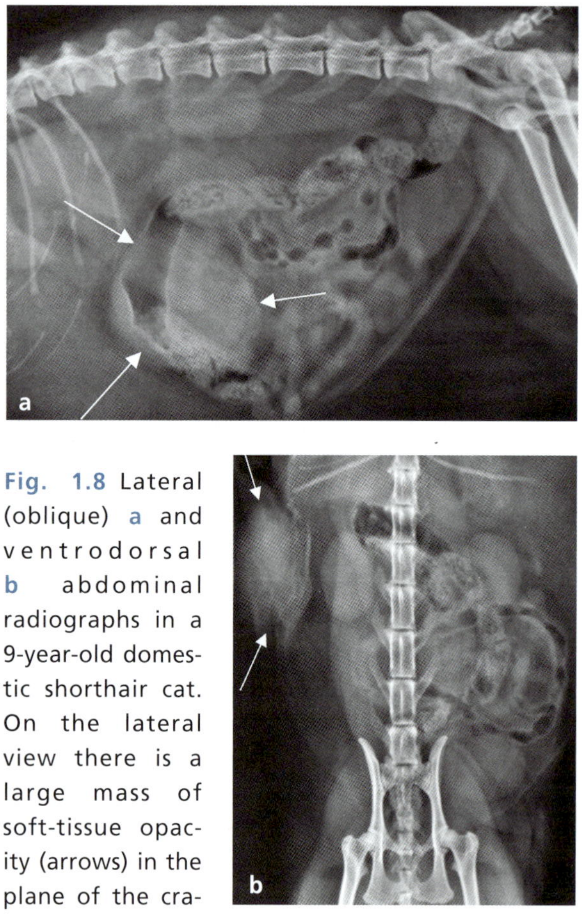

Fig. 1.8 Lateral (oblique) a and ventrodorsal b abdominal radiographs in a 9-year-old domestic shorthair cat. On the lateral view there is a large mass of soft-tissue opacity (arrows) in the plane of the cranial/mid-ventral abdomen. This lesion is of uncertain organ association. On the ventrodorsal view the mass is associated with the subcutaneous tissues of the right abdominal wall lateral to the right kidney, i.e. it is in extra-abdominal location! Histopathological examination yielded a diagnosis of fibrosarcoma.

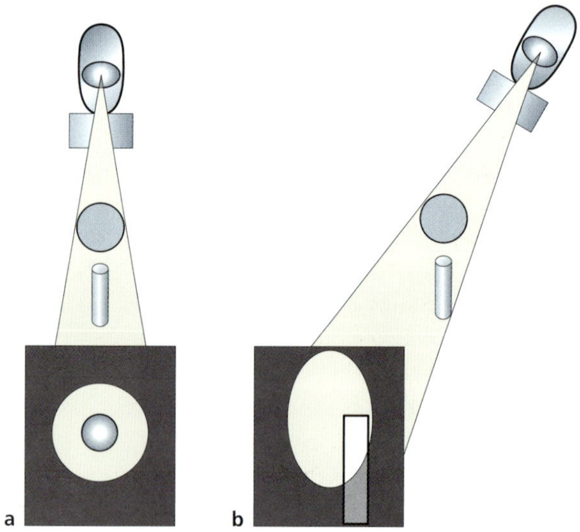

Fig. 1.7 Schematic drawing illustrating the effect of X-ray beam angle on the resultant radiograph. The primary beam in a is in perpendicular orientation to the object and the X-ray film, while it is angled in b. The resultant 'radiographic images' appear markedly different. This illustration of image distortion secondary to an angled primary beam underlines the need for beam collimation to the region of interest. Whole-body survey radiographs are at best of limited diagnostic yield especially in larger patients.

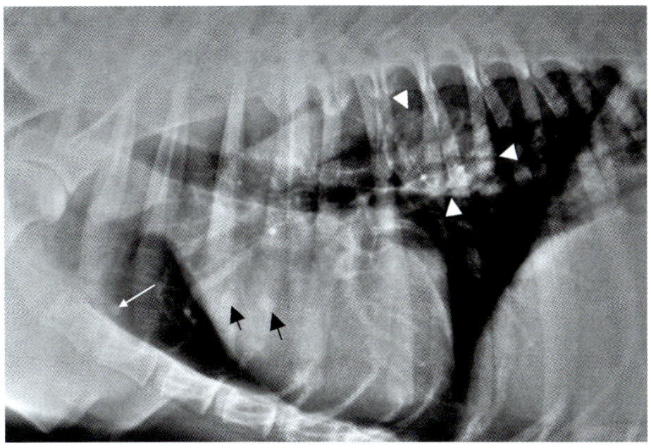

a

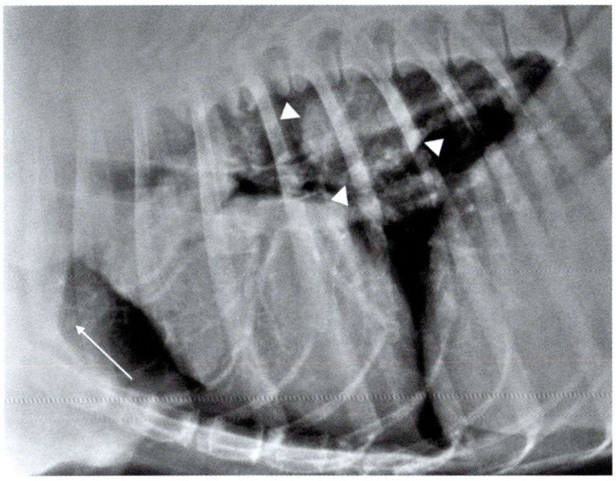

b

Fig. 1.9 Right lateral a and left lateral b thoracic radiographs in a 10-year-old female mixed-breed dog with a diagnosis of mammary tumours. A mass of soft-tissue opacity associated with the left caudal lung lobe (arrowheads) is visible on both views owing to its large size. An additional smaller soft-tissue nodule located between the second and third rib (white arrow) is also visible on both views. However, two additional nodules are only seen on the left lateral view (a; black arrows) and would have been missed if only a right lateral view had been obtained. Their visibility only on the left lateral view indicates that they are located in the nondependent (right) side of the lung. A ventrodorsal or dorsoventral view should always be obtained to complete a radiographic metastatic series. Radiographically suspected pulmonary metastatic disease was confirmed with histopathological examination.

- **Special anatomic considerations**: When obtaining a lateral thoracic radiograph, the dependent lung (adjacent to the plate) collapses and becomes soft-tissue opaque, which will result in loss of visualization of small soft-tissue lesions such as nodules due to silhouetting. Thus, opposite lateral views in addition to a dorsoventral or ventrodorsal projection are essential when evaluating a patient for pulmonary lesions (e.g. preoperative check for metastases or suspicion of aspiration pneumonia) (Fig. 1.9; see also Chapter 9). Additional radiographic projections (e.g. horizontal beam views or tangential views of the thoracic wall) may be needed in a given patient to answer a specific clinical question.
- **Changes that are only visible in a specific projection**: Some (even extensive) changes may only be visible on one specific projection but not others, and in other instances the full extent of an abnormality may be underestimated on one view versus another (Fig. 1.10 and 1.11).

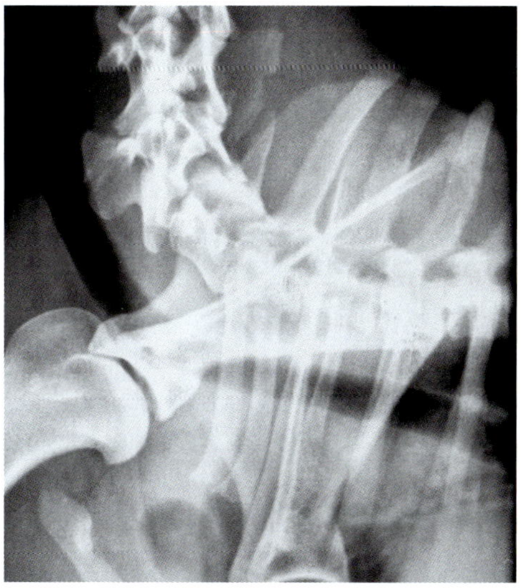

a

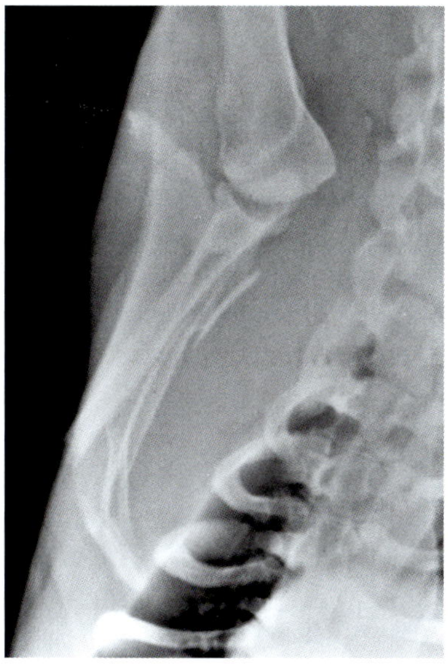

b

Fig. 1.10 Lateral a and caudocranial b radiographs of the scapula in a 2-year-old male neutered mixed-breed dog. A comminuted scapular fracture clearly seen in b is not visible in a even with the benefit of hindsight.

1.6 Radiograph description and interpretation

Choice of the appropriate radiographic examination based on indication, acquisition of high-quality diagnostic radiographs, and complete and accurate evaluation not only test the medical knowledge but also the visual capabilities of the veterinarian, and the examiner has to be familiar with the possibilities and limitations of the technique to maximize its diagnostic utility. In many cases, a diagnosis in a given patient is not solely made on the basis of a radiograph, but radiographs are used to complement patient signalment, history, clinical examination and laboratory findings.

Radiographic interpretation should always occur in a dark room. For conventional radiographs, evaluation should include assessment using a view box and, if needed, a hot lamp. Evaluating radiographs just using the light from a window or a ceiling light is unacceptable. For digital radiographs, a large high-quality computer monitor is a must.

Radiographic interpretation requires a good basic knowledge of normal radiographic anatomy and physiological variants. An anatomy textbook and a radiographic atlas should be at hand. Additionally, a catalogue or collection of normal radiographs that can serve as a comparison if needed is a good idea.

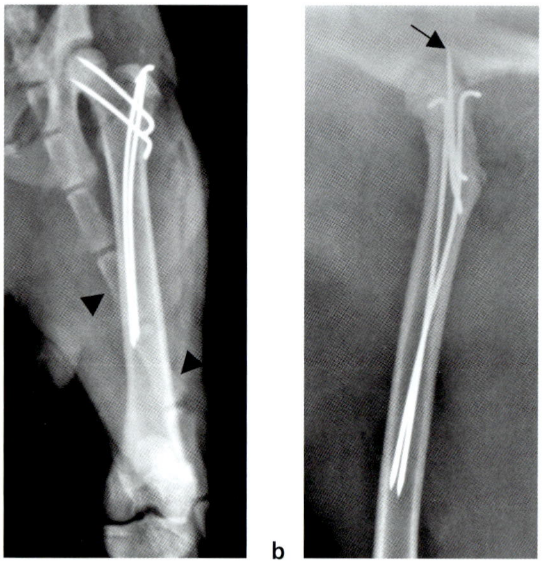

a b

Fig. 1.11 Postoperative radiographs following surgical repair of a femoral neck fracture in a young cat.
a On the craniocaudal view implant placement appears adequate. Note suboptimal radiographic technique with superimposition of the tail (black arrowheads) over the area of interest.
b On the lateral view intra-articular extension of one of the pins placed in the femoral head and neck is evident (arrow). This finding necessitates immediate surgical revision to avoid future severe degenerative joint disease!

The radiographic interpretation should always follow a systematic approach but can be customized to meet individual investigator preferences (e.g. evaluation following organ systems versus evaluation according to body regions). Once a personalized approach has been established it should always be followed. The major goal of this approach is to minimize the risk of incomplete assessment, particularly if a pathological finding is noted early in the course of radiographic interpretation. In particular, inexperienced students and veterinarians tend to summarize radiographic findings with a single 'snapshot' diagnosis (e.g. 'cranial cruciate rupture', 'lung tumour', or 'gastric dilatation and volvulus'). Even after identification of a major abnormality the remainder of the radiographic study should be thoroughly evaluated for the presence of other possibly significant lesions.

The systematic evaluation of a radiograph should begin with a description of available projections and assessment of the technical quality of the study (positioning, technique, artefacts and need for additional views). This should be followed by a complete description of abnormal (and possibly even normal) findings before a final conclusion is reached. If a good radiographic report is relayed over the phone to a veterinarian (or another person with adequate radiographic knowledge), that individual should be able to draw a mental picture without actually having seen the radiographs. Even though a thorough description of radiographs over the phone has lost importance in the age of digital radiography and easy digital transfer of radiographs, the ability to generate a coherent and complete radiographic report remains important.

When interpreting a radiograph the following **Roentgen signs** are taken into account.

- Size: Size measurements can be given as objective measurements (e.g. 2 × 3 cm) or as semiquantitative values in relation to other structures (e.g. three times the length of the vertebral body L2).
- Shape: There are no limits to descriptors that may be used to describe the shape of a structure (e.g. square, lobulated, egg-shaped). The goal is to allow the reader of a radiographic report to generate a mental image of the abnormality in his/her head.
- Opacity: Organs, structures and pathological abnormalities are assigned the aforementioned terms air, fat, soft-tissue, bone or metal opacity.
- Location: The position of a structure on radiographs can be described in different ways. Location within a body cavity (e.g. caudoventral abdomen) or position in relation to adjacent structures and organs (e.g. dorsal to the trachea) are commonly included in a

report. To increase objectivity of the description, listing of distances between an abnormality and nearby structures is very helpful, especially if the lesion is subtle or if recheck radiographs are evaluated by somebody unfamiliar with the initial set of films (e.g. 0.5 cm pulmonary nodule 2 cm dorsal to the sternum at the level of the fifth pair of ribs).

- Margin and contour: Organs and pathological changes are described as sharply marginated or poorly defined, and as having a regular or irregular contour.
- Number: This is used to describe the number of affected organs (e.g. enlargement of one kidney, or pathology in two lung lobes) as well as to list countable pathological abnormalities (e.g. pulmonary nodules or bladder stones).

These Roentgen signs are essential for an accurate description of a radiograph!
Mnemonic: **S**ix **S**ins **O**f **L**onely **M**a**N**iacs.

The following is an example of a detailed radiographic description and diagnostic conclusion. The reader should be able to create a mental image of the abnormalities after reading the report.

Example: Evaluation of abdominal radiographs in a dog

Description: The patient is a small, well-nourished, female spayed middle-aged dog. A right lateral and a ventrodorsal view of the abdomen are available for interpretation. The radiographs are of good diagnostic quality. Within the gastric fundus there are two disc-shaped, round, smoothly marginated and metal opaque structures of 1.8 and 2.6 cm diameter, respectively. The liver, spleen, left kidney, urinary bladder, small intestine, colon and visible musculoskeletal structures are normal. The right kidney is obscured and not clearly visualized.
Conclusion: Two metal opacity gastric foreign bodies (coins).

Many veterinarians and radiologists tend to omit a detailed description of normal structures with increasing experience. This is perfectly fine as long as it is ascertained that all structures have definitely been fully evaluated. After completion of the radiographic assessment the findings are used in conjunction with other information (patient signalment, history, clinical and laboratory findings) to establish a diagnosis or a list of reasonable differential diagnoses.

Suggested reading

Hartung K, Ludewig E, Tellhelm B. Röntgenuntersuchung in der Tierarztpraxis. Stuttgart: Enke 2010.

Hecht S. Für Studium und Praxis: Grundlagen der Röntgenbildentstehung und -interpretation. Tierärztl Prax 2003; 31: 132–5.

Papageorges M. Visual perception and radiographic interpretation. In: Thrall DE (ed.). Textbook of Veterinary Diagnostic Radiology. Philadelphia: WB Saunders 2002; 35–42.

Smallwood JE, Shively MJ, Rendano VT, Habel RE. A standardized nomenclature for radiographic projections used in veterinary medicine. Vet Radiol 1985; 26: 2–9.

Thrall DE. Introduction to radiographic interpretation. In: Thrall DE (ed.). Textbook of Veterinary Diagnostic Radiology, 7th edn. St. Louis: Elsevier 2018; 110–22.

Designing a radiographic technique chart

2

Eberhard Ludewig and Silke Hecht

2.1 Introduction

Following the purchase of X-ray equipment, the small animal practitioner is confronted with the problem of having to set up a chart with appropriate exposure parameters. Factors influencing the radiographic technique include patient size, composition of tissues in the region of interest, patient motion, the sensitivity of the available film–screen or digital detector system and use of a grid. It is not possible to produce a technique chart that will work under all circumstances. However, some basic rules exist which will aid the practitioner in obtaining the best possible radiographs using a given system.

2.2 Influence of tube voltage (kVp) and tube current–time product (mAs) on image quality

Radiographic exposure factors include kVp, which determines the energy and thus penetrative capacity of the X-ray beam, and mAs, which is the product of the tube current (mA) and the exposure time (s) and which determines the quantity of X-rays produced. In film–screen radiography the goal is to select an exposure resulting in an appropriate degree of film blackening (optical density, i.e. fraction of light transmitted through the film). Mean optical density should range between 1.0 and 1.4, and all structures of interest should be in the useful range of 0.5 to 2.2 (Fig. 2.1).

2.2.1 Under- and overexposure

In film–screen radiography, the immediate goal of choosing a 'good' kVp and mAs combination is achieving adequate mean film darkening. Underexposure results in a radiograph that is too light overall as a result of a decreased detector dose. On the other hand, overexposure results in excessive film blackening. In both instances diagnostic image information is lost, and in extreme cases radiographs may be non-diagnostic. Film–screen systems leave very little room for variation in exposure settings, and even minor changes have a significant effect on image quality (narrow exposure latitude or dynamic range). Digital radiography systems (storage phosphor systems, flat panel detectors) are much more forgiving and will tolerate fairly large variations in radiographic technique due to their wide dynamic range for exposure. With these systems

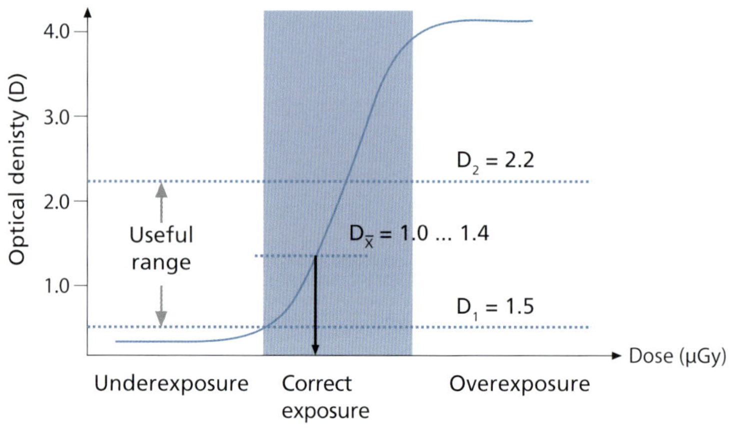

Fig. 2.1 Optical density curve of radiographic film. Exposure should be selected so that the mean optical density (Dx) ranges from 1.0 to 1.4. The useful range, i.e. the range of densities in which structures can be distinguished by the reader, falls between 0.5 and 2.2.

there is no direct association between the radiation dose delivered to the detector and the darkness of the resulting radiographs, and it is (nearly) impossible to overexpose or underexpose a radiograph to the point of necessitating repetition of the study. Nevertheless, the detector dose has an impact on image quality. Underexposed digital radiographs are characterized by a grainy appearance ('noise'), which under extreme circumstances may obscure important structures. Overexposure on the other hand usually goes unnoticed as the change in signal-to-noise ratio with high doses is imperceptible (Fig. 2.2). To ensure adequate image quality, and for radiation safety reasons, exposure parameters should be optimized even when using a digital radiography system. Use of a radiographic technique chart is a practical way to achieve this goal. Furthermore, digital systems are required to indicate a numeric value corresponding to the detector dose (dose indicator).

2.2.2 Motion unsharpness

Unsharpness or blurring caused by involuntary patient motion (e.g. respiration) are common and may limit diagnostic quality of thoracic, abdominal or spinal radiographs (Fig. 2.3). Exposure time should be kept very short (≤ 0.05, preferably ≤ 0.02 seconds) to avoid this problem. A decrease in mAs (and thus exposure time) can be achieved by the following means.

- Decrease in mAs with concurrent 'compensatory' increase in kVp.
- Decrease of the focus-to-detector distance.
- Use of high-speed film–screen combinations with higher sensitivity.
- Use of X-ray equipment capable of producing higher tube currents.

Halving mAs necessitates increasing kVp by approximately 10 kVp.

Exposure point tables are helpful in adjusting exposure parameters.

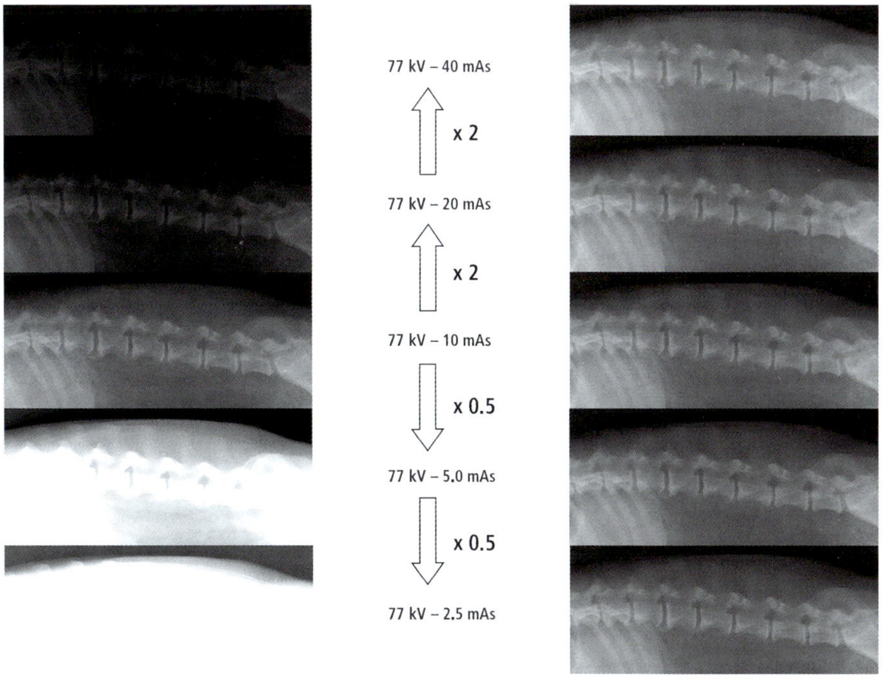

Fig. 2.2 Effect of exposure on image quality with a film–screen system (left) and a digital detector (right). While deviations from optimal technique with a film–screen system result in very light (underexposed) or dark (overexposed) images, variations in technique do not affect image brightness in a digital system. However, image noise increases with decreasing dose (not noticeable on these printed images). This figure also illustrates that overexposure on digital radiographs does not affect image quality and thus is not easily noted. These are serial radiographs of the lumbar spine in a German Wirehaired Pointer. The film–screen system has a sensitivity S=400 (Screen: Kodak Lanex Regular, Film: Kodak T-MAT plus DL; Kodak, Rochester, Great Britain). The digital radiographs were obtained using a photostimulable phosphor plate (Plate: Fuji ST-V, Fujifilm Medical Systems, Tokyo, Japan; Reader: Philips AC 500, Philips Healthcare, Hamburg, Germany). Other factors were left constant (FDD: 110 cm, + grid).

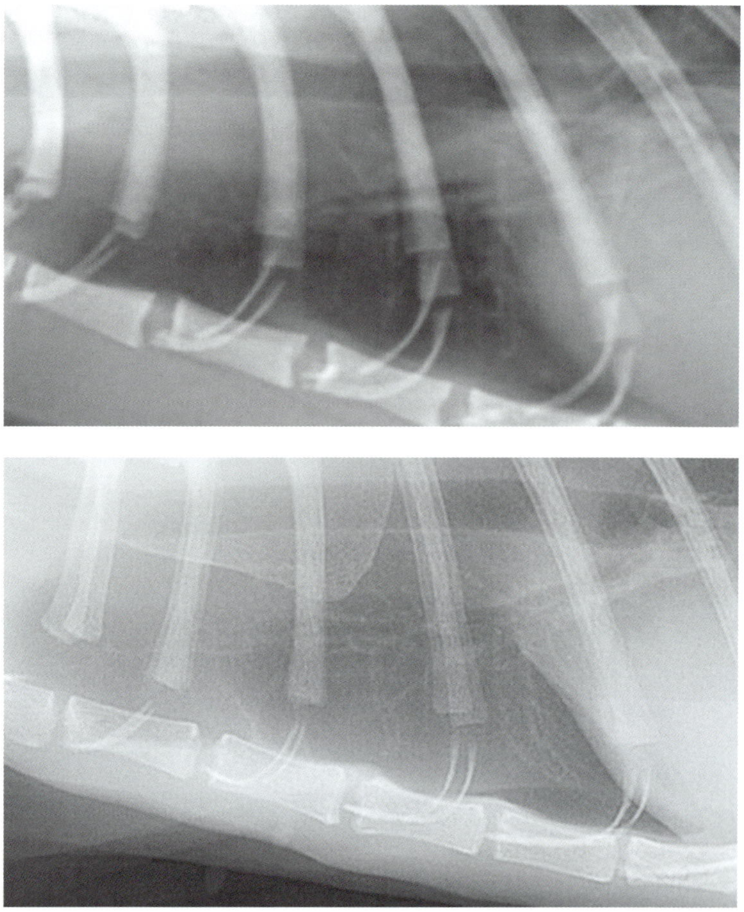

Fig. 2.3 Motion unsharpness/blurring in feline thoracic radiographs collimated to area of interest.
a Peripheral vascular structures are not visible and thus cannot be evaluated for any changes.
b With a decreased exposure time pulmonary vessels are sharply marginated and clearly visible.

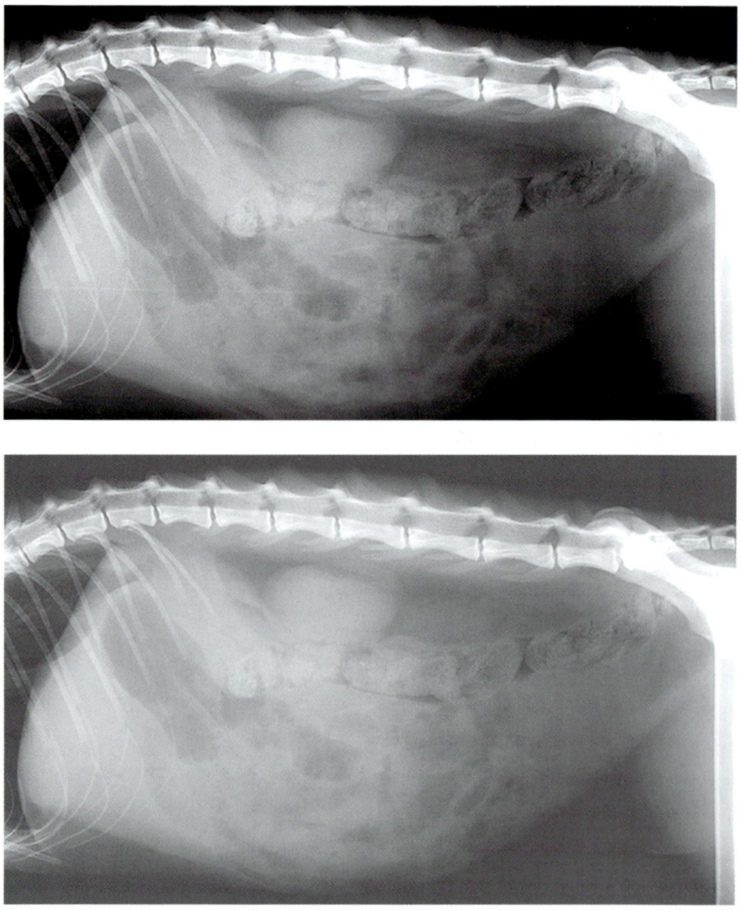

Fig. 2.4 Effect of exposure on greyscale of the image. Both radiographs were obtained using a film–screen system with a sensitivity of S=400. The mean optical density of both radiographs is identical.
a 42 kVp, 8 mAs.
b 52 kVp, 2 mAs.

2.2.3 Display of differences in attenuation

An important basic concept allowing radiographs to be used for diagnostic purposes is that differences in X-ray attenuation between tissues are displayed as different shades of grey on the image (greyscale). This display can be steered by exposure. Important parameters when discussing greyscale are 'dynamic range' (number of all shades of grey displayed on an image) and 'contrast' (relative differences in brightness of neighbouring structures). With increasing kVp values, attenuation differences between tissues decrease due to the higher penetrative capacity of the X-ray beam. In regions where tissues differ significantly in their X-ray attenuation properties (thorax, skeletal system), high kVp values should be used to minimize the effect of differential attenuation by tissues and allow display of the entire spectrum of attenuation differences on the radiograph. Conversely, in regions with low object contrast (abdomen), low kVp values should be used

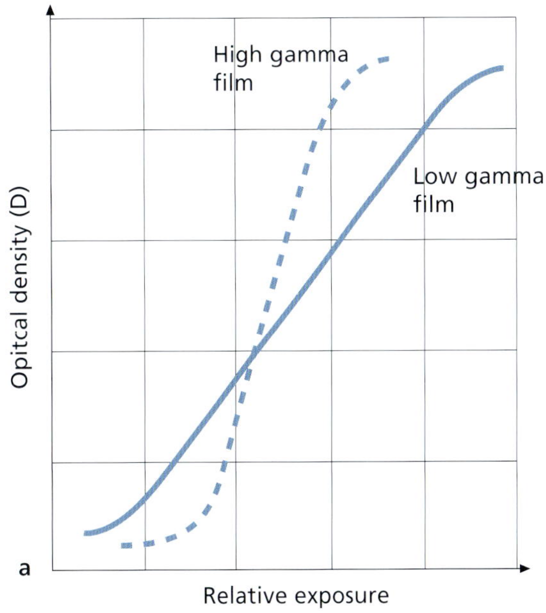

a

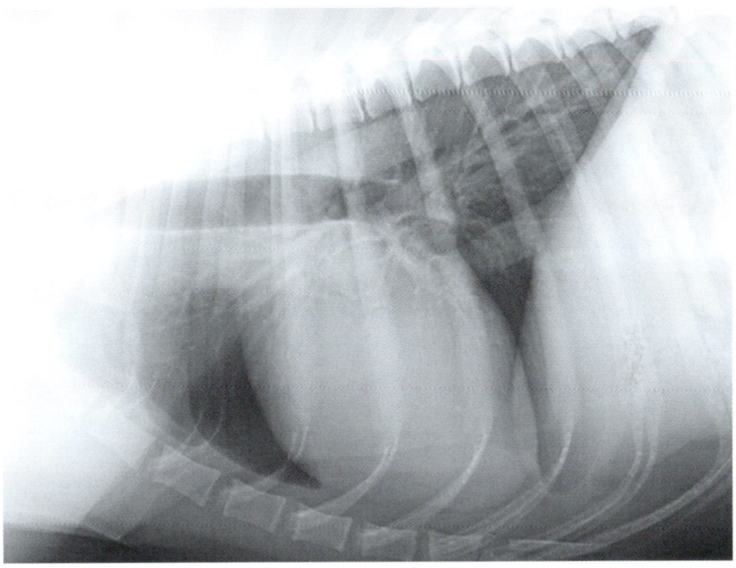

b

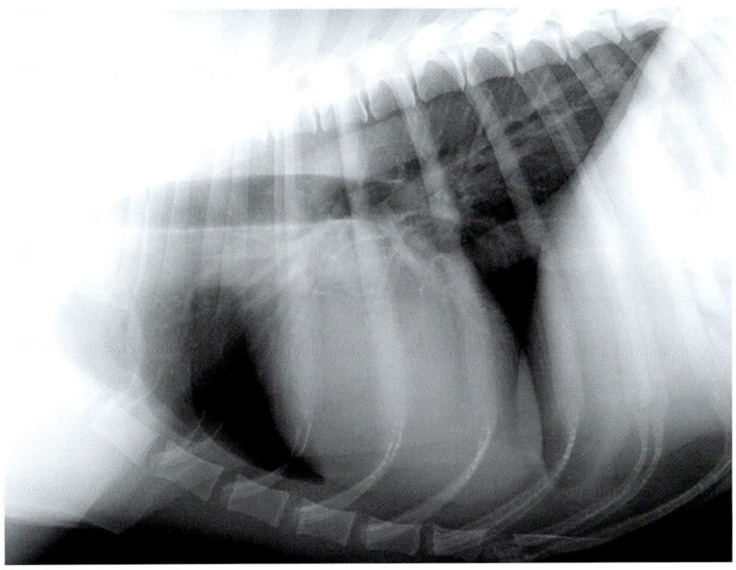

c

Fig. 2.5 Greyscale changes dependent on the optical density curve (gradient) of a radiographic film.
a Optical density curves of a 'steep' and a 'shallow' film. With a steep curve, more absorption values are included in the same shade of grey. This results in high contrast and little exposure leeway (low latitude).
b Radiograph obtained using a 'shallow' film. The thorax is characterized by high inherent contrast (range of X-ray attenuating structures from low to high). By using a film and technique aimed at a decrease in image contrast, regions with a low density (lung) can be evaluated as well as structures with a high density (mediastinum, spine).
c Radiograph obtained using a 'steep' film. Pre-existing large attenuation differences between structures are accentuated, resulting in decreased image information (in this case especially affecting the lung).

to accentuate minor attenuation differences between tissues. In both instances mAs has to be adjusted accordingly. In small animal radiography tube voltage typically ranges between 40 and 100 kVp.

> Tube voltage (kVp) affects greyscale. High kVp values result in a decrease in image contrast (Fig. 2.4).

The potential to steer the image greyscale by manipulating exposure parameters is somewhat limited as several additional factors have to be taken into account when choosing kVp (patient size, sensitivity of detectors, etc.). Another important way to adjust contrast and dynamic range is to use radiographic film with differences in density curve steepness (Fig. 2.5).

2.3 Film–screen systems and digital radiography

In film–screen systems the light output yielded by intensifying screens depends on the thickness of the screen's phosphor layer. Thick layers (high-speed screens) result in a higher light yield, but a certain degree of image blur is unavoidable due to light scatter. With thinner screens there is less light scatter and the resultant image is sharper. However, thin screens require an increase in exposure time to result in the same degree of film blackening (high-detail screens) compared to thicker screens. Manufacturers provide a 'sensitivity value' (S) indicating the dose requirements of a given film–screen system. This value is standardized and allows comparison between systems produced by different manufacturers (Table 2.1). For radiographs in small animal patients, high-speed film–screen systems (sensitivity approximately 400) are used for larger patients and for regions in which respiratory motion is of concern to allow short exposure times. High-detail film–screen systems (sensitivity approximately 100) are used to image small structural changes in thinner body regions. Under certain circumstances use of especially detailed systems (mammography film, non-screen film) may be indicated and goes along with an increase in exposure factors and radiation dose. Care should be taken to always use matching film–screen combinations. As properties of radiographic screens change over time, the same exposure may lead to different radiographic results. Thus, concurrent use of older and newer screens in the same practice is not advisable.

Table 2.1 Image detector dose and limit of spatial resolution of film–screen systems (according to DIN 6868-50).

Sensitivity (S-value)	Dose requirement (μGy)	Limit of spatial resolution (line pairs/mm)
800	1.25	2.0
400	2.50	2.4
200	5.00	2.8
100	10.00	3.4
50	20.00	4.0
25	40.00	4.8

> Film–screens systems with a sensitivity (S) of 100 and 400, respectively, differ by a factor of four in their intensifying properties. A film–screen system with a sensitivity of 100 requires a fourfold increase in mAs to achieve the same film blackening compared with a 400 system.

In a similar way to conventional film–screen systems, digital detectors also differ in their dose efficiency (see section 3.1.3; Fig. 3.2). The 'detective quantum efficiency' (DQE) describes the detector's ability to convert X-ray quanta to image information. It is defined as the quotient of the square of the signal-to-noise ratio (SNR) at the detector exit to the square of the SNR at the detector entrance:

$$DQE\ (f) = (SNR_{exit})^2(f) : (SNR_{entrance})^2(f)$$

DQE is influenced by image detail (spatial frequency, f). As system unsharpness and noise have a greater effect at higher frequencies, imaging of smaller details (i.e. higher frequencies) is more dependent on DQE than imaging of larger structures. Using an identical exposure, detectors with a high DQE produce a higher SNR compared to detectors with a low DQE. Alternatively, to maintain a constant SNR, systems with a high DQE allow dose reduction compared to systems with a lower DQE.

2.4 Grids

The purpose of grids is to avoid scatter radiation produced in the patient reaching the detector, which decreases image contrast. As scatter radiation contributes to the degree of film blackening (or signal generation using a digital detector), and as some primary X-rays are absorbed by the grid, use of a grid necessitates an increase in exposure. Therefore, it is important to determine which circumstances require the use of a grid. Basically, a grid is necessary when patient thickness exceeds 10 cm in regions with a high soft-tissue component and 15 cm in regions with a high gas component. For smaller structures, use of a grid is to be avoided to ensure short exposure times and decrease radiation dose to patient and personnel. Digital detectors with high DQE exhibit significant dose-saving potential. Even with larger patient thicknesses, low exposure settings can be applied. This results in less scattered radiation. Under these circumstances it may not be necessary to use a grid.

Use of a grid necessitates an increase in exposure factors. The grid factor determines how much exposure has to be increased (Table 2.2).

Grid factors (Bucky factors) typically range between 3 and 7. The grid factor depends on the grid ratio, in other words the ratio between the height of the lead strips and the distance between two strips. Grids used in veterinary radiography typically have a grid ratio ranging from 5:1 to 12:1.

2.5 Focus-to-detector distance

In contrast to large animal radiography, the focus-to-detector distance (FDD) is typically kept constant for small animal radiographs. However, a change in FDD is sometimes necessary even in small animal radiography (e.g. for horizontal beam radiographs). With an increase in distance between the X-ray tube and the detector, fewer X-ray quanta reach the detector. Specifically, the intensity of the X-ray beam is inversely proportional (squared) to the distance from the source (inverse square law; see also Chapter 4) necessitating an adjustment in exposure factors.

When changing the focus-to-detector distance (FDD) the new mAs value can be determined by simply using the following formula:

$$mAs_{new} = (FDD_{new})^2/(FDD_{old})^2 \times mAs_{old}$$

2.6 Practical application

Several factors affect the choice of optimal exposure parameters:

- patient: region, thickness, condition
- focus-to-detector distance
- sensitivity of film–screen system or DQE of digital detector, respectively
- grid: yes/no; if yes: grid factor
- generator
- collimation
- overlying bandage material.

The effect of several of these image factors on quality has been discussed above.

When designing a chart with optimized exposure parameters, most of these variables should initially be kept constant, and only body region and thickness should be modified.

For thoracic and abdominal radiographs patient thickness is measured using calipers.

The common method of guessing body size based on 'experience' is inappropriate and commonly dissatisfactory. Using visual inspection alone it is virtually impossible to determine a 3 cm difference in a dog's thickness (requiring either doubling or halving of the exposure!).

Even though relatively straightforward exposure point tables are available (Tables 2.3 and 2.4), recalculation of exposure parameters for every single patient is not practical. The solution is to develop a radiographic technique chart listing all relevant exposure factors for a given region and thickness. This can easily be accomplished in small animal practice. A table is generated using well exposed radiographs (of past patients or cadavers if available) in which region thickness and exposure factors were documented as a starting point. Missing exposure parameters for other body regions or patient sizes can be calculated using exposure point tables and filled in over time. To obtain initial test radiographs the following rule can be used.

Table 2.2 Correction factors to adjust radiographic technique according to the grid ratio.

Grid ratio	Increase in mAs (multiplied by original value)	Increase in kVp (added to original value)
5:1	2	6–8
8:1	3	8–10
12:1	4	12–15
16:1	4.5	15–20

Notes: It is important to modify either mAs or kVp, not both at the same time! Modified from Curry et al. 1990.

Important rules:

1. Exposure should be doubled with an increase in body thickness:
   - 3 cm for the abdomen
   - 5 cm for the thorax
2. Doubling of the detector dose can be achieved by:
   - doubling mAs OR
   - increasing kVp by 10.

Table 2.3 Technique chart: adjustment in exposure points to correct for changes from the initial situation.

kV	Points	mAs
–	−10	0.1
–	−9	0.125
–	−8	0.16
–	−7	0.2
–	−6	0.25
–	−5	0.32
–	−4	0.4
–	−3	0.5
–	−2	0.63
–	−1	0.8
40	0	1
41	1	1.25
42	2	1.6
44	3	2
46	4	2.5
48	5	3.5
50	6	4
52	7	5
55	8	6.3
57	9	8
60	10	10
63	11	12.5
66	12	16
70	13	20
73	14	25
77	15	32
81	16	40
85	17	50
90	18	63
96	19	80
102	20	100
109	21	125
117	22	160
125	23	200
133	24	250
141	25	320
150	26	400
–	27	500
–	28	630
–	29	800
–	30	1000

Note: Excerpt from: 'Aufnahmehelfer für die Röntgendiagnostik' ('Diagnostic Radiology Technique Aid'), Siemens Medical Technology.

Voltage:

kVp = (Thickness of body part (cm) × 2) + FDD (in inches or in cm/2.5) + grid factor

kVp Example:

Dog measuring 13 cm in thickness, FDD 100 cm, grid factor 3 (for a grid ratio of 8:1)

kVp value: $(13 \times 2) + 100/2.5 + 3 = 69$ kVp

The exposure time is chosen to achieve the following mAs values while using the highest possible mA:

Sensitivity (S) 200: 10 mAs

Sensitivity (S) 400: 5 mAs = (Thickness of body part (cm) × 2) + FDD (in inches or in cm/2.5) + grid factor

Now well exposed radiographs are possible simply by measuring patient thickness and consulting the technique chart for appropriate exposure parameters. An example of a simple custom-made technique chart is shown in Table 2.5.

Exposure parameters for both front and hind distal extremities (distal to humerus and femur) are fairly similar for patients of a comparable size. Thus, in the same animal the same technique can usually be used for radiographs of carpus and tarsus or stifle and elbow. Craniocaudal views typically require an increase in exposure parameters compared to lateral views due to an increase in thickness of the area of interest.

Modern radiographic equipment is equipped with an automated phototimer system (automatic exposure control; AEC) which only requires the operator to choose the tube voltage and a 'density factor'. These phototimers operate by measuring the actual amount of radiation exiting the patient and automatically terminating exposure once the desired exposure is reached. If used appropriately, these systems significantly decrease time and effort needed to consistently produce well exposed radiographs.

Neither a complete technique chart nor automatic exposure control guarantee perfectly exposed radiographs every time. Exposure parameters often have to be adjusted to address patient variables and produce an acceptable result (e.g. adiposity or cachexia; Table 2.6). Additionally, errors in film processing can result in radiographs that are too dark or too light, a problem especially prevalent with manual development (see Chapter 3).

Table 2.4 Exposure point table to determine mAs and kVp values using exposure points.

Exposure range	± 1 Exposure point (EP)			
Patient thickness	In general: ± 1 cm equals ± 1EP Exception: thorax ± 1.5 cm equals ± 1 EP			
Current–time product (mAs) 1 EP from each value to the next	Double or half mAs product: ± 3 EP 6.4 10 16 25 40 64 100 160 250 400 mAs 5 8 12 20 32 50 80 125 200 320			
Tube current (kVp)	40 — 50 — 60 — 70 — 80 — 90 — 100 — 110 — 120 kVp 6 5 3 3 3 2 1 1 ± EP 'Middle kVp range'			
Focus-to-film distance	0.5 0.7 1.0 1.4 20.0 m −6 − 3 ± 0 + 3 + 6 EP			
Screens	S = 25 + 9 EP S = 100 + 3 EP S = 200 ± 0 EP (Reference) S = 400 − 3 EP S = 800 − 6 EP			
Grids	High selectivity c.g. Pb 12/40	Medium selectivity e.g. Pb 8/40	Low selectivity e.g. Pb 5/50	No grid
	± 0 EP (Reference)	−1 to −2 BP	−2 to −4 EP	−4 to −6 EP
Generators	6-Pulse generator	12-Pulse generator	2-Pulse generator	
	± 0 EP (Reference)	−1 EP	+2 EP	
Collimation	Small field size compared to large: ± 0 to +4 EP (dependent on object thickness, grid and collimation)			

Table 2.5 Example of a radiographic technique chart for dogs used in small animal practice.

Thickness (cm)	11–12	13–14	15–16	17–18	19–20	21–22	23–24	25–26	27–28
Abdomen			60/10	70/10					
Spine			64/12						
Thorax					64/10				

Notes: Exposure parameters in kVp/mAs. Other factors such as focus–detector distance, film–screen system and grid must be known and kept constant.

Table 2.6 Adjustment of exposure parameters.

Decreased exposure	Increased exposure
Weight loss/cachexia Increased gas content (pneumothorax, pneumoperitoneum, emphysema, negative contrast study, gastric dilatation volvulus, etc.) Osteopenia Others	Adiposity Increased amount of fluid or other opaque material (pleural effusion, pulmonary oedema, ascites, subcutaneous swelling, positive contrast study, etc.) Bandage or cast material Others

Suggested reading

Bushberg JT, Seibert JA, Leidholdt EM, Boone JM. The Essential Physics of Medical Imaging. Philadelphia: Lippincott Williams & Wilkins 2002.

Curry TS, Dowdey JE, Murry RC. Christensen's Physics of Diagnostic Radiology, 4th edn. Philadelphia: Lippincott Williams & Wilkins 1990.

DIN (Deutsches Institut für Normung). DIN 6868-50: Sicherung der Bildqualität in röntgendiagnostischen Betrieben, Abnahmeprüfung an medizinischen Röntgeneinrichtungen für Aufnahme, Durchleuchtung und Filmverarbeitung. Berlin: Beuth Verlag, June 1990.

Dixon RT. Construction of a radiographic technique chart. Austr Vet J 1967; 43: 588–9.

Hartung K, Ludewig E, Tellhelm B. Röntgenuntersuchung in der Tierarztpraxis. Stuttgart: Enke 2010.

Hecht S. Für Studium und Praxis: Die richtige Belichtung des Röntgenbildes. Tierärztl Prax 2002; 30: 238–42.

Laubenberger T, Laubenberger J. Technik der medizinischen Radiologie. Köln: Deutscher Ärzte-Verlag 1999.

Morgan JP. Techniques of Veterinary Radiography. Ames: Iowa State University Press 1993.

Siegel EL, Kolodner RM. Filmless Radiology. New York: Springer 2001.

Ticer JW. Radiographic Technique in Veterinary Practice. Philadelphia: WB Saunders 1984.

Watters JW. Development of a technique chart for the veterinarian. Compend Contin Educ Pract Vet 1980; 2: 568–71.

Radiology physics and artefacts 3

Eberhard Ludewig and Silke Hecht

3.1 Generation of a radiograph

Artefacts are structures visible on a radiograph which do not correspond to patient anatomy and may render a radiograph of limited or nondiagnostic quality. To understand radiographic artefacts and their remedies it is important to have a basic knowledge of X-ray production, principles of radiographic exposure, and function of both film–screen and digital radiography systems.

3.1.1 X-ray production and interaction with the patient

The goal of this chapter is to provide a very brief overview of basic physical principles important for daily radiographic diagnostics and understanding of artefacts. For a more detailed description of the physics of radiology the reader is referred to specific literature.

X-rays are a form of high-energy (short-wave) radiation produced in an X-ray tube. A cathode is heated to the point of releasing electrons, which are accelerated towards an anode due to the voltage applied between the two components. After colliding with the anode the electrons slow down, a process which produces X-rays (braking and characteristic radiation) and heat. The anode is made of tungsten and may have a stationary or rotating design. Rotating anodes have a higher capacity due to more efficient heat dissipation and a smaller focal point. The energy (quality) and quantity of X-rays produced is determined by the tube voltage and the tube current–exposure time product, respectively (see Chapter 2).

Following bombardment of the anode with electrons, the X-rays produced exit in all directions, and many of them are absorbed by the tube housing. Only X-rays exiting the tube via a window can be used for radiographic exposure. The size of the tube outlet can be adjusted by means of collimators (i.e. the radiographic field is 'collimated' to the area of interest).

Possible interactions of X-rays with the patient include absorption and scatter (change in direction) of X-rays. Scattered X-rays may maintain their original level of energy or lose some of it while being deviated from their original path. Scatter radiation has two disadvantages: it results in additional detector exposure which decreases image contrast, and radiation scattered in other directions contributes to radiation exposure of people present in the vicinity of the patient. Absorption of the X-ray beam results in loss of energy. Different materials (bone, soft tissue, fat, gas) result in different degrees of X-ray attenuation. X-rays transmitted through the patient are registered by the image detector, and differential absorption of X-rays in tissues provides image contrast on the resultant radiograph (see Chapter 1).

3.1.2 Film–screen systems

Radiographic cassettes with integrated film–screen systems are commonly used for radiographic examination of small animal patients. The front surface of the cassette is designed to maximize X-ray transmission, while the back surface is relatively radiation absorbent. A window on the back of the cassette allows focal exposure of the film to imprint patient information.

Even though different types of films and screens may differ in design details, their basic construction follows the same principles. The X-ray film consists of a base layer coated on one or both sides with radiographic emulsion. An adhesive layer connects the emulsion to the base, and an outer protective layer ('super coat') guards the film from mechanical influences. As radiographic film is light sensitive it has to be kept in the dark until it has been developed (in a darkroom, or within a film cassette). Radiographic emulsion consists of silver halide crystals (predominantly silver bromide, also silver iodide) which are arranged as a network (lattice).

Intensifying screens are located within the radiographic cassette and are in close contact with the radiographic film. Their function is to convert incident X-rays into visible light, which has an intensifying effect as radiographic film is significantly more sensitive to light than to X-rays. Approximately 95% of film darkening is caused by fluores-

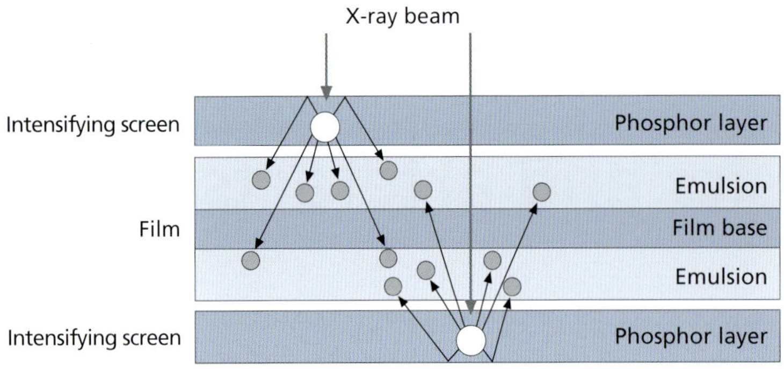

Fig. 3.1 Diagram of film exposure using film–screen systems.

cent light produced by screens, while direct X-ray exposure only contributes approximately 5%. Use of intensifying screens results in a significant decrease in radiation dose (Fig. 3.1; see also Chapters 2 and 4). The most important component of an intensifying screen is the phosphor or scintillating layer, which consists of fluorescing crystals from the group of rare earth elements (rare-earth screens). Intensifying properties of a screen depend on the size of these crystals and the thickness of the phosphor layer (see Chapter 2).

1. Radiographic exposure results in a cascade of reactions in the silver bromide lattice of the radiographic film. The end result of this process is the 'latent image'.
2. X-ray exposure removes electrons from bromine ions.
3. Free electrons are trapped at 'sensitivity specks' (crystal imperfections) in the lattice.
4. These collections of negative charges attract positively charged silver ions, which are subsequently reduced to metallic silver.

The aggregates of silver ions transform the sensitivity specks in the emulsion to 'latent image centres' which constitute the starting point of subsequent film processing.

Following exposure, radiographic film is processed in a darkroom. During manual film processing, radiographs are affixed to metal frames, submerged in tanks filled with chemicals and water, and finally hung up to dry. As chemical processes depend on ambient temperature, lower temperatures result in increased film processing times. With manual development, replenishment of chemicals also has to be done by hand.

With automatic processing, the film is transported using an intricate system of rollers through several tanks filled with chemicals and then a hot air dryer. As chemicals used in this process are kept at a higher temperature (35 °C) than the ones used for manual processing, the time needed for film processing is significantly shortened (90 seconds). Replenishment of chemicals occurs automatically.

Even though manual and automatic film processing differ with regards to the exact composition of chemical solutions, duration of the procedure and resultant artefacts, some basic principles are identical.

Development During development the process of silver reduction initiated during film exposure is continued, which results in amplification of the latent image. The most important component of the developer solution is a reducing agent (phenidone, hydroquinone, metol, etc.). Additional components are activators, hardeners, preservatives, restrainers and water. With manual development, the film has to be washed following this step, while it is directly advanced to the fixer tank during automatic processing.

Fixing During this step silver halide crystals that were not exposed (and thus, not developed) are removed from the emulsion. This ensures that the resulting radiograph can be viewed by light without further film darkening and allows long-term storage of the radiograph without risk of image degradation. The most important component of the fixer solution is the clearing agent (hypo; ammonium or sodium thiosulphate). Other components are activators, hardeners, preservatives and water.

Washing Following development and fixing the film has to be thoroughly washed to remove all remaining chemicals adhering to the film surface.

Drying After the radiograph has been dried it can be handled and used for interpretation.

3.1.3 Digital radiography

Digital radiography utilizes electronic media for radiographic image capture, processing, display and storage. While conventional radiographic film fulfils all these tasks (it is a 'Jack of all trades'), the steps are handled by independent technical units in digital radiography.

In digital radiography four individual steps are required for image generation.

- Step 1: Signal acquisition.
- Step 2: Signal processing.
- Step 3: Image presentation.
- Step 4: Image transfer and archival.

This has several advantages.

- It is possible to customize systems to specific requirements for individual users. Images produced by other modalities (e.g. ultrasound, MRI, CT, endoscopy) can be saved and linked in a common archive.
- Network integration allows rapid distribution of images (even over large distances). Archiving digital image data leads to a significant decrease in cost compared with expenses incurred for film purchase, film development and storage.
- Image interpretation using a monitor can improve diagnostic results. An important advantage compared with conventional film–screen systems is the large latent greyscale range of digital images, which allows optimization of image display based on information received by the detector.

Ultimately, image quality is determined by the weakest link in the image chain.

There are different ways to **capture** large format digital radiographs (Fig. 3.2). Differences in technical concepts of image generation result in differences in dose efficiency, achievable image quality and potential for artefacts. Compared to film–screen systems, digital detectors are able to register a much larger number of attenuation differences. Spatial resolution of digital systems is limited by pixel size. Large format digital detectors can achieve a spatial resolution comparable to high speed film–screen systems at best.

Both photostimulable phosphor (PSP) detector systems (computed radiography; CR) and flat panel detectors (direct digital radiography; DDR) are used in veterinary practice. **PSP screens** (storage phosphors, imaging plates) are flexible polyester screens which are contained in cassettes similar to those used in film–screen radiography. They are especially useful for mobile applications. Following exposure, the latent image information is stored on the imaging plate and is later retrieved and digitized by means of a CR read-out unit. The plate is then erased and can immediately be reused for additional image acquisitions. The read-out process only takes seconds.

Flat panel detectors consist of an active matrix of electronic elements which cover the entire detector area. Individual components correspond to individual pixels in the resultant image. Each detector element consists of a receptor and a relay unit. In indirect detection flat panel systems, incident X-rays are initially converted to visible light by an X-ray intensifying screen, analogous to the process in film–screen radiography. Depending on the type of detector, different scintillators may be used. Photodiodes serve as sensors and convert light photons into electrical signals (Fig. 3.3a). In direct detection flat panel systems, the step of optical conversion is omitted and X-rays interact directly with thin-film transistor (TFT) arrays covered by a layer of photoconductor material (commonly selenium). X-ray interactions in the photoconductor layer release electrons, which migrate to the underlying detector elements (which are posi-

System	Principle	Scintillator	Dose efficiency
Storage phosphor systems	Powder structure	BaFX:Eu $^{2+}$	++
	Needle crystal structure	CsBr:Eu $^{2+}$	+++
	Double-sided read-out	BaFBrI	+++
Flat panel detectors	Direct	Se	+++
	Indirect	Gd_2O_2S	+++
		CsI	++++
CCD systems	Optical coupling	Gd_2O_2S	+
		CsI	+
	Slit scanner	CsI	++

Fig. 3.2 Summary of image registration in digital radiography.

tively charged compared to a thin electrode on top of the selenium layer) where they are recorded (Fig. 3.3b). Integrated control and data channels ensure appropriate spatial registration in pixel elements. Even though wireless flat panel detection systems have been developed, mobile applications for shock-proof units are thus far limited due to their weight and high cost.

Another important step in the digital imaging chain is the signal **processing**. Mathematical algorithms used for this step significantly affect image quality. Processing achieves improved image contrast and resolution, harmonizes image impression and suppresses image noise. Insufficient processing can result in artefacts or loss of relevant image information.

Lastly, image quality depends on the quality of the monitor used for **image display**. Suitability of a monitor for radiographic interpretation is determined by its size, matrix, maximum luminance and contrast ratio.

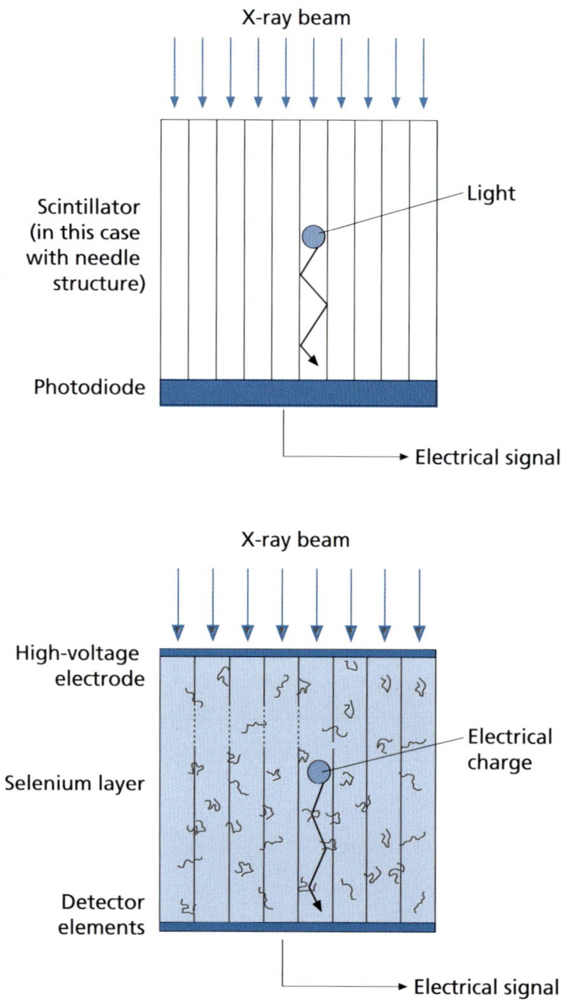

Fig. 3.3 Structure of flat panel detectors.
a Opto-direct (indirect detection) flat panel detectors.
b Electro-direct (direct detection) flat panel detectors.

3.1.4 Grids

As inappropriate use of a grid is a frequent cause of radiographic artefacts, this section will briefly cover basic rules for grid usage and common mistakes. Scatter radiation that reaches the image detector causes a diffuse veil which reduces image contrast and causes unsharpness. Use of an antiscatter grid greatly reduces the amount of scatter radiation reaching the detector. Grids consist of multiple thin lead septa (grid bars) aligned with the primary beam which absorb X-ray photons arriving with oblique incident angles. The interspaces between the lead lamellae (made of carbon fibre, for example) do not attenuate incident X-rays. Grid bars and interspaces are protected from external damage by a firm cover of aluminium or plastic. X-rays that exit the patient's body without having undergone a change in direction travel between lead lamellae through the permeable interspaces and reach the detector (see also Chapter 2).

Grids are categorized according to the orientation of the lead lamellae. Focused grids in which the lead septa are increasingly angled from the centre to the periphery are most common. The slant of the grid bars is aligned with the convergence of the X-ray beam at the focal point. Diverging primary beam quanta can reach the periphery of the film, which assures homogeneous distribution of the X-ray beam across the detector area (Fig. 3.4). The lead septa of a stationary grid are visible as very fine regularly spaced lines on a radiograph (Fig. 3.5). If the grid moves during the exposure (Potter-Bucky grid), the grid lines become blurred.

3.2 Artefacts

3.2.1 Importance of artefacts

Artefacts are components of the image that do not correspond to real structures. As a result, real existing structures

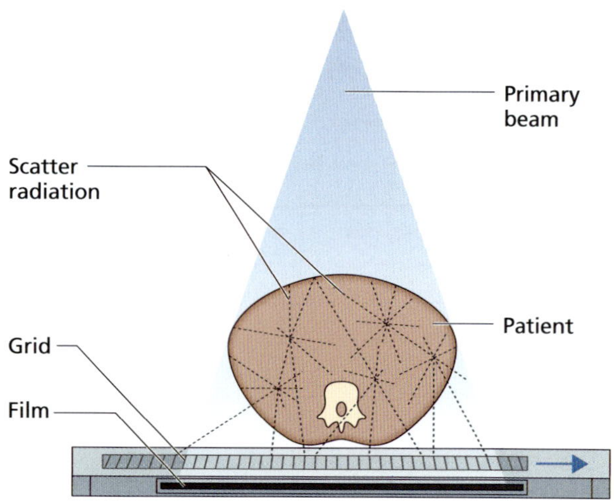

Fig. 3.4 Grid function. The lead lamellae are oriented parallel with the primary beam direction and absorb scatter radiation incident at an oblique angle.

may be masked, or artefacts may mimic structures not present in reality. This definition may be expanded to include real artefactual factors (e.g. dirt in the patient's fur) and poor image quality which compromise diagnostic image information. Artefacts are important for the following reasons.

- They decrease diagnostic quality of a radiograph and can lead to misdiagnoses or oversight of actual lesions.
- They come at a cost of time and money. Repeat radiographs necessitate additional expenses for material and personnel.
- They increase radiation exposure to personnel if the patient is positioned manually for repeat radiographic examinations.

Artefacts are common, and it is important to develop a systematic approach to the problem. The goal is to prevent artefacts before they occur.

3.2.2 Assessment of image quality – recognition of artefacts

Each radiographic interpretation begins with the evaluation of technical image quality. This includes recognition, description and assessment of artefacts.

- How is the radiograph labelled? Unequivocal identification of a radiograph includes the name of the client and the animal, the date of birth, the breed, the veterinary practice or clinic and the date of examination. A laterality marker is also necessary (especially for radiographs of extremities). Incomplete or faulty image labelling can result in confusion and mistakes.
- How was the image generated? Image appearance and quality can vary considerably, not only when comparing analogue and digital radiographs but also within these systems.
- If artefacts are present: Is it possible to identify the underlying cause?
  - Is the artefact only present when a specific cassette is used?
  - Is the artefact localized to only one area of the radiograph (e.g. dark or light spot, sharp or unsharp margination) or is it spread across the entire image (e.g. image brightness, image contrast, streaks, lines, arrangement of changes)?
  - Is the artefact limited to the patient, or does it extend beyond patient boundaries?

3.2.3 Causes of artefacts

Artefacts can occur at any stage of image generation (Table 3.1).

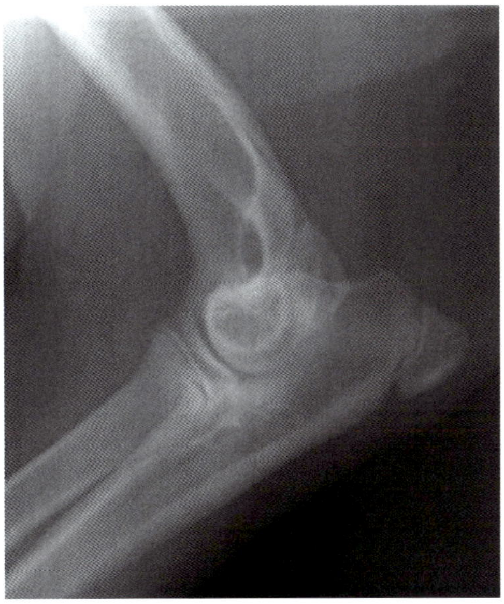

Fig. 3.5 Grid lines. Lines on the radiograph are caused by use of a stationary grid.

Artefacts generated before image registration

Artefacts caused by patient factors Regions of increased opacity can be caused not only by metallic material (Fig. 3.6) but also by wet or dirty fur (Fig. 3.7) and by bandage material (Fig. 3.8).

Artefacts caused by mistakes in grid usage Possible grid artefacts are illustrated in Figure 3.9. Inappropriate positioning of the grid may result in absorption of primary beam radiation (Fig. 3.10) or result in visible opaque grid lines on the radiograph (Fig. 3.11).

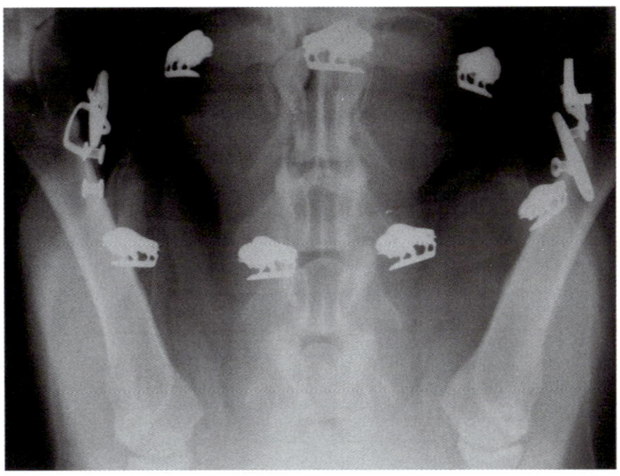

Fig. 3.6 Collar. The collar was not removed prior to radiographic exposure. A full evaluation of the cervical spine is not possible.

Table 3.1 Classification of artefacts according to the time of occurrence during image generation.

Classification			Causes
Artefacts related to the patient			Collar Bandage material Dirt on fur coat Wet hair Ultrasound gel Identification microchips
Artefacts related to exposure technique	Technique factors		Overexposure Underexposure Double or multiple exposure Increased exposure time
	Grid use		Failure to use grid with large patient size Grid decentring Tilted grid Upside-down grid Wrong distance (too small or large)
	Positioning		Positioning errors Errors with centring and collimation Extreme patient dyspnoea or unrest
Artefacts generated during image registration and processing	Film–screen systems	Cassette errors	Light entry Defective compressive foam layer Dirt on screen Screen or film defects
		Errors during development	Fogged or old film Exhausted chemicals Time spent for development, fixing and washing too short or too long Incomplete mixing of chemicals Temperature differences in tank Damage to the film emulsion Static electricity
	Digital radiography	Detector errors	Mechanical or thermal damage PSP plates: Defective read-out unit Flat panel detectors: Detector array loss, missing or wrong calibration
		Errors during image processing	Malfunction during processing steps (field recognition, histogram analysis, filter applications) Lack of appropriate filters Choice of inappropriate filters Use of inappropriate look-up table (LUT)

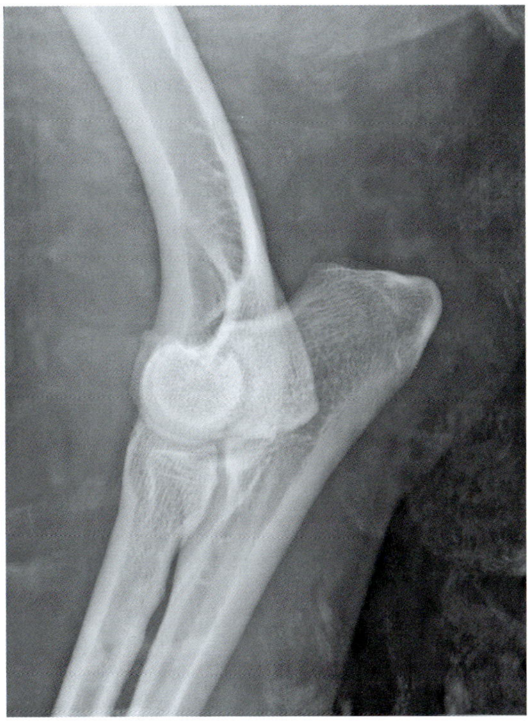

Fig. 3.7 Wet hair. In this long-haired dog with wet fur, cloudy regions overlie the area of interest and limit image interpretation.

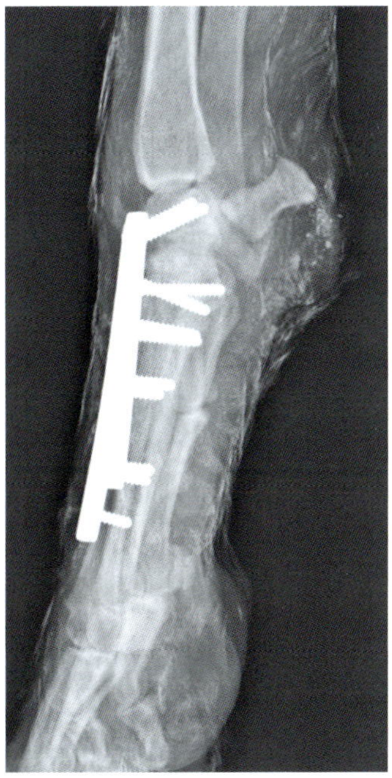

Fig. 3.8 Bandage material. Overlying bandage material and residual ointment stains interfere with evaluation of healing (callus formation, evidence of infection). However, evaluation of implant position and bone alignment is possible.

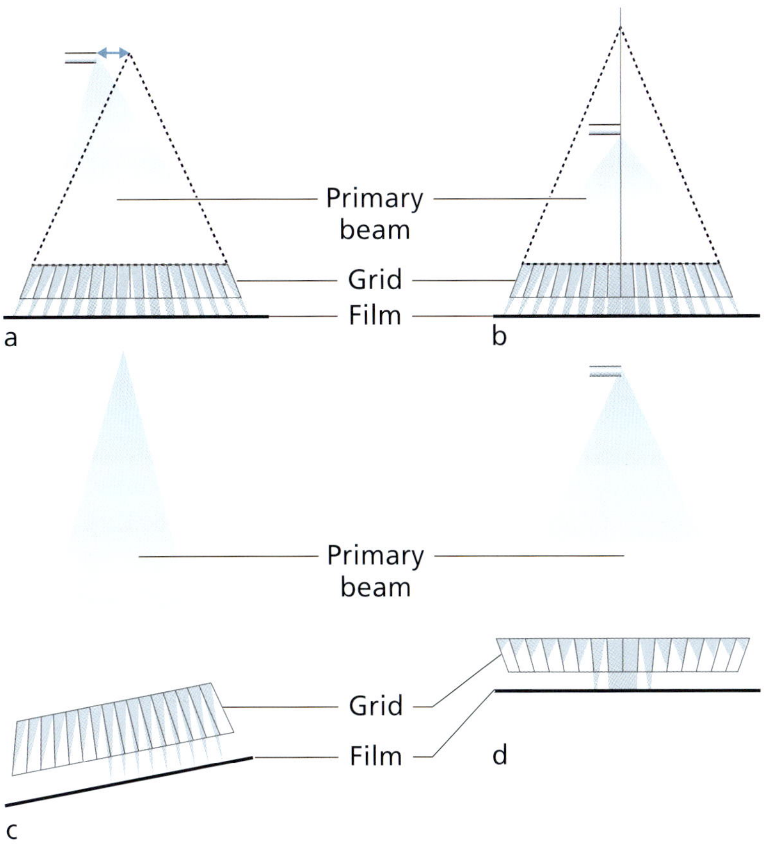

Fig. 3.9 Mistakes with grid usage.

a Lateral decentring of the grid in relation to the X-ray tube (or vice versa). This results in homogeneous attenuation of the X-ray beam across the film.

b Grid-focus decentring. X-rays in the middle of the field remain parallel to the grid lamellae while primary radiation is increasingly absorbed towards the periphery. The film is centrally well exposed while peripheral areas are underexposed. An increased distance would yield similar effects.

c Off-level grid decentring. This grid malposition can lead to relatively homogeneous attenuation of the X-ray beam across the entire film or can, as shown here, result in increasing underexposure from one end of the film to the other.

d Upside-down grid. An upside-down focused grid permits uninhibited X-ray transmission in the centre of the area of collimation while radiation in the periphery of the field is almost completely absorbed.

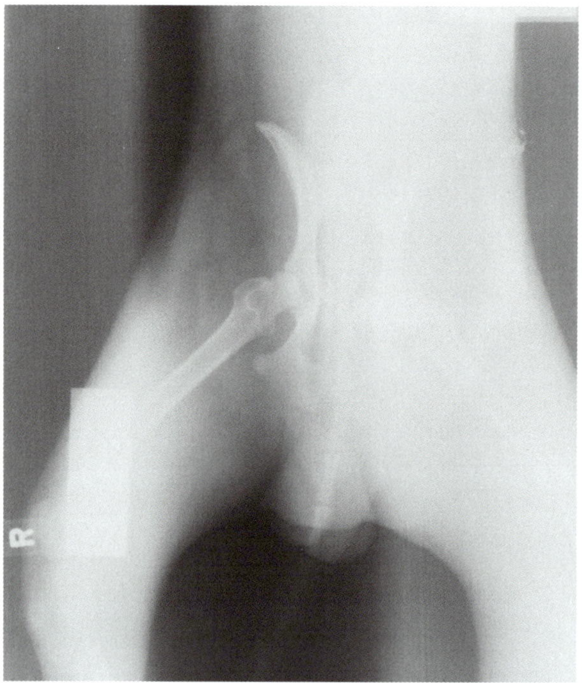

Fig. 3.10 Grid artefact. The significant attenuation of the X-ray beam in the periphery with near normal film exposure in the centre and visible grid lines is characteristic for an upside-down focused grid (see also Fig. 3.9d).

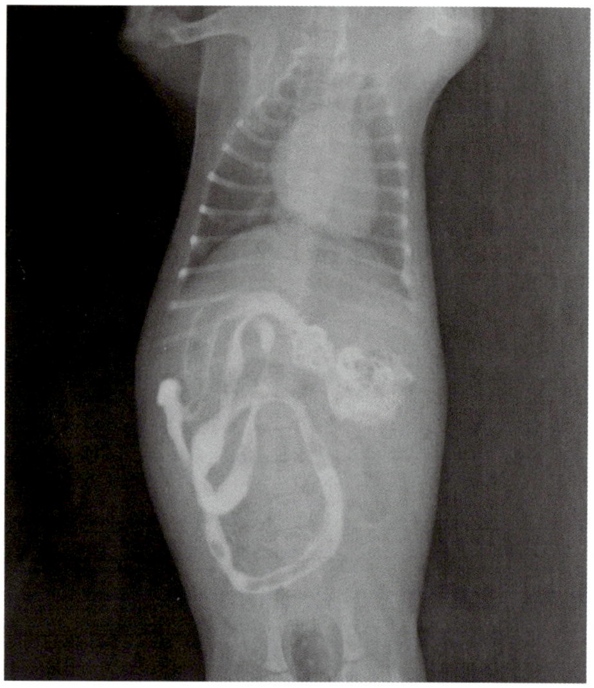

Fig. 3.11 Grid artefact. The grid was not centred properly. There is increased attenuation of the primary beam with increasing distance from the tube (see also Fig. 3.9a).

Double exposure Double exposures always lead to unexpected and new insights (Fig. 3.12).

Motion unsharpness Patient motion or physiological organ movement during radiographic exposure leads to blurred images especially with long exposure times (Fig. 3.13).

Specific artefacts in film–screen radiography

Exposure errors

As film–screen systems only have a narrow exposure range, **overexposed** and **underexposed** films can be easily recognized based on image brightness. An underexposed film appears too bright (see also section 2.2 and Fig. 2.2). However, the film around the patient is, typically, adequately darkened (except in cases of extreme underexposure). Overexposure results in excessive film darkening. In contrast to underexposed films, overexposed radiographs may still have some diagnostic yield if evaluated using an

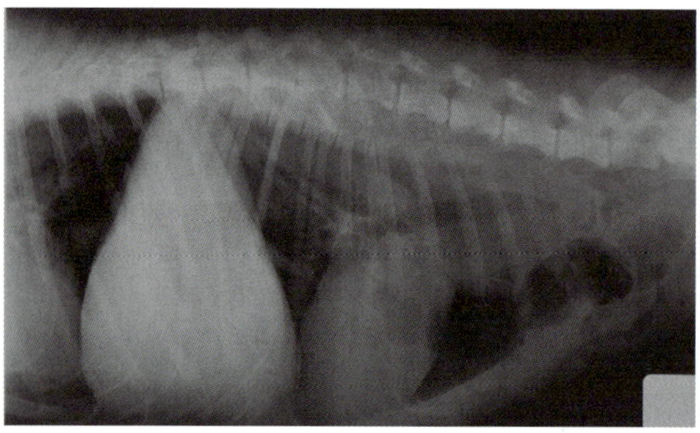

Fig. 3.12 Double exposure. Lateral thoracic and abdominal radiographs were exposed on the same film. The radiograph is too dark, and this patient's anatomy is definitely not normal!

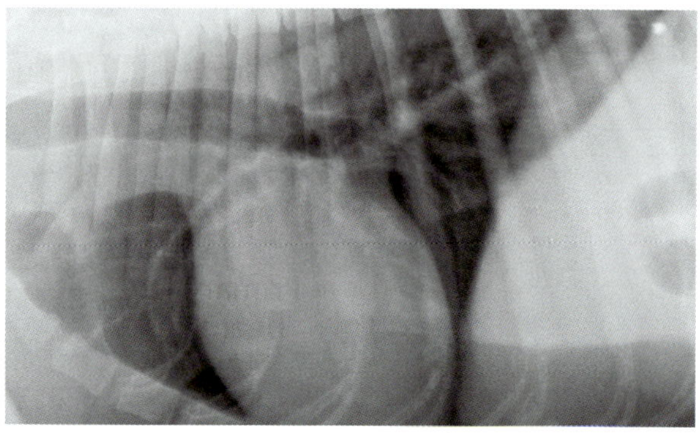

Fig. 3.13 Motion artefact. The caudal thorax and cranial abdomen are blurred due to respiratory motion (panting) during exposure.

intense light source (hot lamp). Exposure errors are typically the result of an inappropriate choice of technique factors. Mistakes in grid operation or malfunction of the X-ray equipment are much less common.

Excessive scatter radiation may result from failure to use a grid and can result in **decreased image contrast**.

Excessively dark radiographs may also be the result of **double exposure**. In this case, structures of different body regions (in the case of failure to replace the film in the cassette before taking the next radiograph (see Fig. 3.12), or a double silhouette of the patient (in the case of inadvertent double exposure), will also be recognized on the film.

Motion unsharpness is remedied by a decrease in exposure time (see Chapter 2).

ARTEFACTS RELATED TO THE FILM–SCREEN SYSTEM

Use of a radiographic cassette upside down results in structural parts of the cassette being visible on the resultant radiograph. If the back of the cassette contains lead, the radiograph will also be underexposed (Fig. 3.14). Damage to the cassette can markedly interfere with image quality. A defective closure mechanism allows entry of visible **light**, which will result in complete blackening of the exposed area of film. A defect in the **compressible foam layer** located within the cassette behind the intensifying screen will cause an unsharp region in the area where the film loses immediate contact with the screen. **Dirt or foreign material** located between the intensifying screen and the film appears as white, sharply marginated structures on the resultant radiograph (Fig. 3.15). Similarly, **mechanical damage** to the intensifying screen and film will be reflected on the radiographic image. **Old film** will have decreased contrast compared to new material.

ARTEFACTS RELATED TO FILM PROCESSING

The risk of causing artefacts or even completely ruining a radiograph during film processing is high, and extreme care should be taken to avoid this problem. Flawless film development is possible both with manual and automated processing techniques.

LOSS IN IMAGE CONTRAST A possible reason for this during manual development is the use of exhausted developer fluid and a compensatory increase in development time. The increased contact time between developer fluid and radiographic film results in reduction of all crystals in the emulsion (exposed or unexposed). The radiograph will appear homogeneously grey. A decrease in image contrast can also result from film exposure in the darkroom, for example when red light of the wrong wavelength is used, when the red light lamp is positioned too close to unexposed films, or when the darkroom is compromised by light leaks. The degree of loss in film contrast can vary from minor fogging to complete film blackening (Fig. 3.16, Fig. 3.17).

OVERDEVELOPMENT AND UNDERDEVELOPMENT These processing mistakes may affect the greyscale of a radiograph and should be distinguished from underexposure and overexposure. This can be accomplished by taking advantage of the fact that patient data are imprinted on the film after and independently of radiographic film exposure, while film development affects both equally. With overexposure, excessive film darkening is limited to the area of the film exposed during the radiograph. Patient information imprinted separately is of adequate density. With overdevelopment, the

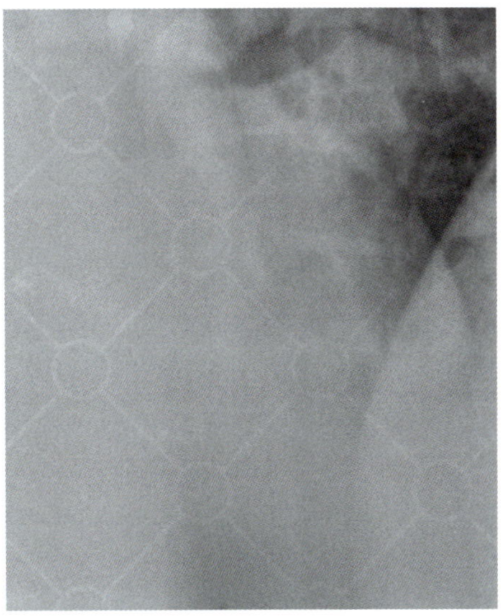

Fig. 3.14 This artefact is caused by acquisition of a radiograph through the back of a cassette.

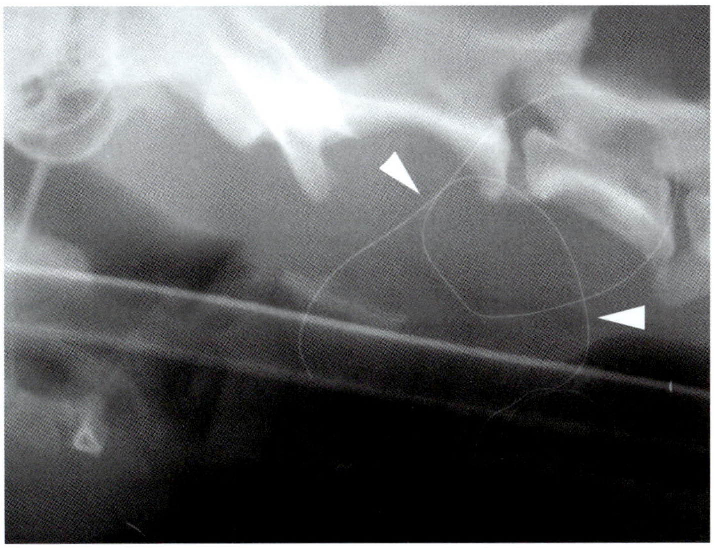

Fig. 3.15 This sharply marginated curvilinear opaque structure on the radiograph (arrowheads) is caused by a long hair located within the radiographic cassette.

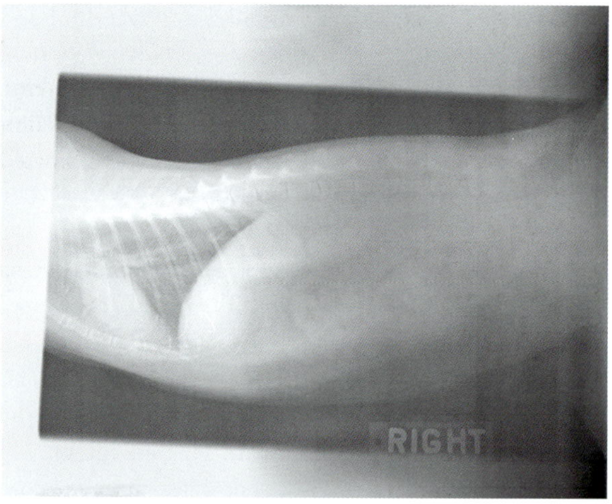

Fig. 3.16 Film fog. This film was left in the darkroom and was subject to an extended period of red light exposure before development. The red light source was located to the right of the film. On this side, fog affects both exposed and unexposed regions of the film including the metallic marker.

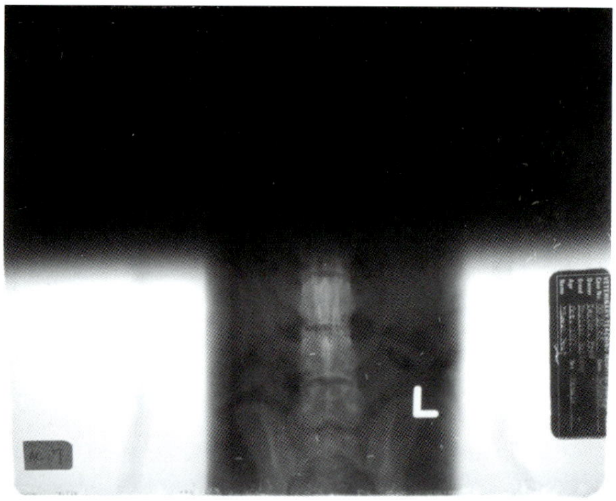

Fig. 3.17 Complete blackening of part of a film. The door to the darkroom was opened when only one third of the film had entered the automated developer. The remaining two thirds are completely exposed and black.

entire X-ray film (including imprinted patient information) is too dark. The imprinted patient information can also aid in distinguishing underexposure and underdevelopment. With film underexposure the corner of the radiograph with the separately imprinted patient information is of adequate density (Fig. 3.18a). With underdevelopment the patient information is too light as is the rest of the film (Fig. 3.18b).

Incomplete fixation With incomplete fixation, a portion of film emulsion is retained. Film regions outside the collimated area have a milky appearance when inspected against a light source. Adequately fixed film appears clear and transparent.

Incomplete washing Incomplete washing following film development leads to transfer of some residual developer fluid into the fixation bath, which subsequently becomes

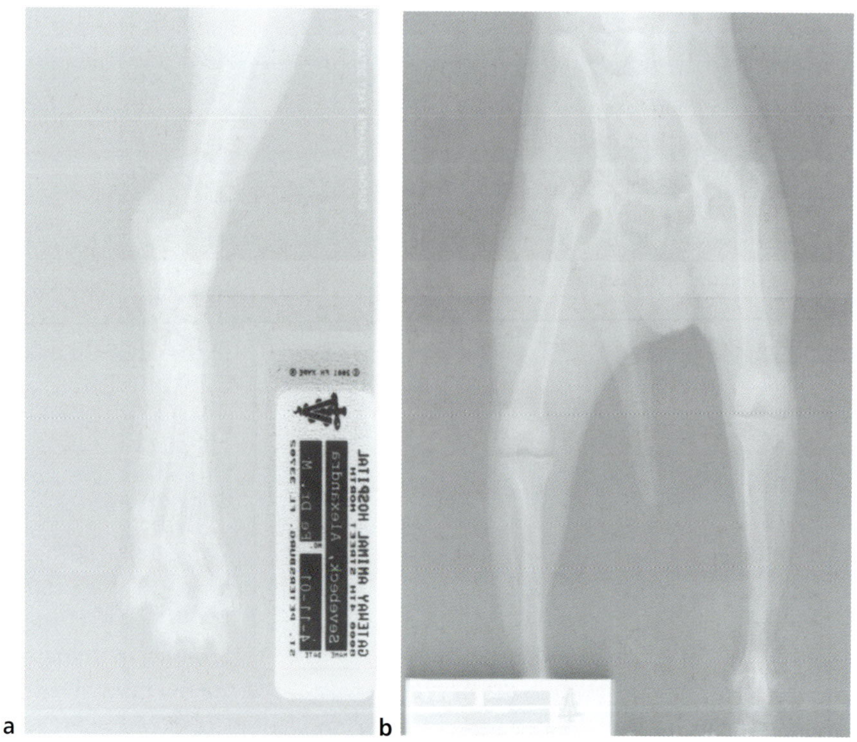

Fig. 3.18 Underdevelopment versus underexposure.
a Underexposure results in very light and usually nondiagnostic radiographs. Note that the separately imprinted patient information is clearly visible and well exposed.
b Underdevelopment also results in very light and usually nondiagnostic radiographs. Note that in these cases the radiograph and patient information are equally affected.

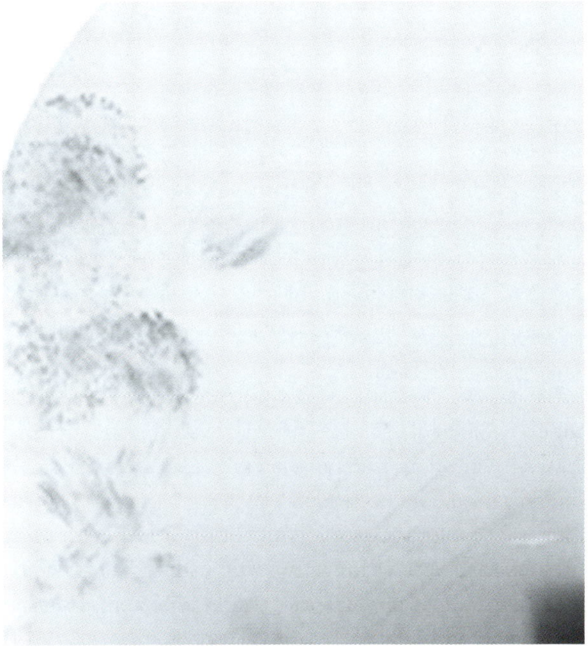

Fig. 3.19 Black fingerprints on these radiographs are caused by developer fluid on the fingers of the examiner.

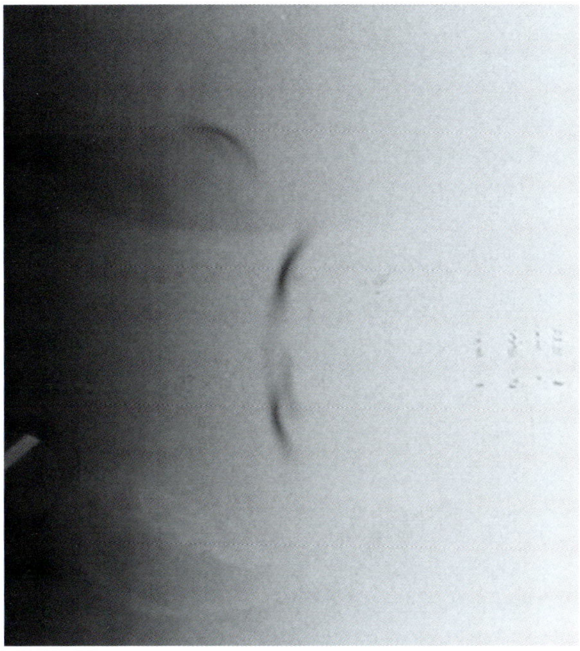

Fig. 3.20 This focal dark crescent caused by impression of a fingernail is a very common artefact.

dysfunctional. Incomplete washing following fixation results in oxidation of fixer retained on the film. These radiographs are characterized by brown discoloration, a metallic gleam and a characteristic 'chemical' smell.

SPOTS AND SCRATCHES, LINES, CLOUDS, FLASHES AND THUNDER

SPOTS These may be caused by:

- handling of undeveloped film with wet or oily fingers (Fig. 3.19)
- air bubbles adhering to the film
- water splashes on the film surface
- film kinks (e.g. caused by finger nails) (Fig. 3.20).

Direct contact or adhesion of two films during development or fixation leads to mirrored, clear or milky spots on the films or complete regional loss of the emulsion layer (Fig. 3.21). Close inspection of the abnormal areas in reflected light or palpation of the film may aid in identification of the specific underlying cause of the artefact.

SCRATCHES AND LINES When using an automatic processor, small, regularly spaced film scratches oriented in the direction of the rollers are common and are caused by the receiving mechanism of the machine. 'Irregular' scratches are a result of mechanical damage of the film emulsion. Increased pressure from automatic processor rollers results in regular black lines which typically extend over the entire length or width of the radiographic film. Their orientation with respect to the direction of film transport will aid in determining which exact part of the processor is causing the problem.

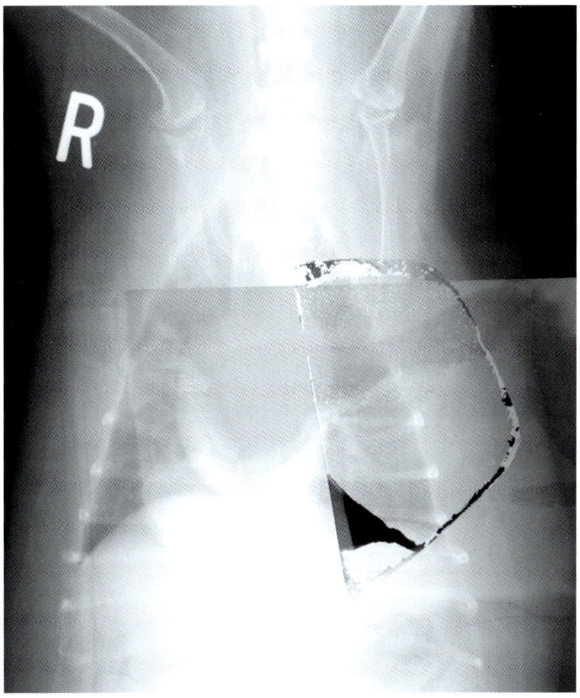

Fig. 3.21 Extensive defects of the emulsion layer and sharply marginated milky regions result from contact of two films during development ('kissing defects').

Clouding 'Clouds' are typically caused by insufficient mixing of the developer fluid and increased concentration of developer at the bottom of the tank compared with the surface. If the developer liquid is not stirred at all before a film is inserted, the part of the radiograph closer to the bottom of the tank is overdeveloped and very dark. Developer concentration decreases towards the tank's surface and the film developed in this part of the tank is lighter. Stirring but incomplete mixing of developer fluid results in streaky lighter and darker regions on the radiograph (Fig. 3.22).

Flashes Electrical discharge (static electricity) results in focal film exposure and thus blackening. These artefacts are of characteristic shape and often resemble tree-like branching structures (Fig. 3.23).

Thunder associated with film development has to our knowledge not been reported to date.

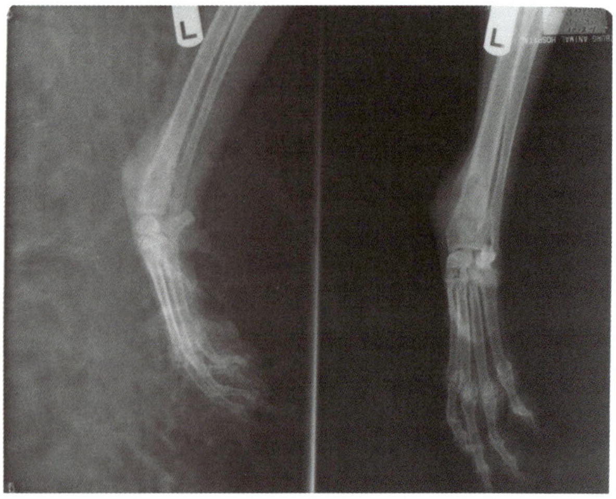

Fig. 3.22 Clouds. Cloudy brighter and darker regions on the left hand radiograph are caused by insufficient mixing of developer fluid or different temperature layers within the tank (manual development).

Specific artefacts in digital radiography

Many artefacts, for example motion or grid artefacts or those caused by foreign material blocking the beam path, will have the same effect on digital as on conventional radiographs. Other artefacts are specific to digital radiography. In general, identification of the underlying cause (and thus finding remedies for the problem) is more complicated than with film–screen artefacts even for experienced radiologists. In this chapter only common artefacts in digital radiography will be covered.

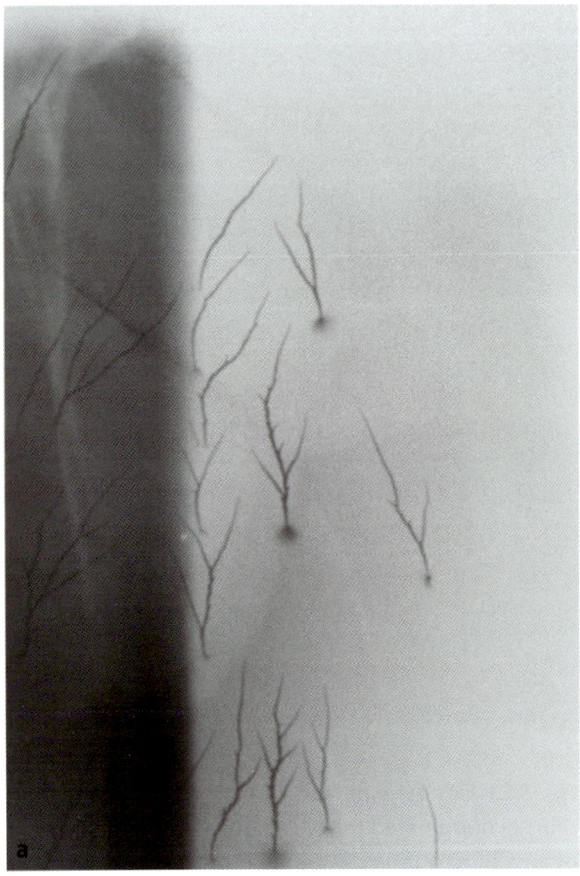

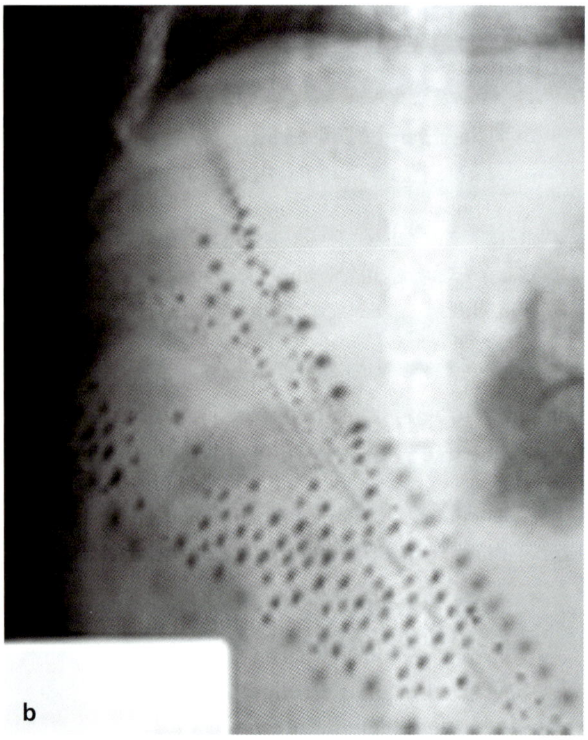

Fig. 3.23 Static electricity due to electrical discharges.
a Tree-like branching artefacts.
b Rounded smudge or spot densities.

Exposure errors As previously mentioned, **underexposure** leads to increased image noise and subsequently to a decrease in image detail (Fig. 3.24). **Extreme overexposure** also negatively affects image quality. The detector reaches a state of saturation, and signal differences are no longer registered. The image is homogeneously grey, and small details are not visible even when modifying the window settings. In some flat panel detectors, parts of the detector construction become visible (Fig. 3.25). To correct these problems, the radiograph has to be repeated using a lower dose. In cases of inadequate collimation (field too small or too large) the histogram provides the wrong pixel values for image processing (see **'Errors in signal processing'** below).

Detector errors – storage phosphor systems Dirt and dust accumulation on the plate over time is somewhat unavoidable but is easily remedied by regular cleaning of the plate with specific solutions. Scratches and cracks are more critical as they cannot be fixed and require replacement of the plate. Imaging plates with needle crystal structure (see Fig. 3.2) are shock sensitive, and dropping these plates can render them unusable. Artefacts can also be induced by plate readers due to imprecision of the read-out laser beam or receptors of luminescence, or if the imaging plate is not completely erased following the read-out process.

Detector errors – flat panel detectors Malfunction of detector elements can to some degree be compensated for electronically. Extensive detector array loss may necessitate replacement of the detector. Errors in calibration can result in regions of a different greyscale or in linear streaks at the contact zones between individual detector elements. Incomplete read-out is also possible with flat panel detectors, resulting in ghost images on subsequent radiographs ('memory artefacts'). Flat panel detectors used in a mobile setting are at risk of mechanical damage and resultant image artefacts.

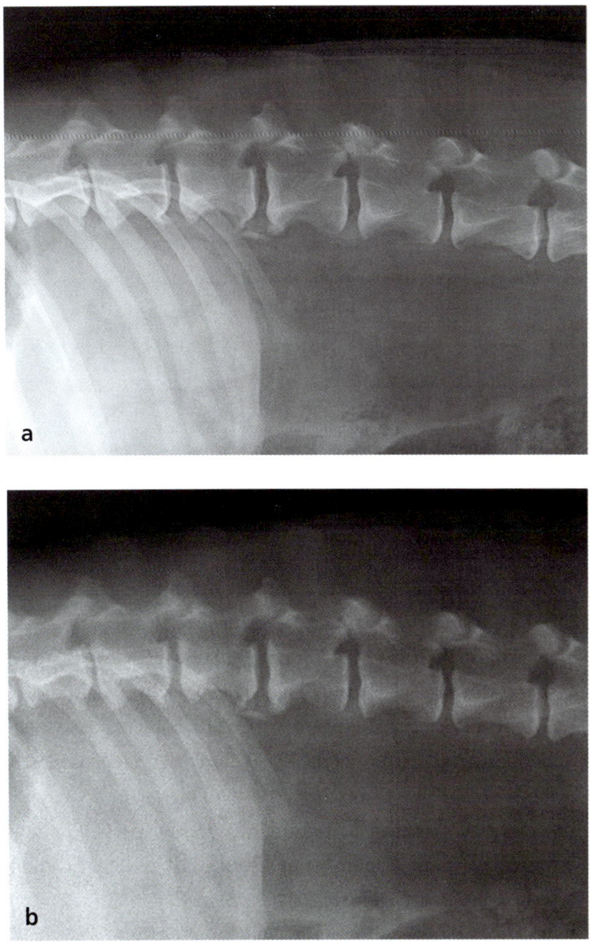

Fig. 3.24 Underexposure on a photostimulable phosphor detector system.

a Optimal exposure.

b Exposure obtained with reduction to 1/16 of the dose used for the initial radiograph in (a). The vertebral trabecular structure cannot be evaluated due to image noise.

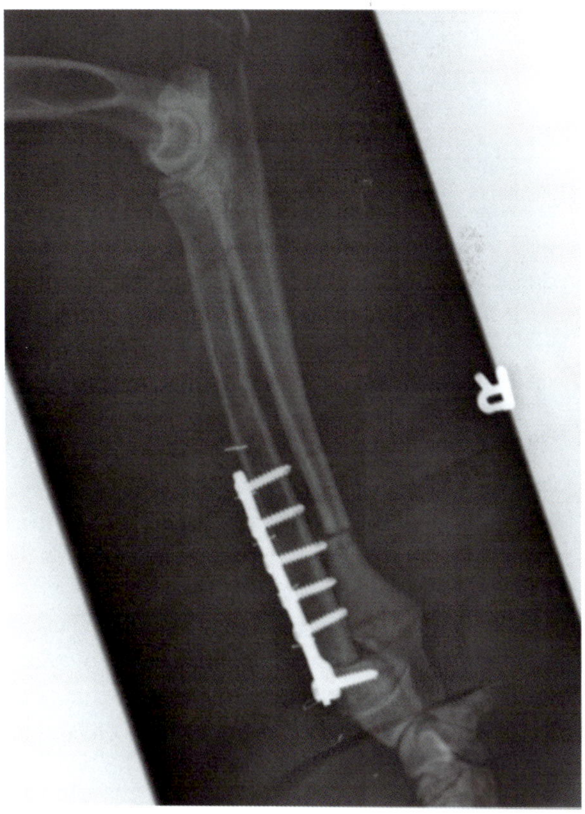

Fig. 3.25 Extreme overexposure on a flat panel detector. The soft tissues of the limb and the trabecular structure of the bones are not visible. Additionally, lighter and darker squares are noted in the background. This 'plank artefact' results from oversaturation of the flat panel detector.

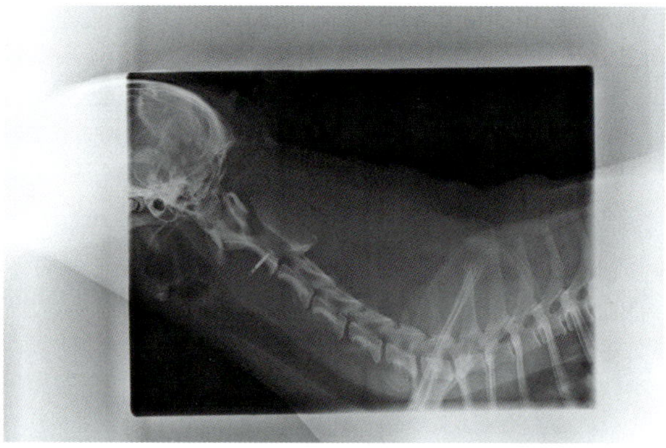

Fig. 3.26 Error during field recognition. This image essentially reflects raw data. The patient's body contour is visible outside the collimated area as detectors are able to register very small amounts of radiation aside from the primary beam. The visualization of body parts outside the primary beam is attributable to extrafocal radiation and radiation that has passed through the collimator leaves. The first step in image processing is the correct identification of the exposed field. If this does not happen all shades of grey (including many white and light grey shades) are used for further calculations. The resultant image is extremely low in contrast.

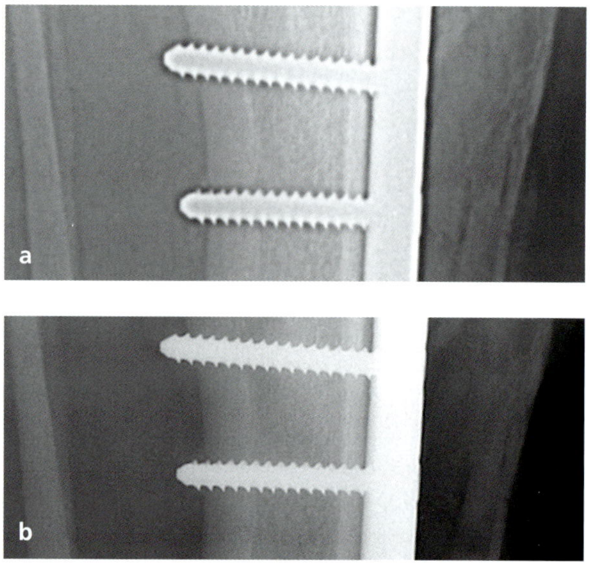

Fig. 3.27 Überschwinger artefact.
a The regional lucencies around the screws as well as between the plate and cortex are artefactual secondary to an error in image processing. This artefact can mimic implant loosening.
b This artefact is remedied by changing image processing parameters.

Errors in signal processing These artefacts are common. Image processing involves three separate steps (field recognition, histogram analysis, accentuation of structures). As these occur successively, early mistakes are propagated throughout the process. An error in automatic recognition of the exposed field means that the subsequent histogram analysis is based on wrong assumptions (Fig. 3.26). The greyscale used to display pixel values is too large or too small, significantly reducing image contrast. A similar effect can occur when the exposed field only constitutes a very small part of the entire detector area. This can be avoided by using the smallest imaging plate possible. Actual signal processing serves to generate image information. Mathematical algorithms process the pixel values from the histogram to represent the entire greyscale of a specific region while concurrently enhancing regional contrast and suppressing image noise. A typical artefact occurring during a specific type of signal processing ('unsharp mask filtering') is called the 'Überschwinger artefact' and results in a radiolucent halo sign around metallic implants (Fig. 3.27).

Errors in image display Use of an inappropriate 'look-up table' (LUT) can interfere with contrast display and image brightness. This error can easily be corrected using computer post-processing.

Suggested reading

Bushberg JT, Seibert JA, Leidholdt EM, Boone JM. The Essential Physics of Medical Imaging. Philadelphia: Lippincott Williams & Wilkins 2002.

Cesar LJ, Schueler BA, Zink FE, Daly TR, Taubel JP, Jorgenson LL. Artefacts found in computed radiography. Br J Radiol 2001; 74: 195–202.

Curry TS, Dowdey JE, Murry RC. Christensen's Physics of Diagnostic Radiology, 4th edn. Philadelphia: Lippincott Williams & Wilkins 1990.

Drost WT, Reese DJ, Hornof WJ. Digital radiography artefacts. Vet Radiol Ultrasound 2008; 49: 48–56.

Hartung K, Ludewig E, Tellhelm B. Röntgenuntersuchung in der Tierarztpraxis. Stuttgart: Enke 2010.

Hogge JP, Palmer CH, Muller CC, Little ST, Smith DC, Fatouros PP, de Paredes ES. Quality assurance in mammography: artifact analysis. Radiographics 1999; 19: 503–22.

Krupinski EA, Williams MB, Andriole K, Strauss KJ, Applegate K, Wyatt M, Bjork S, Seibert JA. Digital radiography image quality: image processing and display. J Am Coll Radiol 2007; 4: 389–400.

Laubenberger T, Laubenberger J. Technik der medizinischen Radiologie. Köln: Deutscher Ärzteverlag 1999.

Ludewig E, Werrmann A, Kamm KF, Oechtering G. Digitale Projektionsradiographie – eine Übersicht zu Begriffen und Prinzipien. Prakt Tierarzt 2007; 88: 593–603.

Mattoon JS. Digital radiography. Vet Comp Orthop Traumatol 2006; 19: 123–32.

Sweeney RJ. Radiographic Artifacts: Their Cause and Control. Philadelphia: Lippincott 1983.

Ticer JW. Radiographic Technique in Veterinary Practice. Philadelphia: WB Saunders 1984.

Willis CE, Thompson SK, Shepard SJ. Artifacts and misadventures in digital radiography. Appl Radiol 2004; 1: 11–20.

4

Applied radiation safety

Silke Hecht

The goal of this chapter is to discuss practical aspects of radiation safety which can be applied in small animal practice. Legal aspects of radiation protection and radiation safety (including definitions, dose limits and regulations) vary between different countries and are beyond the scope of this textbook.

There are two basic types of possible radiation exposure in radiography (Fig. 4.1).

Primary beam radiation This refers to radiation emitted directly from the X-ray tube. It is transmitted through the patient and results in exposure of the X-ray film or digital detector. The primary beam is high in energy and able to penetrate lead gloves. The examiner's hands or other body parts should never be included in the collimation and exposed to the primary beam (Fig. 4.2 and Fig. 4.3).

Secondary (scatter) radiation Interaction of the useful (primary) beam with an object (housing of the X-ray tube, patient, X-ray table) results in divergence (scatter) of a proportion of the X-rays. Scattered X-rays are attenuated to a variable degree compared to the primary beam and may spread in any direction. Scattered X-rays may be reflected again after hitting the floor, wall or table and result in exposure of the examiner and/or X-ray film. A primary goal of radiation safety in small animal practice is avoidance/minimization of scatter radiation.

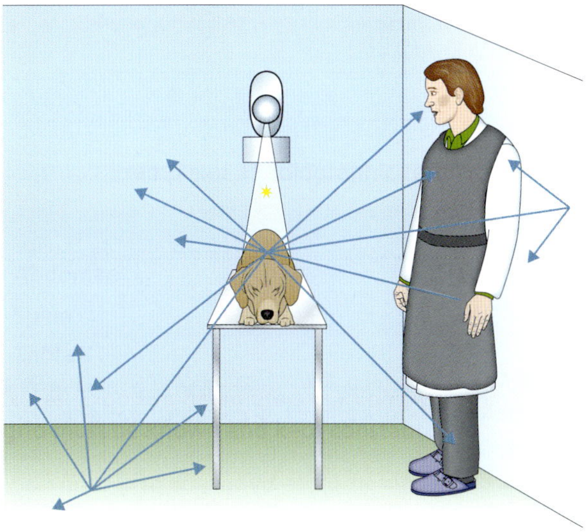

Fig. 4.1 Schematic illustration of different types of radiation exposure. The primary beam (*) exits the X-ray tube. Secondary (scatter) radiation is caused when X-rays are deflected, e.g. in the X-ray tube housing, within the patient or the examination table. Scattered X-rays may be reflected again from the floor or wall and result in additional exposure of the examiner.

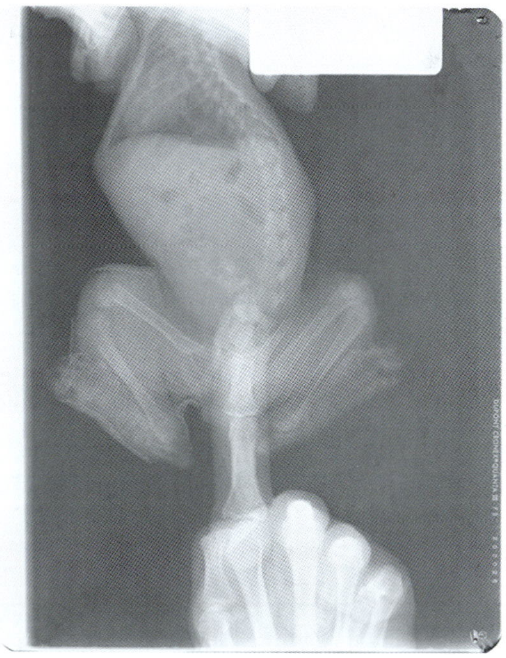

Fig. 4.2 Unprotected human hand in the primary beam. This is completely unacceptable! The radiograph is nondiagnostic due to severe obliquity in positioning and superimposition of the patient with human fingers.

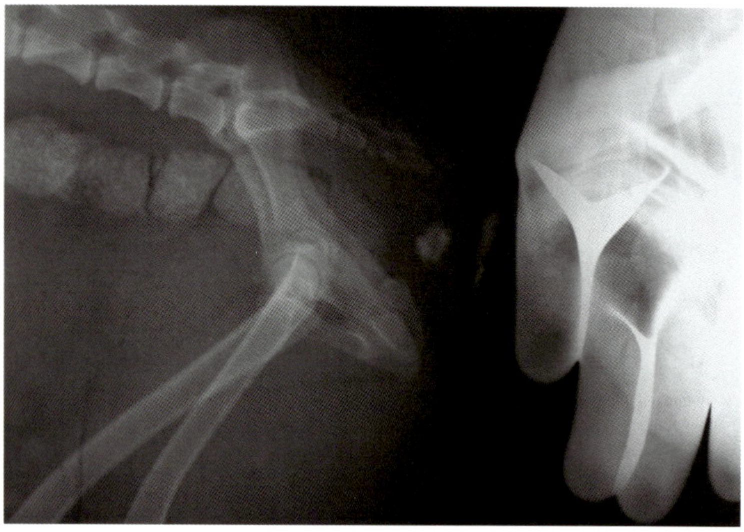

Fig. 4.3 Examiner's hand with lead glove included in the collimation of the primary beam. The radiographer wears appropriate protective clothing; however, it is important to note that this does not provide protection from the primary beam! Note that the examiner's digits are faintly visible behind the outline of the lead glove.

Scatter radiation can be reduced by the use of intensifying screens and grids, and by appropriate collimation of the primary beam.

Radiation exposure can be minimized by adhering to the **ALARA** (**as low as reasonably achievable**) concept. The three principles of ALARA are time, distance and shielding.

- **Time**: The amount of radiation absorbed is proportional to the exposure time. Practical ways to reduce the time spent in close proximity to the X-ray beam include the following.
  - Avoidance of unnecessary duplication of radiographs. For example, a complete radiographic series of a broken leg in an awake dog following trauma may be avoided if preoperative radiographs under general anaesthesia (and without personnel present in the X-ray suite) are scheduled for the following day.
  - Limitation of number of individuals in the X-ray suite. For example, training of students or technicians does not require their presence in the room during the actual image acquisition.
  - Rotation of personnel between different services may aid in reducing the time assigned to radiology in larger practices.
  - Obtaining radiographs under sedation or anaesthesia is not only beneficial from a radiation safety perspective, it also results in a reduced stress level for the patient and markedly improved quality of the resulting radiographs (decreased motion artefacts, adequate positioning, decreased patient resistance). Positioning aids may include ropes, foam wedges, sand bags and/or V-troughs (Fig. 4.4 and Fig. 4.5).

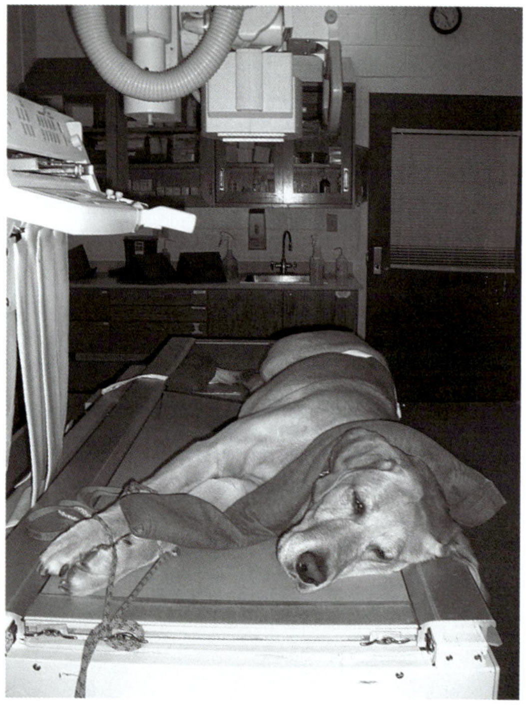

Fig. 4.4 Appropriate use of positioning aids when obtaining radiographs of a sedated patient. The extremities are secured with ropes and the head and neck are held in place by means of a sand bag. Thoracic and abdominal radiographs were obtained in this patient without any personnel present in the room.

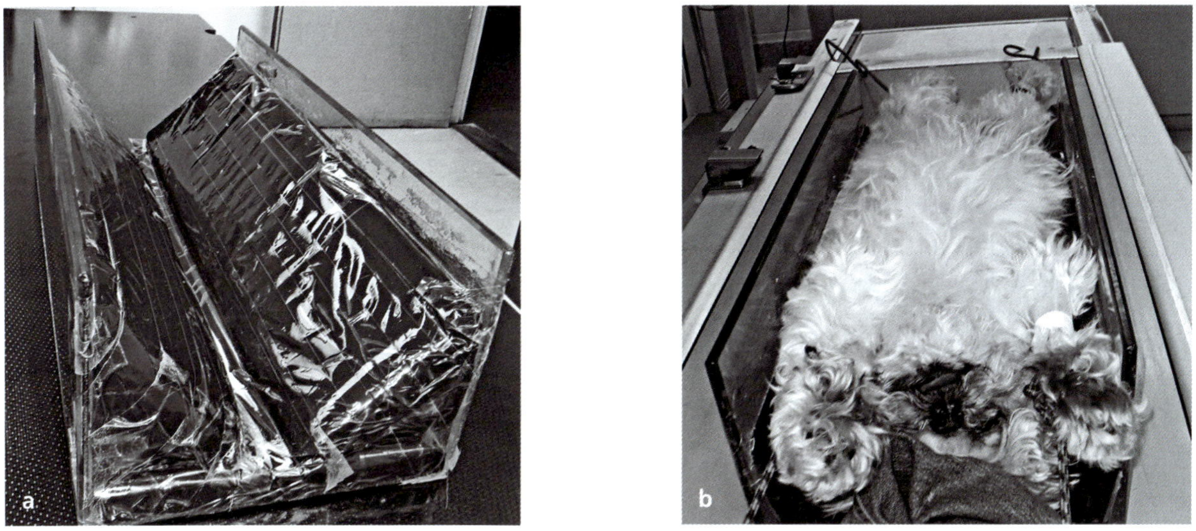

Fig. 4.5

a V-trough used as positioning aid for ventrodorsal views of the thorax, abdomen, spine and pelvis. This custom-made device consists of three Plexiglas sheets which were assembled in a U-shaped fashion and subsequently padded with foam wedges.

b Positioning of a sedated dog for a ventrodorsal thoracic radiograph using a V-trough. Straight patient positioning is much easier than placing the dog on the hard and flat X-ray table. Note use of ropes to fix the legs in place, and sand bag placed to stabilize the head. Radiographs in this patient were obtained without any personnel present in the room.

Practical tips for positioning aids

Ropes: When attached to the distal extremities of sedated or anaesthetized animals, ropes can be used to extend the patient's legs and tie them to the table, minimizing superimposition with the area of interest. They are also useful for straight patient positioning (especially in dorsal recumbency) and to achieve appropriate positioning for extended radiographs, for example of the coxofemoral or scapulohumeral joints. Based on our experience, ropes used for various sports activities (such as climbing or sailing) are well suited for patient positioning purposes. They are available in different diameters and can be cut to any length. They are unlikely to cause skin abrasions or get entangled in the patient's fur due to their smooth surface. They are durable and designed to allow easy tying and untying of knots. Finally, the modern synthetic materials used for these ropes (e.g. nylon) are often easier to clean and disinfect than natural materials such as hemp.

Foam blocks and wedges: These can be purchased at home improvement supply or hobby stores and can be cut to any size and shape. Optimally, they should be covered with plastic for improved durability and to allow appropriate cleaning and disinfection. A more expensive alternative is purchase of X-ray positioning kits available online or in medical supply stores.

Sand bags: These can be manufactured easily and cheaply by cutting off the legs of old trousers (preferably jeans) and filling them with sand (e.g. from home improvement stores). It is important not to overfill the bags as this will decrease their flexibility. When using sand bags for small animal positioning, sand is distributed into the periphery of the bag, and the central (lighter, empty) part is placed on top of the patient (Fig. 4.4). The patient is effectively tethered to the table but not squashed by the heavy sand bag. It is important to note that sand is radiopaque, and that a sand bag should not be superimposed with the area of interest.

V-troughs: These are extremely valuable for patient positioning in dorsal recumbency (i.e. for ventrodorsal views of the thorax, abdomen, spine and pelvis). The patient's spine is wedged in the deepest part of the 'V', resulting automatically in fairly straight positioning. Using a trough made from or padded with foam minimizes patient discomfort, and many animals tolerate positioning in a trough better than being directly placed on a cold, hard X-ray table. V-troughs of variable sizes are available online and from medical supply stores. Alternatively, boxes of different sizes (at least two, one for large and one for small patients) can be manufactured by a talented handyman in the practice (or the family) from Plexiglas, for example, and subsequently covered with foam (Fig. 4.5). For custom-built troughs it is advisable to obtain radiographs of the material to be used prior to assembly to ascertain adequate X-ray transmission. Wood should be avoided as a building material for positioning aids due to the risk of splintering.

- **Distance**: After exiting the X-ray tube, the X-ray beam spreads out. The intensity of radiation decreases with distance from the tube following the inverse square law (Fig. 4.6). In practice, this means that doubling the distance from the X-ray tube will quarter the dose to the examiner. With three times the original distance, the original radiation dose is decreased to 1/9.

  - Any person not involved in patient positioning but remaining in the room during the radiographic procedure (e.g. anaesthetist with a highly critical patient) can reduce their radiation dose by taking a step backwards.
  - If an animal has to be held during the radiographic procedure, the radiation dose to the examiners can be decreased by placing them at the respective ends of the X-ray table with their arms extended rather than at the sides of the patient.
  - When obtaining horizontal beam radiographs (large animal radiology, some special thoracic and abdominal projections, orthopaedic 'skyline' views), use of a cassette holder allows the distance between the examiner and the primary beam to be increased.

- **Shielding**: Different types of shielding can be used to protect personnel from X-ray exposure.

  - Some components of the X-ray room design (e.g. wall thickness) are dictated by national/regional radiation safety regulations. During daily operations it is important to be mindful and take advantage of structural features intended to provide radiation protection (e.g. close doors to the room during image acquisition, stand behind mobile lead walls if presence in the X-ray room is required, etc.).
  - Protective clothing should be worn by any person present in the radiographic suite during image acquisition. This includes at least a lead gown and lead gloves and, if available, a thyroid shield and lead goggles. While protective wear does not provide adequate shielding from the primary beam, it protects the examiner from scatter radiation. Older lead gowns, in particular, are prone to breaking, and protective wear should be handled with utmost care and hung up rather than folded. Small breaks or defects in lead shields may not be apparent upon visual inspection, and regular X-ray examination of protective clothing (without the examiner in the room!) is indicated for early damage detection (Fig. 4.7).

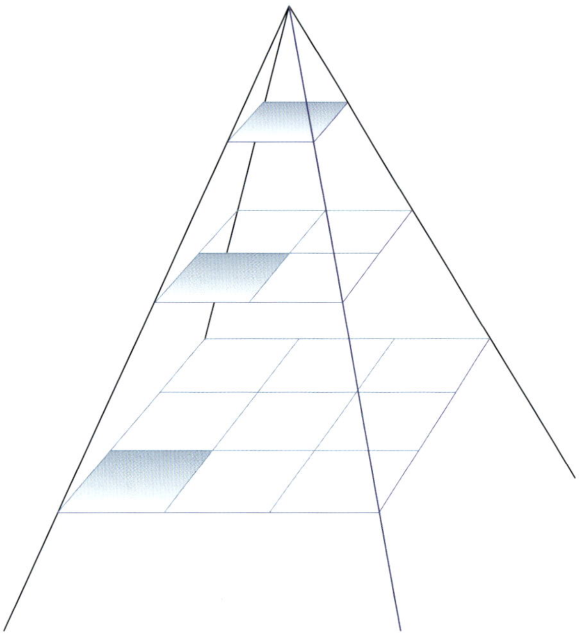

Fig. 4.6 Inverse square law. The radiation dose decreases with the square of the distance, i.e. the dose to the examiner is reduced to 1/4 when doubling the distance to the X-ray tube.

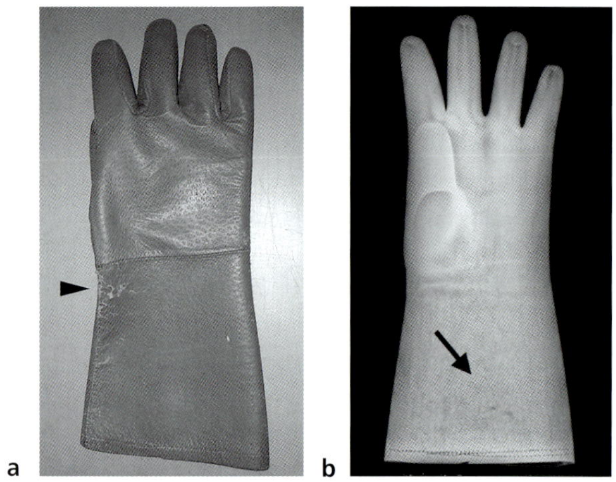

Fig. 4.7 Evaluation of a protective lead glove.
a Upon visual inspection there is evidence of small superficial defects at the level of the examiner's wrist (arrowhead).
b Radiographic examination does not show evidence of defect in the lead layer in the area of concern. However, small rents are noted at the level of the examiner's forearm (arrow).

> The radiation dose to the examiner is determined by the time spent in the X-ray room, the distance to the X-ray tube, and shielding.

In addition to these general basic principles of applied radiation safety, digital radiography has added a complicating factor. As described in Chapters 1 through 3, the detector dose (i.e. exposure) cannot be immediately detected by inspection of the radiograph. An overexposed radiograph may appear very similar to a radiograph obtained with adequate exposure factors, and even recurrent or persistent errors in radiographic technique may go unnoticed. Systematic overexposure of radiographs results in a significant increase in radiation dose to personnel in the room. A possible solution is continued use of a radiographic technique chart. Attention should also be paid to dose indicators by which digital radiography manufacturers provide an indication of the estimated exposure to the detector.

Suggested reading

Bushberg JT, Seibert JA, Leidholdt EM, Boone JM. The Essential Physics of Medical Imaging. Philadelphia: Lippincott Williams & Wilkins 2002.

Hartung K, Ludewig E, Tellhelm B. Röntgenuntersuchung in der Tierarztpraxis, 2nd edn. Stuttgart: Enke 2010.

Ludewig E, Gensler A, Oechtering G, Gosch D. Ergebnisse dosimetrischer Untersuchungen in der Kleintierpraxis: Welchen Einfluss haben der Abstand und die Position des Untersuchers zum Patienten? Berl Münch Tierärztl Wochenschr 2010; 123: 506–15.

Statkiewicz Sherer MA, Visconti PJ, Ritenour ER. Radiation Protection in Medical Radiography. St. Louis: Mosby 2002.

5 Advanced diagnostic imaging

Silke Hecht and Federica Morandi

The body of knowledge and literature pertaining to advanced imaging in veterinary patients has undergone rapid growth in recent years. The purpose of this chapter is to provide a very brief overview of the basic principles of these technologies. The reader is referred to specific articles and textbooks on these topics for more detailed information.

5.1 Ultrasonography (ultrasound)

5.1.1 Basic principles

Ultrasound has properties similar to audible sound but has a frequency above the human hearing range (i.e. above approximately 20 kHz). The frequency used for imaging of small animal patients ranges from approximately 3 to >15 MHz (depending on equipment, patient size and body area evaluated). The higher the **frequency** of the ultrasound transducer, the better the **resolution** of the image but the lower the **penetration depth** of the beam. Practically, this means that ultrasonographic evaluation of the abdomen in a medium-sized dog may be performed with a 5–10 MHz transducer, while ultrasonographic evaluation of superficial structures (e.g. thyroid gland) may require a frequency at or above 15 MHz.

Ultrasound waves are produced by special crystals (**piezoelectric elements**) in the ultrasound transducer and are then transmitted into the patient in the form of a rectangular or fan-shaped beam. Boundaries within the patient (organ surfaces, vessel borders, cellular structures, etc.) reflect part of the ultrasound beam back towards the transducer. Reflected ultrasound waves received by the transducer are converted to electrical impulses and reconstructed into two-dimensional greyscale images.

The degree of reflection differs between different types of boundaries. The **greyscale** of a substance or organ on the ultrasound image corresponds to its degree of ultrasound beam reflection.

- Fluid that is low in cells and protein (e.g. urine, bile, transudate) does not reflect ultrasound waves and appears black (**anechoic**) on the resultant ultrasound image. Ultrasound waves are transmitted through the fluid-filled regions, and visualization of structures in the far field is possible.
- Mineralized and bony structures as well as gas-filled organs (lung, intestine) constitute the other end of the spectrum. Most of the incident ultrasound waves are absorbed or reflected at the surface of these structures, and they appear bright (**hyperechoic**) on the resultant ultrasound image. Structures in the far field cannot be evaluated due to lack of ultrasound beam transmission.
- Soft-tissue structures (most organs) contain numerous small (cellular and other) surfaces which partially reflect and partially transmit ultrasound waves and which have an **intermediate echogenicity** on the resultant ultrasound image.

An ultrasound examination results in a two-dimensional picture in which various shades of grey indicate the degree of ultrasound beam reflection occurring at different organ surfaces. This basic type of ultrasonography is called **B-mode** (B = brightness). An ultrasound image is generated in a matter of milliseconds, allowing evaluation of structures in real time.

Another important ultrasonographic technique is the **Doppler mode** (colour Doppler, power Doppler and spectral Doppler). Reflectors moving towards or away from the transducer (e.g. flowing blood) differ from stationary tissues and can be detected and characterized.

M-mode (M = motion) captures motion over time and is predominantly used in echocardiography.

A-mode (A = amplitude) is occasionally used in ophthalmology. Rather than in the form of an image, ultrasound beam reflection is displayed as a straight line with occasional peaks occurring at the level of reflective interfaces. This technique allows accurate measurements of the distance between two reflectors (e.g. anterior and posterior lens capsule).

5.1.2 Advantages and disadvantages

Advantages

- Ultrasonography equipment is increasingly available in small animal practice and is **easily accessible** compared to other advanced imaging technologies.
- General anaesthesia is generally not needed, even though sedation is helpful in many cases.
- The evaluation is performed in **real time** and allows assessment of moving structures (blood flow, sedimentation of contents in fluid-filled structures, gastrointestinal tract motility, etc.).
- **Soft tissues and fluid can be distinguished**, which is a great advantage of ultrasound over radiographs. Identification of bladder tumours, differentiation of intraluminal fluid from a thickened intestinal wall, and identification of gestational chambers in the case of a radiographically enlarged uterus are only a few examples of additional information gained with ultrasonography over radiographs.
- An ultrasonographic examination is not associated with ionizing radiation and is (to the best of our knowledge) a **very safe** imaging procedure. In veterinary medicine this is important, not only from the patient's, but also the examiner's perspective.
- Structures not visible on abdominal radiographs are easily imaged by means of ultrasound (adrenal glands, pancreas, lymph nodes, abdominal vessels, etc.).
- Ultrasonography allows guided **fine-needle aspiration or biopsy** in real time and is useful in monitoring subsequent complications, such as haemorrhage.
- In recent years there has been an increase in the use of ultrasound guidance for **minimally invasive therapeutic procedures**, such as ethanol ablation of parathyroid tumours or drainage of abdominal abscesses.

Disadvantages

- Even more so than radiographic examination, ultrasonography is highly dependent on the **quality of the equipment** and the **examiner's experience level**.
- Ultrasound waves cannot penetrate bone, metal or gas, and ultrasonographic examination of the thorax or intrapelvic structures, for example, is limited. This is in contrast to radiography, which takes advantage of differences in radiographic opacity between metal, bone, soft tissues, fat and air.
- In contrast to radiography, an ultrasonographic image does not provide global information but only shows a **limited view of a small section of the area under investigation**. This has the following implications.
  - The examiner has to be able to create a **mental three-dimensional image** of the patient's anatomy derived from multiple small cross-sectional ultrasound images.
  - Lesions may be missed even with a thorough examination technique and many years of experience. For example, evaluation of the liver in deep-chested dogs and evaluation of a gas-filled gastrointestinal tract are notoriously difficult.
  - Interpretation of images saved or printed by another examiner is difficult or impossible. Determination of the organ of origin of a lesion (e.g. lymph node vs. pancreas), or even identification of the body region (e.g. cranial mediastinal vs. abdominal mass) may be impossible for somebody who did not perform the examination or was not at least present during the procedure.

5.1.3 Applications in small animal practice

ABDOMEN Abdominal ultrasonography is probably the most common application of this technology in small animal practice and (with a few limitations) allows evaluation of all abdominal organs (Fig. 5.1).

THORAX Ultrasonography can be used for evaluation of the heart (echocardiography) and other thoracic structures. Intrathoracic structures cannot be assessed if they are obscured by air (lung, pneumothorax) or overlying osseous structures. However, an ultrasonographic examination may provide valuable information if pathological processes, such as pleural effusion or thoracic mass lesions, provide a suitable 'acoustic window' for ultrasound waves to enter the thoracic cavity (Fig. 5.2).

MUSCULOSKELETAL SYSTEM Ultrasonography is an excellent technique for evaluation of soft tissues (such as muscles, tendons and ligaments) and larger joints. Bone lesions may also be amenable to ultrasonographic investigation unless obscured by overlying strongly hyperechoic intact cortical bone (Fig. 5.3). Ultrasound is used increasingly not only for diagnostics but also for minimally invasive treatment (e.g. stem cell injections or ultrasound-guided retrieval of embedded foreign material).

HEAD AND NECK Ultrasonography plays an important role in the diagnostic workup of many diseases in the head and neck region. Ocular ultrasound is used routinely for the evaluation of intraocular as well as retrobulbar

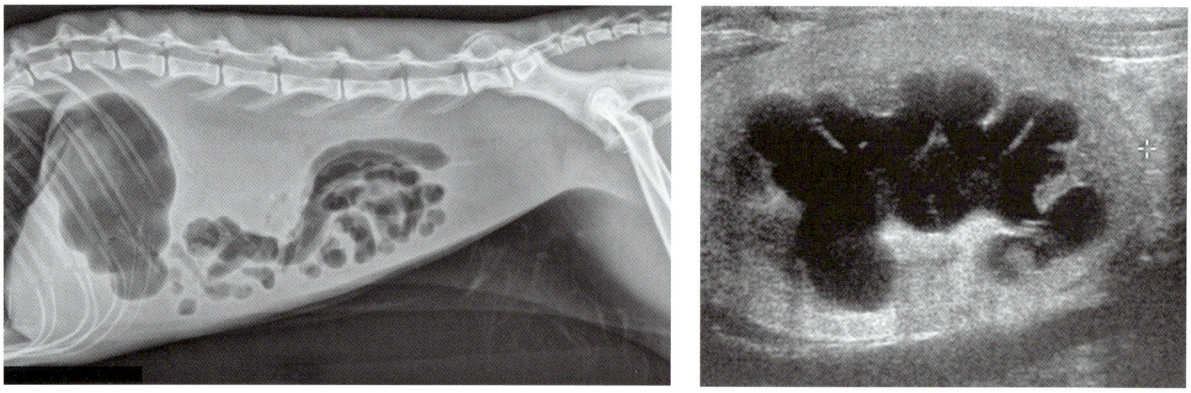

a b

Fig. 5.1

a Lateral abdominal radiograph in a cat with loss of peritoneal and retroperitoneal detail due to abdominal and retroperitoneal effusion. Abdominal structures are not clearly delineated with the exception of gas-filled intestinal segments.

b This sagittal ultrasound image of the right kidney shows moderate to marked dilatation of the renal pelvis (recognized as anechoic region in the centre of the kidney). The proximal ureter was also dilated and contained hyperechoic material. Similar changes were seen on the left. Final diagnosis was bilateral hydronephrosis and hydroureter due to ureteral obstruction as well as right ureteral rupture.

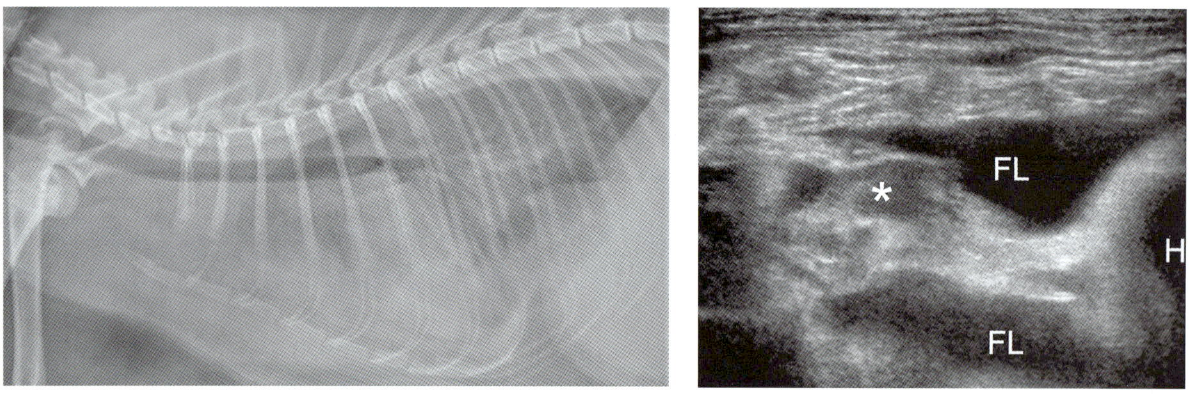

a b

Fig. 5.2 Pleural effusion in a young cat.

a Only a limited evaluation of thoracic structures is possible on this lateral thoracic radiograph due to superimposition of pleural effusion.

b This ultrasound image was obtained by placing the transducer on the lateral cranial thoracic wall. Pleural effusion (FL) is noted bilaterally in the thoracic cavity. An enlarged sternal lymph node (*) is associated with the cranial mediastinum. Aspiration of this lymph node under ultrasound guidance yielded a diagnosis of granulomatous inflammation of undetermined cause (H = heart).

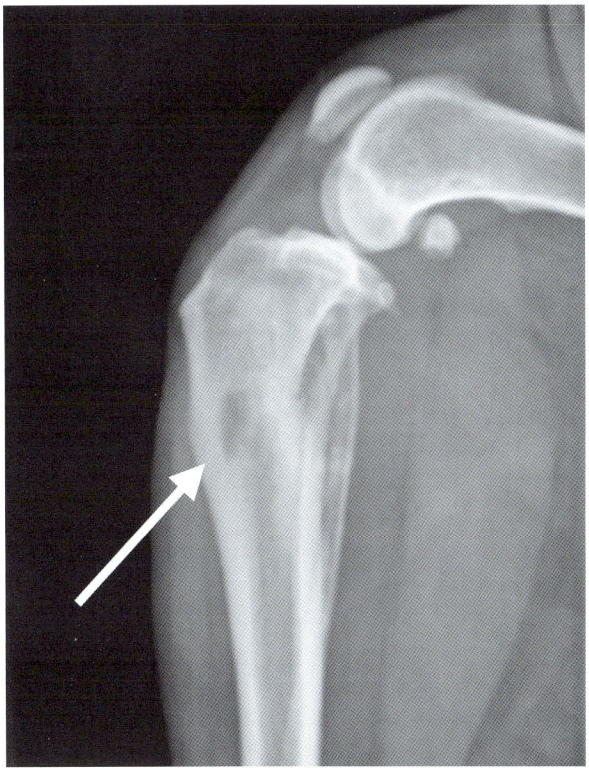

a

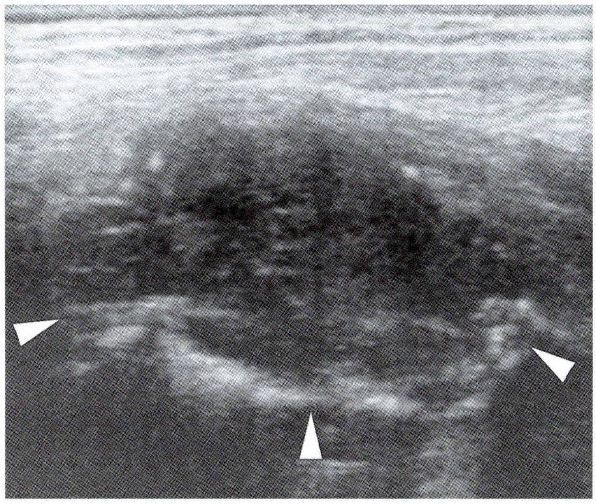

b

Fig. 5.3 Lytic lesion of the proximal tibia.

a The lateral radiograph shows an oval, relatively well-defined radiolucent lesion associated with the proximal tibia (arrow). There is also mild sclerosis of the adjacent bone, periosteal reaction associated with the caudal tibia, and intracapsular soft-tissue swelling of the stifle joint. Ultrasound was recommended to identify a region amenable for ultrasound-guided fine-needle aspiration.

b This ultrasound image shows an approximately 2 cm diameter soft-tissue mass of intermediate echogenicity with destruction of the underlying cortex of the tibia (arrowheads). Cytological diagnosis was undifferentiated sarcoma.

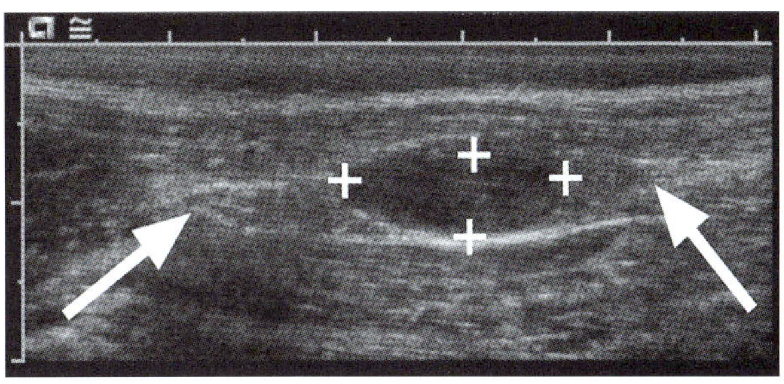

Fig. 5.4 Parathyroid tumour in a dog with hypercalcaemia. The ultrasound image was acquired with the transducer positioned parasagittally (to the left of the trachea) on the mid-ventral neck. The thyroid gland (arrows pointing towards the cranial and caudal pole) appears as a fusiform structure which is fairly isoechoic to surrounding tissues. A hypoechoic nodule is associated with the centre of the thyroid gland (+). Histopathology was consistent with a diagnosis of parathyroid adenoma.

disease processes. Ultrasound is also helpful in the evaluation of mass lesions in the head and neck region as well as in the evaluation of patients with thyroid and parathyroid conditions (Fig. 5.4). Occasional applications for ultrasound imaging in neuroradiology include diagnosis of select intracranial diseases (specifically, hydrocephalus), ultrasound-guided aspiration of superficial spinal lesions (e.g. tumours or abscesses), and intraoperative ultrasound (see below).

OTHER APPLICATIONS In addition to body regions listed above, ultrasound can be used to evaluate any other superficial structure (e.g. subcutaneous tissues, mammary gland and scrotum). Intraoperative ultrasound is uncommonly performed in small animal practice but may be useful in the identification of, for example, a small pancreatic tumour (insulinoma), a deep-seated liver lesion, or a lesion within the brain or spinal cord (Fig. 5.5). Contrast-enhanced ultrasound is a fairly new technique allowing improved visualization of vascular structures as well as improved detection and characterization of lesions of various parenchymal organs. Finally, ultrasound is gaining importance in minimally invasive interventions such as ultrasound-guided drainage of cavitary lesions (abscesses, pseudocysts), ablation of parathyroid adenomas, for example, and intracavitary chemotherapy.

5.2 Nuclear medicine (scintigraphy)

5.2.1 Basic principles

With nuclear scintigraphy, a radioactive substance (**radiopharmaceutical**) is administered to a patient, and the distribution of this substance within the body is monitored by means of a detector system (gamma camera). There are two major differences compared to other imaging techniques. Scintigraphy is not only a morphological but also a **functional imaging technique**, and the patient, rather than an X-ray tube or other piece of equipment, serves as the **source of radiation**.

Numerous different radioactive isotopes (**radionuclides**) may be used for scintigraphic imaging. The most common type used in human and veterinary medicine is technetium-99m (99m-Tc), which is characterized by good imaging properties (emission of relatively low energy gamma rays), favourable chemical properties and a short half-life (6 hours). Depending on the type of scintigraphic examination to be performed, the radionuclide can be coupled to a variety of molecules (**ligands or tracers**) which differ in their biochemical properties and metabolic pathway in the body. The combination of the radioactive radionuclide and the ligand is called a **'radiopharmaceutical'**. The radiopharmaceutical used for a procedure is selected depending on the organ of interest and may accumulate in that organ, for example

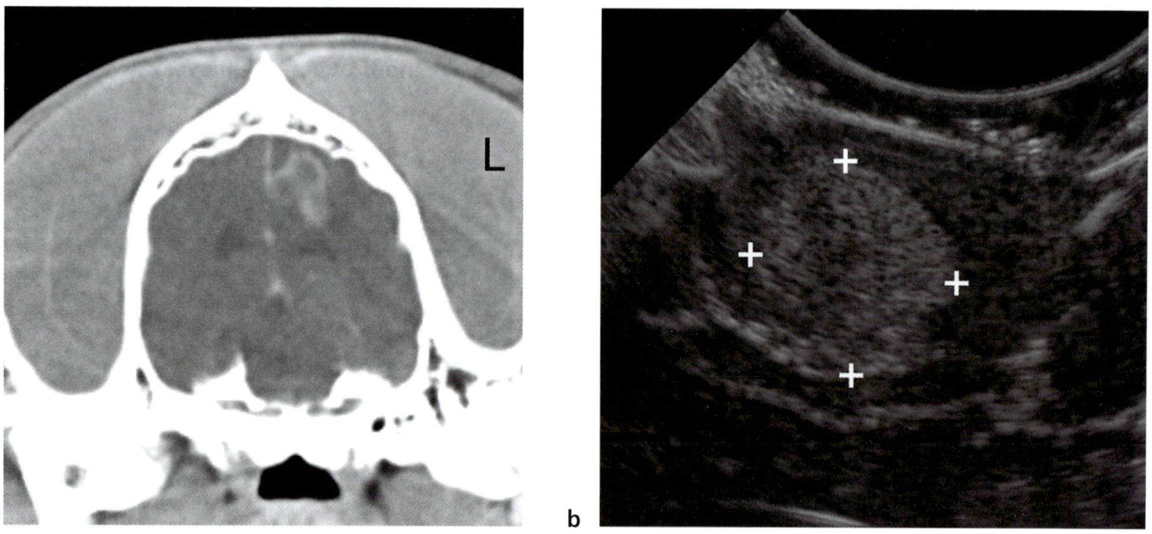

a b

Fig. 5.5 Intra-axial brain tumour in a dog.
a On this transverse CT image, following administration of intravenous contrast medium, there is a lobular, irregularly shaped ring-enhancing lesion associated with the left parietal lobe. There is a subtle decrease in attenuation of adjacent brain parenchyma suggesting brain oedema. The left lateral ventricle is mildly compressed, and there is a midline shift of the falx towards the right.
b Intraoperative ultrasound during craniotomy shows a homogeneously hyperechoic mass lesion (+) surrounded by hypoechoic brain parenchyma. The mass was surgically resected. Histopathology yielded a diagnosis of oligodendroglioma.

due to filtration (kidney), surface adsorption (bone), active transport (thyroid gland), or capillary blockage (lung).

The time of data acquisition varies depending on the examination. Imaging may be performed immediately following administration of the radiopharmaceutical, minutes or even hours later. Data may be captured as **static images** (e.g. skeletal scintigraphy) or **dynamic datasets** which provide information about the path of the radiopharmaceutical within the body, organ function and metabolic abnormalities (e.g. renal scintigraphy).

Images are captured using a gamma camera. A static acquisition results in a two-dimensional picture (black and white or colour-coded) of radiopharmaceutical distribution within the body. The higher the concentration of radiopharmaceutical in a given region, the more activity will be registered at that site. With a dynamic acquisition, successive individual images are recorded as a 'film'. Subsequent **post-processing** is possible. For example, regions of interest may be selected in successive images to record varying concentrations of the radiopharmaceutical in that area (uptake – excretion) over time. Quantitative measurements are also possible.

Special forms of nuclear medicine include positron emission tomography (**PET**) and single photon emission computerized tomography (**SPECT**). With these techniques, the patient is surrounded either by a ring of detectors (**PET**), or the detector(s) rotate(s) around the patient (**SPECT**). Both techniques allow improved anatomic visualization and localization of the radiopharmaceutical compared to conventional scintigraphy. In recent years, fusion of PET detector systems with other cross-sectional imaging modalities (computed tomography, CT; magnetic resonance imaging, MRI) has resulted in an increased use of PET technology. These modern **PET-CT** and **PET-MRI** scanners allow anatomically accurate display of radiopharmaceutical accumulation in different organs without superimposition of surrounding structures. ^{18}F-fluorodeoxyglucose (FDG) is the most common radiopharmaceutical used for PET diagnostics. It is a glucose analogue, and its distribution pattern can provide valuable information in the evaluation of metabolic processes, especially in oncology. Conventional PET scanners have become virtually obsolete since the introduction of PET-CT and PET-MRI. SPECT is predominantly used for cardiology applications in human medicine, and is not routinely used in veterinary patients. PET-CT and PET-MRI have shown promising results in preliminary veterinary studies, but at this point are limited to few specialty institutions.

5.2.2 Advantages and disadvantages

Advantages

- Nuclear medicine allows evaluation of normal and abnormal organ function, while other imaging procedures provide mostly morphological information.
- Static and dynamic data acquisitions are possible.
- Quantitative measurements are possible (e.g. renal function, liver function).
- Scintigraphy has a very high sensitivity and may detect functional anomalies before morphological changes are evident on other imaging studies (e.g. early detection of bone metastases before lesions are detected on radiographs).
- PET-CT and PET-MRI: Fusion of morphological (CT or MRI image) with functional (PET) information with excellent anatomic resolution.

Disadvantages

- Scintigraphy is limited to academic institutions and specialty hospitals due to the necessity for **expensive specialized equipment** and **stringent radiation safety regulations**.
- With the exception of modern fusion imaging (PET-CT and PET-MRI), scintigraphic images are characterized by **poor anatomic resolution** compared to other imaging procedures.
- The patient serves as the source of radiation, and the examination can result in a relatively **high radiation dose** to both the animal and the examiner.
- Although state regulations vary, the patient must remain **confined or isolated** until radiation emission falls below the legal limits. In many cases this means an overnight stay, in others up to several days.
- In contrast to their very high sensitivity, some scintigraphic techniques have **very low specificity**. For example, a bone lesion may be found very early; however, different types of bone lesions (tumour, osteomyelitis, fracture) appear similar and cannot be distinguished on a bone scan.

5.2.3 Applications in small animal practice

SKELETAL (BONE) SCINTIGRAPHY This technique is mostly used to evaluate animals with lameness of undetermined cause and to screen oncology patients for bone metastases (Fig. 5.6).

THYROID SCINTIGRAPHY This technique is most commonly used in the diagnostic workup of patients (mostly cats) with hyperthyroidism, and much less commonly in patients with hypothyroidism. Other indications include suspected ectopic thyroid tissue, screening for metastatic disease from thyroid carcinoma, evaluation of cervical mass lesions, and recheck examinations in patients treated for various thyroid diseases.

RENAL SCINTIGRAPHY Various scintigraphic methods have been developed to evaluate the kidneys. Today, morphological renal scintigraphy has largely been replaced by abdominal ultrasound. Similarly, excretory scintigraphy to evaluate patients with suspected ureteral obstruction has largely been replaced by ultrasound and CT. Scintigraphic evaluation of renal function (global and individual glomerular filtration rate; GFR) is probably the most common renal scintigraphic technique used in small animal patients today (Fig. 5.7). Following injection of the radiopharmaceutical and a 6 minute dynamic data acquisition, regions of interest are drawn over the area of both kidneys (Fig. 5.7a). Time intensity curves derived from the dynamic data provide information on radioactive material present within each kidney throughout the time of the study. GFR is determined subsequently from these data using a specific computer program (Fig. 5.7b).

PULMONARY SCINTIGRAPHY This technique can be used in the diagnosis of pulmonary thromboembolism but has largely been replaced by CT angiography.

LIVER SCINTIGRAPHY Hepatobiliary scintigraphy allows evaluation of liver function and may be used for the diagnosis of biliary obstruction. A more common indication for the use of scintigraphy in small animal medicine is the evaluation of patients with suspected portosystemic shunt. Radiopharmaceutical is injected into the spleen (or, in an older technique, deposited into the rectum), and its distribution in the body is monitored (Fig. 5.8).

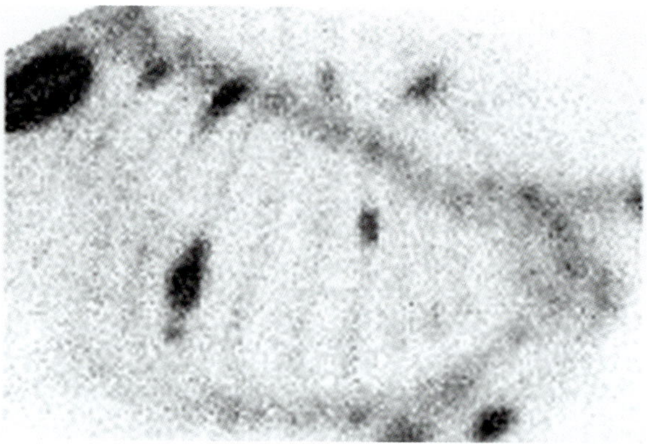

Fig. 5.6 Skeletal scintigraphy in a dog. There is multifocal increased radiopharmaceutical uptake associated with several ribs, vertebrae and forelimbs. Ultimate diagnosis was metastatic osteosarcoma. Note that, in contrast to other imaging modalities, scintigraphic images are displayed as acquired from the point of view of the camera. On this image acquired in right lateral recumbency, the patient's head is oriented to the right.

Fig. 5.7 Renal scintigraphy in a normal dog.
a The dorsal static image was acquired following completion of the dynamic data acquisition. The kidneys have increased radiopharmaceutical uptake and appear darker than surrounding tissues.
b Determination of the glomerular filtration rate (GFR). A dynamic data acquisition is performed for 6 minutes over regions of interest drawn in the area of both kidneys. Both renal curves are very similar. After an initial spike (arterial peak, arrow) there is a gradual increase in renal activity. The curve begins its descent with the start of the excretory phase. Global GFR in this patient was 4.28 ml/min/kg. Individual GFR was 2.03 (right kidney) and 2.24 ml/min/kg (left kidney), respectively. The background activity adjacent to the kidneys (background 1 and 2, respectively) are subtracted from renal measurements during this procedure.

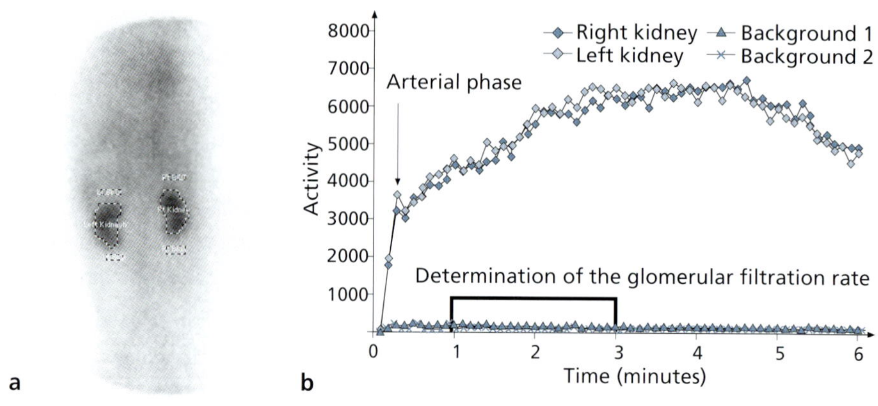

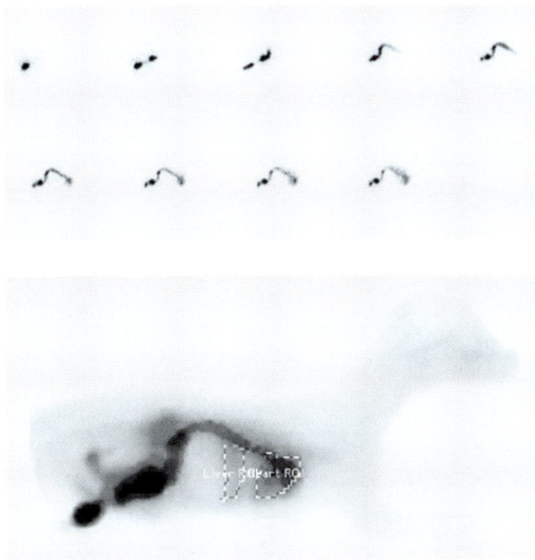

Fig. 5.8 Scintigraphic diagnosis of a portosystemic shunt in a dog. The radiopharmaceutical was injected into the spleen under ultrasound guidance.
a The dynamic acquisition shows distribution of radiopharmaceutical for 20 seconds after the injection. The radiopharmaceutical bypasses the liver and reaches the heart first. A static image (not shown) was acquired for improved shunt classification following completion of the dynamic study.
b Fusion of the static and dynamic datasets illustrates the course of the radiopharmaceutical from the spleen dorsally and cranially, through the splenic vein into the portal vein. From here it connects directly to a large vessel entering the heart from caudally. The presumptive diagnosis of congenital portacaval shunt was confirmed surgically.

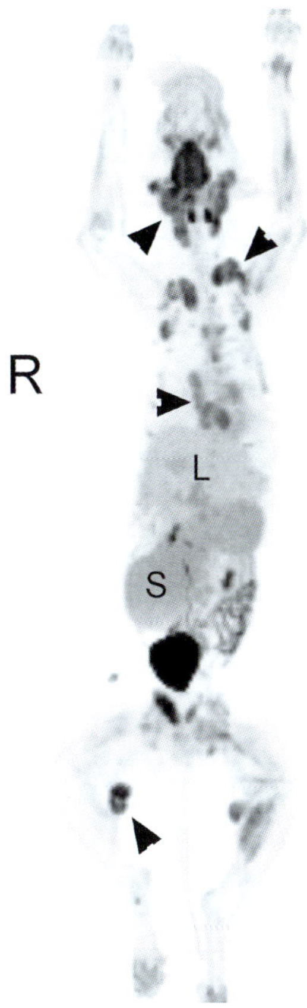

Fig. 5.9 Dorsal whole-body PET obtained approximately 1 hour after intravenous injection of 18F-FDG in a 6-year-old male neutered mixed-breed dog with systemic lymphoma. Enlarged lymph nodes with markedly increased 18F-FDG uptake are visible throughout the body, including mandibular, prescapular, sternal, cranial mediastinal, right, left and central tracheobronchial, hepatic, gastric, sublumbar, inguinal and popliteal lymph nodes (arrowheads). The spleen (S) and liver (L) are increased in size, and the spleen has increased, mottled uptake. The focal area of intense, increased uptake in the liver, near the gallbladder neck, is considered normal, and is frequently observed in normal dogs. Normal areas of 18F-FDG uptake include the brain, renal pelves and urinary bladder. Incidental uptake is noted in the gastrointestinal tract (a common finding in dogs) and the musculature of the limbs (especially the left gastrocnemius region), the latter related to muscle spasm/contraction.

GASTROINTESTINAL SCINTIGRAPHY Intravenous injection of a radiopharmaceutical coupled to erythrocytes may aid in the identification of a bleeding gastric or intestinal ulcer. This technique and other gastrointestinal nuclear medicine studies are rarely performed in veterinary patients.

PET, PET-CT, PET-MRI As mentioned above, these techniques are currently limited to human and few specialty veterinary hospitals. Because FDG is a glucose analogue, its distribution pattern reflects glucose metabolism and can aid in the evaluation of metabolic processes especially in oncology patients (Fig. 5.9).

OTHER APPLICATIONS As with ultrasonography, there are few limitations to scintigraphic applications. Cardiovascular scintigraphy is uncommonly performed in veterinary medicine. Scintigraphy of the central nervous system (CNS) has largely become obsolete since the introduction of CT and MRI. Lymphoscintigraphy may aid in identification of lymphatic obstruction and tributary lymph nodes in oncological cases. Mucociliary scintigraphy can be used to diagnose ciliary dyskinesia. Receptor antagonist scintigraphy for identification of endocrine tumours has unfortunately yielded disappointing results in veterinary patients and is not commonly used at this point.

5.3 Computed tomography (CT)

5.3.1 Basic principles

Computed tomography utilizes **X-rays** for image generation, and many basic radiographic concepts described in Chapters 1 through 3, such as X-ray production and differential attenuation of X-rays in different tissues, apply. However, there are some important differences.

- The X-ray tube is not fixed but **rotates** around the patient.
- The X-ray beam does not spread out in all directions but is **collimated** to a certain slice thickness (typically <1–10 mm).
- The X-ray beam is transmitted through the patient and received by **detector rows** rather than an X-ray film or digital plate. The data are then transmitted to a computer and converted into images using complex mathematical algorithms.

The result is a **cross-sectional image of the patient** in which structures with different X-ray attenuation are displayed in various shades of grey. As in radiographs, denser materials (e.g. bone) are displayed in a brighter tone (hyperattenuating, hyperdense) than less attenuating structures (e.g. lung).

Older generation CT scanners acquire one single image after the other, which is time-consuming. Modern CT scanners have multiple rows of detectors, and the examination of a small animal thorax or abdomen can be completed in few seconds. This shortening of the examination time is probably less important in veterinary than in human medicine as patients are typically heavily sedated or anaesthetized. However, it is very helpful for studies of the vascular system (e.g. evaluation for pulmonary thromboembolism or portosystemic shunt) and in any case where multiplanar or three-dimensional (3-D) image reconstructions are desired. A decrease in examination time is also advantageous if a patient is sedated rather than anaesthetized. Compared to radiographs, CT images display structures **without superimposition** and have a greater ability to **differentiate structures of similar or equal radiographic opacity,** such as soft tissues and fluid. With computed tomography, water is assigned a density of 0 HU (**Hounsfield units,** named after one of the inventors of CT). The relative density of all other substances is calculated in comparison with water density. This provides an objective measure of object density in addition to mere subjective evaluation, and may aid in identification of, for example, CNS-associated haemorrhage, subtle contrast enhancement in an organ or lesion, diffuse osteopenia, etc.

Different density ranges can be accentuated following image acquisition by manipulating CT images in dedicated viewing software or picture archiving and communication system (PACS). A so-called **soft-tissue window** allows assessment of soft tissues and provides the ability to identify relatively small differences in density. A **bone window** is used to evaluate osseous structures, and a **lung window** is applied for evaluation of pulmonary parenchyma.

The CT examination can be combined with intravenous administration of iodinated contrast medium. **Contrast enhancement** is identified in most normal organs, and parenchymal lesions may be characterized by an increased or decreased contrast uptake in comparison with normal tissue, depending on their vascularity. When imaging the CNS, contrast enhancement is identified in vascularized lesions which have disrupted, or originate outside the blood–brain barrier. Many **conventional contrast procedures** (excretory urography, angiography, portography, myelography) can be combined with CT, which enhances their diagnostic capabilities.

5.3.2 Advantages and disadvantages

Advantages

- CT has gained popularity in veterinary medicine and is now available not only in academic medical centres but also many private (specialty) hospitals.
- It is a **cross-sectional** imaging technique: images allow evaluation of the area of interest without superimposition of surrounding structures. The evaluation of, for example, the cranial vault or contents within the vertebral canal thus becomes possible.
- The examination is **fast**, especially if using a multislice scanner.
- The operator of the equipment is located outside the scan room, so there is **no radiation exposure** to the examiner.
- Image manipulation following data acquisition (**windowing**) permits improved evaluation of structures of different density.
- Administration of intravenous contrast medium aids in identification of lesions with a different degree of enhancement or pattern compared to adjacent tissue.
- An **objective quantitative determination** of density of a certain substance or region is possible.
- CT can be combined with conventional contrast procedures, which enhances their diagnostic capabilities.
- Images can be reconstructed into sagittal, dorsal and oblique planes or into 3-D images, which can provide additional morphological information.
- The thickness of acquired slices can be modified to

enhance imaging of very small structures (e.g. small bony lesions such as fragments of the medial coronoid process) or cover a large area in a short time (e.g. entire abdomen in a dog with haemoabdomen).
- CT is more sensitive than radiographs for many indications (e.g. pulmonary metastasis check).
- Lesions inaccessible for ultrasound or fluoroscopy-guided sampling may be amenable for **CT-guided fine-needle aspiration or biopsy**.

Disadvantages

- A CT examination is typically **more expensive** than radiographs, and a decision about which imaging test to perform should include a cost–benefit analysis.
- The examination requires **heavy sedation or general anaesthesia** to prevent patient motion and artefacts.
- The **radiation dose to the patient** is significantly higher compared to conventional radiography. For example, the radiation dose received during thoracic CT is approximately 50 times the dose received in the frame of a three-view radiographic study.
- Compared to MRI, CT is **limited in the evaluation of soft-tissue structures** including brain and spinal cord.
- In contrast to MRI, CT is **not a true multiplanar imaging modality** as image planes are determined by the position of the X-ray tube and detectors within the machine. However, additional planes can be reconstructed from the initial data set and, with multislice scanners, are of excellent quality.
- Certain **artefacts** may limit the diagnostic quality of the scan (e.g. beam hardening resulting in dark streaks in the caudal fossa of the head).

5.3.3 Applications in small animal practice

Skeletal system Due to its excellent spatial resolution that allows visualization even of small bony structures, CT is the modality of choice in many orthopaedic conditions such as elbow dysplasia (Fig. 5.10). Multiplanar and 3-D reconstructions are possible and may be very helpful for surgical planning, for example in cases of complex pelvic or skull fractures, or in correction of angular limb deformities.

Nervous system Even though MRI is considered the gold standard for most indications in neuroimaging, CT may yield a diagnosis in many cases. CT may even be preferred in trauma patients or if a bone lesion (e.g.

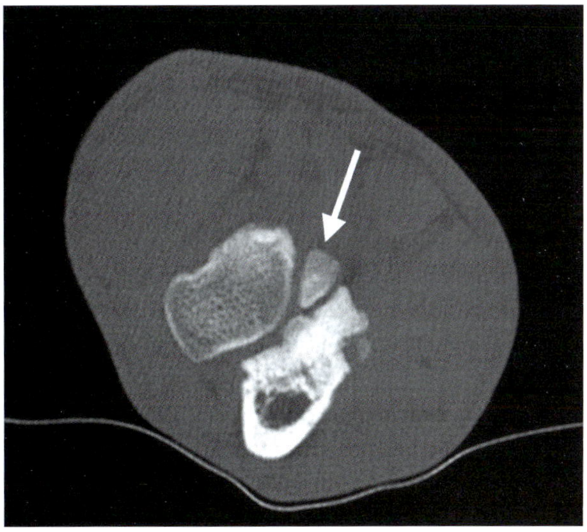

Fig. 5.10 Fragmentation of the medial coronoid process in a dog. This transverse CT image (slice thickness 1 mm, displayed in a bone window) shows an isolated bone fragment originating from the medial coronoid process (arrow). This bone fragment is of decreased attenuation compared to parent bone and has rounded margins. The adjacent region of the ulna is increased in attenuation (sclerosis), has an irregular contour and multifocal periarticular osteophytes (degenerative joint disease). Note that use of a bone window facilitates differentiation of cortex and medulla, while surrounding soft tissue and fat are fairly homogeneously hypodense.

congenital vertebral anomaly) is suspected. Contrast medium administration and post-contrast image acquisition is required in most patients undergoing brain CT to identify or fully evaluate a lesion (see Fig. 5.5a). Several common spinal conditions are readily identified without contrast medium administration (e.g. vertebral fracture or extrusion of mineralized intervertebral disc material; Fig. 5.11). However, other cases (e.g. herniation of nonmineralized disc material or intramedullary lesions such as tumours) may require intravenous contrast medium administration and/or combination with myelography. CT-guided aspiration or biopsy of a spinal lesion is occasionally performed.

Skull, nose, paranasal sinuses, tympanic bulla and orbit CT is an excellent imaging modality for imaging the fine bony detail and air-filled spaces of these structures (Fig. 5.12).

Thorax CT is also an excellent modality for evaluation of the lungs and other thoracic structures. CT has been proven to be more sensitive than conventional radiographs in the identification of pulmonary metastases (Fig. 5.13). It is also

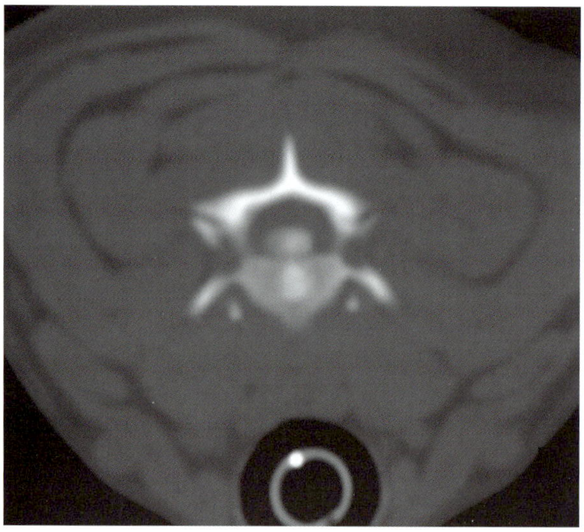

Fig. 5.11 Intervertebral disc extrusion in a dog. The transverse CT image at the level of the C2–3 intervertebral disc space (slice thickness 3 mm, bone window) shows mineralized disc material within the ventral aspect of the vertebral canal, resulting in marked compression of the spinal cord. Note that evaluation of the spine has to be performed both in a bone and soft-tissue window, as less attenuating structures (e.g. non-mineralized disc material, haemorrhage, surrounding soft tissues) cannot otherwise be distinguished.

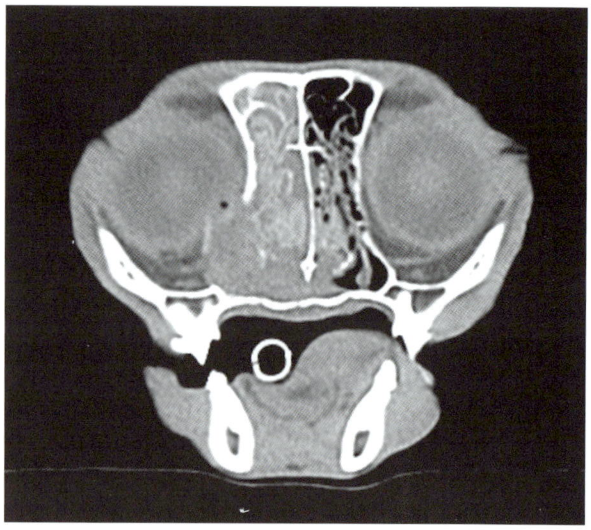

Fig. 5.12 Nasal tumour (lymphoma) in a cat. The transverse CT image (slice thickness 2 mm, soft-tissue window) shows a soft-tissue attenuating mass lesion within the right nasal cavity resulting in destruction of normal nasal turbinates, displacement of the nasal septum towards the left, invasion of the left nasal cavity and invasion into the right orbit with lysis of the orbital wall. Note that the soft-tissue window not only permits differentiation between bone, soft tissues and retro-orbital fat, but also between the lens of the eye and the adjacent hypodense globe. As for the spine, a CT study of the head must also be evaluated in both a soft-tissue and a bone window for adequate assessment of all structures.

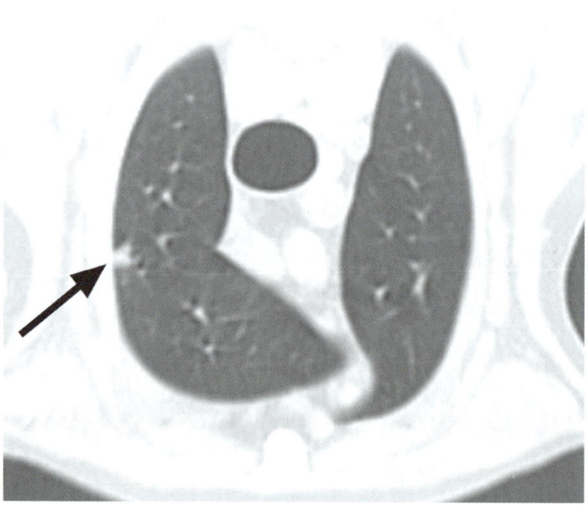

Fig. 5.13 Pulmonary metastasis in a dog. A large right caudal pulmonary mass (pulmonary carcinoma) had been identified on previous radiographs, and CT was performed prior to thoracotomy and lung lobectomy to evaluate the patient for metastases to thoracic lymph nodes and/or lung. Based on thoracic radiographs in three views, there was no evidence of pulmonary metastases. The transverse CT image (slice thickness 2 mm, lung window) shows a small subpleural soft-tissue attenuating nodule in the right cranial lung lobe (arrow).

helpful in the evaluation of intrathoracic lymph nodes, mediastinal mass lesions, diaphragmatic lesions and the thoracic wall. The cardiovascular structures can be evaluated by means of CT angiography, which may aid in diagnosis of vascular ring anomalies or pulmonary thromboemboli, for example. Finally, CT is well suited to monitor needle placement for fine-needle aspiration or biopsy of deep-seated intrathoracic lesions that cannot be visualized by means of ultrasonography due to superimposition of aerated lung parenchyma.

Abdomen In many small animal patients an adequate evaluation of the abdominal cavity can be performed by means of ultrasonography, which is cheaper and more readily available in small animal practice than CT. However, abdominal CT is gaining popularity due to its improved accuracy in identification of abdominal lesions in large dogs, speed of examination, and potential to be combined with intravenous contrast medium administration and/or conventional contrast procedures. CT is advantageous compared to ultrasound in the evaluation of (large) abdominal masses, including vascularity, vascular invasion and resectability (Fig. 5.14). It is an excellent modality for the diagnosis of vascular anomalies (e.g. portosystemic shunt) and congenital urinary tract disorders (e.g. ectopic ureters). CT can be used to guide fine-needle aspiration or biopsy of deep-seated abdominal lesions not accessible for other methods of tissue sampling. These are only a few examples of possible applications of abdominal CT in small animal veterinary medicine. It is likely that within the next few years this technique will become as important as it is in human medicine.

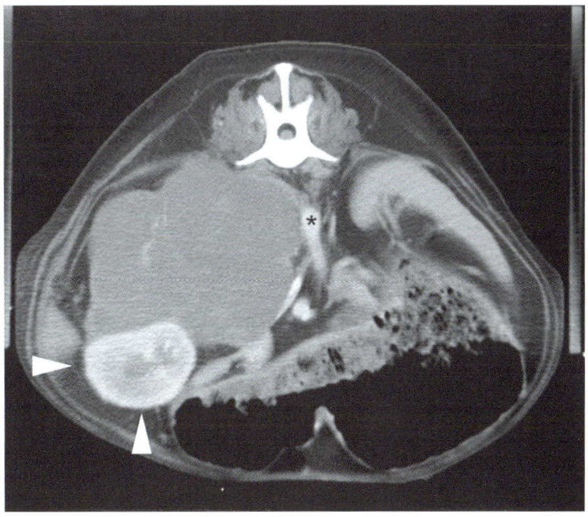

Fig. 5.14 Large right adrenal tumour (adenocarcinoma) in a dog. This transverse CT image acquired following intravenous administration of positive contrast medium demonstrates a very large mass in the right dorsal abdomen. The right kidney (arrowheads) is ventrally displaced and is deformed due to tumour infiltration into the renal capsule. The tumour abuts the abdominal aorta (*).

OTHER APPLICATIONS Despite limitations in imaging of soft-tissue lesions, CT can be successfully used in the diagnosis and characterization of contrast-enhancing lesions, for example in the neck, extremities and body wall (Fig. 5.15). It is helpful for obtaining CT-guided tissue samples and for treatment planning (e.g. deciding between surgical resection and radiation therapy).

5.4 Magnetic resonance imaging (MRI)

5.4.1 Basic principles

Simply put, magnetic resonance imaging (or nuclear magnetic resonance imaging) involves **imaging of protons** (specifically, **hydrogen** protons). These are characterized by a positive charge and rotation/spin around their axis (similar to a spinning top). As these protons (**'spins'**) are moving charges, they produce a small magnetic field in their environment. This is of course very weak for individual protons, but the strength of neighbouring protons oriented in the same direction adds up.

Fig. 5.15 Tumour (fibrosarcoma) of the hind limb in a dog. The transverse CT image acquired following intravenous contrast medium administration shows a ring-enhancing mass (M) embedded within the left thigh musculature. The mass extends into the pelvic canal (arrow). The diagnosis was made based on ultrasound-guided fine-needle aspiration.

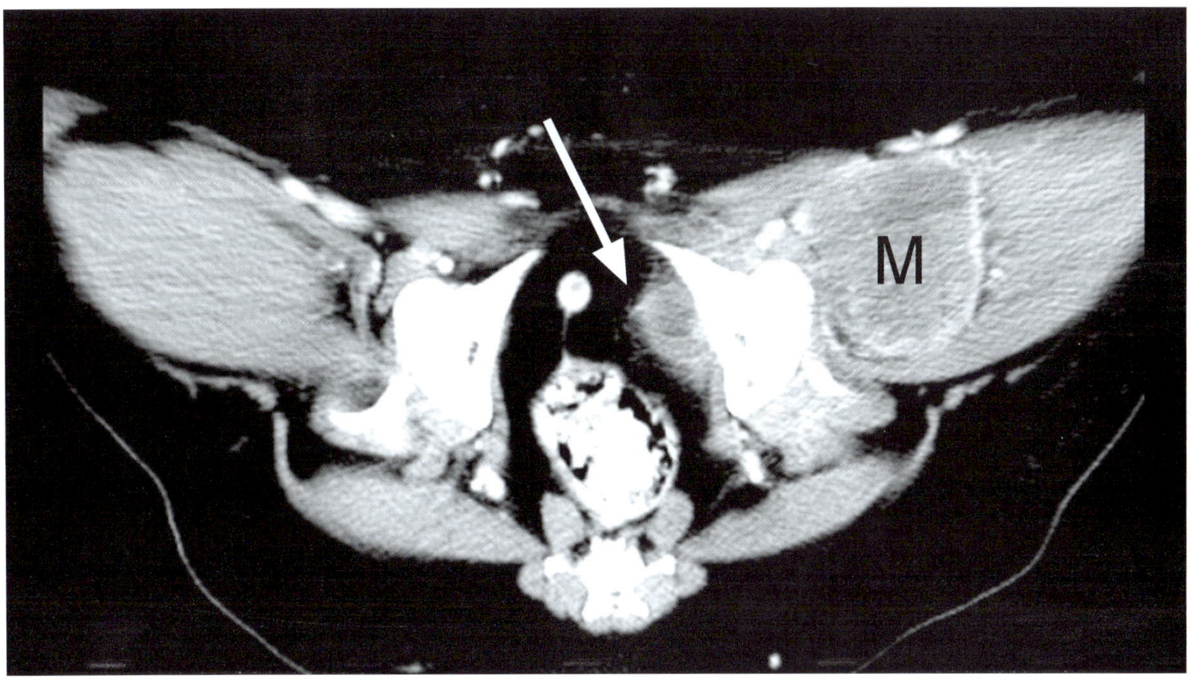

When the protons are exposed to a **strong external magnetic field** (i.e. when the patient is positioned within the MRI scanner), most protons align with the main magnetic field and assume a wobbling motion (**'precession'**). This is again comparable to a spinning top which not only spins around its own axis but starts wobbling under the influence of gravity.

The protons can be kicked out of alignment with the main magnetic field by sending in **electromagnetic radiofrequency (RF) pulses**. The strength and duration of the pulse determines the degree to which the protons change position (e.g. 90°). As mentioned above, when the spins are in alignment with each other they cause a magnetic field on their own. Following the radiofrequency pulse, this magnetic field has a different orientation from the main magnetic field (e.g. with a 90° RF pulse the net vector of the spins is perpendicular to the main magnetic field). At this point, the protons precess in unison and are able to **induce a signal in a receiver coil** (MR signal). This is the basis of MR image generation.

Initially, all protons are in similar alignment and thus produce the same signal, regardless of whether they are contained in fat, water or soft tissues. Something has to happen so that different tissues can be distinguished on MR images. This is where so-called **relaxation** comes into play: after the radiofrequency pulse is switched off, the protons leave their high-energy position and realign with the main magnetic field. This results in a decrease of signal strength in the receiver coil. This process is called **longitudinal relaxation** (also called spin–lattice relaxation, **T1 relaxation**). In addition, signal intensity decreases when the unified front of protons precessing together loses its coherence, and proton motion becomes uncoordinated. Essentially, this can be envisioned as protons bumping into each other. This process also results in a decrease in intensity of the MR signal. This process is called **transverse relaxation** (also called spin–spin relaxation, **T2 relaxation**).

Protons contained in different tissues are characterized by different relaxation times. Fat has short relaxation times, water has long relaxation times and soft tissues are intermediate. The art and magic of MRI lies in the ability to manipulate image parameters, so different tissues have different imaging characteristics and can be recognized on MR images. Important **imaging parameters** include the following.

- The **time of repetition (TR)** of successive radiofrequency pulses.
- The **time of echo (TE)**, i.e. the time between the pulse and the generation of the MR signal.
- Multiple other factors including the **flip angle** and **application of additional pulses** also affect the signal intensity of different tissues on MR images. Modification of these and other parameters results in generation of different MR sequences. The two most basic, yet very important, MR sequences are T1- and T2-weighted images:
  - T1-weighting:
    - Fluid is dark.
    - Fat is bright.
    - Soft tissues are of variable shades of grey.
  - T2-weighting:
    - Fluid is bright.
    - Fat is variable.
    - Soft tissues are of variable shades of grey.

MRI is very **sensitive in detecting an increase in mobile proton content** of a tissue. On a T2-weighted image of the brain, the cerebrospinal fluid (CSF)-filled ventricles and subarachnoid space are physiologically bright (hyperintense). Abnormal fluid-filled lesions (cysts) also have a high signal intensity. In addition, parenchymal lesions which are solid but have an increased content of mobile hydrogen protons (e.g. oedema, tumour, inflammation) will also be T2 hyperintense and can thus be distinguished from surrounding tissues.

There are **numerous additional MRI sequences** which allow, for example, the selective suppression of fat (short tau inversion recovery sequence, **STIR**), the selective suppression of fluid (fluid-attenuated inversion recovery sequence, **FLAIR**), or exhibit signal loss in the presence of certain blood degradation products (**T2***). Intravenous contrast medium administration results in enhancement in regions of increased vascularity, and, for the CNS, in regions with an absent or damaged blood–brain barrier. Unlike radiography and CT, which utilize iodinated contrast media, MRI uses specific paramagnetic substances.

Like CT, MRI is a **cross-sectional imaging technique**. The steps described above (application of radiofrequency pulses, relaxation, image reconstruction from the MR signal) occur in pre-selected slices, which unlike CT can be obtained in any orientation (transverse, dorsal, sagittal and oblique).

5.4.2 Advantages and disadvantages

Advantages

- MRI is a **cross-sectional/tomographic modality** which allows acquisition of slices without superimposition of other structures over the area of interest.
- Images can be obtained in **any orientation** (transverse, dorsal, sagittal and oblique).
- MRI is characterized by **excellent soft-tissue contrast**, and in this regard is superior to radiography and CT.
- Depending on the imaging system, large areas of the body can be included in the scan field of view.
- MRI **does not use ionizing radiation** and, at least at this point in time, appears to be a very safe imaging procedure.
- The availability of multiple sequences allows **selective enhancement or suppression of specific substances** like fat, haemorrhage or fluid.

Disadvantages

- MRI equipment is **expensive** and is typically limited to larger hospitals and specialty institutions.
- The examination requires **general anaesthesia**.
- Depending on the system, the ability to resolve small structures and image patients of a small size is limited.
- The time needed for MRI examination is **long**. Depending on the system, acquisition of a single sequence may take several minutes, and typically several sequences are needed to establish a diagnosis. Depending on the MRI system available, the indication, patient size and the number of sequences acquired, study duration may range anywhere from 20 to 90 minutes for the head and 15 to 120 minutes for the spine.
- Presence of **ferromagnetic material** (certain metals) in the area of interest results in artefacts which may be so severe that the entire MRI study is nondiagnostic. Examples of metal which may be present in small animal patients include surgical implants (these may or may not be ferromagnetic), identification microchips and ballistic projectiles. To the best of our knowledge, severe complications or death following migration of metallic material has not been reported in veterinary patients. This is in contrast to human medicine where migration of intracranial aneurysm clips or shrapnel fragments has been reported to have potentially fatal consequences.
- Image generation in MRI is based on the **presence of mobile protons**. Evaluation of regions of low mobile proton density (lung, cortical bone, nasal cavity) is limited. A possible counterargument is that pathological processes result in an increase in proton content in these structures, increasing the diagnostic yield of MRI.

a b c d

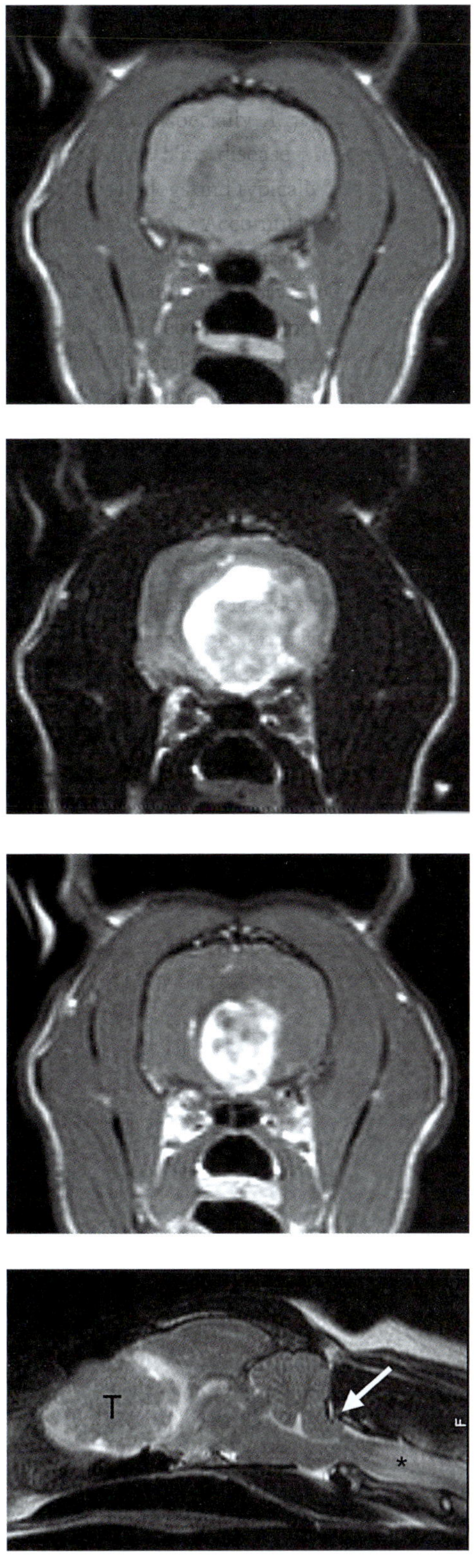

Fig. 5.16 Brain tumour (meningioma) in a cat. Transverse MR images acquired at the border between frontal and parietal lobes show a large intracranial mass lesion.
a The lesion is indistinct and mildly hypointense to surrounding brain parenchyma on a T1-weighted image.
b The lesion is hyperintense and heterogeneous on a T2-weighted image, with a strongly hyperintense rim along the dorsal and right aspect.
c Following contrast medium administration, the ventral aspect of the mass is characterized by strong and heterogeneous contrast enhancement. Note that the region of the mass which was strongly hyperintense on the T2-weighted image (b) is non-enhancing, indicating a cystic component.
d Additional information is gained on this sagittal T2-weighted image. The tumour (T) extends from the olfactory bulb to the level of the margin between the frontal and parietal lobes and in its rostral aspect involves the entire height of the cranial vault. Secondary to the intracranial mass effect, the cerebral sulci are attenuated, and there is herniation of the cerebellum into the foramen magnum (arrow). There is also evidence of subtentorial herniation of brain parenchyma with compression of the rostral margin of the cerebellum. There is increased signal intensity to the cranial cervical spinal cord (*), consistent with syrinx formation.

5.4.3 Applications in small animal practice

NERVOUS SYSTEM MRI is considered the gold standard for evaluation of most brain disorders in humans and animals (Fig. 5.16 and 5.17). Even though myelography and CT are very good imaging modalities to evaluate the bony structures of the spine and intervertebral discs, MRI is superior in evaluating the spinal cord and adjacent soft tissues (Fig. 5.18).

SKULL, NOSE, PARANASAL SINUSES, TYMPANIC BULLA AND ORBIT Even though MRI is inferior to CT in the evaluation of small bony structures, most regions of the head can be adequately evaluated by means of MRI (Fig. 5.19). MRI is superior to CT in the evaluation of soft-tissue lesions (e.g. in the retro-orbital space).

a

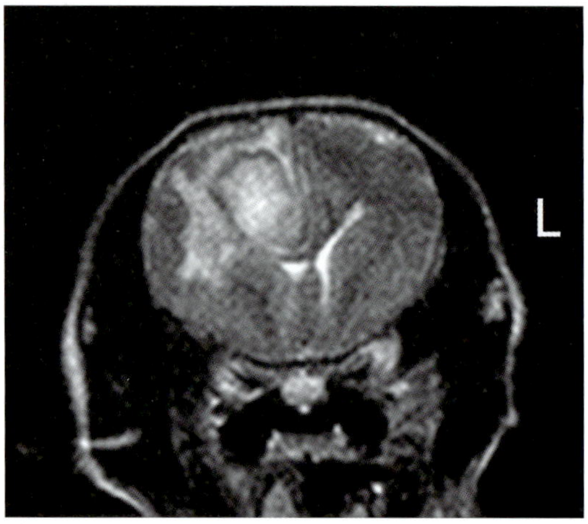

b

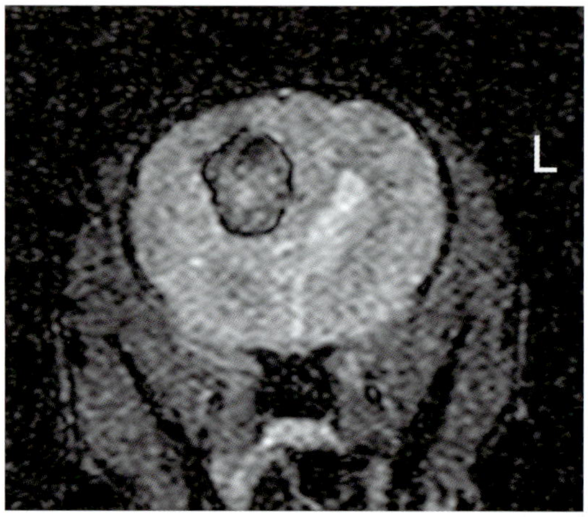

Fig. 5.17 Intracranial haemorrhage (haemorrhagic stroke) in a dog.
a On this T2-weighted transverse image there is an oval intra-axial mass associated with the right cerebral hemisphere. The mass lesion is heterogeneously hyperintense and surrounded by hyperintense finger-like projections along the white matter tracts. There is compression of the right lateral ventricle and midline shift towards the left. (L = left).
b On this transverse T2*-weighted image the mass lesion is generally moderately hypointense, with a strongly hypointense rim. This is characteristic for a haemorrhagic lesion. The surrounding finger-like T2 hyperintense projections are less well defined, are not associated with signal attenuation, and are consistent with vasogenic oedema (L = left).

a

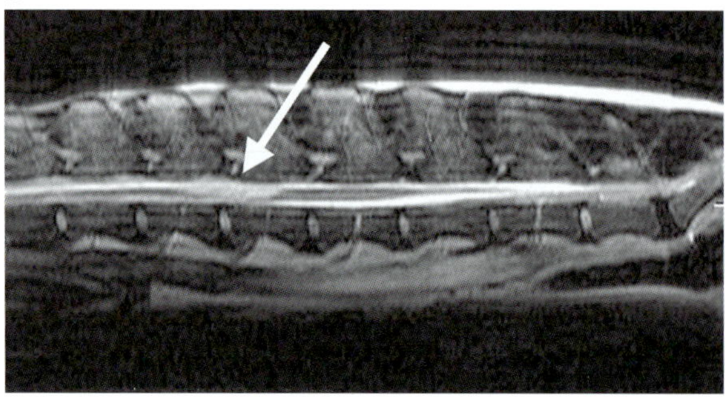

b

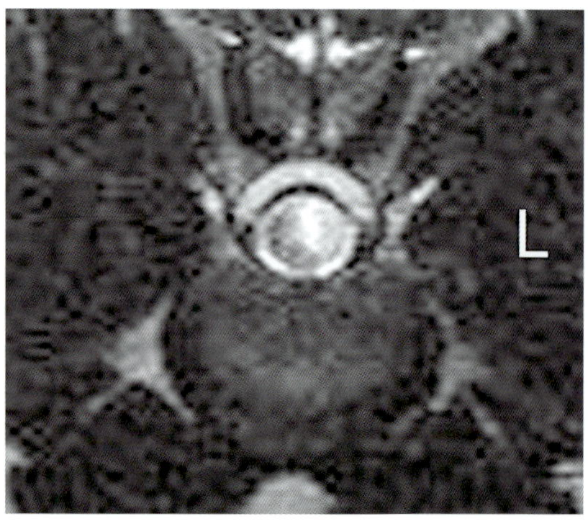

Fig. 5.18 Fibrocartilaginous embolism in a dog.
a On the sagittal T2-weighted image there is a region of hyperintensity within the spinal cord at the level of the second and third lumbar vertebrae (arrow).
b On the transverse T2-weighted image at this level, the left half of the spinal cord is hyperintense compared to the normal right half (L = left).

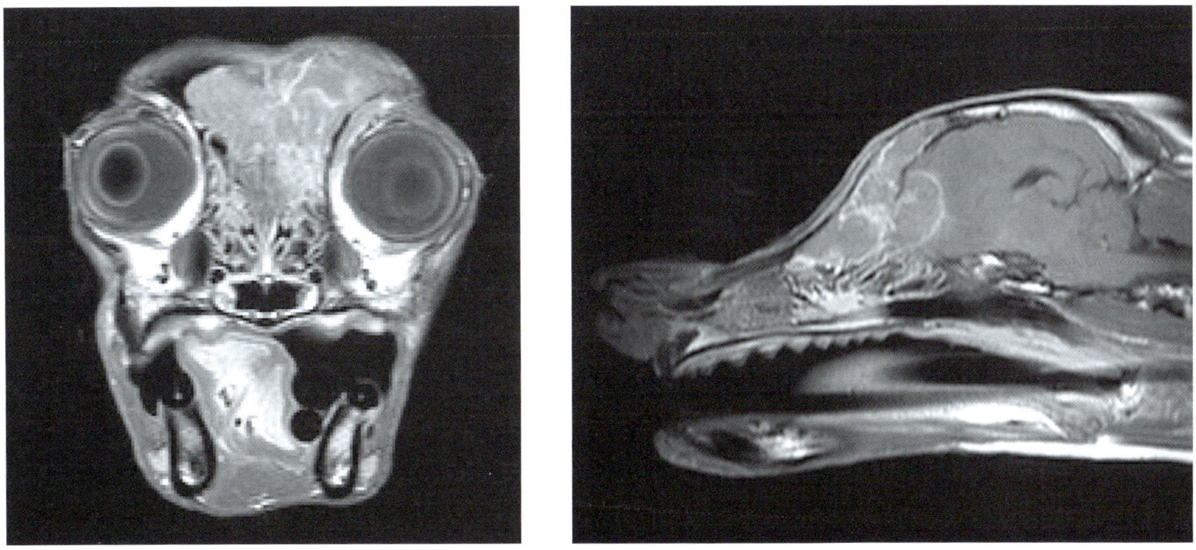

a b

Fig. 5.19 Nasal tumour (adenocarcinoma) in a dog. Transverse a and sagittal b T1-weighted MR images following contrast medium administration show a large heterogeneous mass associated with the left dorsal nasal cavity and frontal sinus, which results in destruction of surrounding bone, including the cribriform plate, and extension into the cranial vault.

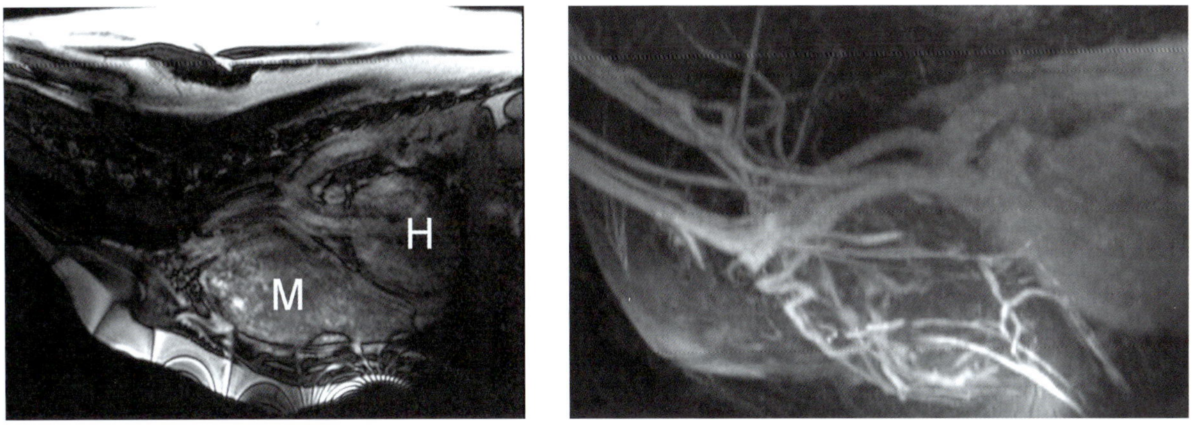

a b

Fig. 5.20 Cranial mediastinal mass (thymoma). The initial diagnosis was made based on thoracic radiographs and ultrasound-guided biopsy of the mass. MRI was performed for surgical planning.

a On this sagittal image (sequence: 'True FISP') a large mass (M) is visible within the cranioventral thorax. The lesion appears fairly well demarcated and results in displacement of the heart (H) and the large mediastinal vessels caudally and dorsally.

b Magnetic resonance angiography (MRA) was performed and shows marked vascularization of the mass, but no evidence of mass invasion into adjacent large vessels. Based on the imaging findings, surgery was considered feasible. The mass was resected without surgical complications.

Musculoskeletal system Despite its limitations in resolving small bony structures, MRI is gaining importance in orthopaedic imaging of small animal patients. Abnormalities which may be detected with MRI include bone contusions and microfractures, inflammatory or neoplastic bone lesions, and injuries or infiltrative disorders of soft tissues (ligaments, tendons, muscles, connective tissue).

Other applications Due to its excellent soft-tissue imaging properties, MRI has great potential for evaluation of the abdomen. However, abdominal MRI is at this point rarely performed in veterinary patients. Other possible applications of MRI include surgical planning for infiltrative soft-tissue tumours, tumour staging and diagnosis of vascular anomalies (e.g. portosystemic shunt). MRI is inferior to CT in the evaluation of the thorax due to the duration of the examination, increased risk of motion artefacts, and poor lung imaging capabilities. However, MRI can be used successfully for evaluation of mediastinal structures and the thoracic wall (Fig. 5.20).

Suggested reading

Barr F, Gaschen L. BSAVA Manual of Canine and Feline Ultrasonography. Gloucester: British Small Animal Veterinary Association 2011.

Daniel GB, Berry CR. Textbook of Veterinary Nuclear Medicine. American College of Veterinary Radiology 2006.

Gavin PR, Bagley RS. Practical Small Animal MRI. Ames: Wiley Blackwell 2009.

Hecht S, Adams WH. MRI of brain disease in veterinary patients part 1: Basic principles and congenital brain disorders. Vet Clin North Am Small Anim Pract 2010; 40: 21–38.

Hecht S, Adams WH. MRI of brain disease in veterinary patients part 2: Acquired brain disorders. Vet Clin North Am Small Anim Pract 2010; 40: 39–63.

Hecht S, Da Costa R. Principles and application of magnetic resonance imaging (MRI). In: Dewey CW, da Costa RC (eds). Practical Guide to Canine and Feline Neurology, 3rd edn. Ames: Wiley Blackwell 2016.

Hecht S, Thomas WB, Marioni-Henry K, Echandi R, Matthews AR, Adams WH. Myelography vs. computed tomography in the evaluation of acute intervertebral disc extrusion in chondrodystrophic dogs. Vet Radiol Ultrasound 2009; 50: 353–9.

Kalender WA. Computed Tomography. München: Publicis MCD Verlag 2000.

Koechli VD, Marincek B. Wie funktioniert MRI? Berlin: Springer-Verlag 1998.

Kremkau FW. Diagnostic Ultrasound: Principles and Instruments. Philadelphia: WB Saunders 2002.

Leblanc AK, Daniel GB. Advanced imaging for veterinary cancer patients. Vet Clin North Am Small Anim Pract 2007; 37: 1059–77.

Mai W. Diagnostic MRI in Dogs and Cats. Boca Raton: CRC Press, Taylor and Francis Group 2018.

Nyland TG, Mattoon JS. Small Animal Diagnostic Ultrasound. Philadelphia: WB Saunders 2002.

Penninck D, d'Anjou MA. Atlas of Small Animal Ultrasonography, 2nd edn. Ames: Wiley-Blackwell 2015.

Robertson I, Thrall DE. Imaging dogs with suspected disc herniation: Pros and cons of myelography, computed tomography, and magnetic resonance. Vet Radiol Ultrasound 2011; 52: 81–4.

Schwarz T, Saunders J. Veterinary Computed Tomography. Ames: Wiley-Blackwell 2011.

Tidwell AS, Jones JC. Advanced imaging concepts: A pictorial glossary of CT and MRI technology. Clin Tech Small Animal Practice 1999; 14: 65–111.

Wisner E, Zwingenberger A. Atlas of Small Animal CT and MRI. Ames: Wiley Blackwell 2015.

Head

6

Randi Drees

6.1 Anatomy and indications

6.1.1 Skull

ANATOMY The skull is divided into the cranium and facial bones including the jaw. Due to the complex anatomical configuration of the skull, osseous structures typically appear superimposed on conventional radiographs. A comparison of bilateral symmetry and application of multiple projections or possibly cross-sectional imaging (computed tomography, CT; magnetic resonance imaging, MRI) are therefore essential. The anatomic proportions of the skull vary between feline and canine species as well as between individual breeds (e.g. short- and long-nosed breeds). The cranial vault contains the brain, which is not visible on conventional radiographs. Impressions of the cerebral gyri on the inner skull result in a marbled radiopacity, which is best seen on lateral views. Imaging of the brain requires cross-sectional imaging (CT or MRI) and is described elsewhere. The caudal part of the cranium is formed by the occipital bone. Its foramen magnum constitutes the connection to the vertebral canal, and its articular processes articulate with the first cervical vertebra.

INDICATIONS Trauma, mass lesions/swelling, and suspicion of congenital malformation (foramen magnum, hydrocephalus).

6.1.2 Nasal cavity and paranasal sinuses

ANATOMY The boundaries of the nasal cavity are formed by the maxilla, incisive, nasal and palatine bones. The right and left sides are divided by the sagittal nasal septum and the vomer bone. The nasal cavity connects caudoventrally to the nasopharynx and is separated from the cranium by the sickle-shaped ethmoid bone. The ethmoid and the maxilla give rise to the ethmoid and nasal turbinates, respectively. Dogs and cats have a paired frontal sinus which is connected to the caudal nasal cavity. Nasal cavity and frontal sinuses physiologically contain air, resulting in characteristic contrast on a radiograph.

INDICATIONS Nasal discharge, mass lesions/swelling, suspicion of foreign body or trauma.

6.1.3 External, middle and inner ear

ANATOMY The external ear canal is air-filled and thus can be distinguished from adjacent soft tissues. Only the very medial portion of the ear canal is bony and embedded in the temporal bone. The tympanic membrane, which forms the border to the middle ear, is not visible on radiographs. The middle ear is located within the temporal bone, and its air-filled cavity (tympanic bulla) is visualized on radiographs as a thin-walled rounded structure. Its connection to the nasopharynx via the Eustachian tube is not radiographically visible. An evaluation of the inner ear is only possible using cross-sectional imaging modalities.

INDICATIONS Radiographic evaluation of the auditory apparatus is indicated when clinical signs of otitis and neurological symptoms such as head tilt or vestibular disease are present.

6.1.4 Temporomandibular joints

ANATOMY Aided by a meniscus, the articular process of the mandible forms an articulation with the temporal bone rostral to the tympanic bulla. The coronoid process of the mandible is located medial to the zygomatic arch and, in healthy animals, it does not contact this structure. The retro-articular process of the temporal bone is located caudal to the joint. Radiographic evaluation includes assessment of joint surfaces and joint space as well as the relationship between the coronoid process and the zygomatic arch.

INDICATIONS Difficulty or pain when opening or closing the mouth during eating and mastication, trauma, and clinically visible asymmetry.

6.1.5 Dental structures

ANATOMY The teeth of dogs and cats are brachydont and consist of the tooth root embedded in the alveolar bone and the crown, which is located in the oral cavity. Dentin and enamel appear radiographically as mineral opaque structures, while the pulp cavity is of soft-tissue opacity. Teeth in young animals are characterized by a wide pulp cavity and an open pulp canal (apical foramen) at the apex of the tooth root. The pulp cavity and canal progressively mineralize with age and appear narrower. With progressive mineralization, developing permanent teeth are visible radiographically, starting at approximately 12 weeks of age, and should be fully erupted by 7 months in the dog and 6 months in the cat, respectively (Table 6.1). The dental formulas for milk (deciduous) and permanent teeth are listed in Table 6.2. Teeth are anchored in the alveoli of the maxilla and mandible by radiolucent Sharpey fibres (periodontal membrane). Thus, mineralized teeth are separate from the opaque lamina dura (fine cortex of the alveolar bone) by a radiolucent line (Fig. 6.1). Increasing sclerosis of the trabecular alveolar bone in older animals results in decreased visibility of the margins of the lamina dura compared to young animals. The bone between teeth is called the alveolar crest or alveolar septum and appears increasingly flat in older animals. This should be recognized as a physiological change and not be mistaken for periodontal disease.

INDICATIONS Trauma, swelling/masses, periodontal disease and loose, missing or supernumerary teeth. The radiographic examination is part of a routine dental workup. This examination can be performed using special dental radiographic equipment if available.

6.1.6 Soft tissues

ANATOMY The nasal cavity and pharynx are typically mostly air-filled. Radiographically, mass lesions or foreign bodies can be visualized due to their increased opacity compared to the radiolucent surrounding passages.

INDICATIONS Suspected obstruction of the upper airways and foreign bodies are the main indications for a radiographic examination.

Table 6.1 Timing of tooth eruption in dogs and cats. Variations occur depending on the breed and size of the patient.

	Deciduous teeth (weeks)		Permanent teeth (months)	
	Puppy	Kitten	Puppy	Kitten
Incisor teeth	3–4	2–3	3–4	3–4
Canine teeth	3	3–4	4–6	4–5
Premolar teeth	4–12	3–6	4–6	4–6
Molar teeth			5–7	4–5

Table 6.2 Dental formulas in dogs and cats.

	Dog	Cat
Deciduous teeth	i3c1p3 -------- = 28 i3c1p3	i3c1p3 -------- = 26 i3c1p2
Permanent teeth	I3C1P4M2 ------------ = 42 I3C1P4M3	I3C1P3M1 ------------ = 30 I3C1P2M1

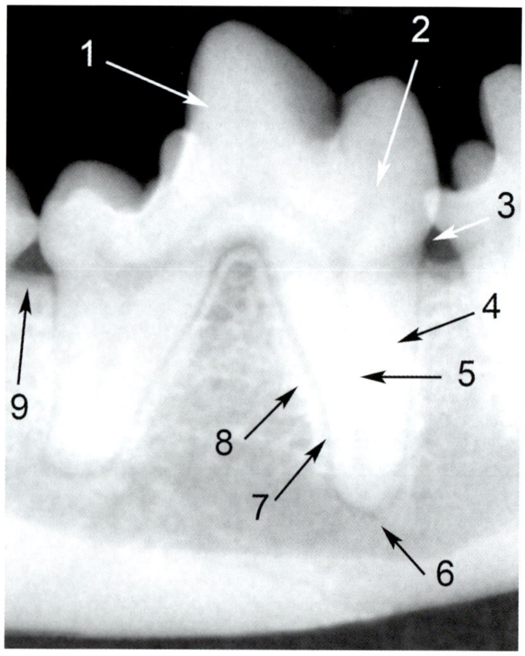

Fig. 6.1 Normal dental structure of a mandibular premolar tooth in a dog. 1 Crown, 2 Pulp cavity, 3 Tooth neck (transition between cementum and enamel), 4 Tooth root, 5 Root canal, 6 Apex, 7 Periodontal membrane, 8 Lamina dura, 9 Alveolar crest. (Courtesy of Christopher Snyder, UW Madison, USA)

6.1.7 Salivary glands

ANATOMY Dogs and cats have four paired salivary glands (parotid, zygomatic, mandibular and sublingual salivary glands) as well as multiple smaller glands in the oral mucosa. These are not normally distinguishable from adjacent soft tissues.

INDICATIONS Swelling or abscessation in the area of a salivary gland and bite wounds to the neck.

6.2 Radiographic technique and positioning

Radiographs of the head require exact patient positioning and are therefore usually acquired under anaesthesia or deep sedation. In most instances, multiple projections are necessary. Use of a grid may be required depending on the thickness of the region of interest.

- **Lateral projection with closed or open mouth**: A closed-mouth radiograph is useful for examination of the nose, frontal sinuses and cranium. Keeping the mouth wide open by means of a radiolucent device (e.g. wooden mouth gag) results in ventral movement of the mandibular coronoid processes, which would otherwise be superimposed with the parietal and frontal parts of the cranium (Fig. 6.2, 6.3 and 6.4).
- **Ventrodorsal (VD) projection with closed or open mouth**: The patient is positioned in dorsal recumbency and the head is positioned without rotation so that it forms a straight line with neck (Fig. 6.5a, 6.6 and 6.7). This projection is mostly aimed at the examination of the cranium, zygomatic arches and temporomandibular joints (see Fig. 6.33). Open-mouth radiographs allow evaluation of the nasal passages and teeth of the upper dental arcade (Fig. 6.5b; see Fig. 6.22).

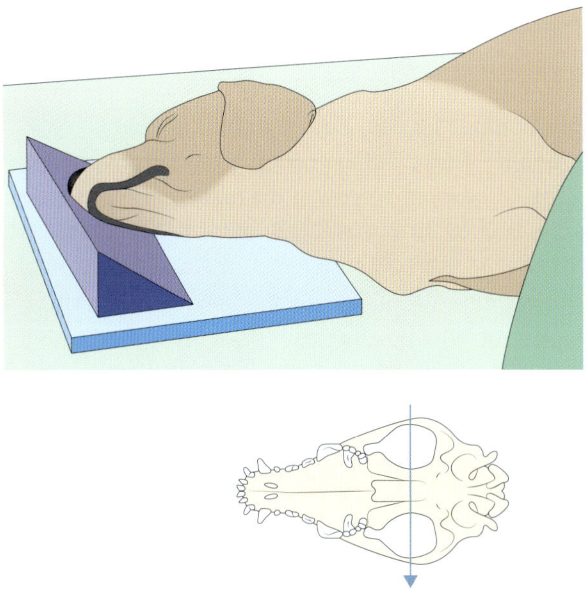

Fig. 6.2 Positioning for a lateral projection of the head with closed mouth. The head should be projected exactly in a laterolateral direction. To achieve a symmetric radiograph, nose and mandible have to be supported by radiolucent material (cotton or foam).

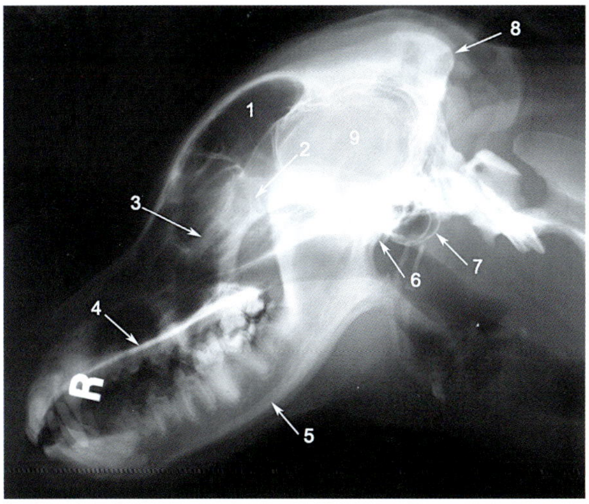

Fig. 6.3 Lateral radiograph of the head in a 5-year-old Labrador Retriever. Paired structures such as the tympanic bullae or left and right halves of the mandible should be projected on top of each other. 1 Frontal sinuses, 2 Cribriform plate, 3 Ethmoid turbinates, 4 Hard palate, 5 Mandible, 6 Temporomandibular joint, 7 Tympanic bulla (middle ear), 8 Occiput, 9 Cranium (R = right).

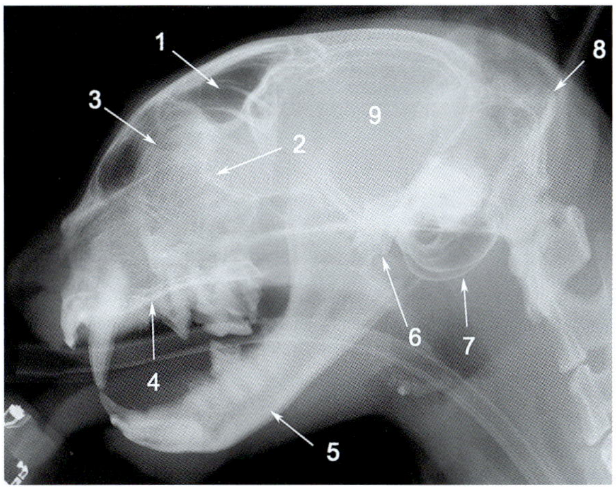

Fig. 6.4 Lateral radiograph of the head in a 2-year-old cat. 1 Frontal sinuses, 2 Cribriform plate, 3 Ethmoid turbinates, 4 Hard palate, 5 Mandible (note missing M1), 6 Temporomandibular joint, 7 Tympanic bulla (middle ear), 8 Occiput, 9 Cranium.

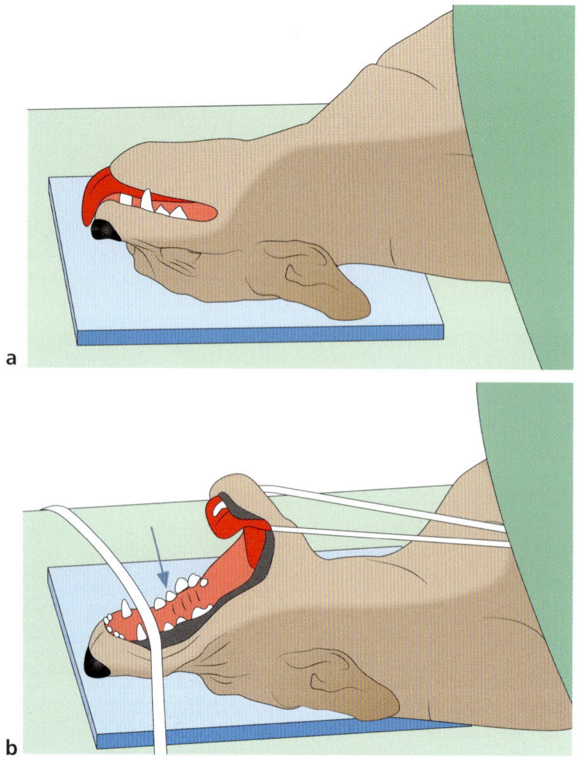

Fig. 6.5 Positioning for ventrodorsal projections of the head with a closed and b open mouth: The palate should be oriented parallel to the tabletop to avoid distortion of anatomic structures on the radiograph. For the open-mouth projection b, the mouth is opened as far as possible using ropes or radiolucent mouth gags. The tongue and tracheal tube are affixed to the mandible. The X-ray beam is angled approximately 20° caudally (arrow) to avoid superimposition.

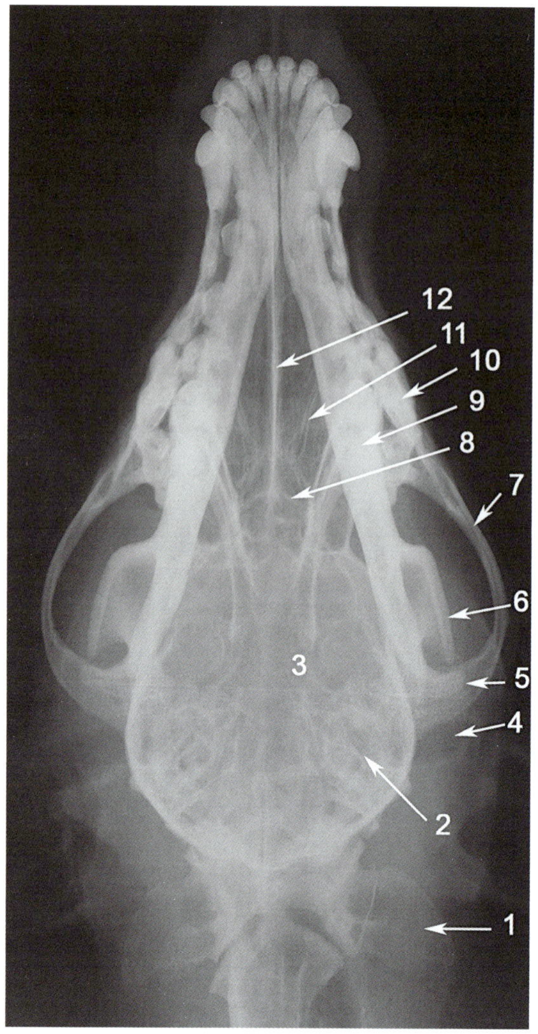

Fig. 6.6 Ventrodorsal radiograph of the head in a 14-year-old Sheltie. Mandible, nasal septum and zygomatic arches can be used to ensure symmetric positioning. 1 Atlas, 2 Tympanic bulla (middle ear), 3 Cranium, 4 External ear canal, 5 Temporomandibular joint, 6 Coronoid process of the mandible, 7 Zygomatic arch, 8 Cribriform plate, 9 Body of the mandible, 10 Maxilla, 11 Ethmoid turbinates, 12 Nasal septum. Note the appearance of the temporomandibular joint (5) in this projection: the wide base of the triangular articular process of the mandible articulates with the articular surface of the temporal bone, which appears flat.

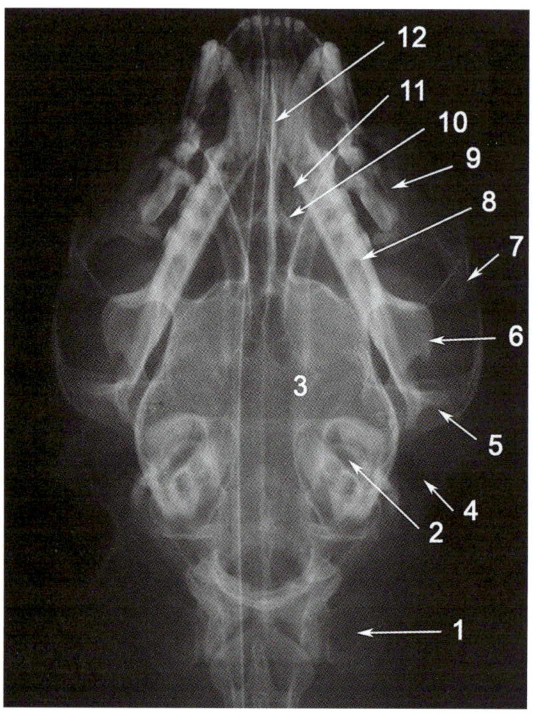

Fig. 6.7 Ventrodorsal radiograph of the head in a 2-year-old cat. 1 Atlas, 2 Tympanic bulla (middle ear), 3 Cranium, 4 External ear canal, 5 Temporomandibular joint, 6 Coronoid process of the mandible, 7 Zygomatic arch, 8 Body of the mandible, 9 Maxilla, 10 Cribriform plate, 11 Ethmoid turbinates, 12 Nasal septum.

- **Dorsoventral (DV) projection**: The head and neck are aligned straight without rotation, with the patient positioned in sternal recumbency. This projection allows assessment of the mandible, temporomandibular joints, zygomatic arch, cranium and region of the middle ear (Fig. 6.8). Positioning for a DV projection of the head is usually easier than for a VD projection and is often preferred.
- **Oblique lateral projections with closed or open mouth**: For individual display of the temporomandibular joints and tympanic bullae, the patient is positioned in lateral recumbency with the mouth closed, and the tip of the nose is slightly elevated (Fig. 6.9 and 6.10). To image the dental arcades of the upper and lower jaw, the mouth is opened wide and rotated along the long axis (Fig. 6.11 to 6.14).

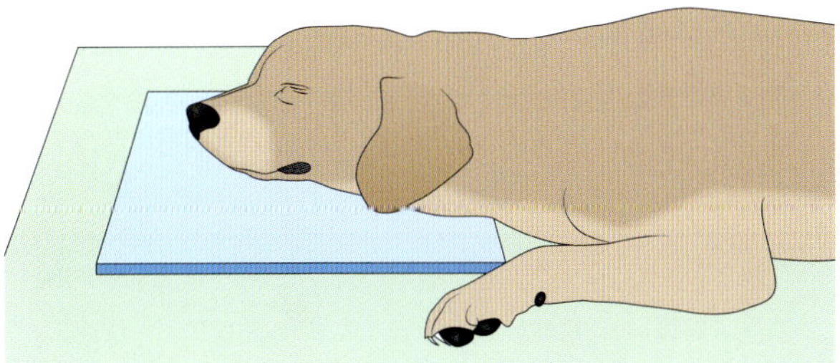

Fig. 6.8 Positioning for the dorsoventral (DV) projection. As straight alignment of the head is easier in this position, symmetric radiographs are more readily obtained on DV than ventrodorsal (VD) radiographs. However, the resultant images are of slightly lower diagnostic quality for dorsal and rostral structures (nasal cavity and frontal sinuses) due to increased distance from the film compared to a VD view and resultant magnification unsharpness.

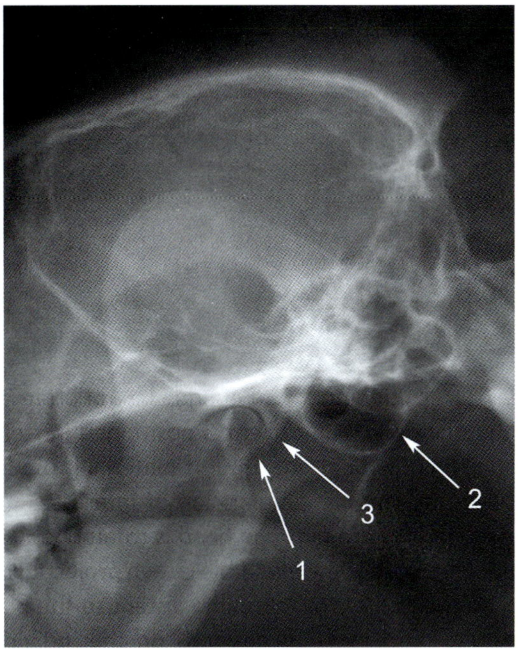

Fig. 6.10 Oblique lateral radiographs of the temporomandibular joint (1) and the tympanic bulla (2) in a dog. The rounded articular process of the mandible communicates with the concave joint surface of the mandibular fossa. The retro-articular process (3) prevents a caudal luxation.

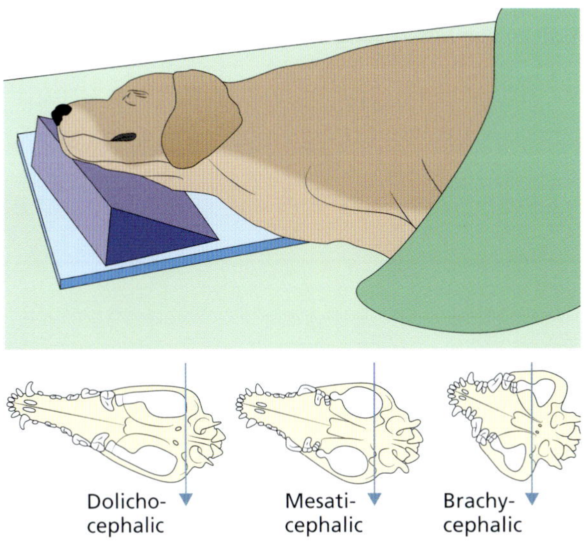

Fig. 6.9 Positioning for the oblique lateral projection aimed at imaging of the individual temporomandibular joint and tympanic bulla. How far the tip of the nose has to be elevated depends on the patient's conformation.

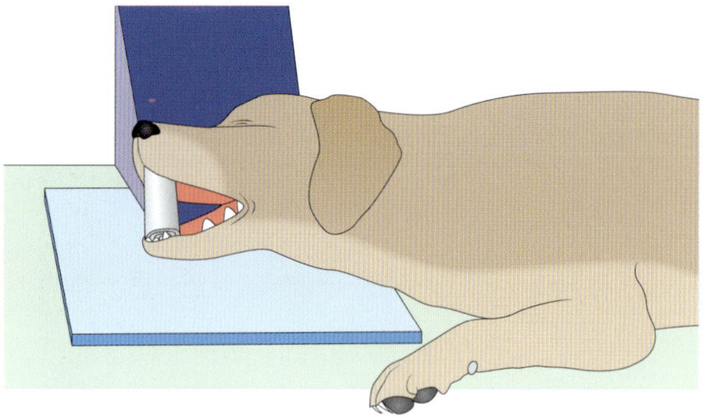

Fig. 6.11 Positioning for an oblique lateral projection of the mandible. The patient is positioned in sternal recumbency. Radiolucent support material is used for positioning. The mandibular side of interest is positioned close to the film, the head is rotated, and the dependent part of the mandible is seen projected dorsally to the half of the mandible distant to the plate. The degree of rotation depends on the individual patient's head shape. Care has to be taken that the central beam is aimed at the region of interest and that the tongue is not superimposed.

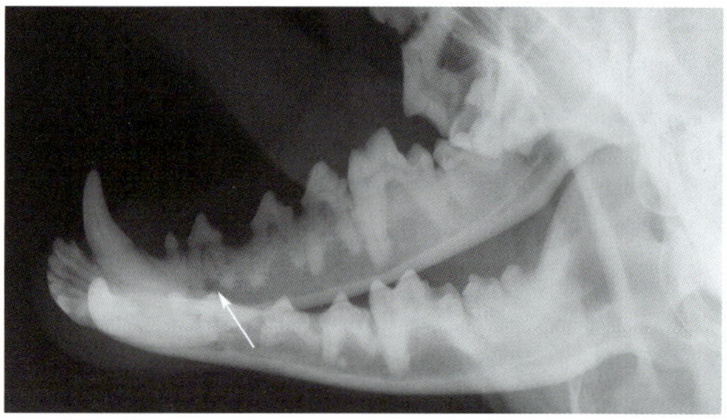

Fig. 6.12 Oblique lateral radiograph of the mandible for evaluation of the mandibular dental arcade in a dog. Separate radiographs are necessary for evaluation of the left and right parts of the mandible. The middle mental foramen (arrow) is visible as a focal lucency ventral to the tooth root of the second premolar tooth and should not be confused with an apical lesion.

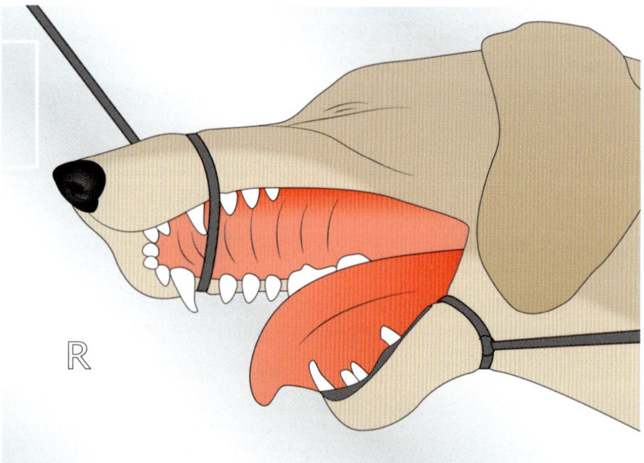

Fig. 6.13 Positioning for an oblique lateral projection of the upper jaw. The head of the patient is rotated towards the side to be projected. The degree of rotation depends on the individual patient's head shape. The side of interest is positioned close to the film and is projected ventrally to the non-dependent side. Care has to be taken that the central beam is aimed at the region of interest and that the tongue is not superimposed.

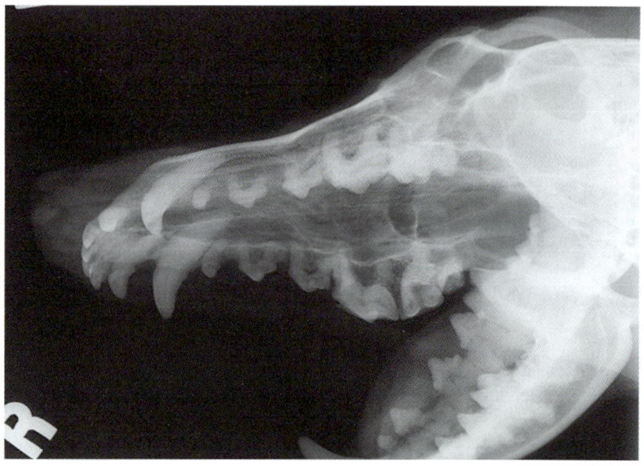

Fig. 6.14 Oblique lateral radiograph of the maxilla in a dog. Separate radiographs are necessary for evaluation of the left and right side (R = right).

- **Intraoral projection (DV and VD)**: This technique allows evaluation of the incisors and canine teeth, the osseous structures of the rostral head, and the rostral nasal cavity. The X-ray film is positioned within the oral cavity. Optimally, a non-screen, high-detail film is used for these projections (Fig. 6.15 and 6.16; see also Fig. 6.23 and 6.31).
- **Rostrocaudal projections with closed or open mouth**: Rostrocaudal projections can be helpful in the evaluation of different anatomic structures. Using a frontal projection, the frontal sinuses are displayed separately (Fig. 6.17a; see also Fig. 6.32). The rostrocaudal projection with open-mouth allows visualization of the tympanic bullae, the first cervical vertebra, and the dens of the axis (Fig. 6.17d; see also Fig. 6.28). The occipital bone and foramen magnum are best evaluated using a fronto-occipital projection (Fig. 6.17c and 6.18). In cats, an extended rostro 10° ventral-dorsocaudal projection can be used to image the tympanic bullae (Fig. 6.17d).

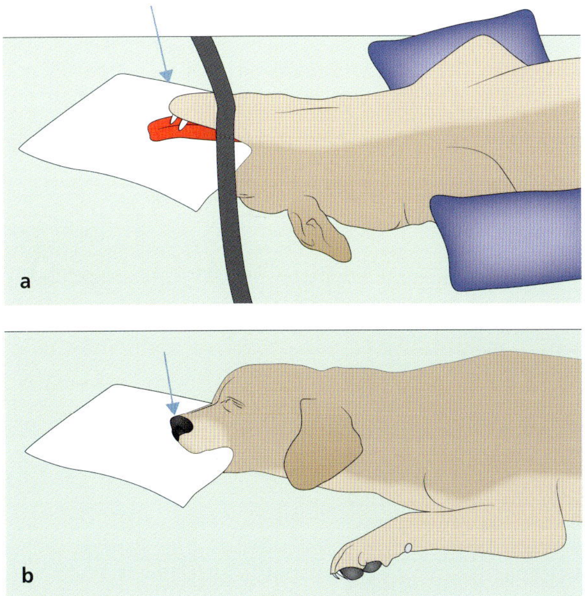

Fig. 6.15 Positioning for a ventrodorsal (a) and a dorsoventral (b) intraoral projection. The film is positioned between the incisive bone/maxilla and the mandible, and the tongue is located ventral to the film. With both techniques, the X-ray beam should be aimed towards the incisors with a slight caudal angle (arrow) to achieve an angle approximately perpendicular to the tooth roots.

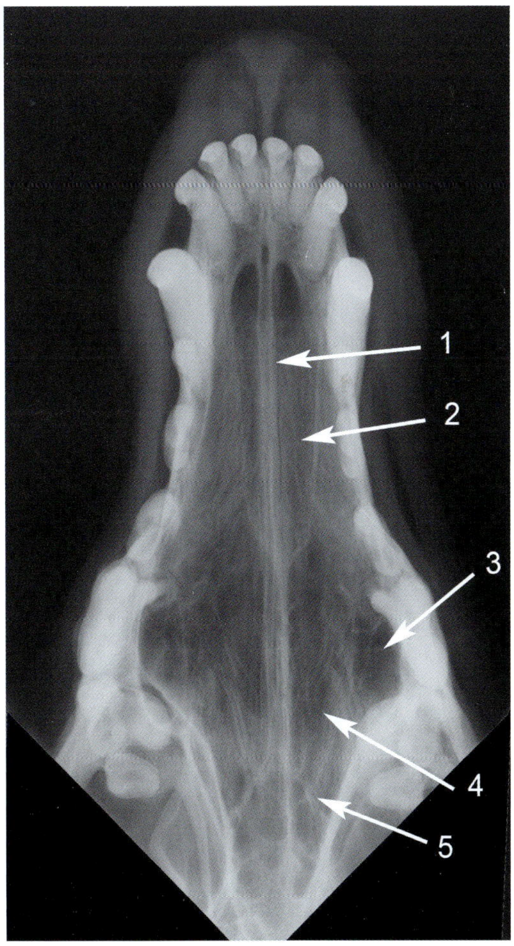

Fig. 6.16 Intraoral radiograph of the incisive bone and maxilla in a dog. 1 Nasal septum, 2 Maxillary turbinates, 3 Maxillary recess, 4 Ethmoid turbinates, 5 Cribriform plate.

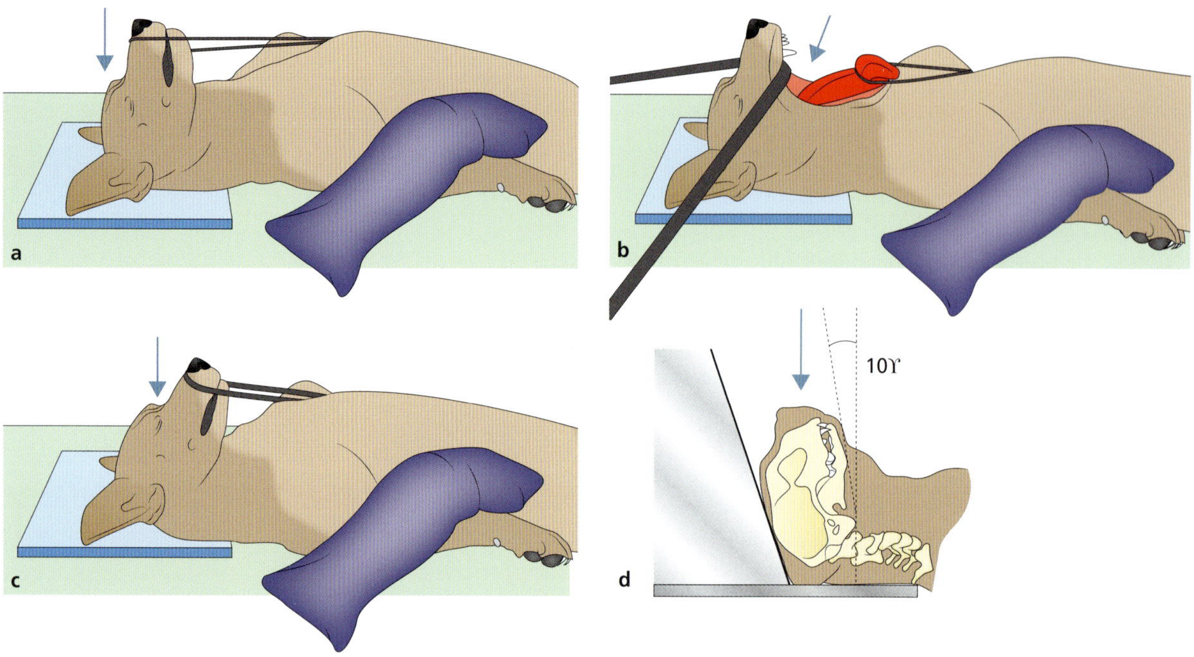

Fig. 6.17a For rostrocaudal projections, the patient is usually positioned in dorsal recumbency. For the frontal projection the head is angled 90° to the spine, and the X-ray beam is aimed at the frontal sinuses.

b For the rostrocaudal projection of the tympanic bullae and the first two cervical vertebrae, the patient is positioned similarly, but the mouth is opened as far as possible. The X-ray beam is aimed into the open mouth, perpendicular to the pharynx and bisecting the angle between the palate and the mandible. The tongue and tracheal tube should be affixed to the mandible.

c The fronto-occipital projection for visualization of the foramen magnum is performed with the mouth closed. The head is flexed approximately 45–60° with respect to the spine, and the central beam is aimed between the eyes.

d For the extended rostro 10° ventral–dorsocaudal projection of the tympanic bullae in the cat, opening of the mouth is not necessary.

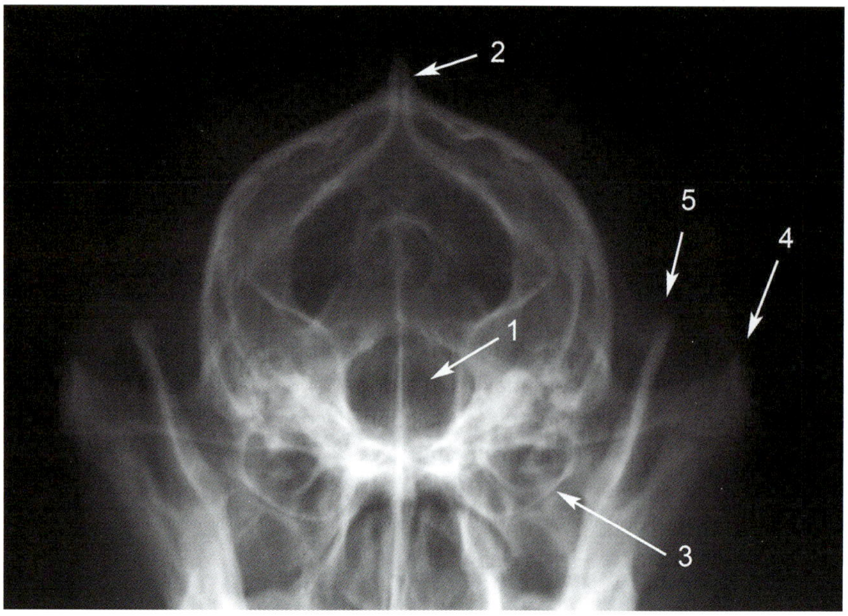

Fig. 6.18 Normal fronto-occipital projection for visualization of the foramen magnum. 1 Foramen magnum, 2 Occipital crest, 3 Tympanic bulla, 4 Zygomatic arch, 5 Coronoid process of the mandible.

6.3 Diseases of the head

6.3.1 Congenital diseases

Hydrocephalus

The term hydrocephalus denotes the congenital or acquired excessive accumulation of cerebrospinal fluid within the calvarium. The congenital form has been reported in multiple toy dog breeds (Maltese, Yorkshire Terrier, Chihuahua, Toy Poodle, Pug and others) and in Siamese cats.

RADIOGRAPHIC FINDINGS If hydrocephalus develops after skeletal maturation it does not usually result in radiographic changes. With congenital hydrocephalus, a relatively large size and domed shape of the calvarium, thinning and diminished contouring of the cortical bone, and persistent open fontanelles are noted (Fig. 6.19). A previously used contrast procedure to evaluate ventricular size (ventriculography) has become obsolete since ultrasound and cross-sectional imaging have become available.

Occipital dysplasia ('keyhole' malformation)

This congenital malformation of the occipital bone results in enlargement of the foramen magnum mostly dorsally and may be associated with cerebellar herniation. This disorder is predominantly found in toy-breed dogs as well as Cavalier King Charles Spaniels and in association with other congenital diseases such as hydrocephalus or atlanto-occipital malformation.

RADIOGRAPHIC FINDINGS Dorsal enlargement of the foramen magnum is noted, typically resulting in a keyhole shape. As the defect is commonly covered by a radiolucent fibrous membrane, this radiographic finding does not necessarily indicate cerebellar herniation.

Temporomandibular joint dysplasia

This malformation results in flattening or incongruence of the joint surfaces of the temporomandibular joints and represents a predisposition for subluxation (see 'Temporomandibular joint (sub)luxation' below).

RADIOGRAPHIC FINDINGS Flattening or incongruence of the joint surfaces of the temporomandibular joints can be seen (Fig. 6.20).

Mucopolysaccharidoses

This group of lysosomal storage diseases is inherited via an autosomal recessive trait and has a high prevalence in Siamese cats.

RADIOGRAPHIC FINDINGS Changes affecting the skull include shortened nasal turbinates, aplasia or dysplasia of the frontal sinuses, and shortening of the upper jaw. Radiographs of the remainder of the skeleton show epiphyseal dysplasia, generalized osteoporosis, pectus excavatum and vertebral malformations (see section 7.3.10).

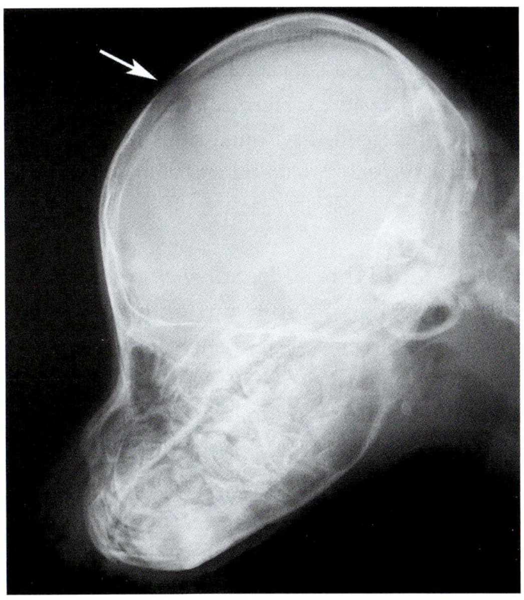

Fig. 6.19 Hydrocephalus in a 3-month-old Chihuahua puppy. The calvarium appears subjectively enlarged and is of homogenous opacity. The normally visible impressions of the cerebral gyri are absent and the fontanelle is open (arrow).

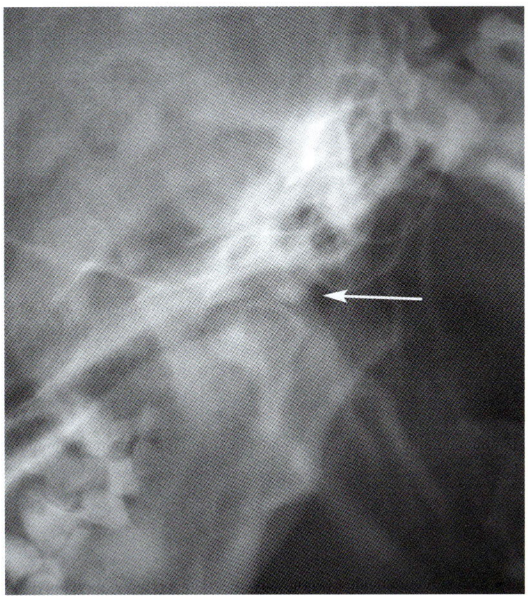

Fig. 6.20 Temporomandibular joint dysplasia in a 9-year-old Beagle. Flattening of the articular fossa (arrow) predisposes to subluxation.

6.3.2 Metabolic diseases

Primary or secondary hyperparathyroidism

Primary hyperparathyroidism may be caused by adenomas or carcinomas as well as uni- or bilateral adenomatous hyperplasia of the parathyroid gland. Secondary hyperparathyroidism results from calcium and phosphorus imbalances due to inappropriate nutrition or dysregulation of retention/excretion in renal disease. Both causes result in increased production of parathyroid hormone and mobilization of calcium from skeletal structures. Secondary fibrous osteodystrophy can result in regional thickening of the affected bones.

RADIOGRAPHIC FINDINGS The major radiographic finding is a decrease in bone opacity. Highly metabolically active tissues are predominantly affected (jaw in juvenile and adult animals and the entire skeleton in young animals). A reduction in radiographic opacity of the lamina dura may be the first radiographic sign (Fig. 6.21).

6.3.3 Neoplasia

Nasal tumours

Nasal tumours are an important differential diagnosis in older patients presenting usually with unilateral haemorrhagic nasal discharge. These tumours are often unilateral and tend to develop in the caudal nasal cavity. Dogs are more commonly affected than cats. **Carcinomas** (adenocarcinoma, squamous cell carcinoma or undifferentiated carcinoma) are most common; **sarcomas** (fibrosarcoma, chondrosarcoma, osteosarcoma, haemangiosarcoma or undifferentiated sarcoma) are less common. Both groups of tumours are locally invasive and can metastasize to the regional mandibular lymph nodes. Depending on the stage of the disease and the invasiveness, the caudal border of the nasal cavity (cribriform plate) may be disrupted and the tumour may extend into the cranial vault. In this case, patients commonly present with central nervous system symptoms. Lymphoma is the most common nasal tumour in cats. Obstructive rhinitis and sinusitis may develop secondary to nasal tumours. At this point, the most effective treatment option is external beam radiation therapy, which requires cross-sectional imaging for planning.

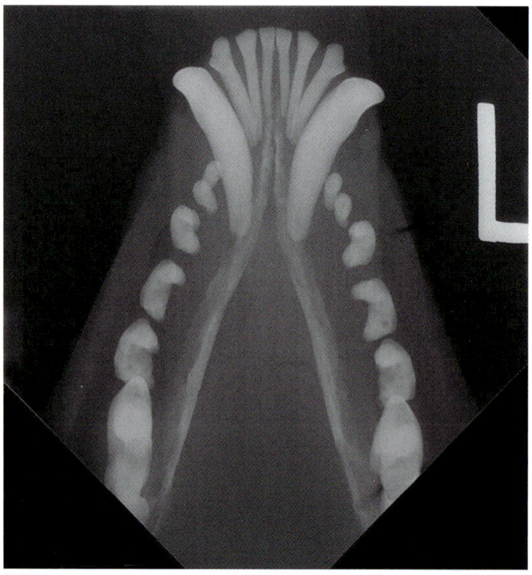

Fig. 6.21 Intraoral ventrodorsal radiograph in an 11-year-old Keeshond with primary hyperparathyroidism due to an adenoma of the parathyroid gland. In this advanced stage of the disease, generalized decreased radiopacity of the mandible with the impression of 'floating teeth' is easily recognized (L = left).

RADIOGRAPHIC FINDINGS Nasal tumours manifest as soft-tissue opacity in the affected nasal cavity. Visible destruction of the fine nasal turbinates and possibly of the osseous boundaries of the nasal cavity allow classification of the lesion as aggressive. The nasal septum may also be destroyed or deviated from midline.

> Mild septal deviations from midline without evidence of a space-occupying lesion in the nasal cavity are normal anatomic variants and should not be mistaken for nasal neoplasia.

An important factor in tumour diagnostics is the assessment of the integrity of the sickle-shaped cribriform plate. Lysis of this structure implies tumour extension into the cranial vault, which is associated with a significantly worse prognosis for the patient (Fig. 6.22). Concurrent ipsilateral soft-tissue opacity in the frontal sinus may result from secondary obstructive rhinitis and sinusitis or tumour invasion.

Soft-tissue tumours of the oral cavity

The most common oral tumours in dogs and cats are squamous cell carcinomas followed by fibrosarcomas and malignant melanomas.

Squamous cell carcinomas in dogs predominantly develop in the rostral aspect of the maxilla. The extent of local invasiveness and osteolysis depends on the histological malignancy grade (Fig. 6.23). Regional or distant metastases are rare. Squamous cell carcinomas in cats are usually associated with a very poor prognosis. They may affect the maxilla or mandible and exhibit locally aggressive behaviour.

Oral fibrosarcomas are common in large-breed dogs and Golden Retrievers. They tend to exhibit locally expansile and aggressive behaviour with osteolysis, despite benign histological categorization (Fig. 6.24).

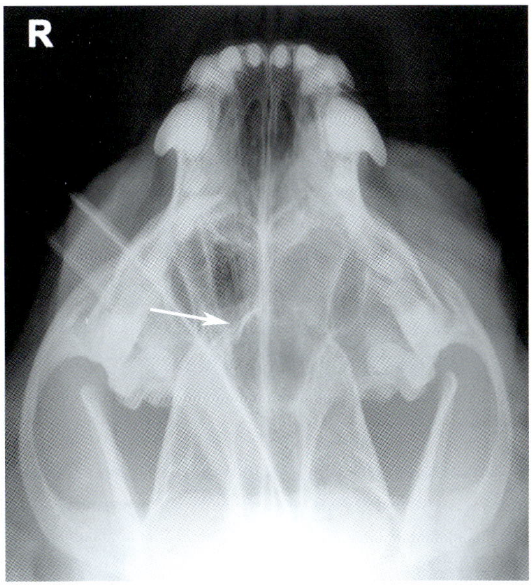

Fig. 6.22 Adenocarcinoma of the left nasal cavity in a 7-year-old Chow-Chow. The ventrodorsal open-mouth radiograph demonstrates increased soft-tissue opacity in the caudal nasal cavity and lysis of the nasal turbinates and cribriform plate. The cribriform plate (arrow) as well as the nasal turbinates on the right are intact (R = right).

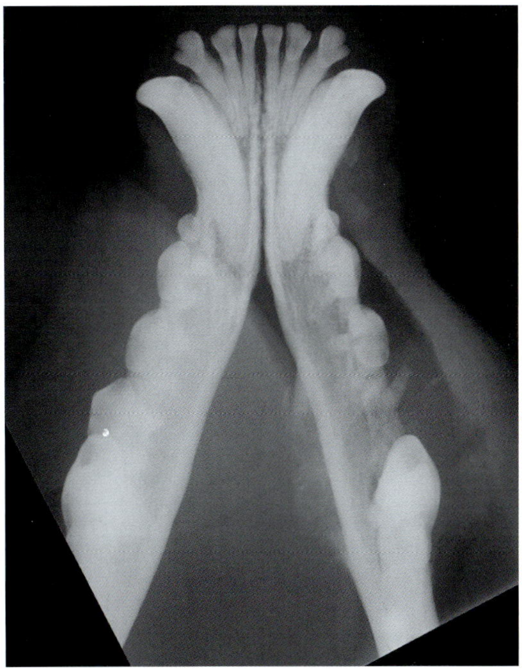

Fig. 6.23 Intraoral radiograph of a squamous cell carcinoma of the mandible in a 12-year-old Labrador. The left mandible is characterized by an aggressive process with lytic and osteoproliferative changes as well as loss of the fourth premolar tooth. The tongue is superimposed with the normal right mandible.

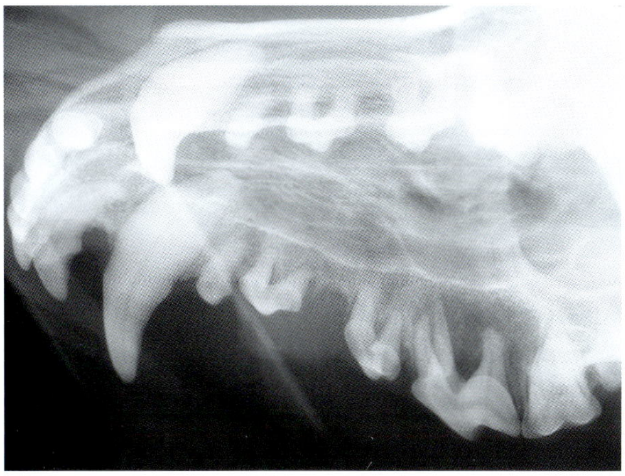

Fig. 6.24 Fibrosarcoma of the maxilla in a 6-year-old Golden Retriever. The focal soft-tissue opacity mass exhibits locally expansile behaviour, displaces the third premolar tooth caudally, and results in mildly irregular lysis of the alveolar septum between the second and third premolar teeth.

Conversely, **malignant melanomas** are more commonly found in small-breed dogs. These tumours are variably locally invasive but tend to metastasize to regional lymph nodes and lung.

Virus induced papillomas are soft-tissue tumours which do not cause radiographic bone lesions.

Polyps can originate from the middle ear or the Eustachian tube and are predominantly found in young cats. These represent benign soft-tissue neoplasms which can lead to upper airway obstruction.

RADIOGRAPHIC FINDINGS Determination of the histological tumour type of oral carcinomas and sarcomas is not possible radiographically but requires cytology or histopathology. Soft-tissue opaque swelling or masses and aggressive bone lesions such as poorly marginated bone lysis and irregular bony proliferation are variable. Polyps do not typically result in bony changes but appear as structures with soft-tissue opacity in the upper airways (pharynx) or the tympanic bulla.

Dental tumours

Epulides derive from periodontal tissue. They are subdivided into three categories: fibromatous, ossifying and acanthomatous. While the former two are generally benign, the latter type exhibits locally aggressive behaviour. Other tumours of dental origin include ameloblastomas, odontomas, cementomas and dentigerous cysts. **Ameloblastomas** are slow growing expansile mass lesions in young dogs which originate from enamel-forming tissue. **Odontomas** are benign tumours of tooth-forming tissues. **Cementomas** are usually self-limiting proliferations of fibrous tissue in the periapical region of the lamina dura which show progressive mineralization. Fluid-filled **dentigerous cysts** are found in the region of the crown of unerupted teeth.

RADIOGRAPHIC FINDINGS Acanthomatous epulides appear radiographically similar to previously described oral soft-tissue neoplasms, with soft-tissue swelling of variable severity and lytic bone lesions (Fig. 6.25). Ameloblastomas typically manifest as large, sometimes multicavitary cysts. Odontomas contain variable amounts of mineralized dental material which is usually surrounded by a radiolucent zone (Fig. 6.26). Cementomas appear as bony structures near a tooth root. They are typically round and may be surrounded by a radiolucent rim. Dentigerous cysts are well-circumscribed expansile cystic structures which occur in association with the crown of an unerupted tooth.

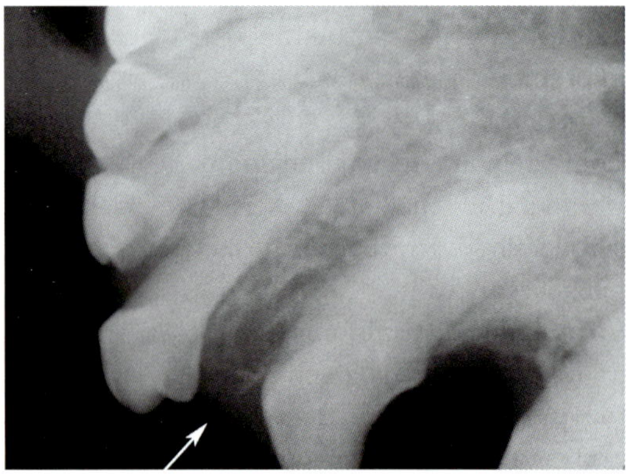

Fig. 6.25 Early stage acanthomatous epulis affecting the incisive bone in a 10-year-old English Setter. Irregularity and focal lysis of the alveolar septum between the second and third upper incisors is noted (arrow). (Courtesy of Jason W. Soukup, UW Madison, USA)

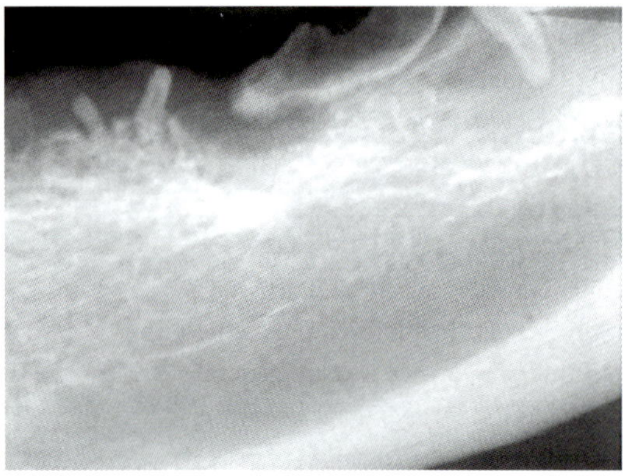

Fig. 6.26 Mandibular odontoma in an 18-month-old Springer Spaniel. Mineralized irregular dental structures are surrounded by a mildly radiolucent zone and soft-tissue swelling. (Courtesy of Jason W. Soukup, UW Madison, USA)

Multilobular tumour of bone (aka multilobular osteochondrosarcoma; MLO)

This is a rare tumour of the skull which is most commonly seen in older large-breed dogs. This tumour type was formerly known as 'chondroma rodens'. Tumours typically develop in the occipital or temporal region; however, other areas of the skull including the orbits, maxilla, mandible and zygomatic arch can also be affected.

RADIOGRAPHIC FINDINGS **MLO** has a characteristic appearance with well-defined margins, marked bony proliferation and little osteolysis. The centre of the tumour has a coarse granular appearance (Fig. 6.27). Cross-sectional imaging is helpful in further characterization of the tumour and to evaluate resectability.

Other tumours

Squamous cell carcinomas of the tympanic bulla are aggressive tumours and often associated with marked bony lysis (Fig. 6.28). Osteosarcomas are the most common primary bone tumours, and approximately 10–15% of cases occur in the region of the skull. Other primary bone tumours occasionally affecting the head include osteomas, chondrosarcomas and chondromas. Osteomas are commonly found in cats and are slow growing benign tumours which predominantly affect the mandible, cranium or frontal sinus.

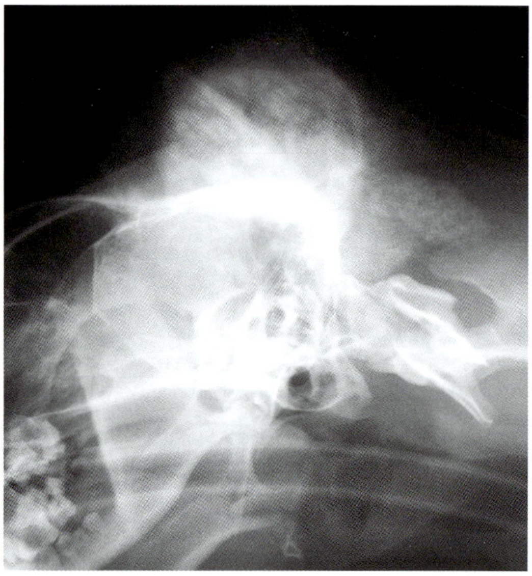

Fig. 6.27 Multilobular tumour of bone in a 6-year-old Labrador Retriever. The tumour originates from the occipital bone and is characterized by a typical osteoproliferative appearance with coarse granular texture and relatively smooth margins. Cross-sectional imaging techniques are necessary to assess the intracranial extent of the tumour and determine resectability.

Radiographic findings In contrast to their often lytic behaviour in the remaining skeleton, osteosarcomas of the skull appear rather mixed osteoblastic–osteolytic (Fig. 6.29). Osteomas are smoothly marginated and well-circumscribed osteoproliferative lesions (Fig. 6.30).

A diagnosis of a brain tumour can usually only be made using cross-sectional imaging techniques. A possible exception is a meningioma with associated mineralization or focal hyperostosis of the adjacent cranium.

> As with other bone and soft-tissue lesions, a radiographic diagnosis of a tumour of the head does not replace cytological or histological determination of the tumour type.

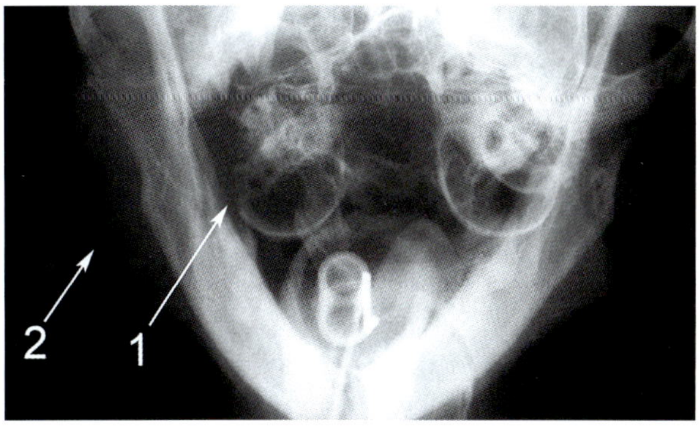

Fig. 6.28 Rostrocaudal open-mouth radiograph in a cat. The bony margins of the right tympanic bulla are partially destroyed by a squamous cell carcinoma (1). Additionally, soft-tissue swelling associated with the tumour is visible adjacent to the right mandibular ramus (2). The left side is anatomically normal.

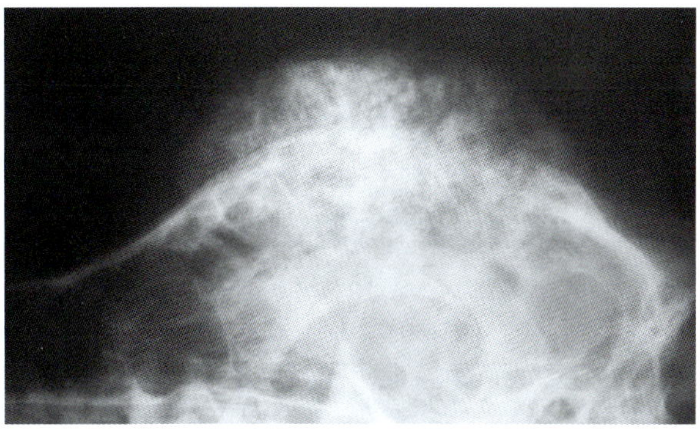

Fig. 6.29 Mixed osteolytic and proliferative changes of the cranium in a 10-year-old Border Collie secondary to osteosarcoma.

6.3.4 Infectious diseases

Mycotic rhinitis

Aspergillus species (especially *A. fumigatus*) can cause a destructive rhinitis. This disease predominantly affects young, long-nosed dogs and typically begins in the rostral aspect of the nasal cavity. Accumulation of excessive secretions in the nasal cavity or frontal sinuses is typically not observed; however, inflammatory hyperplasia of the nasal mucosa is possible. Secondary hyperostosis may develop, especially in the frontal sinus region. Other fungal organisms that may cause mycotic rhinitis in animals exposed to an endemic region are *Penicillium* or *Blastomyces* species. *Cryptococcus neoformans* causes a non-destructive rhinitis which is most commonly seen in cats.

Radiographic findings Aspergillosis typically causes an 'empty nose' appearance. The destructive activity of the organisms causes lysis of the fine nasal turbinates and thus increased lucency in the affected nasal cavity. As there is usually no accumulation of nasal secretions, increased soft-tissue opacity in the abnormal region is absent (Fig. 6.31). The nasal septum is typically intact. Hyperostosis of the frontal bone is common and can be visualized with an appropriate radiographic projection (Fig. 6.32).

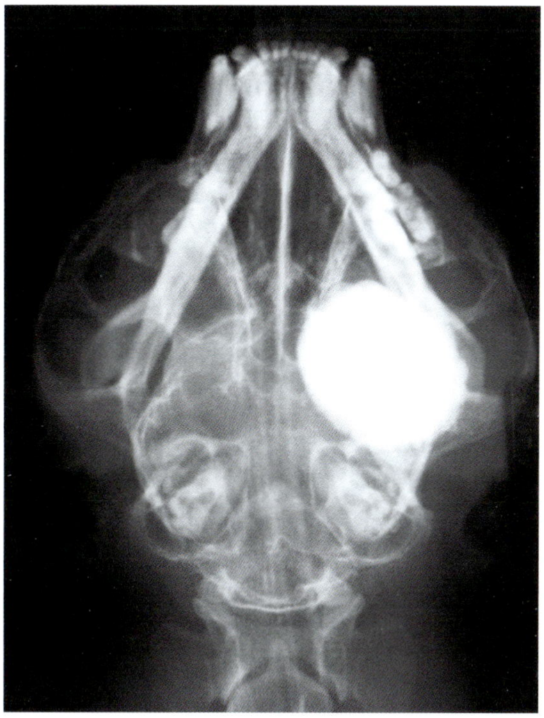

Fig. 6.30 Osteoma associated with the left mandible in a 14-year-old Maine Coon cat. This is a slow growing tumour characterized by smooth and well-defined margins. (From: Schwarz et al. 2002 [Figure 20]; with permission.)

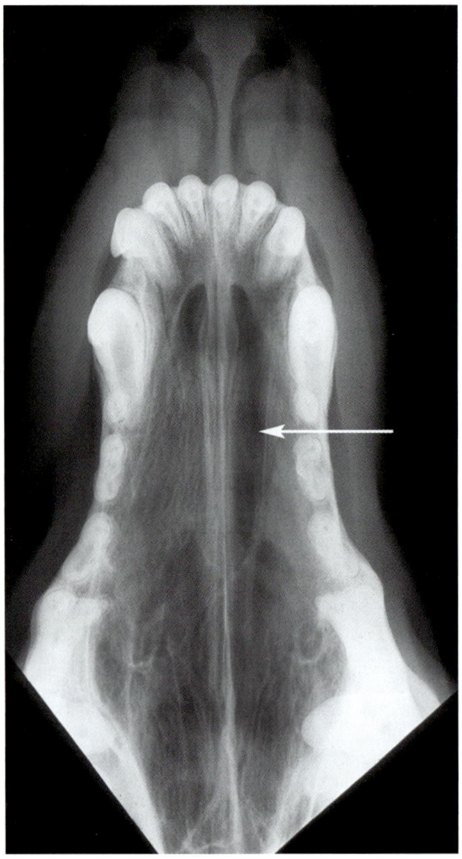

Fig. 6.31 Dorsoventral intraoral radiograph of the nasal cavity in a 4-year-old Labrador with aspergillosis. There is decreased opacity of the left nasal cavity in particular due to loss of the nasal turbinates (arrow). Changes may be bilateral and are most commonly rostral. This picture of an 'empty nose' is typical for a destructive mycotic rhinitis caused by Aspergillus species.

Other types of rhinitis and nasal foreign bodies

Dogs and cats can be affected by **bacterial rhinitis** or by steroid-responsive **lymphocytic–plasmacytic rhinitis**. Both are typically associated with an increased production of nasal secretions which may accumulate in the nasal cavity and frontal sinuses. Depending on the duration and severity of the disease, a variable degree of destruction of fine nasal structures is possible.

Nasal foreign bodies are most commonly found in dogs. These are often radiolucent plant particles such as grass awns which get stuck between the nasal turbinates and incite an acute rhinitis.

RADIOGRAPHIC FINDINGS These types of rhinitis typically result in increased soft-tissue opacity of the nasal cavity and possibly frontal sinuses bilaterally. Depending on the severity and duration of the disease, destruction of the small nasal turbinates is possible. In these cases, differentiation from nasal tumours is difficult and requires advanced imaging (CT, MRI) and biopsy. A radiographic diagnosis of radiolucent plant foreign bodies is only possible if regional rhinitis and mucopurulent nasal discharge cause a focal region of increased soft-tissue opacity within the nasal cavity. On the other hand, identification of radiopaque foreign bodies is straightforward.

Otitis

While a radiographic diagnosis of **otitis externa and media** is possible, otitis interna requires cross-sectional imaging and clinical diagnostics. Otitis externa is associated with increased production of cerumen and inflammatory secretions which accumulate within the normally air-filled external ear canal. Chronic otitis externa, which is predominantly seen in Spaniel dogs and other floppy-eared dog breeds, leads to calcification of the epidermis of the external ear canal. Otitis media is a common sequela of chronic otitis externa and manifests as an accumulation of inflammatory secretions in the normally air-filled tympanic bulla. Depending on chronicity, changes of the osseous bulla wall are also possible.

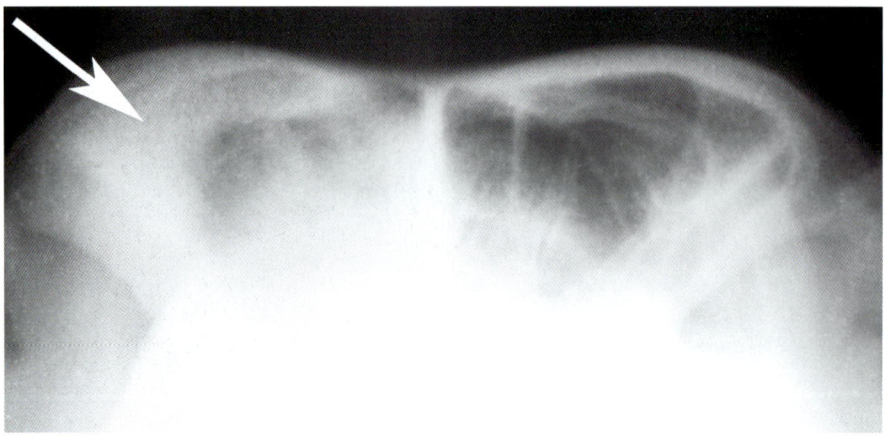

Fig. 6.32 Rostrocaudal projection of the frontal sinuses in a 4-year-old Labrador with hyperostosis of the frontal bone secondary to aspergillosis. The bony margin of the right frontal sinus is thickened (arrow); the left frontal sinus appears normal.

RADIOGRAPHIC FINDINGS Otitis externa is characterized by increased soft-tissue opacity within the normally air-filled external ear canal, and in chronic cases by mineralization of the wall of the external ear canal (Fig. 6.33). Otitis media can be recognized by increased soft-tissue opacity within the tympanic bulla and changes of the osseous bulla wall. Lysis is rather rare; sclerosis/hyperostosis as well as periosteal reaction are more commonly observed. With unilateral disease, comparison with the normal side can be helpful (Fig. 6.34). Differential diagnoses for otitis include a physiological increase in/sclerosis of the temporal bone in older animals (usually bilateral), new bone formation secondary to craniomandibular osteopathy (usually bilateral, see section 6.3.8), and neoplasia (malignant or polyps).

Osteomyelitis

Osteomyelitis can occur secondary to systemic or local infection. Possible causes for osteomyelitis of the head include bite wounds or penetrating foreign bodies with secondary soft-tissue abscessation, infections of the frontal sinuses or nasal cavity, and prior surgical procedures. Biopsy of abnormal tissues may be warranted in some cases to rule out the possibility that the soft-tissue abnormality in fact represents infection and not ulcerated or abscessed tumour tissue.

RADIOGRAPHIC FINDINGS Inflammation of the skull appears similar to osteomyelitis in other areas of the body with irregular lytic changes, often bordered by regions of increased opacity (sclerosis) and periosteal proliferation in the proximity of abnormal soft-tissue swelling (see section 17.2). Bone sequestration is possible (Fig. 6.35).

6.3.5 Trauma

Fractures

Skull fractures represent a diagnostic challenge due to the complex anatomic structure of the head. Additional tangential radiographs are often necessary to delineate

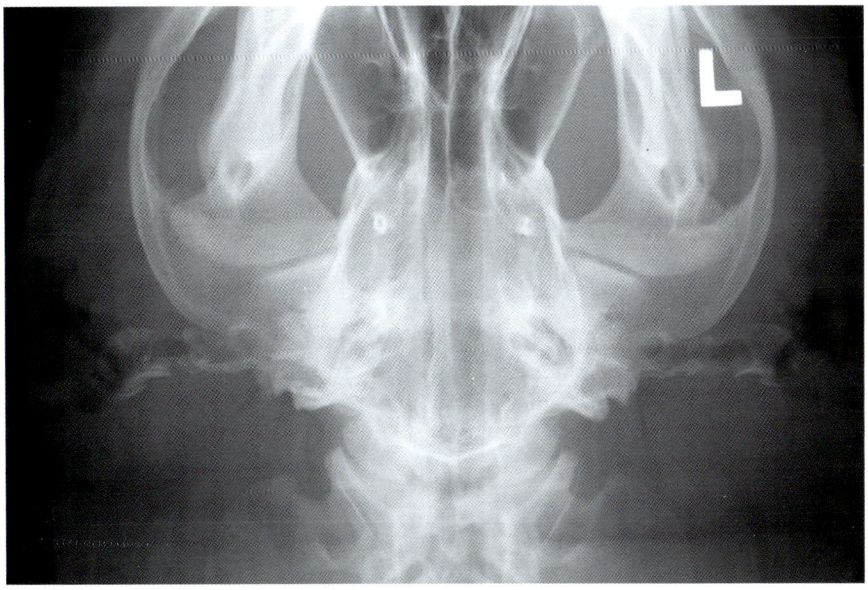

Fig. 6.33 Otitis externa in a 10-year-old Mastiff. There is bilateral mineralization of the wall of the external ear canal with luminal narrowing. Note the normal temporomandibular joints on this ventrodorsal radiograph (L = left).

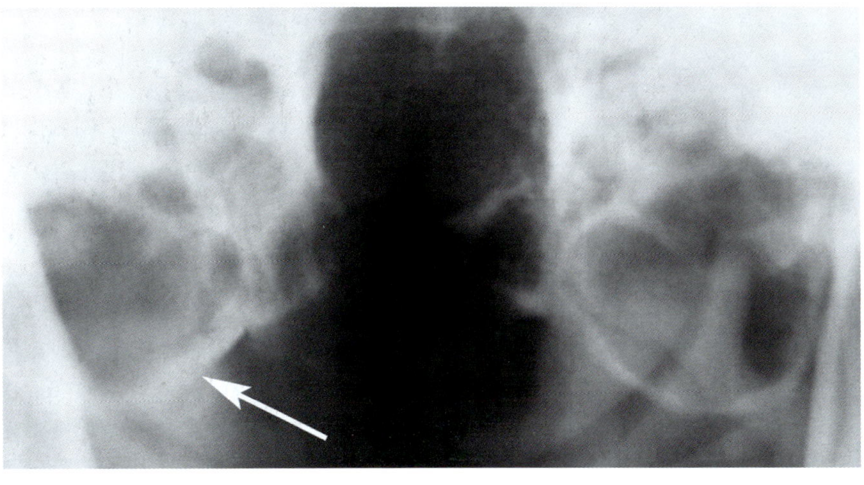

Fig. 6.34 Rostrocaudal open-mouth radiograph in a 5-year-old Irish Setter with right-sided chronic otitis media. The osseous wall of the right tympanic bulla is thickened (arrow), and the lumen is of soft-tissue opacity secondary to accumulation of inflammatory secretions. The left tympanic bulla is normal.

fracture lines. Fractures of the cranium commonly involve multiple bones and may be caused by bite wounds or blunt trauma (falls, hits). Brain trauma without concurrent skull fractures is possible.

> Open fontanelles in some toy-breed dogs (Chihuahua, Yorkshire Terrier, etc.) and fine vascular channels should not be mistaken for fracture lines.

RADIOGRAPHIC FINDINGS Irregular linear defects with minimal displacement of fracture fragments are the most common findings in skull fractures. An interruption in the otherwise smooth curvature of the cranium or identification of bone fragments confirms the diagnosis. Deep dislocation of impression fragments may raise the concern for brain trauma. Fractures involving the nasal cavity or frontal sinus are often associated with subcutaneous emphysema.

With jaw fractures it is important to assess the exact location of the fracture lines, dislocation of fragments and involvement of dental structures. In general, distinction between traumatic and pathological fractures is essential for further treatment planning. Traumatic fractures are characterized by sharp fracture margins (Fig. 6.36), whereas pathological fractures occur secondary to underlying bone weakening (e.g. by tumours or osteoporosis). The diastema is the weakest point of the mandible and predisposed to fractures. Care must be taken to thoroughly evaluate for possible concurrent tooth fractures and (sub) luxations.

Temporomandibular joint (sub)luxation

(Sub)luxation of the temporomandibular joint in dogs and cats typically occurs secondary to external trauma such as motor vehicle accidents or falls from a high elevation (cats). Concurrent fractures of the retro-articular process of the temporal bone, the zygomatic arch and the articular process

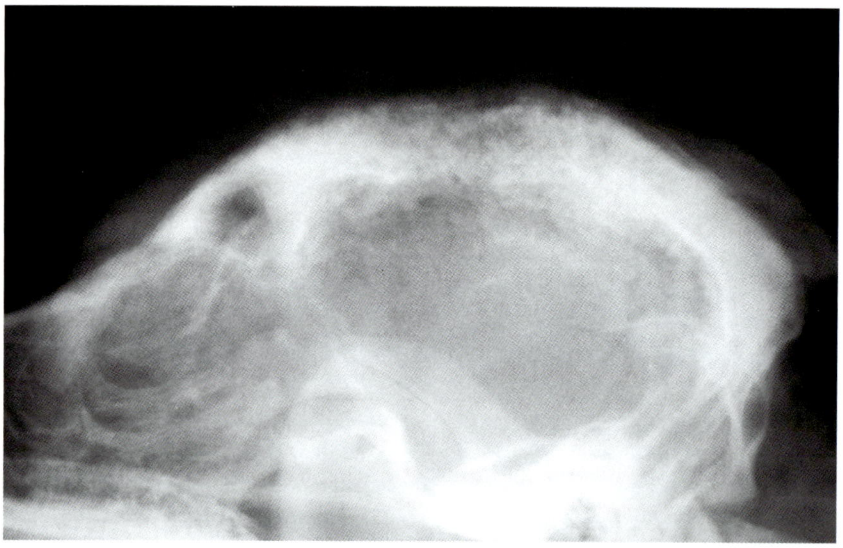

Fig. 6.35 Osteomyelitis secondary to abscess formation following a bite wound in a 3-year-old Labrador. Extensive lytic changes of the calvarium as well as irregular periosteal reaction are noted.

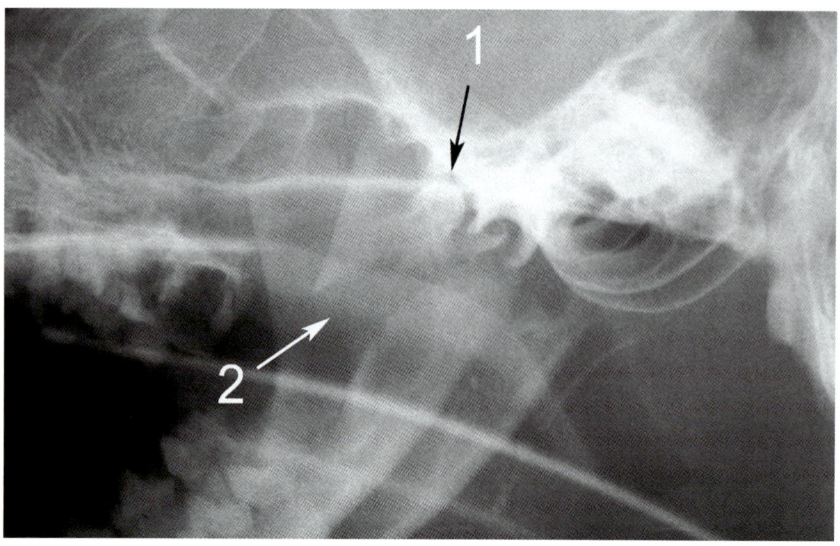

Fig. 6.36 Rostrodorsal luxation of the articular process of the mandible (1) with a horizontal fracture of the coronoid process (2) in an 8-year-old cat following a fall from a window.

of the mandible are common and usually unilateral. A (sub) luxation without concurrent fractures is also possible due to the relatively high lateral mobility of the temporomandibular joints and limited individual motion of both mandibular rami permitted by the symphysis, or if a congenital joint dysplasia causes a pre-existing instability. On clinical examination, affected patients are unable to close the mouth and show increased production of saliva or malocclusion due to lateral displacement of the mandible.

RADIOGRAPHIC FINDINGS The luxation usually occurs in a rostrodorsal direction as the retro-articular process of the temporal bone prevents a ventrocaudal displacement (Fig. 6.36). The coronoid process of the mandibular ramus can concurrently become entrapped by the zygomatic arch, interfering with normal occlusion. To document subtle asymmetry, it can be helpful to compare the position of the coronoid process in relation to the zygomatic arch between the left and right sides.

6.3.6 Diseases of the salivary glands and the nasolacrimal duct

Sialolithiasis

Accumulation of mineral within the salivary glands or salivary ducts is rare in dogs and cats and typically an incidental finding. Mineralization of material within the salivary ducts may possibly occur secondary to chronic sialadenitis.

RADIOGRAPHIC FINDINGS Small, round or linear mineral opaque sialoliths larger than 3 mm may be visible within the region of the salivary gland or salivary ducts.

Sialocele

Sialoceles are defined as accumulations of saliva within the ducts of the salivary glands due to interference with normal drainage. They may occur secondary to trauma during mastication or bite wounds to the neck region. The sublingual salivary gland is most commonly affected; a sialocele of this gland is termed a **ranula**.

RADIOGRAPHIC FINDINGS Depending on the location and size of the lesion, soft-tissue swelling of the affected region may be visible. The salivary ducts can be visualized by means of retrograde injection of positive contrast medium (**sialography**), which allows a diagnosis of ruptures and obstructive lesions. The reader is referred to other resources for a description of this technique.

Salivary duct fistulas

Fistulas of the salivary ducts are usually caused by bite wounds. The parotid salivary gland is most commonly affected.

RADIOGRAPHIC FINDINGS Survey radiographs are unrewarding or non-specific and may show soft-tissue swelling. Retrograde sialography can demonstrate patency or rupture of the duct. Injection of positive contrast medium into the fistulous tract (**fistulography**) may demonstrate the connection to the salivary gland.

Diseases of the nasolacrimal duct

The most common presenting complaint in patients with diseases of the nasolacrimal duct is epiphora. Differential diagnoses include cysts of the orbital adnexa (lacrimal gland or duct, gland of the third eyelid), cysts of the maxilla or nasal cavity, congenital or acquired stenosis or dilatation of the duct, dacryocystitis, or mass lesions blocking the nasolacrimal duct.

RADIOGRAPHIC FINDINGS Survey radiographs are often normal. Possible findings depend on the underlying cause and may include bony destruction, cystic structures, or increased soft-tissue opacity in the region of the expected location of the nasolacrimal duct. Injection of positive contrast medium into the nasolacrimal duct (**dacryocystorhinography**) allows evaluation of the patency of the duct and a diagnosis of obstruction, dislocation, dilatation or rupture. This contrast procedure is rarely performed, and the reader is referred to further literature for additional information.

6.3.7 Dental diseases

Dental tartar

Radiographically visible dental tartar is caused by mineralization of plaques and is commonly associated with periodontal disease. The rough dental surface is usually seen buccally at the level of the gum line. The fourth maxillary premolar and the first mandibular molar, which have nearby terminations of salivary ducts, are commonly affected.

Caries

Caries is rare in dogs and cats. Enamel erosion may expose the pulp cavity, which results in additional endodontal disease.

RADIOGRAPHIC FINDINGS Radiolucent defects of variable size are noted, associated with the dental enamel. A periapical radiolucent halo indicates a secondary pulpitis.

Tooth resorption (feline osteoclastic resorptive lesions; FORL)

This disease is common in cats and rare in dogs. Tooth resorption initially occurs at the level of the gum line and progresses to the root and/or crown. The aetiology is not completely understood. It is theorized that this disease is the result of increased osteoclastic activity, leading to the name 'feline osteoclastic resorptive lesions'.

RADIOGRAPHIC FINDINGS Depending on the stage of the disease, the tooth root and/or crown are resorbed to a variable degree (Fig. 6.37). Secondary periodontal disease with loss of the alveolar septum or alveolar crest between the tooth roots of the premolar and molar teeth, and pathological dental fractures are possible.

Periodontal disease

Periodontal disease affects the supporting tissues of the tooth and is associated with clinically evident local gingivitis. Bacterial pathogens are usually involved. Chronic renal diseases and associated uremic gingivitis may also lead to periodontal disease. A radiographic evaluation complements the clinical dental examination.

RADIOGRAPHIC FINDINGS In advanced stages, osteolysis becomes visible. The alveolar bone adjacent to the affected tooth undergoes resorption; changes affect the alveolar septum and the alveolar crest between the tooth roots of premolar and molar teeth. Additional possible findings include widening of the periodontal membrane, loss of the lamina dura (starting at the corona), cavitation, resorption or loss of teeth, and pathological dental fractures (Fig. 6.38).

Horizontal symmetric regression of the alveolar crest alone is usually associated with physiological ageing and should not be confused with periodontal disease.

Apical diseases and tooth root abscesses

Infections of the pulp cavity usually communicate with the apical periodontal tissue and result in regional osteomyelitis. Infections limited to the apical region are thus categorized under endodontal diseases. Older dogs are most commonly affected. Infection of the fourth maxillary premolar tooth may result in a fistula which typically opens ventral to the eye. Radiographic examination is necessary in these cases, as the endodontal part of the tooth cannot be evaluated clinically with an intact crown.

RADIOGRAPHIC FINDINGS Focal osteomyelitis with resorption of the periapical alveolar bone results in a radiolucent halo surrounding the tooth root (Fig. 6.39). Additional radiographic abnormalities near the tooth root may include widening of the radiolucent periodontal membrane, sclerosis of the alveolar bone, loss of the lamina dura or tooth root resorption. A possible differential diagnosis is a periapical cyst, which appears as a radiolucent region with a radiopaque sclerotic rim.

Tooth fractures

Tooth fractures commonly result from external trauma or chewing on hard structures. Opening of the pulp cavity carries a risk of secondary endodontitis.

RADIOGRAPHIC FINDINGS A diagnosis of small and non-displaced fractures may be difficult. Obviously luxated fractures, or fine linear fractures and fissures of the affected tooth may be visible above or below the gingiva. Depending on the angle of the incident X-ray beam, the fracture may appear as a single or multiple radiolucent

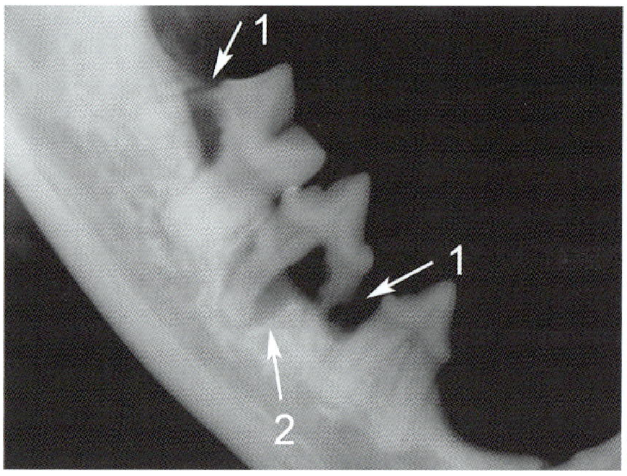

Fig. 6.37 Feline osteoclastic resorptive lesions (FORL) of the mandible in a 6-year-old Abyssinian cat. There is obvious resorption of the roots and necks of several teeth (1). Additionally, periodontal lucencies are noted (2). (Courtesy of Jason W. Soukup, UW Madison, USA)

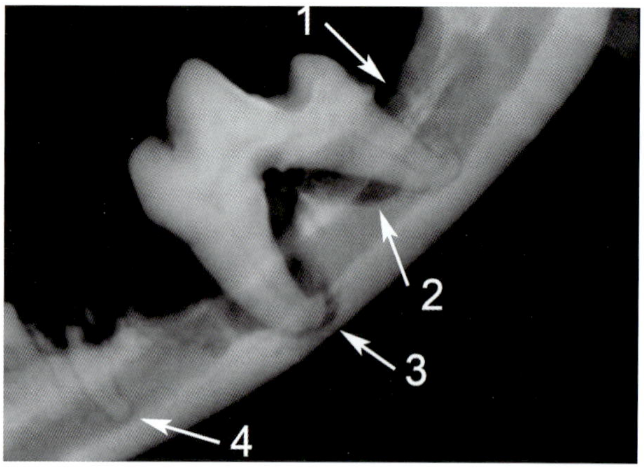

Fig. 6.38 Advanced periodontitis of the mandible in a 9-year-old Miniature Schnauzer. There is extensive horizontal (1) and vertical (2) lysis of the periodontal and alveolar bone; the periapical region (3) is also affected. In addition, a tooth fracture with complete luxation and persistent tooth root remnant is noted (4). (Courtesy of Jason W. Soukup, UW Madison, USA)

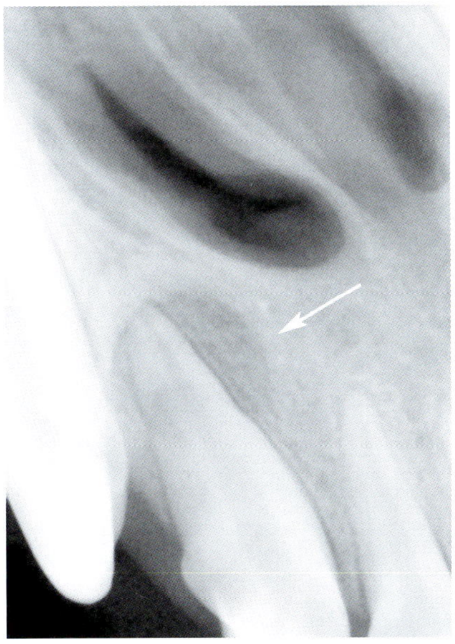

Fig. 6.39 Tooth root abscess of the third upper incisor in a 4-year-old Collie. The tip of the tooth root is surrounded by a radiolucent halo (arrow). (Courtesy of Jason W. Soukup, UW Madison, USA)

fracture lines, and multiple projections with changes in the incident beam angle may be needed for full evaluation. Other possible findings include retained tooth root fragments.

6.3.8 Other diseases

Craniomandibular osteopathy (CMO)

CMO is a proliferative bone disease of young terrier dogs (West Highland White, Scottish, Cairn, Boston and other terrier breeds) but may on occasion be seen in other breeds (Labrador Retriever, Doberman). An autosomal recessive trait has been shown in West Highland White Terriers. Affected animals present at 3–8 months of age with swelling of the mandible. Clinically, patients may exhibit difficulty eating, pain when opening the mouth and chewing, and fever. The disease is self-limiting, the aetiology is thus far unknown. If similar changes are found in dogs of other breeds or age groups, a bone biopsy is indicated to rule out bone tumours or osteomyelitis. In addition to the mandible, the tympanic bulla, petrous temporal bone and calvarium are most commonly affected.

RADIOGRAPHIC FINDINGS Increased radiopacity and periosteal proliferation is noted, which is usually bilateral and mildly irregular to palisading (Fig. 6.40). In some cases, the metaphyses of the long bones of the extremities may show changes similar to those seen with hypertrophic osteodystrophy. The disease period may last months. In the healing phase of disease, the newly formed bone is remodelled, and a thickened cortex remains visible.

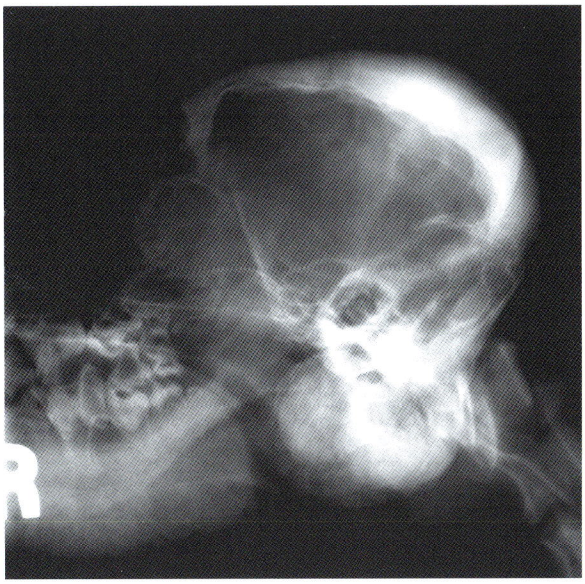

Fig. 6.40 Craniomandibular osteopathy (CMO) in a 7-month-old Cairn Terrier. Radiographic abnormalities include palisading new bone formation associated with the ventral margin of the mandible and the tympanic bullae as well as thickening of the calvarium (R = right).

References and further reading

Assheuer J, Sager M. MRI and CT Atlas of the Dog. Berlin: Blackwell 1997.

Forrest L. The cranial and nasal cavities – canine and feline. In: Thrall DE (ed.). Textbook of Veterinary Diagnostic Radiology, 6th edn. Philadelphia: WB Saunders 2012.

Gelatt KN, Cure TH, Guffy MM, Jessen C. Dacryocystorhinography in the dog and cat. J Small Anim Pract 1972; 13: 381–97.

Hecht S. Für Studium und Praxis: Die Röntgenuntersuchung des Kopfes. Tierärztl Prax 2003; 31: 194–8.

Morgan J, Doval J, Samii V. Head, mandible, nasal passages, paranasal sinuses, and maxillary region, dental studies. In: Radiographic Techniques. The Dog. Hannover: Schlütersche 1998; 53–94.

Mulligan TW, Aller MS, Williams CA. Atlas of Canine and Feline Dental Radiography. Trenton: Veterinary Learning Systems 1998.

Owens JM, Biery DN. Skull. In: Cann CC (ed.). Radiographic Interpretation for the Small Animal Clinician. Baltimore: Williams & Wilkins 1999; 105–25.

Schwarz T, Saunders J. Veterinary Computed Tomography. Ames: Wiley-Blackwell 2011.

Schwarz T, Weller R, Dickie AM, Konar M, Sullivan M. Imaging of the canine and feline temporomandibular joint: a review. Vet Radiol Ultrasound 2002; 43: 85–97.

Wallack ST. The Handbook of Veterinary Contrast Radiography. Solana Beach, CA: San Diego Veterinary Imaging Inc 2003.

Wisner E, Zwingenberger A. Atlas of Small Animal CT and MRI. Ames: Wiley-Blackwell 2015.

7

Spine (neuroradiology including contrast procedures)

Silke Hecht and Federica Morandi

Survey radiographs of the spine and myelography still play an important role in veterinary medicine despite increasing availability and improved diagnostic capabilities of advanced imaging technologies (computed tomography and magnetic resonance imaging). Survey radiographs are helpful in the evaluation of bony structures, while myelography allows evaluation of changes within the vertebral canal.

7.1 Anatomy and indications

7.1.1 Anatomy

Introduction

The spine in dogs and cats consists of seven cervical vertebrae (vertebrae cervicales, C), 13 thoracic vertebrae (vertebrae thoracicae, T), seven lumbar vertebrae (vertebrae lumbales, L), three sacral vertebrae (vertebrae sacrales, S) and a variable number of caudal vertebra (vertebrae caudales, Cd).

Each **vertebra** consists of a ventral body and a dorsal arch, which can be subdivided into lateral pedicles and a dorsal lamina. The vertebral body (ventral) and the vertebral arch (lateral and dorsal) border the vertebral canal, which contains the spinal cord.

Bony protuberances on the vertebrae (vertebral processes) develop differently in different regions of the spine. Generally, the following types are found:

- spinous process
- transverse process
- articular process
- mammillary process
- accessory process.

The dorsal gaps between adjacent vertebral arches (interarcuate spaces) are narrow. Lateral notches associated with the pedicles form intervertebral foramina which allow passage of the spinal nerves. With the exception of the first and second cervical vertebrae and the fused sacral vertebrae, vertebral bodies are separated by intervertebral disc spaces and the **intervertebral discs**. Dorsolaterally, adjacent vertebrae articulate via their articular processes. Intervertebral discs consist of a central nucleus pulposus and surrounding annulus fibrosus. A schematic anatomic drawing of a vertebra is found in Figure 7.1.

The spine is stabilized by multiple long and short ligamentous structures (Fig. 7.2). For a detailed description of the anatomy and function of the different spinal ligaments the reader is referred to anatomy textbooks. **Ligaments** important from the standpoint of pathophysiology and imaging will be briefly covered in this chapter. The dorsal longitudinal ligament is located within the vertebral canal dorsal to the vertebral bodies and, among other functions, helps confine the intervertebral discs to the intervertebral disc spaces. In the cranial thoracic spine (T2–T9 in cats, T2–T10 in dogs), this long ligament is supported by several short ligaments traversing the vertebral canal and connecting the heads of opposite ribs (intercapital ligaments). Dorsally, the vertebral arches are connected by the ligamentum flavum. Several short ligaments support the mobile atlantoaxial joint (see 'Cervical spine', below).

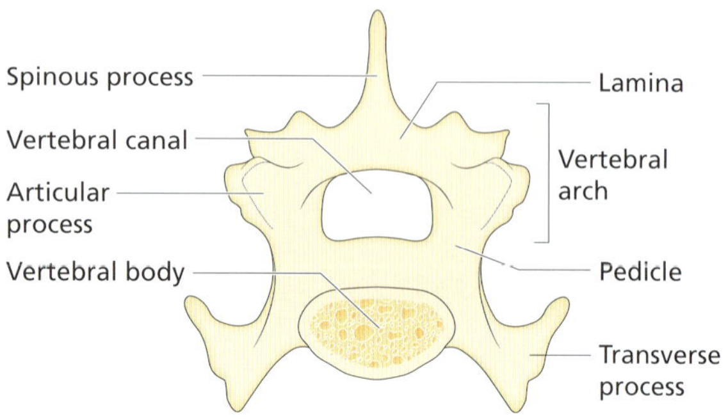

Fig. 7.1 Schematic drawing of a vertebra.

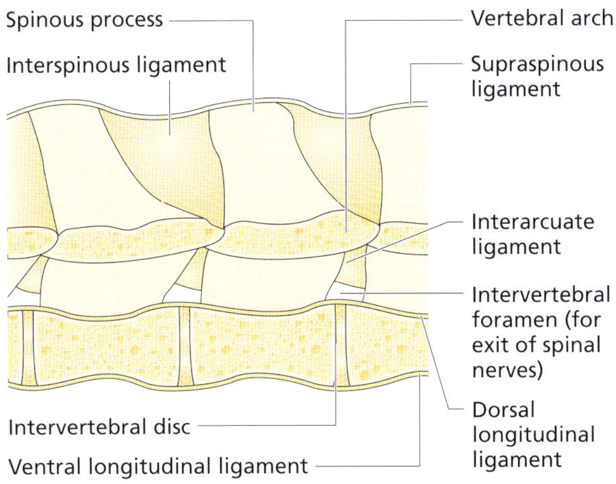

Fig. 7.2 Schematic drawing of some important anatomic structures of the vertebral column.

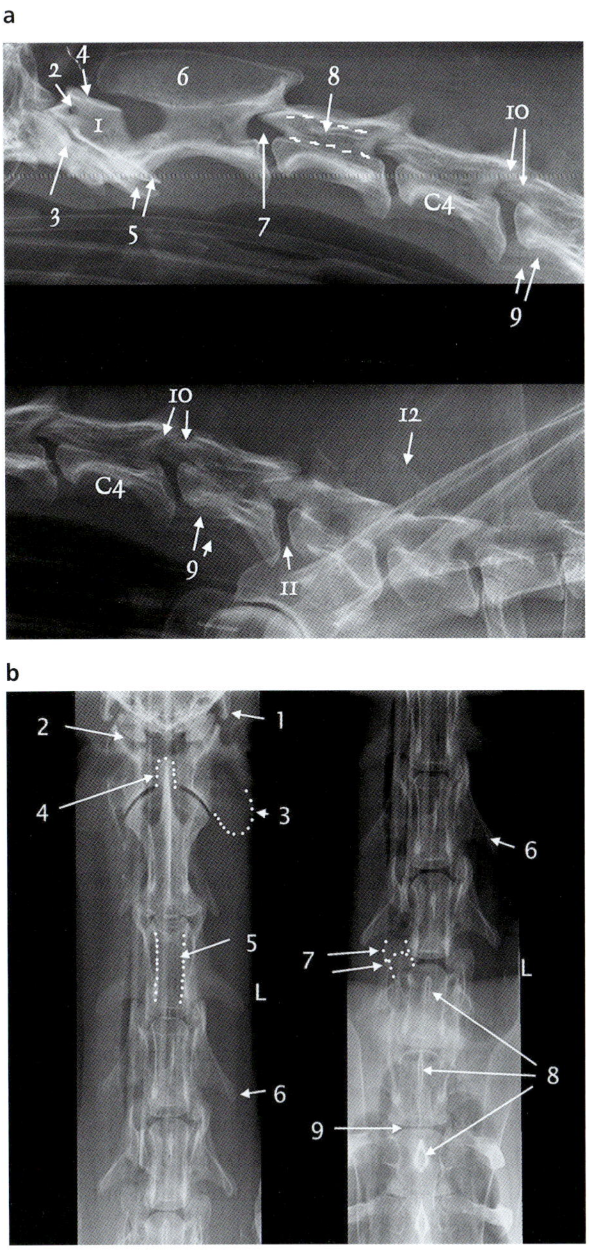

Cervical spine

The cervical spine is characterized by some noteworthy anatomic modifications (Fig. 7.3). Transverse foramina associated with the base of the first through sixth cervical vertebrae form the transverse canal that parallels the vertebral canal and contains nerves and vessels.

The first cervical vertebra (**atlas**) is ring-shaped, with a thin ventral body and wide transverse processes (wings; alae atlantis). The cranial part of the wing of the atlas is perforated by the lateral vertebral foramen, which allows passage of the first cervical spinal nerve. Dogs and cats are lacking an alar foramen present in other species, but instead have a focal notch in the cranial margin of the wings of the atlas (incisura atlantis). A distinct spinous process and typical articular processes are absent. The atlas articulates with the occipital condyles cranially (fovea articularis cranialis), and with the dens of the second cervical vertebra caudally (fovea dentis).

The second cervical vertebra (**axis**) is the longest cervical vertebra. It is characterized by a very large spinous process that extends both cranially and caudally beyond the length of the vertebral body. This spinous process articulates caudally with the third cervical vertebra by means of paired caudal articular processes. Cranially, the axis articulates with the atlas by means of a median long bony protrusion (dens). The atlas and axis are connected by strong ligamentous structures (apical ligament of the dens and paired alar ligaments). Additionally, the dens is held in place by a transverse ligament. The transverse pro-

Fig. 7.3 Radiographs of the cervical spine in a dog.
a Lateral view: 1 Vertebral canal at the level of the atlas, 2 Lateral vertebral foramen of the atlas, 3 Occipital condyles and atlanto-occipital joint, 4 Dorsal arch of the atlas, 5 Wings of the atlas (both sides superimposed), 6 Spinous process of the axis, 7 C2–3 intervertebral foramen, 8 Vertebral canal at the level of C3 (ventral margin formed by vertebral body, dorsal margin formed by vertebral arch), 9 Transverse processes of the fifth cervical vertebra, 10 Articular facet joints formed by articular processes of C4 and C5, 11 C5–C6 intervertebral disc space, 12 Spinous process of the seventh cervical vertebra (C4 = fourth cervical vertebra).
b Ventrodorsal view: 1 Left paracondylar process of the occiput, 2 Right atlanto-occipital joint, 3 Left transverse process (wing) of the atlas, 4 Dens of the axis (superimposed with the cranial edge of the spinous process of the axis), 5 Vertebral canal at the level of C3, 6 Left transverse process of C4, 7 Right C5–6 articular facet joint, formed by articular processes, 8 Spinous processes, 9 C7–T1 intervertebral disc space (L = left).

cesses of the axis are relatively thin and extend caudally beyond its caudal margin.

While the vertebral bodies of the third through seventh cervical vertebrae decrease in length from cranial to caudal, their spinous processes increase in length and have increased angulation. The intervertebral disc spaces between most cervical vertebrae are relatively even in width, with the exception of the intervertebral disc spaces C2–3 and C7–T1, which are physiologically narrowed.

The transverse processes of the sixth cervical vertebra are developed as wide laminae which extend ventrally beyond the margin of the vertebral body (Fig. 7.4). The seventh cervical vertebra has small articular surfaces associated with its caudal body (foveae capitis), which articulate with the first pair of ribs.

Thoracic spine

The thoracic vertebrae (Fig. 7.5) are relatively short and plump and increase in length from the level of T10 caudally. They articulate with each other by means of their dorsal articular processes. Joint surfaces located cranial and caudal on the vertebral bodies (foveae capitis cranialis and caudalis) allow articulation with the rib heads. Additionally, the tubercles of the ribs communicate with the short transverse processes of the thoracic vertebrae. T13 only articulates with the last pair of ribs and thus only has one paired cranial joint surface. The thoracic vertebrae are characterized by tall and narrow spinous processes which decrease in height from cranial to caudal and have increasing caudal angulation from T1 to T10. At the level of T11 (**anticlinical vertebra**), spinous process angulation changes to cranial. The T10–11 intervertebral disc space is narrowed compared to adjacent intervertebral disc spaces, and the shape of the articular process joint differs from the cranial thoracic spine (Fig. 7.6). Mammillary and accessory processes present on the caudal thoracic vertebrae do not have radiographic importance.

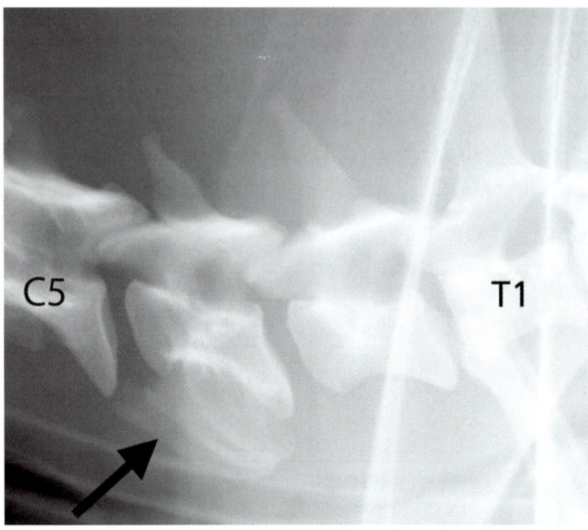

Fig. 7.4 Collimated view of a lateral radiograph of the caudal cervical spine in a dog. The sixth cervical vertebra is characterized by modified transverse processes which form plate-like laminae that extend ventrally beyond the vertebral body (arrow). Note also that the seventh cervical vertebra is relatively short, and that the C7–T1 intervertebral disc space is narrowed compared to adjacent intervertebral disc spaces (C5 = fifth cervical vertebra, T1 = first thoracic vertebra).

> The intervertebral disc spaces C2–3, C7–T1 and T10–11 are physiologically narrowed compared to adjacent intervertebral disc spaces. This can lead to an erroneous diagnosis of intervertebral disc disease.

Lumbar spine

The lumbar vertebrae (Fig. 7.5) slightly increase in length from L1 through L6, but L7 is markedly shorter than the remaining lumbar vertebrae. The intervertebral foramina of the lumbar spine have a characteristic 'horse head' appearance. The lumbar spinous processes are angled cranially. The transverse processes are also oriented cranially and extend beyond the level of the intervertebral disc spaces to approximately the level of the mid body of the cranially located vertebrae. The articular processes and articular facet joints are visible dorsal to the intervertebral foramina. Mammillary processes associated with the cranial articular processes are not of radiographic importance. On the other hand, accessory processes associated with the cranial lumbar vertebrae are visible on lateral radiographs. They extend from the vertebral arches caudally to superimpose with the intervertebral foramina and should not be confused with pathological abnormalities such as mineralized intervertebral disc material within the vertebral canal (Fig. 7.7). Most lumbar vertebrae have smooth ventral margins. However, especially in large dogs, the ventral margins of the third and fourth lumbar vertebrae may be irregularly marginated (Fig. 7.8). This is a physiological change caused by attachment of the diaphragmatic crura on these vertebral bodies.

Sacrum

Three sacral vertebrae are fused to form the short and wide sacrum (Fig. 7.5). Two wide sacral wings provide the articulation between the spine and the pelvis. The spinous processes are fused to form a single ridge which is easily recognized on radiographs.

Caudal spine

A variable number of caudal vertebrae may be present (Fig. 7.5). These are short, square and only carry rudimentary vertebral processes. The cranial to middle caudal vertebrae occasionally have ventrally located haemal arches and processes which should not be mistaken for spondylosis deformans.

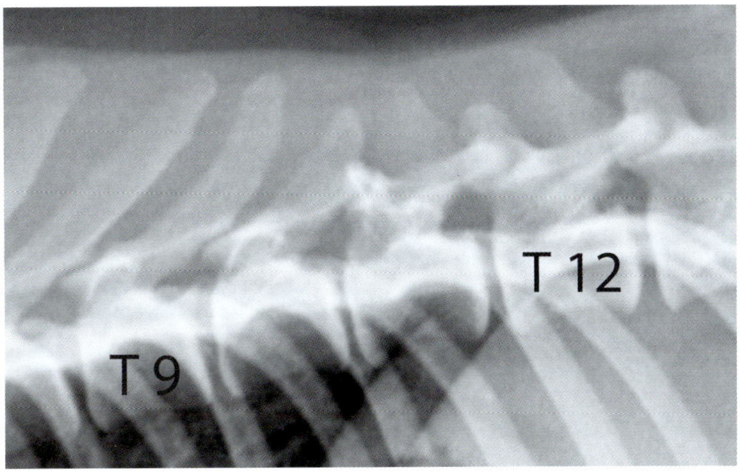

Fig. 7.6 Lateral radiograph of the caudal thoracic spine in a dog. Note change in orientation of the spinous processes, narrowing of the intervertebral disc space and change in shape of the articular processes at the level of T10–11 (anticlinal vertebra).

a

b

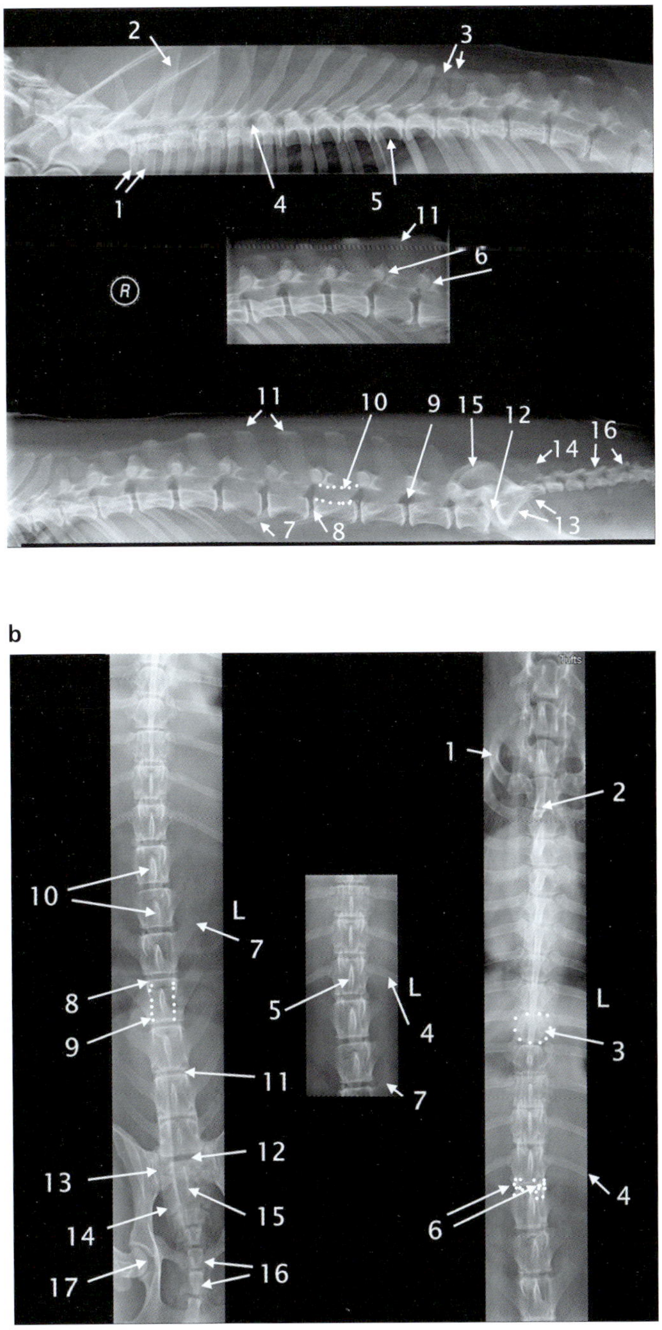

Fig. 7.5 Radiographs of the thoracic, lumbar and sacral as well as part of the caudal spine in a dog

a Lateral view: 1 First pair of ribs, 2 Spinous process of the first thoracic vertebra (T1), 3 Spinous processes T10–11 (anticlinal vertebra, note change in orientation of spinous processes), 4 Intervertebral foramen T4–5, 5 Body of the ninth thoracic vertebra (T9), 6 Articular facet joints L1–2 and L2–3 formed by articular processes, 7 Transverse processes of the third lumbar vertebra (L3), 8 Cranial endplate of L4, 9 Intervertebral foramen L5–6, 10 Vertebral canal at the level of L4 (ventral margin formed by vertebral body, dorsal margin by vertebral arch), 11 Spinous processes of the lumbar vertebrae, 12 L7-S1 intervertebral disc space, 13 Ventral margin of the sacrum, 14 Spinous process of the third sacral vertebra, 15 Iliac crest, 16 Caudal vertebrae (R = right).

b Ventrodorsal view: 1 First right rib, 2 Spinous process of the first thoracic vertebra (T1), 3 Body of the ninth thoracic vertebra, 4 Last (13th) left rib, 5 Spinous process of T13, 6 Articular facet joints T13–L1, formed by articular processes, 7 Left transverse process of the third lumbar vertebra (L3), 8 Cranial endplate of L4, 9 Vertebral canal at the level of L4, 10 Spinous processes of the first and second lumbar vertebrae, 11 L5–6 intervertebral disc space, 12 L7–S1 intervertebral disc space, 13 Right sacral wing articulating with the ilium at the sacroiliac joint, 14 Os penis (projected over vertebral column), 15 Spinous processes of the sacral vertebrae, 16 Caudal vertebrae, 17 Right coxofemoral joint (L = left).

Spinal cord and meninges

The **spinal cord** and its surrounding **meninges** are located within the protective vertebral canal formed by successive vertebral foramina. Important considerations for neurological diagnostics are that eight cervical spinal cord segments are being distributed over only seven vertebrae, and that there is a discrepancy between the location of spinal cord segments and vertebrae in the caudal spine due to spinal cord ascent during fetal development. As a rule of thumb, and leaving aside breed and individual variations, the location of the thoracic and lumbar spinal cord segments T1 through L2 corresponds to the respective vertebral bodies, the lumbar spinal cord segments L3 through L7 are located approximately at the level of the third and fourth lumbar vertebrae, and the sacral spinal cord segments are located approximately at the level of the fifth lumbar vertebra. The terminal portion of the spinal cord (**conus medullaris**) theoretically corresponds to the caudal extent of the surrounding subarachnoid space. While the caudal extent of the subarachnoid space in large-breed dogs is indeed typically located at the level of L5, it may extend to the caudal lumbar vertebrae or even the sacrum in small dogs and cats.

Despite the spinal cord ascent, lumbar and sacral spinal nerves do not exit the vertebral canal until reaching the level of their respective 'normal' intervertebral foramina. They form a bunch of nerves in the caudal vertebral canal which is called the '**cauda equina**' due to its resemblance to a horse tail.

Spinal cord, meninges and subarachnoid space are not visible on survey radiographs. They will be covered later in the chapter under myelography (see section 7.2.3).

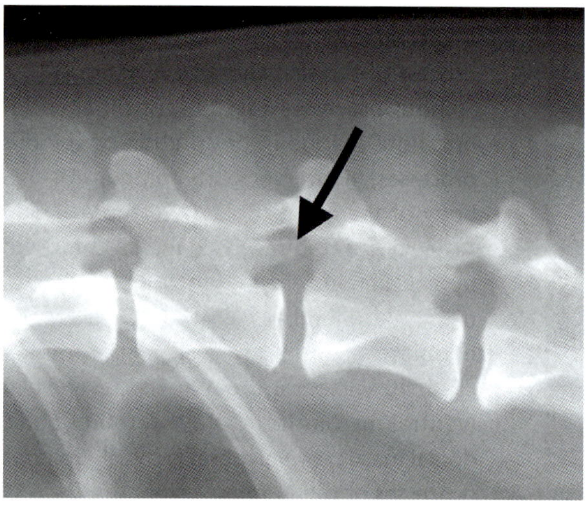

Fig. 7.7 Lateral radiograph of the lumbar spine. Bony protrusions superimposed with the intervertebral foramina (indicated by an arrow at L1–2) are consistent with normal accessory processes and should not be confused with spinal pathology, such as herniation of mineralized intervertebral disc material.

7.1.2 Indications

Indications for radiographic examination of the spine include neurological deficits and pain. Specific indications for a contrast examination of the spine (myelography) are covered in section 7.2.3.

7.2 Radiographic technique and positioning

7.2.1 Technique

A radiographic examination of the spine follows the same basic principles as the examination of other osseous structures: the radiographs should be high in contrast, i.e. a low kVp–high mA technique should be chosen. Exposure time should be as short as possible to minimize risk of motion artefacts. If the thickness of the area of interest exceeds 10 cm (which is the case in most animals), use of a grid is indicated.

In most instances, radiographs are obtained in at least two orthogonal projections (usually right lateral and ventrodorsal). On occasion, and especially with myelography, additional views (left lateral or dorsoventral) or special views (e.g. oblique views or stress views) may be indicated.

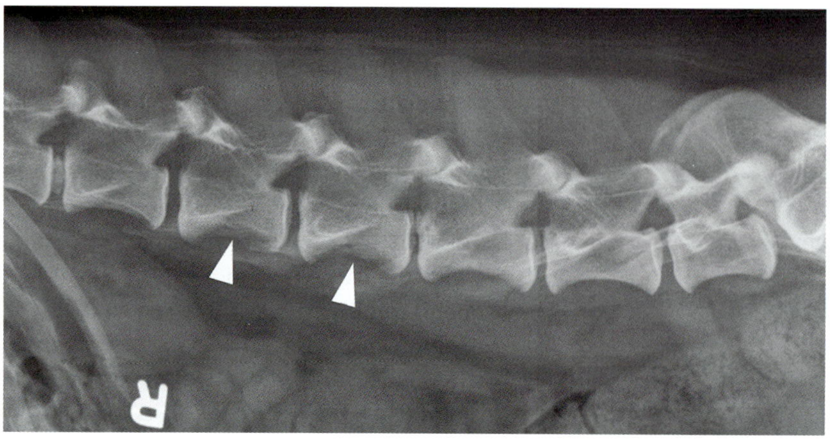

Fig. 7.8 Lateral radiograph of the lumbar spine. The ventral margin of the third and fourth lumbar vertebral bodies is irregularly marginated (arrowheads). This is a physiological change related to the insertion of the diaphragmatic crura on these vertebrae. Note in situ mineralization of the nucleus pulposus at L1–2 and mild degenerative changes of the L4–5 intervertebral disc space (R = right).

7.2.2 Positioning

Perfect positioning is mandatory to allow adequate radiographic evaluation of the spine. Even mild obliquity yields a radiograph that is nondiagnostic for assessment of vertebral anatomy and intervertebral disc space width. Whenever possible, and depending on patient condition and circumstances, spinal radiographs should thus be obtained under sedation or anaesthesia. On a straight lateral view, the vertebral transverse processes and rib heads should be superimposed. On a straight ventrodorsal view, the spinous processes should be superimposed with the mid-vertebral bodies and should appear as ovoid or teardrop-shaped structures.

Collimation to the area of interest is even more important for radiographic evaluation of the spine than for other areas of the body, especially if the radiographic examination is performed for evaluation of suspected intervertebral disc disease. X-rays diverge in the periphery of the radiographic field. This may result in the erroneous impression of intervertebral disc space narrowing or even collapse towards the periphery of the field of view, where X-rays meet the intervertebral disc spaces with an increasing angle compared to the intervertebral disc spaces in the centre of the field of view (Fig. 7.9).

Another consideration when planning a radiographic evaluation of the spine is that body thickness may vary in different areas of the spine even in the same patient. For instance, in large dogs the soft tissues of the caudal neck are often twice as thick as those of the cranial neck. When obtaining ventrodorsal views of the thoracic and lumbar spine the thorax is often markedly thicker than the abdomen. These variations in patient thickness require adjustment of exposure parameters to avoid over- or underexposure.

To account for the divergence of X-rays and variable patient thickness in different areas of the spine, the following radiographic protocol is recommended, and can of course be modified to account for neurological lesion localization and individual circumstances.

- Cervical spine (lesion localization between C1 and T2):
  - Small dogs and cats: one lateral and one ventrodorsal view, centred on the mid region of the cervical spine.
  - Large dogs: two lateral and two ventrodorsal views, centred on the cranial and caudal region of the cervical spine, respectively.
- Thoracic and lumbar spine (lesion localization between T3 and L3): (two to) three lateral and (two to) three ventrodorsal views, centred on the mid-thoracic spine, mid-lumbar spine and thoracolumbar junction, respectively.
- Lumbar spine and sacrum (lesion localization between L4 and S3): one lateral and one ventrodorsal view, centred on the lumbosacral junction.

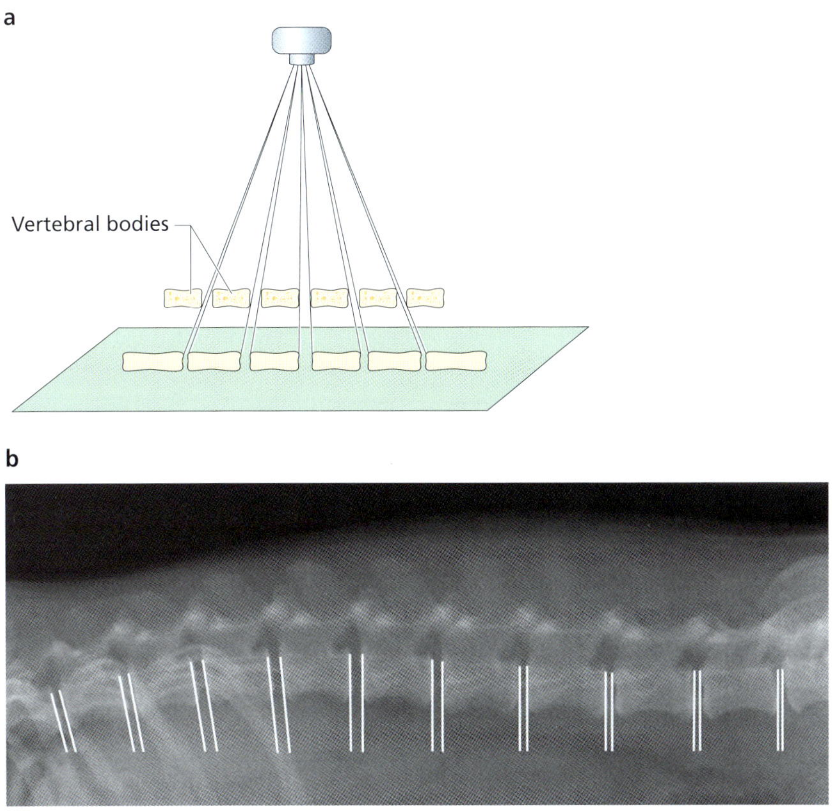

Fig. 7.9 Effect of primary X-ray beam centring on radiographic appearance of intervertebral disc spaces.
a The schematic drawing illustrates the effect of X-ray beam divergence on the projected width of the intervertebral disc spaces. Intervertebral disc spaces in the periphery of the collimated field of view appear increasingly narrow due to the oblique beam angle. This may mimic intervertebral disc disease.
b Lateral radiograph of the lumbar spine in a dog, showing uneven intervertebral disc space width due to divergence of the X-ray beam in the periphery of the collimated field of view.

7.2.3 Myelography

Introduction

Myelography is a contrast examination of the spine that involves injection of positive contrast medium into the subarachnoid space (also known as intrathecal injection). This procedure is not without risk and requires training and experience to perform and interpret. Unlike other contrast procedures easily attempted in practice (e.g. upper gastrointestinal study), myelography should only be performed in practices equipped and able to follow up with neurosurgical procedures if indicated (e.g. if a compressive lesion is identified).

Familiarity with the anatomic relationships between the meningeal layers and their contained spaces is important when performing and interpreting myelograms (Fig. 7.10). The pia mater directly covers the spinal cord. It is separated from the arachnoid membrane by the subarachnoid space which contains cerebrospinal fluid (CSF). The arachnoid membrane is in close contact with the firm outer meningeal layer (dura mater). The subdural space between these meningeal layers is a potential space which is normally completely collapsed. The spinal cord including meninges is surrounded by the epidural space. The subarachnoid space typically ends relatively far cranially (approximately at the level of L5) in large dogs, while it may reach the sacrum in small dogs and cats (see below).

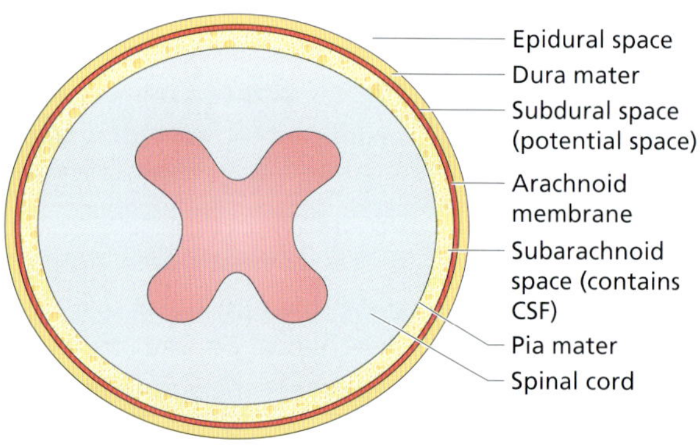

Fig. 7.10 Schematic drawing of the spinal cord and surrounding meninges. The pia mater covers the spinal cord. The arachnoid membrane is closely connected to the overlying dura mater. The CSF-filled subarachnoid space is located between the pia mater and arachnoid membrane. The subdural space between the dura mater and arachnoid membrane is a potential space which is typically of no clinical significance. Within the vertebral canal, the spinal cord and meninges are surrounded by the epidural space.

INDICATIONS

Myelography is indicated when a reason for spinal pain or neurological deficits is not evident on survey radiographs of the spine, if a lesion seen on survey radiographs does not explain the clinical signs, or if several lesions of questionable clinical significance are noted (e.g. several mineralized intervertebral discs). Myelography may also be indicated in cases where survey radiographs clearly show a lesion (e.g. vertebral subluxation or chronic discospondylitis), but further information is desired for optimized treatment planning or prognostication (e.g. determination of an optimal surgical approach, presence and degree of spinal cord swelling, additional complicating factors such as epidural haemorrhage, or determination of whether a compressive lesion is present or not).

CONTRAINDICATIONS

The most important contraindication for myelography is an inflammatory condition within the vertebral canal (meningitis, especially of bacterial aetiology), as the injection of contrast medium can lead to further spread of infectious organisms throughout the subarachnoid space and result in marked worsening in neurological status. A second contraindication is increased intracranial pressure (e.g. in cases of hydrocephalus), as myelography carries the same risks as a CSF tap, including brain herniation in these animals. However, this is a lesser problem in daily practice as these patients typically present with neurological signs referred to the brain rather than spinal cord. Finally, myelography should be avoided in cases of known allergy to iodinated contrast agents (which in our experience is exceedingly rare in veterinary patients).

Use of ionic iodinated contrast agents for myelography has become obsolete since the introduction of nonionic iodinated **contrast media** such as iohexol, iopamidol or iotrolan. They are characterized by low osmolarity and toxicity, which reduces the risk of adverse effects. Iodine concentration in available products typically ranges from 180–350 mg/ml.

Material

The following materials should be prepared when planning a myelography.

- Material for aseptic preparation of the injection site (clippers, scrubbing material).
- Sterile gloves and, depending on personal preference, sterile drapes to cover the patient.
- Water bath: Warm contrast medium has a lower viscosity than cold contrast medium, is easier to inject and distributes more evenly within the subarachnoid space. Warming of the contrast medium can be achieved by placing the bottle in a bath of warm (body temperature) water.
- Tube for CSF collection: When the needle is placed

into the subarachnoid space, CSF flow is usually observed, especially with a cisternal puncture. Collection and analysis of CSF may be indicated depending on the results of the subsequent myelographic study. However, if there is clinical suspicion of (bacterial) meningitis, this must be ruled out prior to the contrast examination.

- Syringe, needle (± filter, ± extension set).
  - These materials should be opened sterilely and only touched by the examiner with gloved hands.
  - Syringe: It is important to be able to feel even slight resistance to injection during the procedure. For this reason, use of low-resistance or loss-of-resistance syringes designed to provide smooth, low-friction plunger action and use of the smallest syringe possible is recommended.
  - Needle: This needle is used to draw up the contrast medium from the bottle. As contamination of the contrast medium with bacteria, talcum powder, glass or rubber particles has to be avoided, a special microbiological filter needle or a conventional needle with filter attachment should be used for this purpose.
  - Extension set: Movement of the needle tip in the vertebral canal following lumbar puncture and successful spinal needle placement in the subarachnoid space can be minimized by attaching a small extension set connected to the syringe. To avoid injection of gas bubbles, the extension line should be prefilled with contrast medium. Connection of the syringe to a tube rather than directly to the spinal needle allows manipulation of the syringe, or attachment of a new syringe, without manipulating the spinal needle. An additional advantage of this technique is that, when performing a myelogram under fluoroscopic guidance, the hands of the examiner are further away from the primary beam than if the syringe is directly connected to the spinal needle. This is desirable from a radiation safety perspective.
- Spinal needles: Myelography requires use of special hollow needles with a bevelled tip and central stylet. The appropriate length and diameter of the needle depend on the size of the patient and the puncture site. A 1.5 inch (3.8 cm) 22-gauge needle is usually sufficient for a cervical injection. Depending on the patient's size, a 1.5–3.5 inch (3.8–8.9 cm) 20- to 22-gauge needle may be used for lumbar injection.
- Contrast medium: As mentioned above, myelograms require use of a nonionic iodinated contrast medium. The amount of contrast medium needed depends on the injection site and the spinal area of interest.
  - Examination of the cervical spine: 0.3 ml/kg (cervical injection) to 0.45 ml/kg (lumbar injection).
  - Examination of the thoracic and lumbar spine: 0.2–0.4 ml/kg (lumbar injection) up to 0.45 ml/kg (cervical injection).
  - Examination of the entire spine: 0.45 ml/kg (independent of the injection site).

If a lumbar injection is performed and fluoroscopy is available to monitor the procedure, contrast medium flow during injection can be observed in real time and the injection can be terminated as soon as the area of interest has filled with a sufficient amount of contrast medium. This allows minimization of the contrast medium dose and thus the risk of adverse effects.

Injection site

With very few exceptions, and depending on personal preference, the examination is performed in lateral recumbency. The injection can be performed following a cervical (cisterna magna) or lumbar (caudal lumbar spine) puncture.

For a **cervical injection** the animal's head is flexed by an assistant and the needle is inserted on the midline, in the centre of a triangle formed by the occiput and the wings of the atlas (Fig. 7.11a). The bevel of the needle is oriented caudally to ensure contrast medium flow towards the neck rather than the head during injection. Successful placement of the needle tip in the subarachnoid space is indicated by an initial characteristic 'pop' sound (more felt than heard) when the needle perforates the ligamentum flavum and dura mater. Subsequently, CSF flow is observed. Injection of contrast medium should be performed slowly (2–3 ml/minute) to minimize the risk of backflow into the cranial vault. Once the injection is complete the patient's head should be elevated for the same reason.

A cervical injection has the following disadvantages.

- The risk of backflow of contrast medium into the cranial vault and the resultant adverse effects is higher than with a lumbar injection.
- The full dose of contrast medium is usually injected, as the degree of filling of the subarachnoid space cannot be easily monitored during injection.
- Many lesions within the vertebral canal will result in increased back pressure to contrast medium injection, and contrast medium flow stops cranial to the area of interest.

In the authors' opinion a cervical injection should be reserved for rare instances where a lumbar puncture is not possible owing to large patient size or anatomic or pathological conditions.

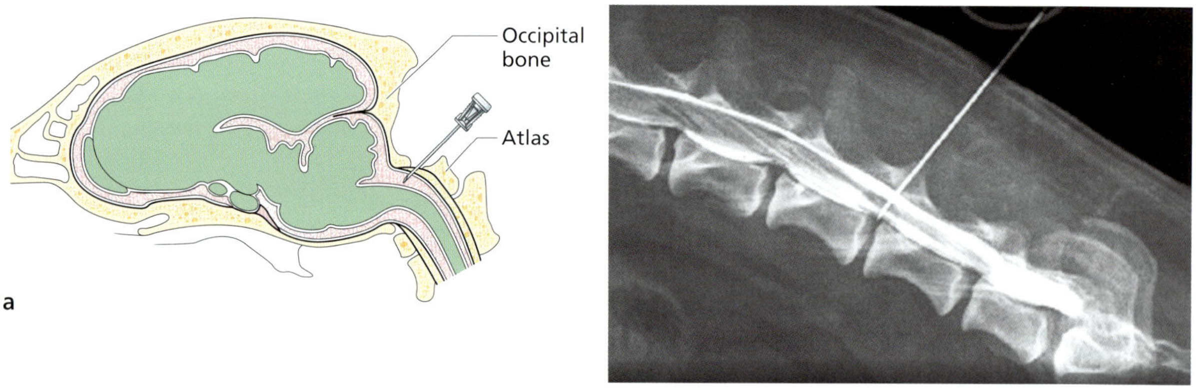

Fig. 7.11 Injection sites for myelography.
a Cervical injection (schematic drawing). The patient's head is flexed, and the spinal needle is inserted into the cisterna magna of the subarachnoid space at the atlanto-occipital space. As neither the head nor the needle can be manipulated during contrast medium injection, fluoroscopic or radiographic verification of needle placement or contrast medium flow is usually impossible.
b Lumbar injection. The needle has been inserted between the fifth and sixth lumbar vertebrae in an oblique cranioventral direction. The needle tip is located in the ventral subarachnoid space. The subarachnoid space in this patient reaches the cranial sacrum.

A **lumbar injection** is usually performed at the level of the fifth / sixth lumbar vertebrae (Fig. 7.11b). In some large-breed dogs, the subarachnoid space may be very short due to the ascent of the spinal cord (see above), necessitating puncture at the level of the fourth / fifth lumbar vertebrae. The interarcuate spaces between the dorsal vertebral arches are narrow but can be widened by flexing the patient's spine, facilitating easier needle placement. Depending on personal preference, the needle is inserted either perpendicular to the spine or in an oblique caudodorsal–cranioventral direction, with cranial orientation of the bevel. With successful advancement of the needle into the ventral subarachnoid space, many animals show a characteristic twitching motion of the hind legs. In many but not all cases a small amount of CSF flow from the needle may be observed following needle placement. The appropriate position of the needle tip can be verified by means of injection of a small test dose of contrast medium and fluoroscopic or radiographic confirmation.

A lumbar injection is also performed slowly, but for different reasons to cervical injection. While there is a lower chance of contrast medium flow to the head, there is a significant risk of contrast medium extravasation into the epidural space or central canal, which will limit the diagnostic quality of the study and in extreme cases may render the examination nondiagnostic.

If adequate equipment is available, the injection should be performed under fluoroscopic guidance. This technique has several advantages.

- Contrast medium injection can be halted once adequate filling of the subarachnoid space has been achieved. This minimizes the dose of contrast medium and the risk of adverse effects.
- As the evaluation is performed in real time, lesions are identified early (during contrast medium injection). Initial radiographs can be targeted at the region of the lesion and can be obtained either during ongoing injection or immediately afterwards. This is important as abnormalities within the vertebral canal (e.g. spinal cord swelling or narrowing of the subarachnoid space) often result in attenuation of contrast medium in the area of the lesion, which subsequently may be difficult to localize and characterize.
- Monitoring the injection in real time allows immediate recognition of complications (such as contrast medium extravasation into the epidural space or central canal) and correction of needle placement.

Procedure

1. General anaesthesia.
2. Acquisition of orthogonal survey radiographs of the spine.
3. Placement of the patient in the desired position and preparation of the injection site (clipping, scrubbing, disinfecting).
4. Preparation of the necessary materials including placement of contrast medium in a warming water bath. Sterility of the procedure can be maximized if an assistant retrieves the contrast medium bottle from the bath and opens it while the gloved examiner draws up the contrast medium immediately prior to injection.

5. Needle placement and contrast medium injection (see above).
6. Acquisition of lateral and ventrodorsal/dorsoventral radiographs, as well as special views if necessary.

Radiographs

Lateral views are acquired for all myelograms. Orthogonal views are usually acquired in a **ventrodorsal** fashion for both the cervical and thoracolumbar regions. However, especially in large-breed dogs, acquisition of a **dorsoventral** view of the caudal cervical spine may be beneficial due to its anatomic conformation resulting in a ventral spinal curvature (Fig. 7.12). If the patient is positioned in dorsal recumbency, the caudal part of the cervical spine is the highest point, and contrast medium flows cranially and caudally under the influence of gravity. If the patient is positioned in sternal recumbency, contrast medium accumulates at the lowest point, i.e. the region of the caudal cervical spine. The effects of gravity on contrast medium distribution can also be exploited in other spinal regions where inadequate contrast medium filling of the subarachnoid space interferes with study evaluation. Elevation of the head and/or the pelvis results in flow of contrast medium to the lower parts of the spine, facilitating improved assessment of these areas. In addition to lateral and ventrodorsal/dorsoventral views, oblique views of the area of interest are often indicated to improve visualization of a lateralized lesion (Fig. 7.13).

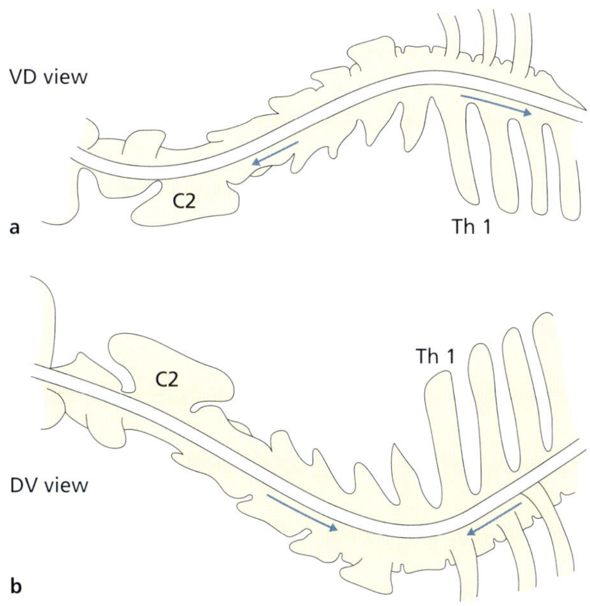

Fig. 7.12 Schematic illustration of the effect of patient positioning on contrast medium distribution during cervical myelography.
a With positioning in dorsal recumbency (i.e. when obtaining a ventrodorsal view), contrast medium follows gravity and accumulates in the lower portions of the spine.
b With sternal positioning (i.e. when obtaining a dorsoventral view), contrast medium accumulates in the region of the caudal cervical spine allowing improved evaluation of this area.

Stress views (flexion or extension of the spine) may aid in the evaluation of dynamic lesions such as those seen with caudal cervical spondylomyelopathy or degenerative lumbosacral stenosis in select cases. However, these techniques carry significant risks, as overt manipulation of an unstable spine can cause additional spinal cord injury and result in exacerbation of clinical signs. Traction radiography of the caudal cervical spine is advocated by some for further characterization of a compressive lesion found on a myelogram. If traction results in partial or complete resolution of a compressive lesion, the lesion is considered, at least in part, to be dynamic in nature. A static compressive lesion will not significantly change under traction. It is important to point out that many neurologists and radiologists disagree on the necessity and diagnostic yield of spinal stress radiographs, and some clinicians consider them obsolete. If stress views are considered in the evaluation of a spinal patient, the risks have to be weighed against the potential benefits.

Other special techniques will be covered in the sections on individual spinal diseases.

Interpretation

PHYSIOLOGICAL FINDINGS

A normal myelogram is characterized by even and homogeneous filling of the subarachnoid space with contrast medium. There should be no evidence of interruption of normal flow of contrast medium, attenuation of the contrast columns, abnormal filling defects or leakage of contrast medium from the subarachnoid space. The contrast columns should be fairly parallel on both the lateral as well as the ventrodorsal views. Normal variations are seen in different regions of the spine which should not be confused with spinal pathology.

Cervical myelogram (Fig. 7.14 to 7.16)

- The subarachnoid space at the level of the first and second cervical vertebrae is relatively wide.
- There is physiological attenuation and mild dorsal deviation of the ventral contrast column at the level of the C2–3 intervertebral disc space.
- The caudal cervical spinal cord is wide (cervical intumescence).
- A serpentine filling defect caused by the vertebral artery is visible within the contrast-filled subarachnoid space on a ventrodorsal view at the level of C1–2.

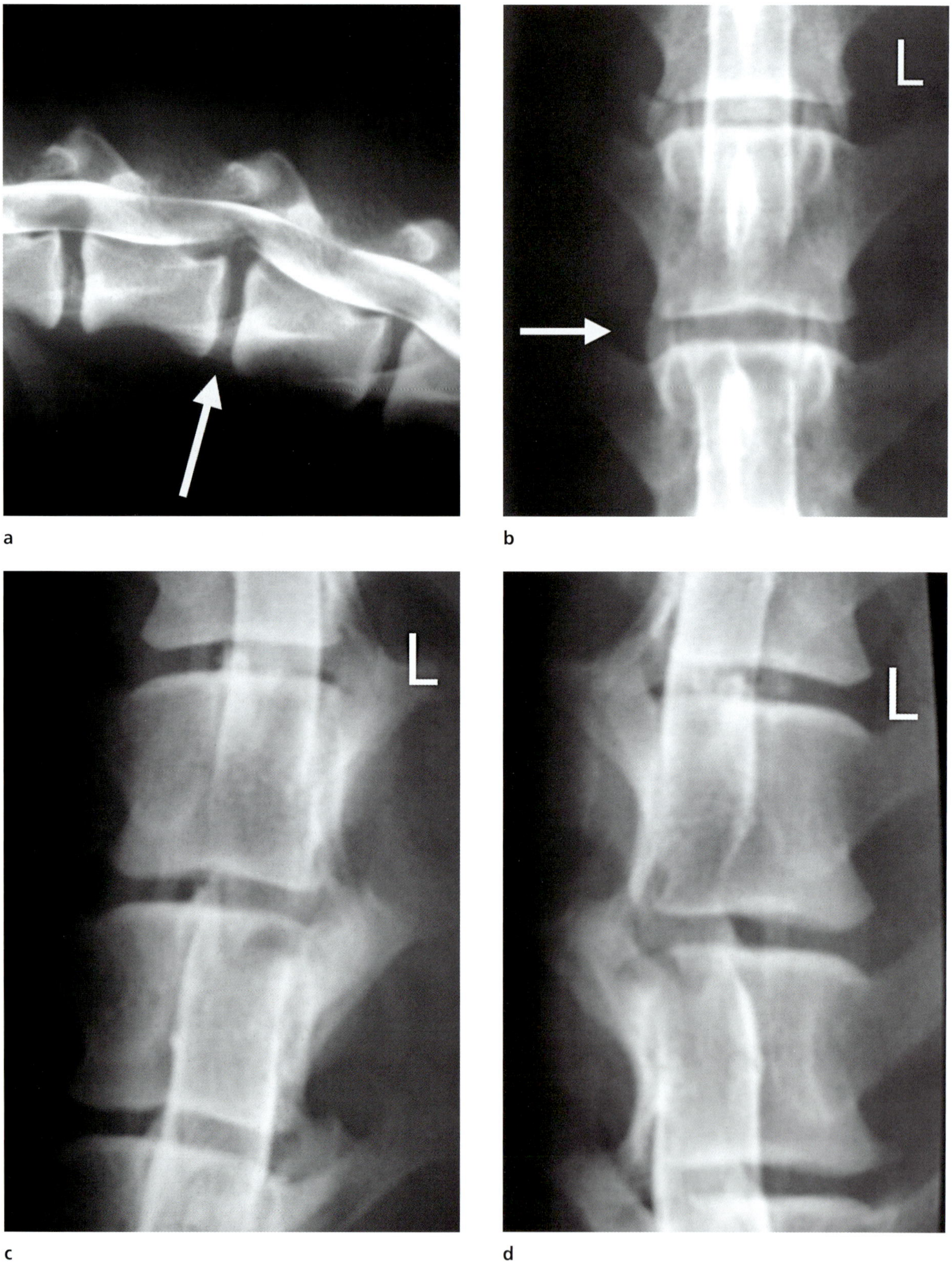

Fig. 7.13 Intervertebral disc herniation in a dog.

a On the lateral view there is dorsal elevation of the ventral contrast column at the level of the L2–3 intervertebral disc space (arrow) with associated attenuation of the dorsal contrast column.

b The ventrodorsal view demonstrates homogeneous attenuation of both contrast columns over this disc space (arrow) without obvious lateralization of the lesion.

c This oblique view highlights the right ventral subarachnoid space.

d This oblique view highlights the left ventral subarachnoid space. An extradural compressive lesion is easily recognized in the left ventral aspect of the vertebral canal. (L = left)

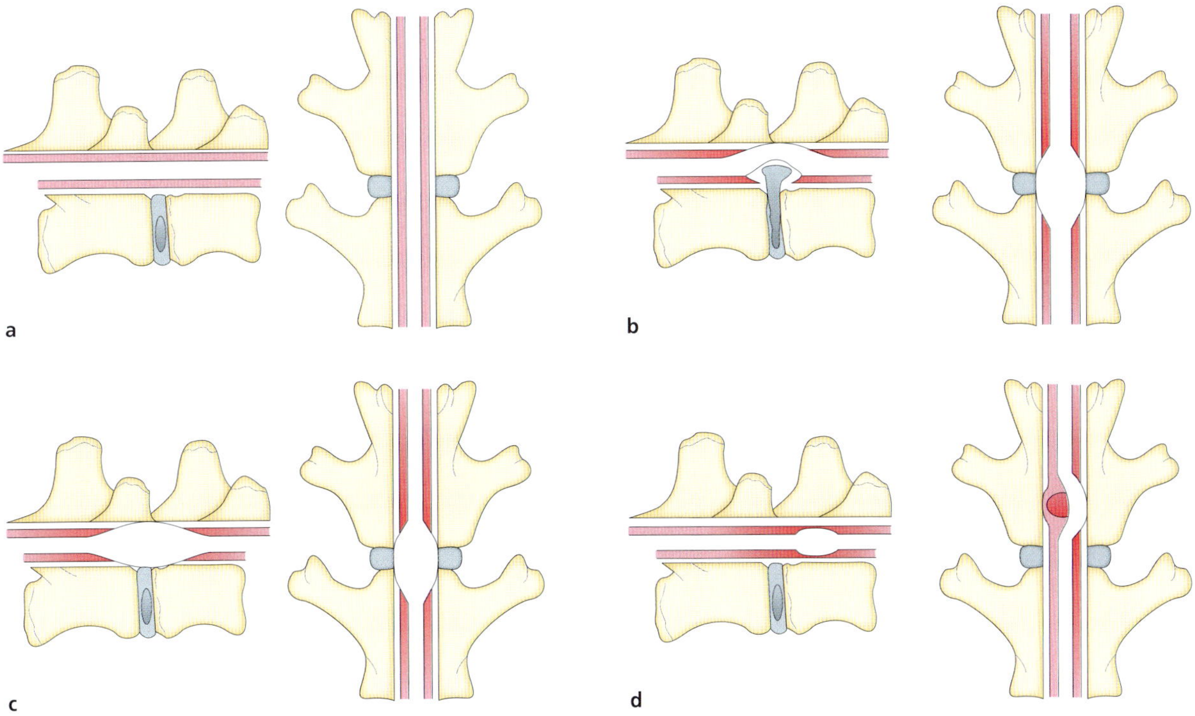

Fig. 7.19 Schematic illustration of possible findings on myelography.
a With a normal myelogram, contrast columns are parallel and of even width.
b An extradural lesion results in displacement of at least one contrast column and possibly in spinal cord compression from the outside seen on at least one view.
c An intramedullary lesion results in spinal cord enlargement visible on all views with associated attenuation of the surrounding contrast columns.
d With an intradural-extramedullary lesion the subarachnoid space is widened adjacent to the lesion and often assumes the shape of a characteristic 'golf tee'.

PATHOLOGICAL FINDINGS

According to their relation to the spinal cord and meninges, spinal lesions can be subdivided into extradural, intramedullary and intradural-extramedullary (Fig. 7.19 and 7.20).

EXTRADURAL LESION This is caused by a structure or accumulation of material outside the dural sac and may or may not result in spinal cord compression. On a myelogram, displacement of at least one contrast column is seen in at least one projection (Fig. 7.20a). In addition to standard lateral and ventrodorsal views, oblique views may be necessary to determine the extradural nature of a lesion (see Fig. 7.13). Numerous conditions can result in extradural lesions including:

- intervertebral disc herniation
- haematoma
- spinal instability (luxation, subluxation or fracture)
- hypertrophy of the spinal ligaments
- neoplasia (originating from vertebrae, epidural space or adjacent structures)
- inflammatory lesion (e.g. discospondylitis)
- bony proliferation (e.g. degenerative joint disease of the articular process joints)
- congenital anomalies / malformations.

INTRAMEDULLARY LESION A lesion within the spinal cord parenchyma results in spinal cord enlargement and subsequently divergence and thinning of the contrast columns visible on all radiographic projections (Fig. 7.20b). Differential diagnoses include neoplastic lesions (e.g. glial tumour, ependymoma, metastases or lymphoma) and benign mass lesions (e.g. granuloma). Focal spinal cord swelling such as seen secondary to fibrocartilaginous embolism or trauma may also cause an intramedullary lesion.

INTRADURAL-EXTRAMEDULLARY LESION This is caused by an abnormal structure or abnormal material within the subarachnoid space, which on a myelogram appears as a filling defect within the surrounding contrast medium (Fig. 7.20c). Focal widening of the contrast column adjacent to the lesion is often compared to a 'golf tee'. Meningiomas and nerve sheath tumours are the most common aetiologies of an intradural-extramedullary lesion. Other differential diagnoses include other tumour types and, less commonly, benign mass lesions such as granulomas or haematomas.

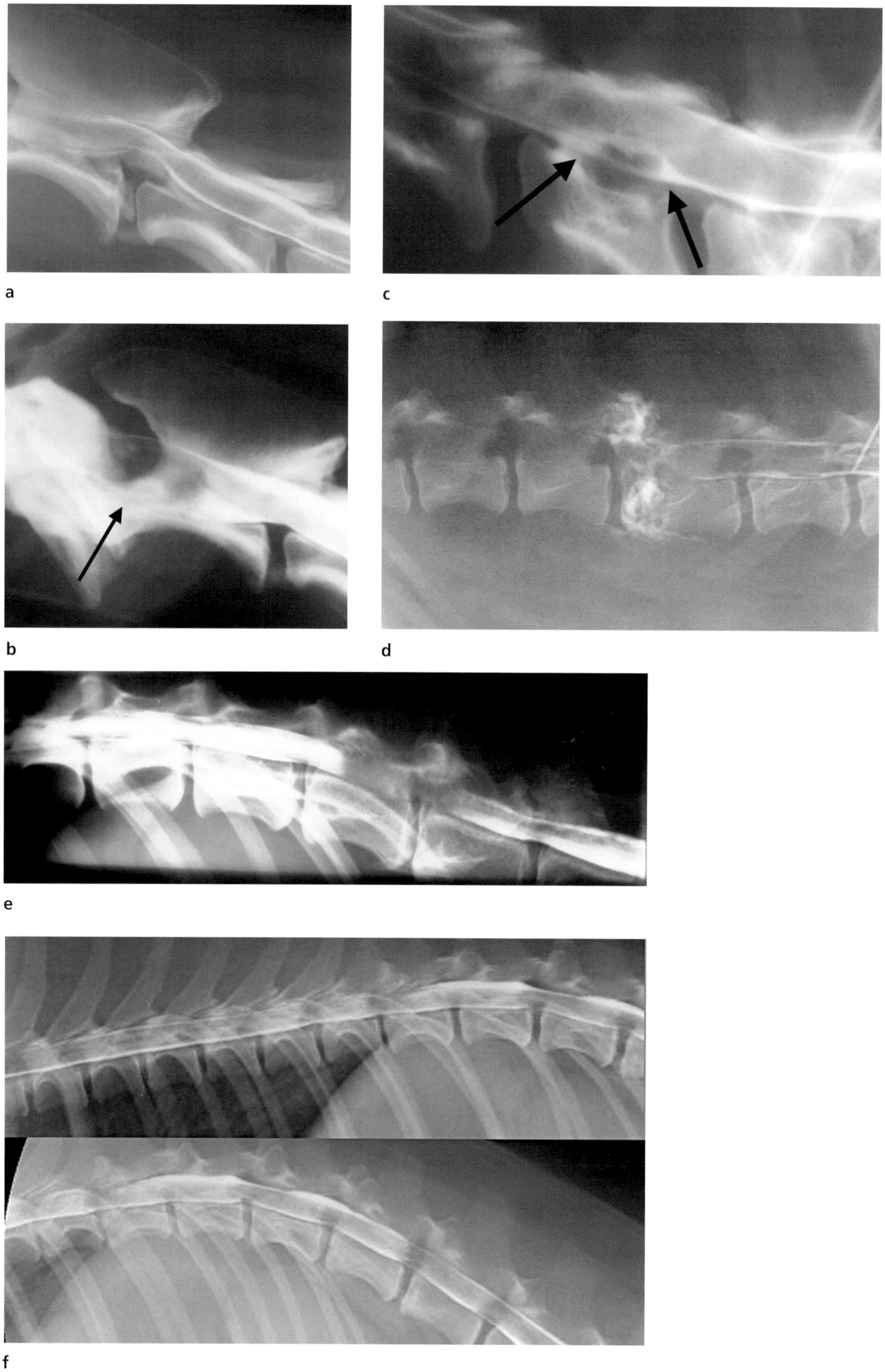
a
c
b
d
e
f

Fig. 7.20 Possible pathological findings on myelography.
a Extradural lesion: On this cervical myelogram, displacement and attenuation of the contrast columns from ventral are noted dorsal to the C2–3 intervertebral disc space. A moderate amount of mineralized disc material remains in situ. These findings are consistent with intervertebral disc extrusion.
b Intramedullary lesion: There is focal swelling of the cranial cervical spinal cord (arrow) with associated attenuation of the adjacent contrast columns. This finding was confirmed on ventrodorsal and oblique views. Spinal cord neoplasia (e.g. glioma) is the most likely differential diagnosis for this finding in this older dog with chronic progressive clinical signs.
c Intradural-extramedullary lesion: There is splitting of the ventral contrast column with a focal mass lesion appearing as a filling defect in the ventral subarachnoid space (arrows). The appearance of the contrast columns is often referred to as a 'golf tee' sign. A neoplastic lesion (e.g. meningioma) is the most likely differential diagnosis for this finding.
d Leakage of contrast medium from the lumbar subarachnoid space in a dog following spinal trauma. This indicates extensive meningeal injury. A vertebral fracture is also noted.
e Contrast medium accumulation within spinal cord parenchyma in a dog. The dog had sustained an acute intervertebral disc extrusion at L2–3 three days prior (note complete attenuation of contrast columns over this disc space). Staining of spinal cord parenchyma with contrast medium is noted cranial to the lesion. This finding is consistent with myelomalacia.
f Multifocal irregular filling defects, particularly associated with the dorsal contrast column in an older dog. These lesions remained static on repeat radiographs obtained during the myelographic procedure. A presumptive diagnosis of chronic adhesive arachnoiditis was made.

> Inadvertent injection of gas bubbles during myelography will result in filling defects within the contrast columns which may mimic intradural-extramedullary lesions. However, unlike true masses, gas bubbles will change shape and position between successive radiographs, allowing differentiation from spinal pathology.

Other possible myelographic findings include the following.

- Extravasation of contrast medium from the subarachnoid space, e.g. secondary to trauma or infiltrative disease processes (Fig. 7.20d).
- Focal dilatation of a contrast column (e.g. due to subarachnoid diverticula, syrinx formation or trauma).
- Accumulation of contrast medium within spinal cord parenchyma, as seen with myelomalacia (Fig. 7.20e).
- Dilatation of the central canal (hydromyelia).
- Adhesions between the pia and arachnoid membrane characterized by multifocal irregular regions of narrowing and filling defects of the contrast columns, e.g. due to chronic adhesive arachnoiditis (Fig. 7.20f).

It is important to keep in mind that a normal myelographic study cannot rule out some diseases of the spinal column, the spinal cord or the meninges. Normal radiographic and myelographic studies are common with the following conditions.

- Subtle intramedullary lesions (e.g. infarcts including fibrocartilaginous embolism [FCE], myelitis, small tumours).
- Noncompressive disorders of intervertebral discs (e.g. disc degeneration and early discospondylitis).
- Subtle vertebral lesions (e.g. nondisplaced fractures or early bone tumours).
- Meningeal disease (e.g. meningitis).
- Degenerative and metabolic conditions (e.g. degenerative myelopathy).

Problems, adverse effects and complications

Problems that may negatively impact the diagnostic quality of a myelographic study include injection of contrast medium into the epidural space (lumbar injection) or the subdural space (cervical injection). Filling of the central canal can occur secondary to a lumbar injection but usually does not interfere with study evaluation. Possible complications and adverse effects of a myelogram may be associated with the technique itself, the patient, or the properties of the contrast medium.

TECHNIQUE With cervical injection, care must be taken that the needle does not touch or, worse, puncture the spinal cord. Direct contact between the needle and the conus medullaris or cauda equina is unavoidable with lumbar injection. However, this mechanical irritation is typically of no clinical significance. Injection of contrast medium into the spinal cord or central canal may result in worsening of the clinical signs. Contamination of the needle and introduction of foreign material (e.g. talcum powder from gloves or glass and rubber particles from contrast medium bottles) must be avoided by all means as these may result in meningitis/ meningoencephalomyelitis, meningeal irritation and meningeal adhesions. The risk of contamination can be minimized by strict adherence to sterility guidelines, use of filter needles and use of powder-free gloves. Procedural adverse effects seen in humans (head and neck pain, nausea and vomiting) are not observed/recognized in dogs and cats which undergo the study under general anaesthesia.

PATIENT Dehydration of the patient is associated with delayed resorption of contrast medium from the subarachnoid space and an increased incidence of adverse effects. Even though this is likely to be a lesser consideration with nonionic contrast media used today, the patient should be adequately hydrated before a myelographic study is performed. Impaired CSF flow within the subarachnoid space due to compressive lesions or meningeal adhesions may also result in delayed resorption of contrast medium.

CONTRAST MEDIUM Adverse effects linked to pharmacological properties of the contrast medium are associated with the following factors: hypertonicity to CSF, ionicity, chemical toxicity and allergenic stimulation. Contrast media used today are nonionic and characterized by decreased osmolarity and toxicity compared to previously used contrast agents. Allergic reactions to myelographic contrast agents seem to be of no concern in veterinary medicine. An increase (or less commonly a decrease) of heart or respiratory rate during injection of contrast medium is common but is usually easily regulated by anaesthetic adjustments. Rapid cervical injection can cause apnoea, which is typically self-limiting. The most common complications following myelography are seizures during the recovery period (reported incidence ranging from 0% to more than 20% using nonionic contrast media). Cervical injection and an increase in dose of contrast medium are associated with an increased incidence of seizures. Other factors that have been associated with increased risk of seizures by some authors include short duration of general anaesthesia and premedication with phenothiazine derivates. Seizures during the recovery period are usually successfully managed medically. Worsening of the clinical signs following myelography is common. Isolated reports of patient death following myelography can be found in the literature.

7.2.4 Other spinal contrast studies

As the subarachnoid space in large-breed dogs commonly terminates cranial to the lumbosacral junction, myelography is of limited value in the diagnostic workup of patients with suspected degenerative lumbosacral stenosis or other (compressive) lesions in the lumbosacral area. Even though injection of contrast medium into the epidural space (epidurography) or into the lumbosacral intervertebral disc (discography) have been used with variable success in the past, these procedures have become obsolete since computed tomography (CT) and magnetic resonance imaging (MRI) have become more readily available in veterinary practice.

7.3 Spinal diseases

7.3.1 Congenital disorders

Many congenital vertebral anomalies encountered, especially in dogs, are commonly incidental findings.

Block vertebrae are characterized by complete or partial fusion of two or more adjacent vertebrae. They result from a defect in somite segmentation during embryological development and may occur anywhere along the length of the spine.

Wedge-shaped malformations and shortening of individual or multiple vertebrae (**hemivertebrae, butterfly vertebrae**) are common, especially in the thoracic spine in certain chondrodystrophic breeds (Bulldogs, Boston Terriers, Pugs) (Fig. 7.21). These malformations can result in kyphosis and, in severe cases, may cause neurological signs, but they are usually an incidental finding.

An **abnormal vertebral number** (e.g. 14 thoracic and 6 lumbar vertebrae) is an occasional observation of no clinical significance. However, when planning spinal surgery, care must be taken to note any abnormalities in vertebral number to avoid a surgical approach at the wrong site.

Transitional vertebrae may be encountered at any transition zone of vertebral column sections and are most commonly noted at the thoracolumbar and the lumbosacral junctions. Transitional vertebrae are characterized by morphological properties of both adjacent spinal sections. For example, lumbarized thoracic vertebrae may have transverse processes instead of normal ribs, or the ribs may be hypoplastic or aplastic. With sacralization of the last lumbar vertebra, one or both transverse processes may communicate with the sacrum (Fig. 7.22), and a normal lumbosacral intervertebral disc may be absent. A lumbarized first sacral vertebra may have one or two transverse processes, and is usually separated from the second sacral vertebra by an intervertebral disc. While thoracolumbar transitional vertebrae are incidental, lumbosacral transitional vertebrae have been associated with an increased risk of hip dysplasia and degenerative lumbosacral stenosis in large-breed dogs. As stated above for abnormal vertebral number, the presence and conformation of transitional vertebrae must be taken into consideration when planning spinal surgery.

Spina bifida is an anomaly resulting from failed or incomplete closure of the neural arch. Bulldogs, Boston Terriers, Pugs and Manx cats are considered predisposed. The disease can be clinically insignificant (**spina bifida occulta**) or may result in clinical signs if spinal cord and/or meninges are involved in the disease process (**spina bifida manifesta**). The condition predominantly occurs in the lumbosacral region of the spine but can be seen in other areas. A radiographic diagnosis is best made on a ventrodorsal view where duplication or absence of one or more spinous processes may be noted (Fig. 7.23). Separation of the vertebral arches may also be seen. Myelography may demonstrate extension of meninges and spinal cord into the defect (**meningocele, myelocele**).

An **abnormal curvature of the spine** (kyphosis, scoliosis or lordosis) is occasionally seen in dogs and cats and is usually an incidental finding.

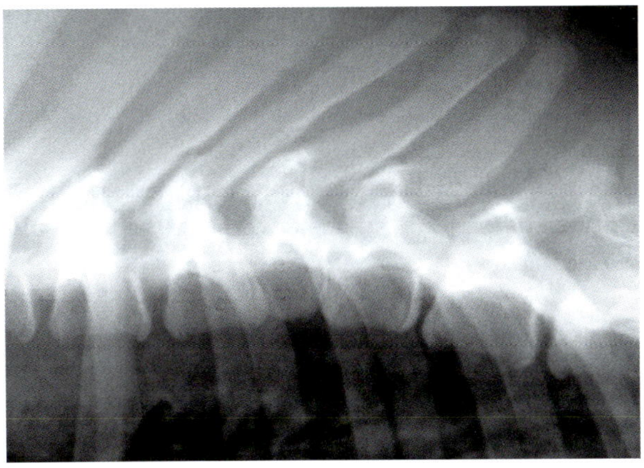

a

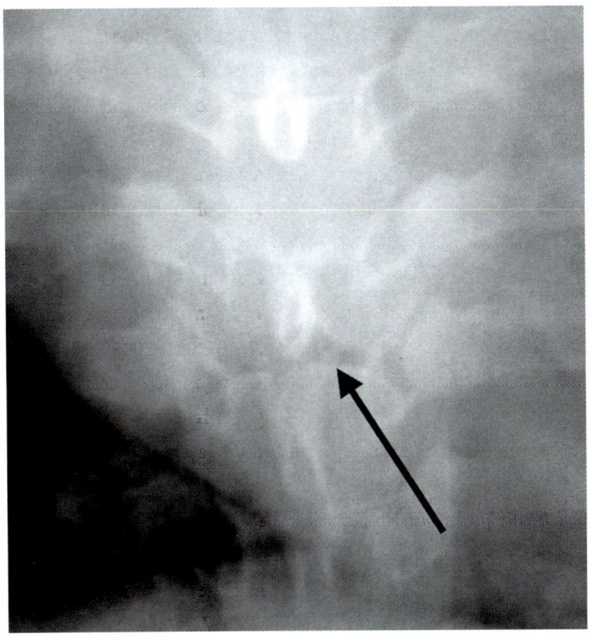

b

Fig. 7.21 Congenital malformation of a thoracic vertebra ('butterfly vertebra') in a Bulldog. This is a common incidental finding in this breed and often not associated with clinical signs.
a The vertebra is foreshortened and wedge-shaped on the lateral view.
b On the ventrodorsal view a median indentation in the caudal vertebral endplate is noted (arrow). Adjacent ribs are in close proximity to each other due to foreshortening of the vertebra.

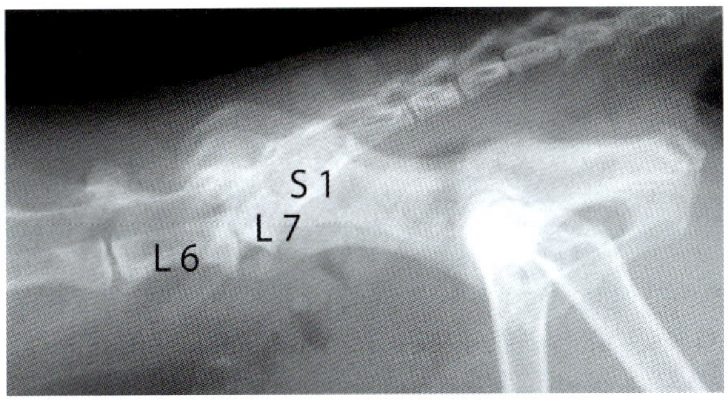

a

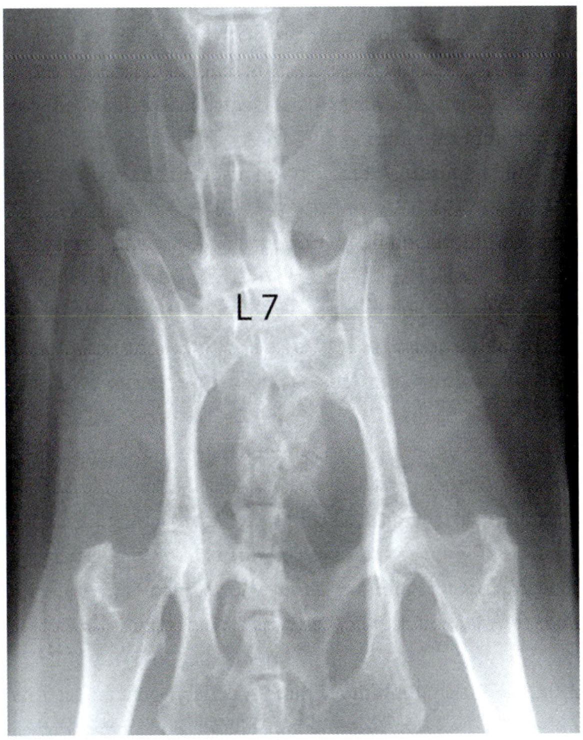

b

Fig. 7.22 Sacralization of the last lumbar vertebra in a cat.
a On the lateral view there is fusion of the seventh lumbar vertebra (L7) with the first sacral vertebra (S1). The intervertebral disc at this level is absent. Note ventral spondylosis deformans at L6–7.
b The lumbosacral junction is asymmetric on the ventrodorsal view. L7 has a left-sided transverse process. The right transverse process is fused with the sacral wing.

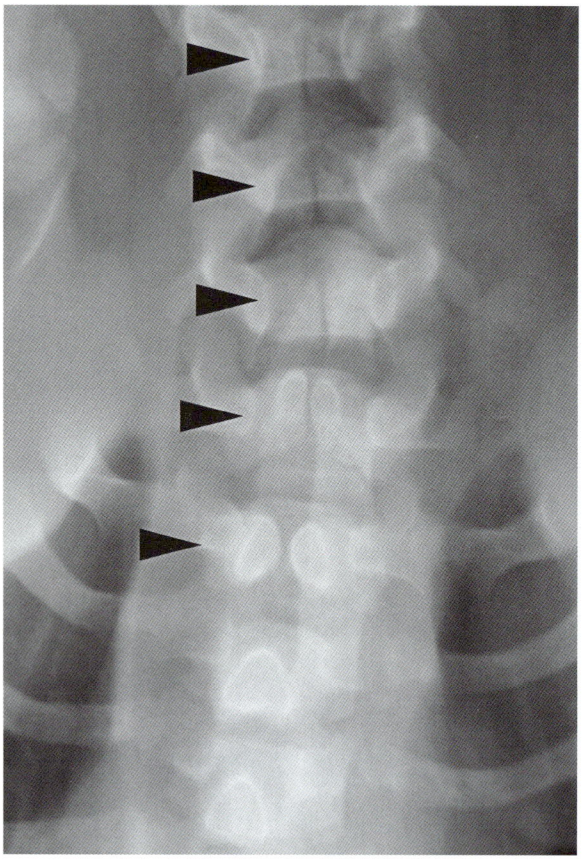

Fig. 7.23 Spina bifida in a dog. The spinous processes and vertebral arches of the caudal cervical and cranial thoracic spine are split on the midline (arrowheads). The vertebrae caudal to this area are normal.

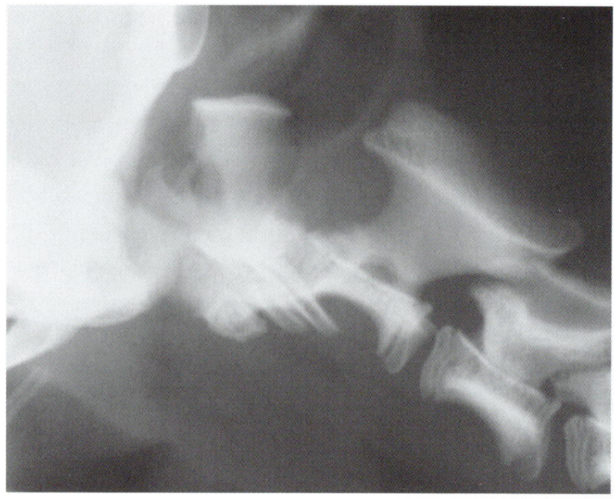

Fig. 7.24 Atlantoaxial instability in a dog. The neutral lateral view of the cervical spine shows a wide gap between the dorsal arch of the atlas and the spinous process of the axis. The intervertebral foramen is abnormally large. On this view the alar wings are superimposed with the dens of the axis, which cannot be evaluated.

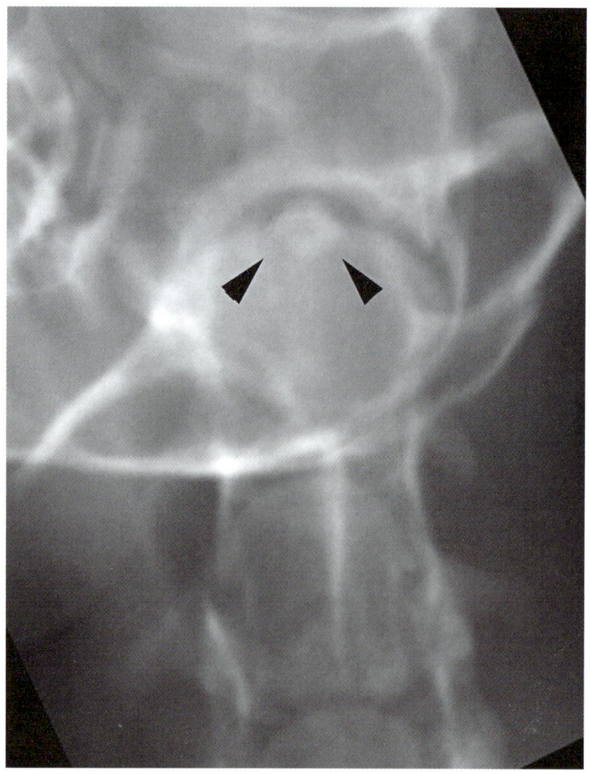

Fig. 7.25 Atlantoaxial instability due to hypoplasia of the dens of the axis in a dog. The rudimentary dens appears as a small focal bony protrusion associated with the cranial endplate of C2 on this ventrodorsal view (arrowheads).

7.3.2 Atlantoaxial instability

Atlantoaxial instability is usually a congenital problem. Miniature and dwarf canine breeds are predisposed. The underlying cause is hypoplasia, malformation or aplasia of the dens of the axis with resultant subluxation of the atlantoaxial joint. A traumatic aetiology is less common but is possible if trauma has resulted in fracture of the dens or injury to the ligamentous structures. Clinical signs are variable and may be acute or chronic intermittent in nature.

Radiographic findings The most common finding is an abnormally large distance between the spinous process of the axis and the dorsal arch of the atlas (Fig. 7.24). These structures should normally overlap. Additional possible findings are subluxation between atlas and axis with resultant narrowing of the vertebral canal or absence/hypoplasia/abnormal angulation or fragmentation of the dens of the axis (Fig. 7.25). This is best evaluated on a ventrodorsal or slightly oblique lateral view. In questionable cases a flexed lateral view of the cervical spine may aid in diagnosis (Fig. 7.26). However, caution must be exercised to avoid damage to the spinal cord and exacerbation of clinical signs.

Any manipulation of the cervical spine including flexion in a dog with suspected atlantoaxial instability has to be performed with extreme caution to avoid further injury and worsening of the clinical signs.

Myelography is usually unnecessary as a diagnosis can be made on survey radiographs. However, it may yield additional information about the presence and degree of spinal cord compression in questionable and chronic cases.

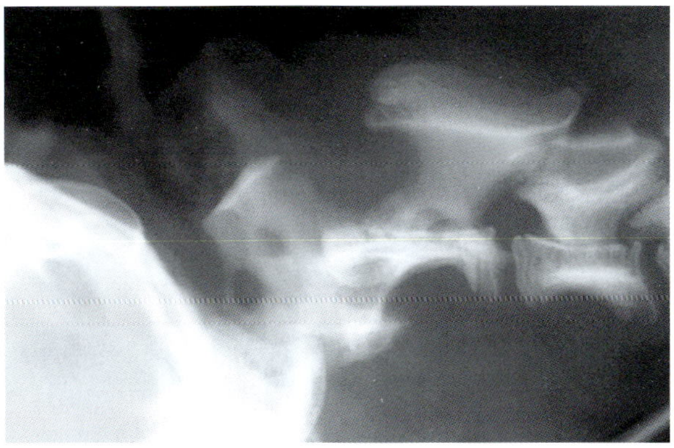

Fig. 7.26 Atlantoaxial instability in a dog. This mildly flexed lateral oblique view accentuates the large distance between the spinous process of the axis and the dorsal arch of the atlas and in addition allows evaluation of the area of the dens, which is now unobscured by the alar wings. The dens is absent in this patient (agenesis).

7.3.3 Degenerative disorders

Spondylosis deformans and diffuse idiopathic skeletal hyperostosis

Spondylosis deformans is an extremely common degenerative disease process affecting the spine, especially in older dogs, and is commonly associated with slowly progressive degeneration of the intervertebral discs. Spondylosis may also occur secondary to spinal instability from various causes (e.g. traumatic subluxation or discospondylitis). Diffuse idiopathic skeletal hyperostosis appears radiographically similar and is a systemic noninflammatory disorder characterized by ossification of soft tissues ventral and lateral to the spine.

Radiographic findings With spondylosis deformans there is new bone formation associated with the insertion site of the annulus fibrosus cranioventral, caudoventral and lateral on the vertebral bodies. This is usually an incidental finding; however, at the level of L7–S1, nerve root irritation by severe lateralized spondylosis deformans is possible. Even though spondylosis deformans can occur with any vertebra, it is most commonly observed in regions of higher mechanical load, i.e. mobility (C5–6, C6–7, T12–13, T13–L1, L7–S1). With early spondylosis, small, hook-like bony projections extend cranioventrally and caudoventrally from the vertebral endplates. Over time, new bone formation may progress and ultimately result in synostosis of neighbouring vertebrae (Fig. 7.27). New bone formation associated with spondylosis deformans is well defined, and the vertebral endplates of affected vertebrae are usually smooth. However, with progressive intervertebral disc degeneration, concurrent intervertebral disc space narrowing and endplate sclerosis are commonly seen, which may or may not be associated with presence of a spinal cord compressive lesion (intervertebral disc herniation).

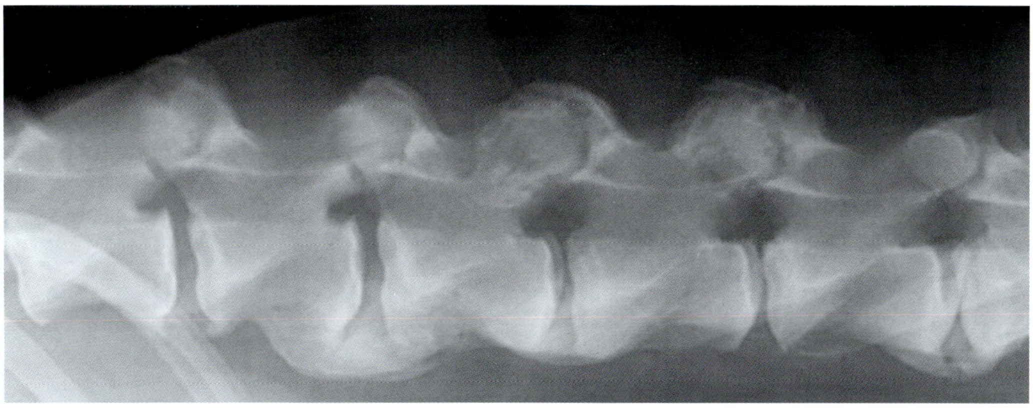

Fig. 7.27 Spondylosis deformans and degenerative joint disease of the articular process joints of the lumbar spine in an older dog. In addition to bony protrusions of variable degrees of severity originating from the cranial and caudal vertebral endplates, periarticular osteophytosis is associated with the articular processes. These changes were incidental in this patient.

Contiguous ossification along the lateral and ventral aspects of the vertebral column over at least three or four adjacent vertebrae with new bone originating from vertebral bodies rather than endplates is commonly seen, for example in Boxer dogs ('bamboo spine') and is indicative of disseminated idiopathic skeletal hyperostosis rather than spondylosis deformans.

Degenerative joint disease of articular facet joints

This is also a common degenerative disease process in older animals and usually not associated with clinical signs. However, if periarticular new bone formation is extensive enough to extend into the vertebral canal, dorsal and lateral spinal cord compression is possible.

RADIOGRAPHIC FINDINGS As with other joints, degenerative joint disease of the spine results in more or less extensive periarticular osteophytosis and irregular margination of the joint surfaces (Fig. 7.27). If new bone proliferation is severe enough to cause spinal cord compression, an extradural lesion will be found on myelography (Fig. 7.28). Severe degenerative joint disease of the lumbar articular process joints may be problematic as it may result in further obliteration of the narrow interarcuate spaces and interfere with needle placement for a lumbar myelogram.

Dural ossification

Meningeal mineralization is occasionally seen in older (especially large-breed) dogs and is usually not associated with clinical signs.

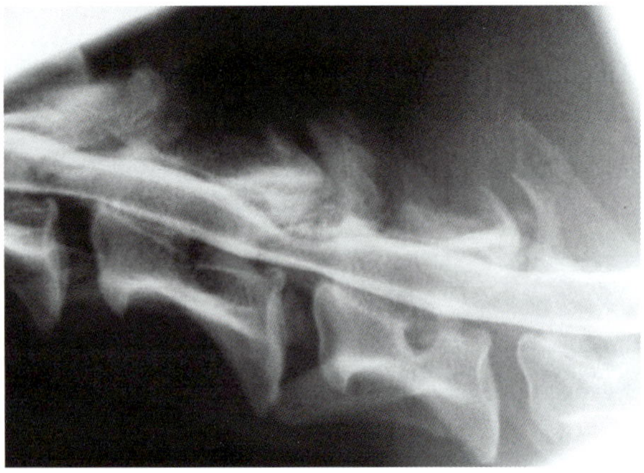

Fig. 7.28 Severe degenerative joint disease of a cervical articular process joint in a dog. The joint space is irregular and poorly visualized. Marked periarticular osteophytosis results in a classic myelographic extradural lesion resulting in spinal cord compression from dorsal. Less severe changes without spinal cord compression are also noted, associated with adjacent articular process joints. (Courtesy of Dr Marc-André d'Anjou)

RADIOGRAPHIC FINDINGS Thin, bone opaque lines are seen in the vertebral canal, delineating the outer margin of the spinal cord, which is normally not radiographically visible. Because of the resemblance to positive contrast medium in the subarachnoid space, this finding is occasionally referred to as an 'auto myelogram'.

7.3.4 Intervertebral disc disease

The intervertebral discs are located between adjacent vertebral bodies and consist of a central nucleus pulposus and a surrounding annulus fibrosus. Displacement of intervertebral disc material from its normal location is termed 'intervertebral disc herniation' (IVDH). Several different types have been reported.

Intervertebral disc extrusion (Hansen type I IVDH)

This type of intervertebral disc herniation is characterized by acute onset of clinical signs, which are often severe. It is most commonly seen in small-breed (chondrodystrophic) dogs but may also affect cats and large-breed dogs. This condition has traditionally been attributed to progressive chondroid degeneration (dehydration and mineralization) of the nucleus pulposus with age.

RADIOGRAPHIC FINDINGS Degenerate mineralized nuclei pulposi appear as smoothly marginated structures of variable mineral opacity in a normal anatomic position (in situ) (Fig. 7.29; see also Fig. 7.8). This is an incidental finding.

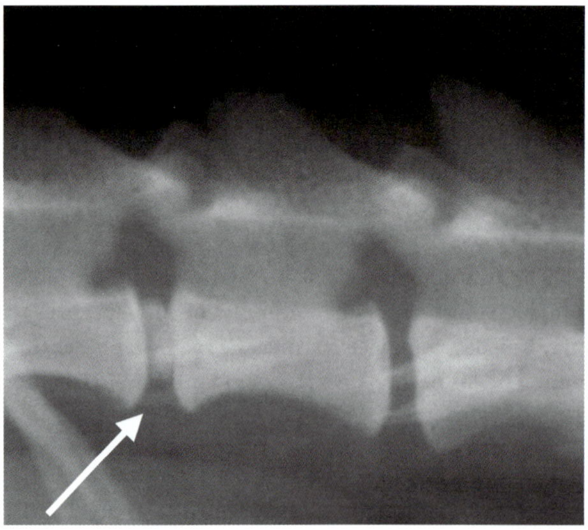

Fig. 7.29 In situ mineralization of a nucleus pulposus in a chondrodystrophic dog. There is smooth focal mineralization in the central area of the degenerate intervertebral disc (arrow). The intervertebral disc space is of normal width, and there is no evidence of abnormal material within the vertebral canal. This is a common finding not associated with clinical signs.

With intervertebral disc extrusion there is an acute rupture of the annulus fibrosus, and some or all of the mineralized nucleus pulposus material explosively enters the vertebral canal. This results in acute spinal cord contusion and often in spinal cord compression caused by herniated intervertebral disc material and associated haemorrhage. This type of disc herniation predominantly occurs in the area of the thoracolumbar junction but can affect any area of the spine.

Radiographic findings Survey radiographs may show generalized or wedge-shaped narrowing of the intervertebral disc space and narrowing of the articular process joint spaces (Fig. 7.30 and 7.31a,b). There is loss of the normal horse head appearance of the intervertebral foramen, which will have a different shape and often a smaller size compared to neighbouring foramina. Extrusion of mineralized material into the vertebral canal may result in a focal region of increased opacity (Fig. 7.30), occasionally resembling a mushroom cloud.

Even if a site suspicious for intervertebral disc herniation is identified on survey radiographs, additional imaging (myelography or, if available, CT or MRI) is indicated to allow evaluation for concurrent spinal cord swelling in addition to the expected finding of an extradural compressive lesion (Fig. 7.31c; see also Fig. 7.13), identify lesions not seen on survey radiographs (including additional sites of disc herniation), allow for surgical planning (length and laterality of a lesion), and to rule out a surgical indication in cases of noncompressive disc herniation (see 'Other types of intervertebral disc herniation', below).

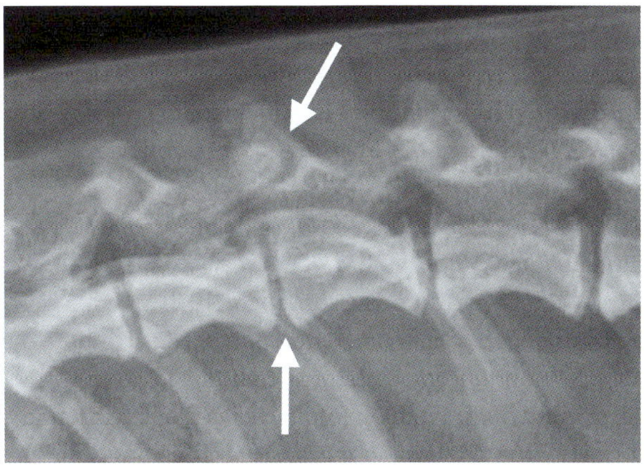

Fig. 7.30 Acute intervertebral disc extrusion in a chondrodystrophic dog. The intervertebral disc space and the joint space of the articular facet joint at T12–13 are narrowed (arrows). The shape of the intervertebral foramen at this level differs from neighbouring foramina and is partially obscured by the presence of mineralized material within the vertebral canal.

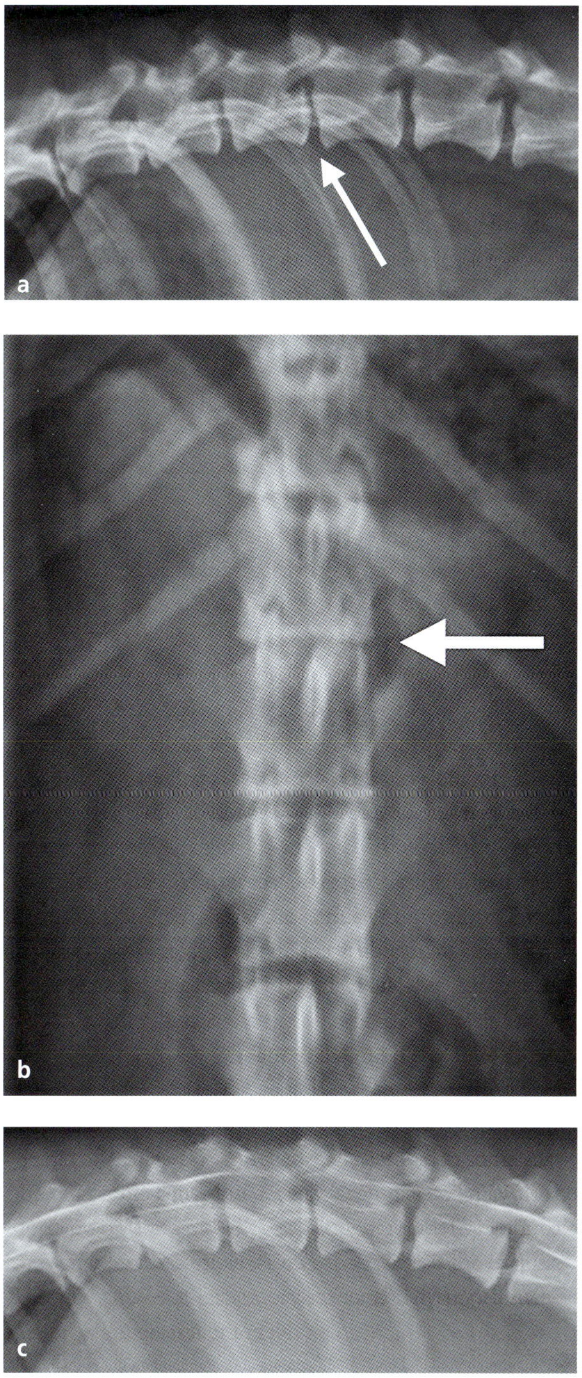

Fig. 7.31 Acute intervertebral disc extrusion in a dog. a, b Lateral and ventrodorsal survey radiographs show wedge-shaped narrowing of the T13–L1 intervertebral disc space (arrow) with a small amount of opaque material visible in the ventral aspect of the intervertebral foramen. Note also in situ mineralization of other thoracolumbar intervertebral discs, most notably at T11–12. c The myelographic study shows elevation of the ventral contrast column at the level of T13–L1. The subarachnoid space and thus the contrast columns are attenuated cranially to the cranial aspect of T13 due to spinal cord swelling and/or extension of extradural compressive material (e.g. haemorrhage).

Intervertebral disc protrusion (Hansen type II IVDH)

This type of intervertebral disc disease is predominantly seen in large-breed dogs and has traditionally been attributed to fibroid degeneration (note that recent literature indicates that intervertebral disc degeneration in both chondrodystrophic and non-chondrodystrophic dogs is characterized by chondroid metaplasia). The annulus fibrosus weakens, its dorsal aspect may protrude more and more into the vertebral canal, and over time this may result in slowly progressive spinal cord compression. Clinical signs are usually chronic and often milder than with intervertebral disc extrusion. As this degenerative disease process typically affects more than one intervertebral disc, identification of the most clinically significant site may be challenging.

RADIOGRAPHIC FINDINGS Narrowing of both the intervertebral disc space and the articular process joints is usually noted. Owing to the chronic nature of the disease process, concurrent degenerative spinal changes are common, and include subchondral sclerosis, irregular margination of vertebral endplates and spondylosis deformans (Fig. 7.32).

Even though radiographic abnormalities are similar to those seen with chronic discospondylitis, changes are usually milder, and there is no evidence of an aggressive bone lesion.

Myelography demonstrates often multifocal extradural lesions dorsal to affected intervertebral discs, usually with rather mild focal attenuation of the contrast columns. Spinal cord swelling with marked attenuation of the contrast columns, seen with acute disc extrusions, is not observed with this condition.

Other types of intervertebral disc herniation

Two types of acute extrusion of non-mineralized disc material have been recently reported. With **hydrated nucleus pulposus extrusion** (HNPE) there is spinal cord compression due to the presence of nondegenerate intervertebral disc material within the vertebral canal. On survey radiographs, narrowed intervertebral disc and joint spaces and an altered shape of the intervertebral foramen may be seen, as with other extrusions. However, there is no evidence of mineralized material within the vertebral canal. A myelogram will demonstrate an extradural compressive lesion. **Acute noncompressive nucleus pulposus extrusion** (ANNPE) is also associated with acute, explosive extrusion of nondegenerate intervertebral disc material. However, in contrast to other types, disc material is distributed within the vertebral canal and does not result in a spinal cord compressive lesion. This type of disc herniation has also been termed **'Hansen type III'** or **'traumatic'** disc herniation. Survey radiographs may show similar abnormalities to those seen with HNPE. A myelographic examination may be normal or may show a focal intramedullary lesion due to spinal cord contusion. In these instances, imaging findings may not allow differentiation from vascular accidents (fibrocartilaginous embolism). Mild focal contrast medium extravasation from the subarachnoid space may be seen if meningeal injury has occurred (Fig. 7.33).

Intradural (intramedullary or intradural-extramedullary) herniation of disc material is uncommon but may pose a diagnostic challenge. Myelography may show an

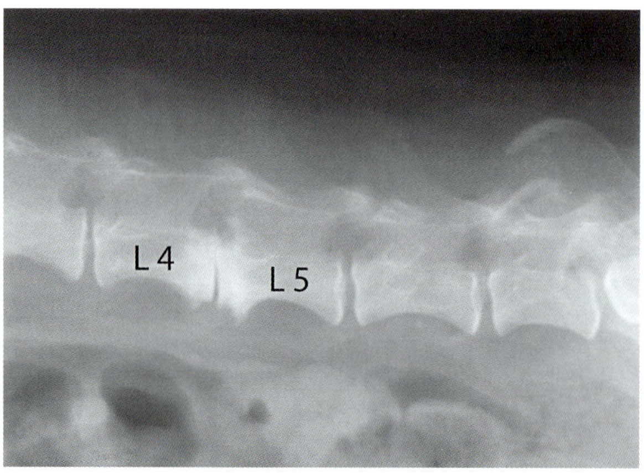

Fig. 7.32 Chronic spinal degenerative changes secondary to intervertebral disc protrusion in a dog. On this lateral radiograph of the lumbar spine, there is near-complete collapse of the L4–5 intervertebral disc space, with subchondral sclerosis, irregular endplate margination and ventral spondylosis deformans. Myelography or cross-sectional imaging would be necessary for full evaluation of the degree of disc herniation and to assess for spinal cord compression.

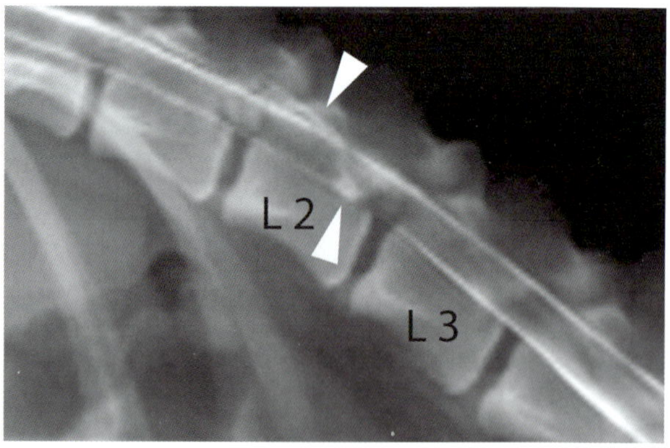

Fig. 7.33 Acute noncompressive nucleus pulposus extrusion in a dog. The L2–3 intervertebral disc space is mildly narrowed and wedge-shaped. There is very mild attenuation of the contrast columns dorsal to this disc space without evidence of a spinal cord compressive lesion. Note mild contrast medium extravasation into the epidural space cranial to the site of disc herniation due to meningeal injury (arrowheads). Post-myelographic CT or MRI could be considered to further evaluate this patient and assess for any spinal cord injury.

intramedullary lesion, intradural-extramedullary lesion and/or contrast medium extravasation into the epidural space or spinal cord parenchyma.

Lateral extrusion of intervertebral disc material (**foraminal disc herniation**) may also be diagnostically challenging and is usually not identified by means of myelography, due to location of the herniated disc material in relation to the subarachnoid space. In rare instances, a (presumptive) diagnosis can be made on survey radiographs; however, CT or MRI are needed for a definitive diagnosis.

The so-called **'Schmorl's node'** is a special type of intervertebral disc disease. It is usually a chronic condition which is very common in humans but less common in animals. With this condition there is progressive intervertebral disc space narrowing, usually slowly over time. The firm nucleus pulposus protrudes into the vertebral endplates, which results in concave defects in the vertebral endplates. This type of intervertebral disc herniation does not result in spinal cord compression and is usually considered an incidental finding.

7.3.5 Cervical spondylomyelopathy (CSM; 'wobbler syndrome')

Cervical spondylomyelopathy (aka wobbler syndrome, cervical vertebral instability, cervical spondylolisthesis, caudal cervical subluxation, caudal cervical malformation/malarticulation and cervical canal stenosis) is a cover term for a variety of developmental and degenerative processes of the caudal cervical spine all of which result in stenotic narrowing of the vertebral canal and static or dynamic compression of the spinal cord. Two major categories are recognized. **Disc associated CSM** predominantly affects middle-aged large-breed dogs. Doberman Pinschers are predisposed. This category includes intervertebral disc protrusion with or without hypertrophy of the dorsal longitudinal ligament and/or the ligamentum flavum. **Osseous associated CSM** is mostly seen in young adult giant-breed dogs (e.g. Great Danes). With this condition there is bony proliferation of the vertebral arch, articular processes and/or articular facets and pedicles.

The following may be seen alone or in combination in dogs with cervical spinal myelopathy.

- Cervical subluxation (Fig. 7.34a).
- Hypertrophy of the ligamentum flavum (Fig. 7.34b).
- Hypertrophy of the dorsal aspect of the annulus fibrosus and/or the dorsal longitudinal ligament (Fig. 7.34b).
- Intervertebral disc protrusion (Fig. 7.34c).
- Malformation and malarticulation of the vertebral bodies, articular process joints and vertebral arches (Fig. 7.34d).

Radiographic findings Depending on the aetiology and chronicity of the process, survey radiographs may reveal stenosis of the vertebral canal, abnormal vertebral shape, subluxation, narrowed and wedge-shaped intervertebral disc spaces as well as sclerosis of the vertebral endplates, spondylosis deformans and degenerative joint disease of the articular facet joints (Fig. 7.35).

Myelography allows assessment of presence, type, severity and extent of a compressive lesion and enables differentiation between static and dynamic lesions. Bony proliferation and herniated intervertebral disc material result in persistent static spinal cord compression (Fig. 7.36), while the degree of spinal cord compression changes with ligamentous hypertrophy or vertebral subluxation if flexion/extension or traction radiographs are obtained (Fig. 7.37 and 7.38). A combination of static and dynamic lesions is possible.

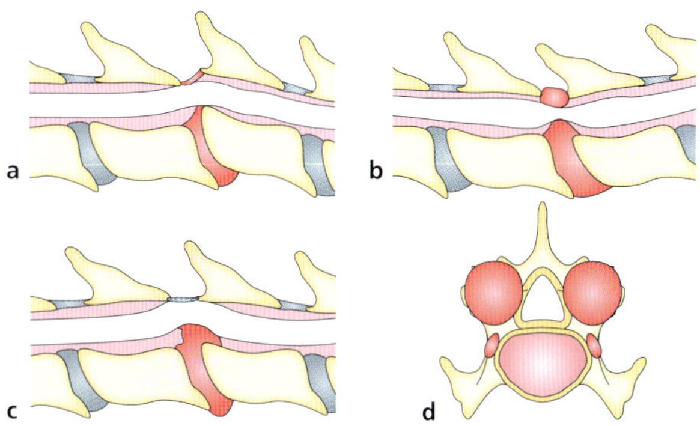

Fig. 7.34 Schematic illustration of possible changes seen with cervical spondylomyelopathy.
a Vertebral subluxation. Malalignment of cervical vertebrae results in compromise of the vertebral canal and spinal cord compression. This is commonly a dynamic lesion which changes if flexion and extension radiographs are obtained.
b Hypertrophy of the ligamentum flavum and the dorsal part of the annulus fibrosus and/or dorsal longitudinal ligament. These abnormalities result in dorsal and/or ventral compression of the spinal cord, respectively. In this example there is hourglass-shaped narrowing of the spinal cord. This type of spinal cord compression often improves with traction (dynamic lesion).
c Intervertebral disc herniation. Intervertebral disc material within the vertebral canal results in static spinal cord compression.
d Malformation and malarticulation of vertebral bodies, articular process joints and vertebral arches. In this example, hypertrophy of the articular processes results in static spinal cord compression from dorsal and lateral. This abnormality is typically not seen on lateral radiographs or a lateral myelogram and requires acquisition of ventrodorsal/dorsoventral and possibly oblique views.

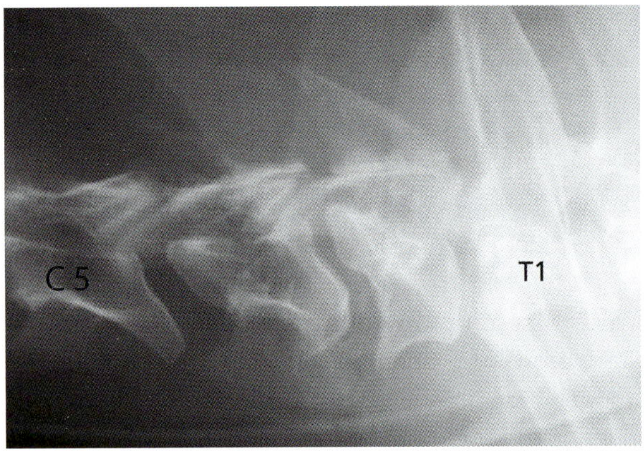

Fig. 7.35 Lateral radiograph of the caudal cervical spine in a dog with chronic caudal cervical spondylomyelopathy ('wobbler syndrome'). The seventh vertebral body is malformed and subluxated craniodorsally, resulting in stenotic narrowing of the vertebral canal. Narrowing of the C6–7 intervertebral disc space and ventral spondylosis deformans are also present. Note that changes in this dog are unusually severe, and that a diagnosis of cervical spondylomyelopathy is usually not possible solely based on survey radiographs.

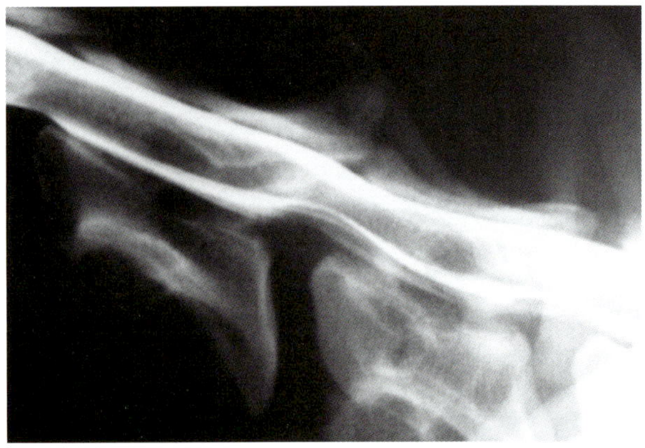

a

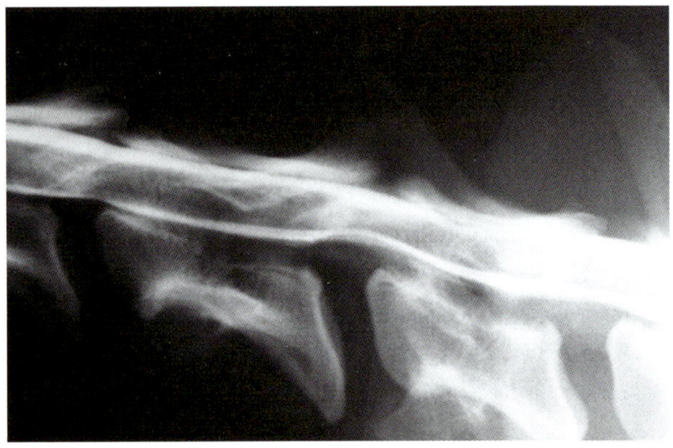

b

Fig. 7.36 Static spinal cord compression due to intervertebral disc protrusion.

a On the neutral lateral view there is a focal extradural compressive lesion at the level of the C5–6 intervertebral disc space.

b Appearance of the lesion and degree of spinal cord compression do not significantly change with traction.

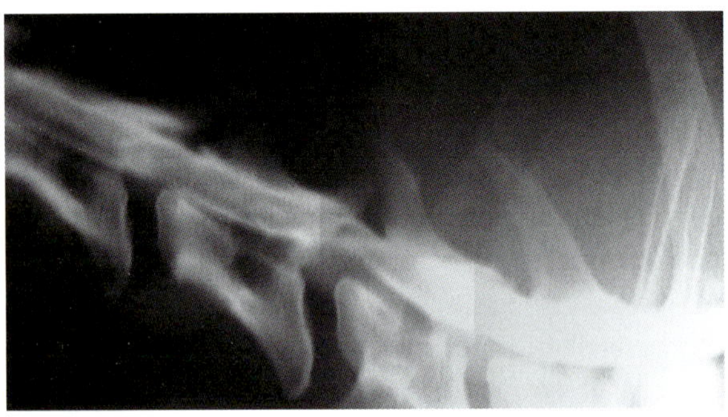

a

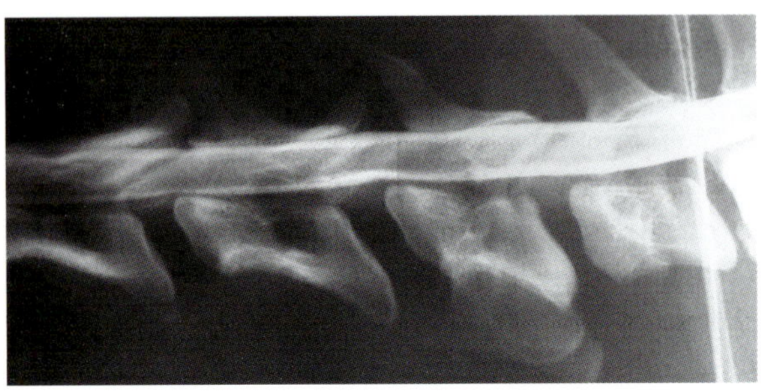

b

Fig. 7.37 Dynamic spinal cord compression due to hypertrophy of the dorsal longitudinal ligament.

a On the neutral lateral view, a focal extradural lesion resulting in marked spinal cord compression is seen dorsal to the C5–6 intervertebral disc space.

b Upon traction there is near-complete resolution of spinal cord compression, consistent with a dynamic lesion.

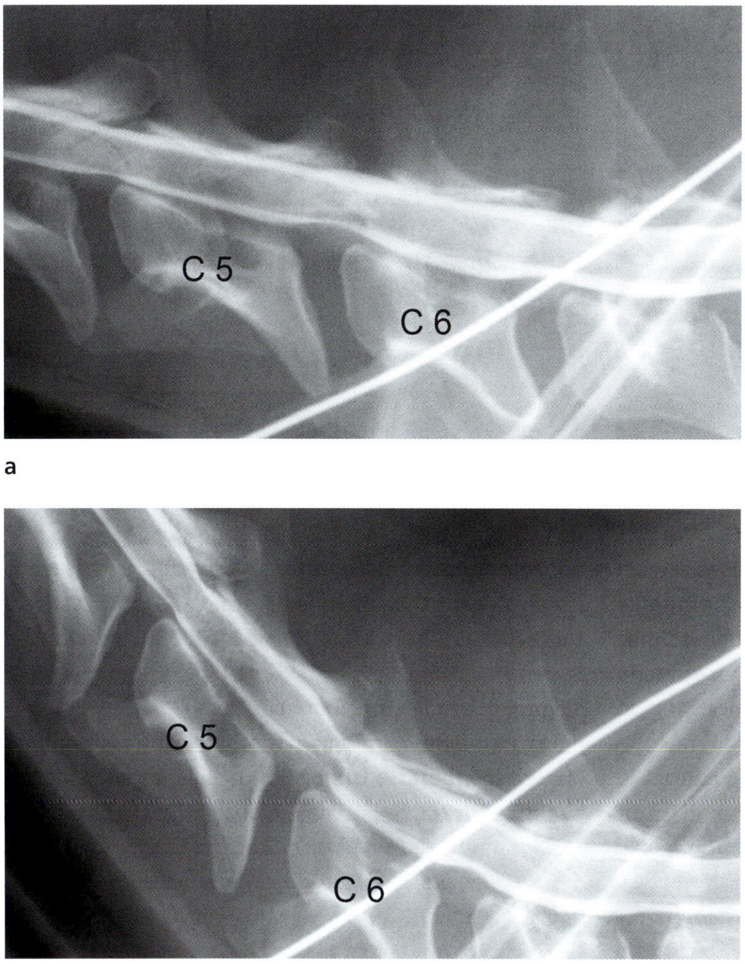

a

b

Fig. 7.38 Predominantly dynamic spinal cord compressive lesion.
a On the neutral view there is evidence of very mild dorsal elevation of the ventral contrast column dorsal to the C4–5, C5–6 and C6–7 intervertebral disc spaces without evidence of significant spinal cord compression.
b This extension view of the cervical spine shows moderate spinal cord compression at C5–6, from both dorsally and ventrally. There remains mild dorsal deviation of the ventral contrast column at C4–5 and C6–7, which is of uncertain significance and may be incidental.

Static and dynamic lesions may differ in regard to therapeutic options and prognosis. Depending on clinician preference, stress views may be acquired in the frame of a myelogram to allow a more detailed assessment of the nature of a compressive lesion. Especially if neutral radiographs do not show a compressive lesion, or if the degree of compression is incompatible with the severity of the clinical signs, flexion and extension radiographs may aid in the identification of a dynamic lesion. If a compressive lesion is identified on neutral views, a traction view may help in lesion classification as static or dynamic. Please note that spinal stress views are controversial and even considered contraindicated by some. As mentioned under atlantoaxial instability above, extreme care must be taken when performing these procedures.

7.3.6 Degenerative lumbosacral stenosis ('cauda equina syndrome')

'Cauda equina' refers to the bundle of nerves located within the lumbar and sacral vertebral canal caudal to the termination of the spinal cord (lumbar, sacral and caudal nerves). Degenerative lumbosacral stenosis (aka cauda equina compression, lumbosacral malarticulation and malformation, lumbosacral disease, lumbosacral stenosis and lumbosacral instability) is a cover term for a variety of dynamic and/or static compressive lesions of the lumbosacral junction. German Shepherd dogs and structurally related breeds are particularly susceptible to this condition. Similar to cervical spondylomyelopathy, degenerative lumbosacral stenosis may also be caused by a variety of abnormalities, as follows.

- Intervertebral disc protrusion.
- Subluxation/instability with ventral displacement of the sacral lamina and with or without new bone proliferation (articular facet degenerative joint disease, lateralized spondylosis deformans).
- Hypertrophy of the spinal ligaments (especially interarcuate and dorsal longitudinal ligament) and synovial joint capsule.
- Malformation of the vertebra, articular processes and/or vertebral arches with resultant spinal stenosis.
- Stenosis of the lumbosacral intervertebral foramina.
- Vertebral anomalies including transitional vertebrae and sacral osteochondrosis.

Other diseases affecting the caudal lumbar spine and lumbosacral junction (e.g. spinal or paraspinal neoplasia, trauma or discospondylitis) can result in clinical signs similar to degenerative lumbosacral stenosis.

RADIOGRAPHIC FINDINGS A radiographic diagnosis of degenerative lumbosacral stenosis is challenging at best. Many dogs, especially older ones, have incidental degenerative changes of the lumbosacral junction. On the other hand, dogs with relatively minor radiographic changes may exhibit severe clinical signs.

Survey radiographs may allow a diagnosis of lumbosacral subluxation, vertebral canal stenosis, change in shape of the intervertebral foramina, ventral and lateral spondylosis deformans, and degenerative joint disease of the lumbosacral articular facet joints (Fig. 7.39a).

As the subarachnoid space terminates cranial to the area of interest in many dogs, myelography is usually of limited value in the evaluation of lumbosacral abnormalities. If the subarachnoid space extends to the level of the sacrum, myelography may be helpful in the identification and characterization of a compressive lesion.

Based on CT studies it is known that the lumbosacral intervertebral disc may occupy a large proportion of the vertebral canal in normal dogs without resulting in clinical signs. Thus, the radiographic findings have to be carefully weighed against a given patient's clinical signs.

Occasionally, flexion and extension radiographs may aid in identification of a dynamic lesion (Fig. 7.39b). Caution should again be exercised when performing stress views.

CT and MRI are advantageous compared to conventional imaging modalities due to their ability to evaluate soft tissues, intervertebral foramina and nerve roots. These cross-sectional imaging modalities should thus be given preference in the diagnostic workup of a patient suspected to have degenerative lumbosacral stenosis. Other previously used radiographic contrast procedures (epidurography and discography) are considered irrelevant today.

7.3.7 Inflammatory conditions of the spine

Inflammatory spinal disorders may affect the intervertebral discs, vertebrae, spinal cord, epidural space and meninges. A diagnosis of advanced/chronic intervertebral disc or vertebral inflammation is possible on survey radiographs. Myelography is uncommonly performed in patients with inflammatory spinal conditions but may allow identification of spinal cord compression in disease processes involving the vertebral canal.

Discospondylitis

Infection of the intervertebral discs and adjacent vertebral endplates is most commonly seen in young adult, large-breed, male dogs, but may affect other animals. Bacterial aetiology is most common (*Staphylococcus aureus*, *Streptococcus* spp., *Brucella canis*, *Escherichia coli*, etc.), although fungal organisms (e.g. Aspergillus spp.) should also be considered, especially in endemic areas. The infection typically occurs via haematogenous spread of septic emboli from a site of prior infection (commonly urogenital tract, heart, teeth or skin). Migration of foreign bodies, bite wounds or iatrogenic contamination (e.g. in the frame of spinal surgery), may also result in discospondylitis. Even though the lumbosacral junction and mid-thoracic spine are most commonly affected, any intervertebral disc may be involved, and the disease process is often multifocal.

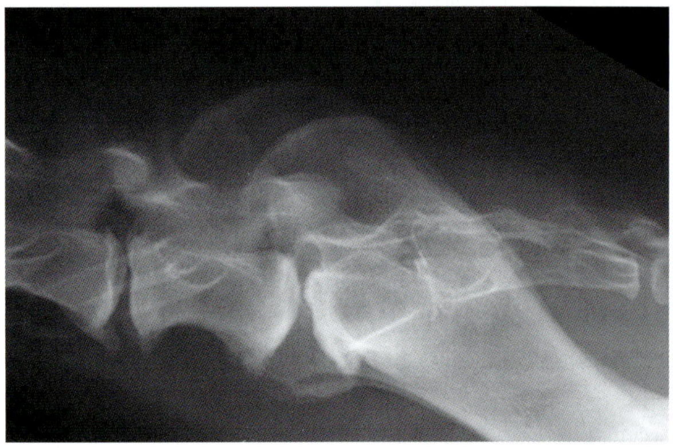

a

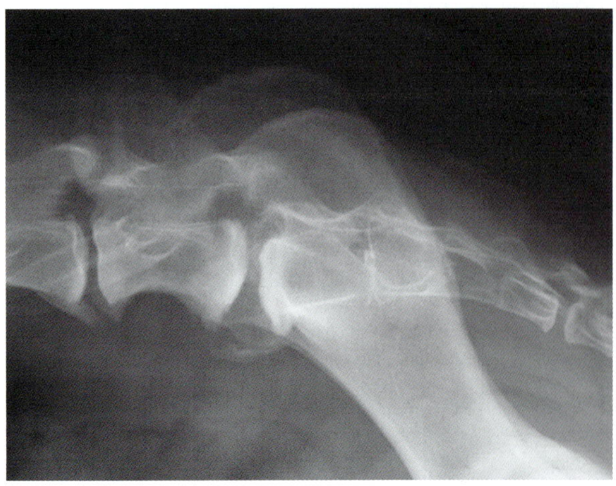

b

Fig. 7.39 Degenerative lumbosacral stenosis in a dog with a transitional lumbosacral vertebra.
a The neutral view shows subluxation at the lumbosacral junction with marked narrowing of the vertebral canal diameter, obliteration of the intervertebral foramen, wedge-shaped narrowing of the intervertebral disc space, vertebral endplate sclerosis and ventral spondylosis deformans.
b The degree of subluxation worsens with flexion of the spine.

Radiographic findings As the infection originates from the intervertebral disc and subsequently spreads to the vertebral endplates, there is often a significant delay between the onset of clinical signs and evidence of radiographic abnormalities (10–30 days!). Early discospondylitis is characterized by irregular lytic changes affecting the endplates of adjacent vertebrae, followed by progressive periosteal proliferation, subchondral sclerosis and narrowing of the intervertebral disc space (Fig. 7.40 and 7.41).

Weakening of the intervertebral disc may result in spinal instability and, in severe cases, subluxation. With chronic discospondylitis the intervertebral disc space often collapses, and there is progressive bridging spondylosis deformans (Fig. 7.41).

Similar to the discrepancy between onset of clinical signs and visibility of radiographic changes, there is also a time delay between clinical improvement and radiographic healing. Even with complete resolution of clinical signs, radiographic abnormalities may progress for several more weeks.

Physitis

Infection of vertebral physes is an occasional finding in young animals with open growth plates. The predilection for large-breed dogs, pathophysiology, clinical symptoms and time course are comparable to discospondylitis.

Radiographic findings Changes are centred on a growth plate rather than the intervertebral disc space but overall are similar to those seen with discospondylitis. The physis is initially widened. Mixed osteolytic and osteoproliferative changes are subsequently noted associated with the adjacent metaphysis and epiphysis. The affected vertebra is often foreshortened, and spinal instability is a possible sequela, as with discospondylitis (Fig. 7.42).

Osteomyelitis

Vertebral osteomyelitis is rather rare. Radiographic changes are similar to those described for the appendicular skeleton (see section 17.2).

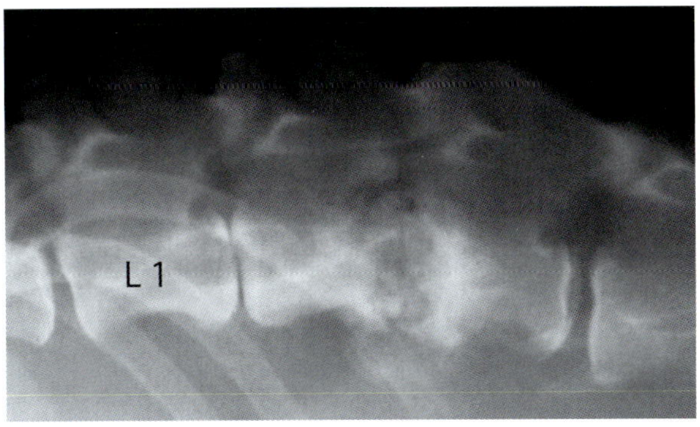

a

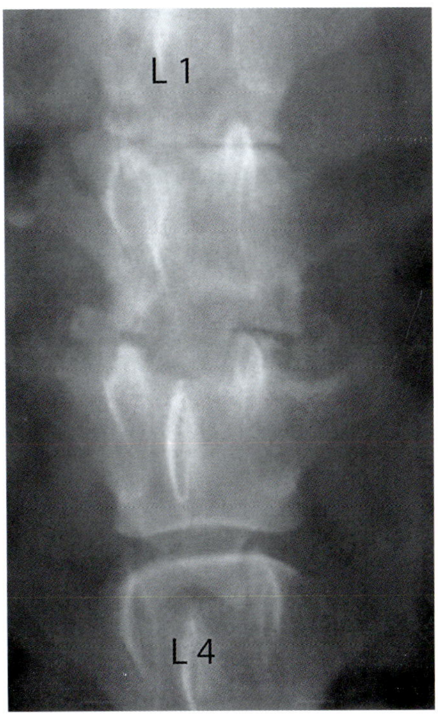

b

Fig. 7.40 Advanced, active discospondylitis in a dog. Lateral a and ventrodorsal b radiographs demonstrate collapse of the L2–3 intervertebral disc space, with moth-eaten lytic regions in the adjacent vertebral endplates and adjacent irregular, heterogeneous vertebral body sclerosis. Early spondylosis deformans formation is noted ventral and lateral to the intervertebral disc space. The intervertebral disc space L1–2 is also narrowed, without evidence of vertebral endplate changes.

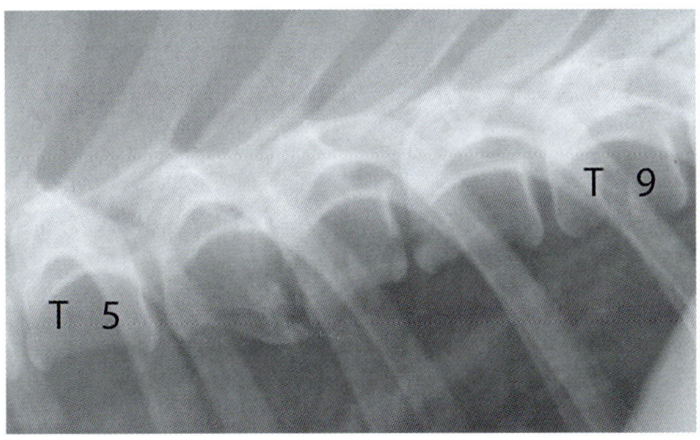

Fig. 7.41 Discospondylitis in a dog. The T6–7 intervertebral disc space is narrowed and ventrally bridged by smooth spondylosis deformans. The vertebral endplates are mildly irregular in contour but sharply marginated. This lesion is chronic and appears inactive. The intervertebral disc space T7–8 is also mildly narrowed and there is mild vertebral endplate lysis on both sides of the disc space. At this point there is no evidence of periosteal new bone formation. These findings are consistent with early, active discospondylitis at this site.

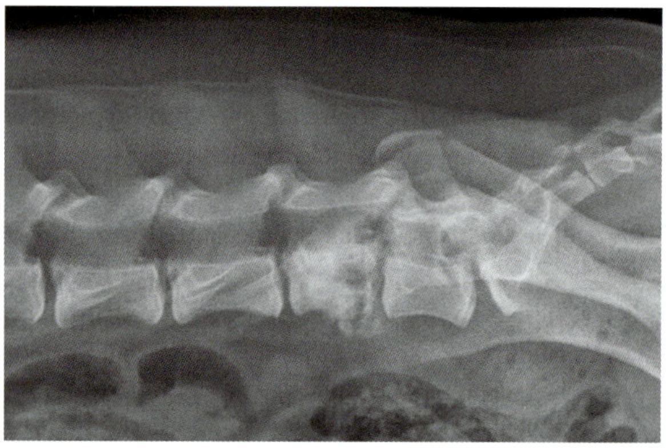

Fig. 7.42 Septic physitis of the caudal physis of the sixth lumbar vertebra in a dog. The physis is irregularly widened, the adjacent vertebral body is sclerotic, and irregular and ill-defined periosteal new bone formation is seen associated with the ventral aspect of the vertebral body as well as in the plane of the vertebral canal. Foreshortening of the vertebra and spinal subluxation are also evident.

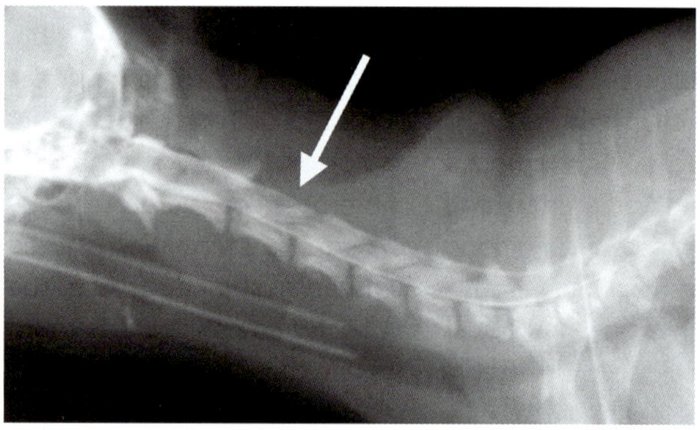

Fig. 7.43 Spinal cord granuloma in a 3-year-old dog. Myelography shows mild spinal cord swelling at the level of C3 and C4 with associated attenuation of the dorsal contrast column (arrow). The suspected intramedullary lesion was confirmed surgically. Histopathology yielded a diagnosis of granuloma of undetermined aetiology.

Myelitis and meningitis

Inflammation of the spinal cord and meninges does not result in radiographic abnormalities visible on survey radiographs.

Myelography is also often normal, especially in acute cases. If the disease process results in spinal cord swelling (e.g. granuloma, syrinx) an intramedullary lesion will be evident (Fig. 7.43). Meningeal adhesions seen in cases of chronic meningitis, or accumulation of inflammatory debris within the subarachnoid space, will result in focal or multifocal attenuation of the contrast columns (see Fig. 7.20f).

> Meningitis and meningomyelitis are contraindications for myelography due to the risk of a massive exacerbation of clinical signs. If there is clinical suspicion of these conditions, a CSF analysis must be performed prior to planning a contrast procedure.

7.3.8 Spinal trauma

Trauma to the spine may result in vertebral lesions and/or injury of the adjacent soft tissues including the spinal cord.

Vertebral fracture and (sub)luxation

These are often visible on survey radiographs (Fig. 7.44). Radiographic findings may include fracture lines, bone fragments, vertebral dislocation, narrowing of the vertebral canal, foreshortening of a vertebral body (compression fracture), abnormal widening of interval vertebral disc or joint spaces, and abnormal alignment between vertebrae. It is important to note that subtle or nondisplaced lesions may not be noted on survey radiographs, potentially necessitating advanced imaging for further evaluation.

Especially if a lesion is not immediately evident on a lateral view, orthogonal radiographs must be obtained (Fig. 7.45). In many cases of spinal trauma, and especially for surgical planning, advanced imaging (CT or MRI) is indicated. Myelography may substitute in select cases if cross-sectional imaging is unavailable. Stress views should be avoided in trauma patients due to the risk of additional injury to the spinal cord in case of spinal instability.

A **myelography** is often unnecessary if a traumatic lesion is visible on survey radiographs. However, it may yield additional information in cases of questionable spinal cord compression, identification of additional lesions not seen on survey radiographs, and determination of presence and degree of spinal cord and meningeal injury (see Fig. 7.20d). Myelography (or cross-sectional imaging) is also indicated if survey radiographs of the spine are normal but there is clinical suspicion of spinal cord injury/compression. Possible findings include extradural compressive lesions (dislocated fracture fragments or epidural haematoma), spinal cord swelling due to intramedullary haemorrhage or oedema, accumulation of contrast medium within the spinal cord due to rupture or myelomalacia, and leakage of contrast medium into the epidural space due to meningeal laceration.

Avulsion of the brachial plexus

This diagnosis is usually made based on clinical examination findings, rather than diagnostic imaging. A ventrodorsal view of the cervical spine may potentially show widening of the intervertebral disc spaces on the side of brachial plexus avulsion due to lack of muscle innerva-

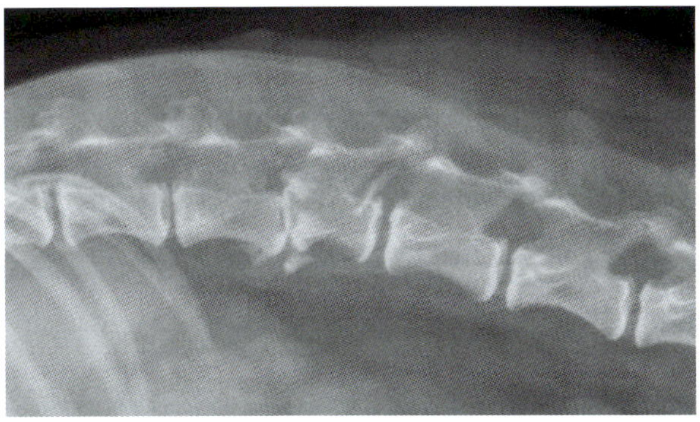

Fig. 7.44 Compression fracture of the third lumbar vertebra and L2–3 subluxation in a dog. The vertebral body of L3 is foreshortened and has an abnormal contour. Numerous small bone fragments are present in the vicinity of the abnormal vertebra. The cranial endplate of L3 is dorsally displaced compared to the caudal endplate of L2 (subluxation), and the intervertebral disc space is collapsed at this level. Note bone fragments superimposed with the L2–3 and L3–4 intervertebral foramina, the exact location of which cannot be determined on this single lateral view.

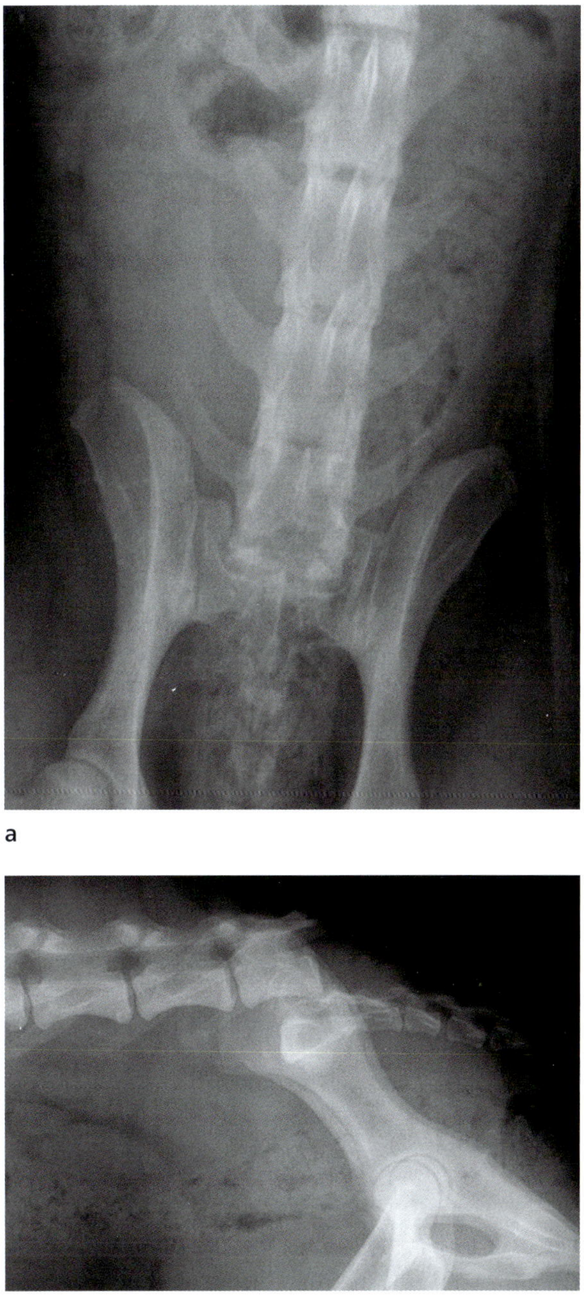

a

b

Fig. 7.45 Lumbosacral luxation with severe displacement. While the lesion is difficult to identify on the ventrodorsal view a, cranial and ventral luxation of the sacrum is clearly evident on the lateral view b. This example underlines the need for two orthogonal projections when evaluating the spine.

tion and resultant decreased muscle tone. Myelography is often inconclusive but in combination with computed tomography may allow visualization of asymmetric filling defects of the subarachnoid space at the site of injury.

7.3.9 Spinal neoplasia

Spinal neoplasms can be subdivided into extradural, intradural-extramedullary and intramedullary, depending on their tissue of origin and location.

Extradural tumours

Most extradural tumours are of vertebral origin. Primary bone tumours such as osteosarcoma, fibrosarcoma, chondrosarcoma or haemangiosarcoma, and some other tumour types (plasma cell tumour) are typically limited to one vertebra (monostotic tumour). Examples of polyostotic spinal tumours include metastases, lymphosarcoma and multiple myeloma. Most vertebral tumours result in osteolytic and/or osteoproliferative changes of the affected vertebra/vertebrae (Fig. 7.46 and 7.47). Secondary pathological (compression) fractures are fairly common. Paraspinal soft-tissue neoplasia or epidural neoplasia of non-bony origin are not visible on survey radiographs. Myelography is helpful in the identification and characterization of an extradural tumour and allows improved evaluation of lesion extent and presence of spinal cord compression.

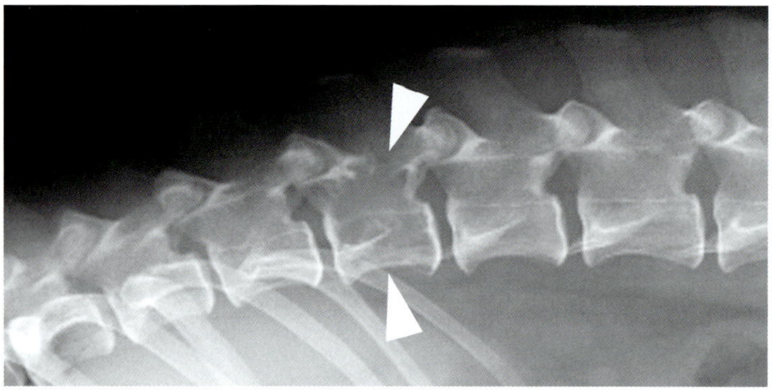

Fig. 7.46 Extensive lysis of the first lumbar vertebra due to a spinal tumour (plasma cell tumour). There is generalized decreased opacity of the vertebral body and arch (arrowheads). The ventral and dorsal margins of the vertebral canal are thin and partially disrupted compared to adjacent vertebrae.

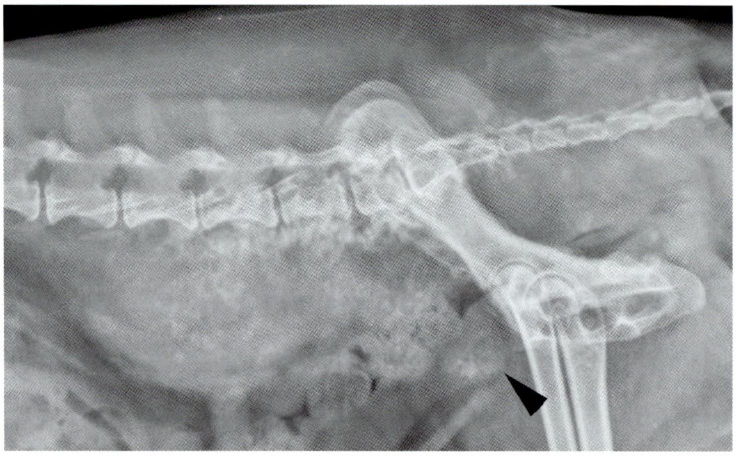

Fig. 7.47 Prostatic carcinoma with metastases to lymph nodes and vertebrae. The prostate is enlarged for a neutered dog and shows mineralization (arrowhead). Extensive, irregularly marginated and variable opacity periosteal new bone formation is associated with the vertebral bodies of the caudal lumbar and the sacral vertebrae. The sublumbar lymph nodes are severely enlarged and mineralized.

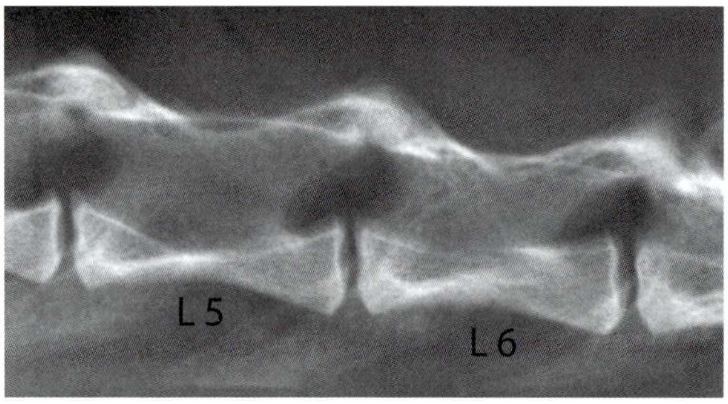

Fig. 7.48 Intramedullary tumour (lymphoma) in a cat. On this lateral view there is evidence of widening of the vertebral canal at the level of the fifth lumbar vertebra, with thinning of the vertebral body due to pressure atrophy and dorsal elevation of the vertebral arch. There is no evidence of an aggressive bone lesion.

Intradural-extramedullary tumours

Meningiomas, nerve sheath tumours and other types of intradural-extramedullary neoplasia do not usually result in visible changes on survey radiographs, with the exception of potential pressure atrophy of a vertebral body and/or vertebral arch adjacent to a slow growing tumour, which may cause focal widening of the vertebral canal or intervertebral foramen on radiographs. Myelography is usually rewarding and demonstrates the classic findings of widening and splitting of the contrast columns with a focal golf tee sign bordering the lesion (see Fig. 7.20c).

Intramedullary tumours

Survey radiographs in gliomas, ependymomas, lymphoma, metastases and other intramedullary tumours are also typically normal. However, as described above for intradural-extramedullary tumours, they may be associated with focal widening of the vertebral canal in the case of a slow growing mass (Fig. 7.48). Myelography shows focal widening of the spinal cord and circumferential attenuation of the subarachnoid space, characteristic for an intramedullary lesion (see Fig. 7.20b).

7.3.10 Other spinal diseases

Numerous genetic, congenital, metabolic, endocrine and nutritional bone diseases may affect the spine and/or other skeletal structures. This section will focus on a few select disease processes that are interesting from a neuroradiology perspective.

Calcinosis circumscripta

This is a fairly rare condition characterized by ectopic soft-tissue mineralization secondary to deposition of calcium salts. It is most commonly seen in young, large-breed dogs. Spinal lesions are less common than abnormalities in other areas (e.g. hind limbs and tongue) but have been reported in association with transverse processes of the cervical spine.

Calcinosis circumscripta is usually an incidental finding; however, compromise of spinal mobility or pressure on adjacent structures (muscles, bones or nerve roots) can result in clinical signs such as pain.

RADIOGRAPHIC FINDINGS A well-circumscribed, round or ovoid, granular bone opacity lesion is associated with the paraspinal soft tissues.

Multiple cartilaginous exostoses (MCE)

These are benign bony proliferations of undetermined aetiology which may develop in association with vertebrae and/or other bones. They are found in young dogs and cats. They are initially fast growing, but growth ceases with skeletal maturity. MCEs originate from the metaphyses of bones formed by endochondral ossification but may be associated with the diaphyseal region at the time of diagnosis due to continued longitudinal bone growth.

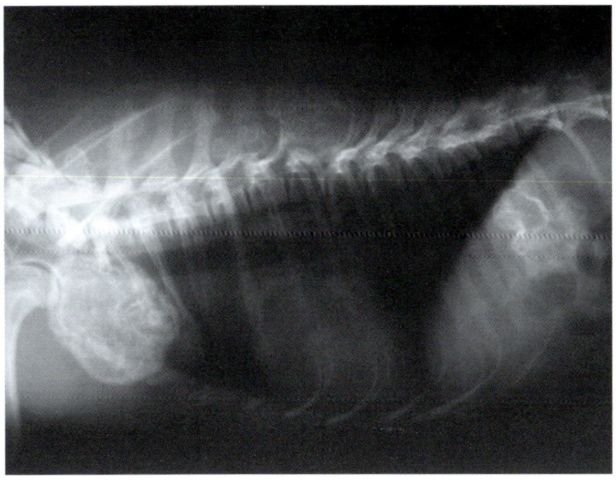

a

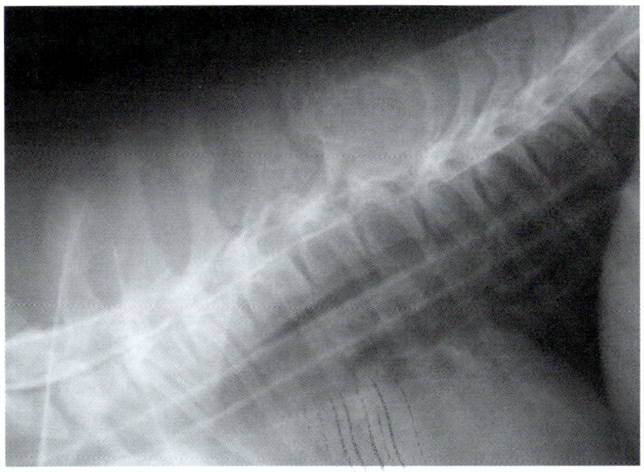

b

Fig. 7.49 Multiple cartilaginous exostoses in an 8-month-old Yorkshire Terrier.

a There are multiple large, expansile, well-circumscribed, cauliflower-like bony masses associated with ribs as well as thoracic spinous processes.

b On myelography there is attenuation of especially the dorsal contrast column in the mid-thoracic spine. This is consistent with an extradural compressive lesion caused by extension of exostosis into the vertebral canal.

RADIOGRAPHIC FINDINGS Exostoses manifest as rounded, expansile, cauliflower-like lesions with a smooth, thin cortical shell. If associated with the spine they may extend into the vertebral canal and result in spinal cord compression (Fig. 7.49).

Osteopetrosis/osteosclerosis

Osteopetrosis is a rare and poorly described condition in dogs and cats resulting from failure of or insufficient osteoclastic bone resorption.

There are several reports of an acquired form of 'osteopetrosis' in cats (e.g. secondary to feline leukaemia virus [FeLV] infection, myeloproliferative diseases, lupus erythematosus, lymphosarcoma). Due to differences in pathophysiology between this condition and osteopetrosis in humans, it is better referred to as 'osteosclerosis'.

RADIOGRAPHIC FINDINGS There is increased radiographic opacity of the medullary cavities of long bones, possibly associated with cortical thickening.

Mucopolysaccharidoses

Mucopolysaccharidoses are a group of genetic lysosomal storage diseases. Different subtypes may result in variable lesions of the musculoskeletal system.

RADIOGRAPHIC FINDINGS Depending on the subtype, affected animals may display facial deformities, signs of generalized epiphyseal dysplasia resulting in growth disturbances and skeletal deformities, osteopenia, vertebral fusion, and spinal cord compression secondary to vertebral bony proliferations.

Congenital hypothyroidism

This rare condition in dogs and cats is characterized by disproportional dwarfism.

RADIOGRAPHIC FINDINGS In addition to abnormalities of long bones, there is evidence of incomplete and delayed ossification of the vertebral epiphyses, with shortening and widening of the vertebral bodies (Fig. 7.50).

Osteopenia

Osteopenia results in decreased radiopacity of bones, often associated with cortical thinning and coarse bone trabeculation. This finding may be associated with a variety of causes including hormonal imbalances (e.g. hyperadrenocorticism, primary or secondary hyperparathyroidism), malnutrition, metabolic conditions and ageing changes (see section 15.5). The abnormalities are often more easily

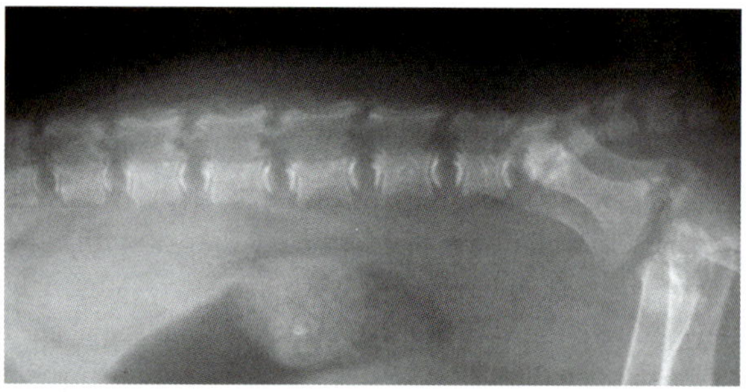

Fig. 7.50 Congenital hypothyroidism in a 6-month-old cat. On this lateral view there is incomplete and delayed ossification of the vertebral epiphyses as well as foreshortening and widening of the vertebral bodies. The physes of the pelvis and femora are open.

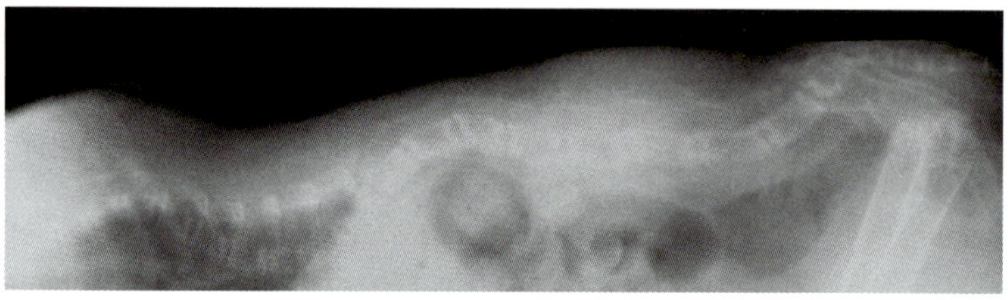

Fig. 7.51 Nutritional secondary hyperparathyroidism in a cat. There is generalized decreased bone opacity with cortical thinning. Foreshortening and deformity of several vertebrae results in spinal kyphosis and scoliosis. Concave defects in corresponding vertebral endplates are caused by pressure from the nuclei pulposi.

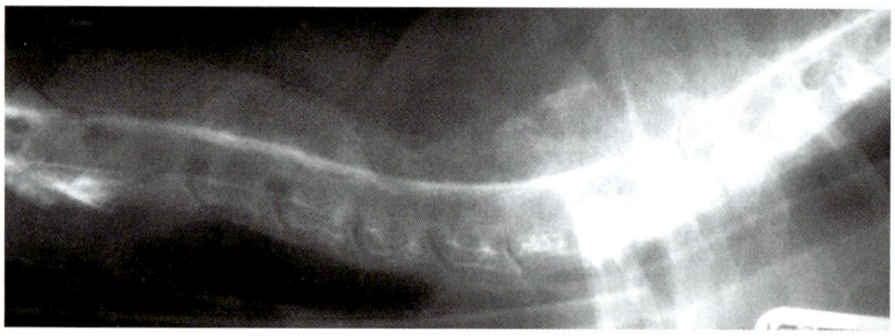

Fig. 7.52 Hypervitaminosis A in a cat. Extensive new bone formation (osteophytosis and enthesophytosis) is noted along the cervical spine, resulting in dorsal vertebral ankylosis. Individual spinous processes of the cervical vertebrae cannot be distinguished due to adjacent bone proliferation.

recognized in the long bones than in the spine. Generalized osteopenia associated with **nutritional secondary hyperparathyroidism**, however, typically results in notable spinal changes. This condition develops in young animals secondary to nutritional oversupply in phosphorus and/or undersupply in calcium (e.g. secondary to a meat-only diet). Malnutrition results in an increased release of parathyroid hormone and subsequent excessive bone resorption.

RADIOGRAPHIC FINDINGS There is generalized decreased bone opacity with cortical thinning (Fig. 7.51). Concurrent multifocal pathological fractures are common. Vertebral microfractures result in shortening and/or deformity of vertebrae, and in turn in an abnormal curvature of the spine (kyphosis, scoliosis, lordosis). Pressure of the firm nuclei pulposi on the thin vertebral endplates results in multifocal smooth indentations resembling Schmorl's nodes (see section 7.3.4).

Hypervitaminosis A

This condition is reported in cats and is related to a nutritional excess in vitamin A (e.g. liver diet). It is rarely diagnosed today.

RADIOGRAPHIC FINDINGS The most significant findings are extensive exostoses and enthesophytes associated with cervical and thoracic vertebrae, which in extreme cases may result in spinal ankylosis (Fig. 7.52). Extensive periarticular new bone formation associated especially with the shoulder and elbow joints is also common.

Joint associated cysts (synovial and ganglion cysts)

Cystic lesions associated with articular process joints are usually incidental, but on occasion may be large enough to extend into the vertebral canal and result in spinal cord compression. They are most commonly seen in the cervical spine of young adult, large-breed dogs (e.g. Bullmastiffs and Great Danes) and may cause clinical signs comparable to cervical spondylomyelopathy.

RADIOGRAPHIC FINDINGS Survey radiographs may be normal or show degenerative joint disease of the articular facet joints. A myelogram may demonstrate one or more extradural lesions originating from the articular processes, resulting in spinal cord compression from dorsolaterally. Cross-sectional imaging is typically necessary for further characterization of the lesions.

Intradural arachnoid (subarachnoid) diverticula

With these lesions there is focal dilatation of the subarachnoid space with accumulation of CSF and resultant spinal cord compression. The exact aetiology is unknown. In many cases the lesions appear to be congenital, while they may also be seen in association with other spinal conditions such as trauma, intervertebral disc herniation, hemivertebrae or articular process dysplasia. Cervical diverticula are more common in larger dogs, and Rottweilers are predisposed. Thoracolumbar diverticula are most commonly seen in small- and medium-breed dogs, and Pugs and French Bulldogs are predisposed.

RADIOGRAPHIC FINDINGS Survey radiographs are unremarkable. On myelography, the lesion manifests as a focal teardrop-shaped dilatation of the subarachnoid space resulting in a variable degree of spinal cord compression. Multifocal diverticula are possible but less common.

Suggested reading

Barone G, Ziemer LS, Shofer FS, Steinberg SA. Risk factors associated with development of seizures after use of iohexol for myelography in dogs: 182 cases (1998). J Am Vet Med Assoc 2002; 220: 1499–1502.

Bray JP, Burbidge HM. The canine intervertebral disk. Part Two: Degenerative changes – nonchondrodystrophoid versus chondrodystrophoid disks. J Am Anim Hosp Assoc 1998; 34: 135–44.

Brearley M. Tumoren des Nervensystems. In: Kessler M (ed.). Kleintieronkologie, 2nd edn. Stuttgart: Parey MVS 2005; 444–56.

Chang Y, Dennis R, Platt SR, Penderis J. Magnetic resonance imaging of traumatic intervertebral disc extrusion in dogs. Vet Rec 2007; 160: 795–9.

Da Costa RC, Parent JM, Dobson H. Incidence of and risk factors for seizures after myelography performed with iohexol in dogs: 503 cases (2002–2004). J Am Vet Med Assoc 2011; 238:1296–300.

Dewey CW, da Costa RC (eds). Practical Guide to Canine and Feline Neurology, 3rd edn. Ames: Wiley-Blackwell 2016.

Gaschen L, Lang J, Haeni H. Intravertebral disc herniation (Schmorl's node) in five dogs. Vet Radiol Ultrasound 1995; 36: 509–16.

Hecht S, Thomas WB, Marioni-Henry K, Echandi R, Matthews AR, Adams WH. Myelography vs. computed tomography in the evaluation of acute intervertebral disc extrusion in chondrodystrophic dogs. Vet Radiol Ultrasound 2009; 50: 353–9.

Johnson KA, Watson ADJ. Skeletal diseases. In: Ettinger SJ, Feldman EC (eds). Textbook of Veterinary Internal Medicine. Philadelphia: WB Saunders 2000; 1887–916.

Jurina K, Grevel V. Spinal arachnoid pseudocysts in 10 rottweilers. J Small Anim Pract 2004; 45: 9–15.

Kirberger RM, Wrigley RH. Myelography in the dog: Review of cases with contrast medium in the central canal. Vet Radiol Ultrasound 1993; 34: 253–8.

Levitski RE, Chauvet AE, Lipsitz D. Cervical myelopathy associated with extradural synovial cysts in 4 dogs. J Vet Intern Med 1999; 13: 181–6.

Lu D, Lamb CR, Targett MP. Results of myelography in seven dogs with myelomalacia. Vet Radiol Ultrasound 2002; 43: 326–30.

Mai W (ed.). Diagnostic MRI in Dogs and Cats. Boca Raton: CRC Press, Taylor and Francis Group 2018.

Roberts RE, Selcer BA. Myelography and epidurography. Vet Clin North Am Small Anim Pract 1993; 23: 307–29.

Robertson I, Thrall DE. Imaging dogs with suspected disc herniation: pros and cons of myelography, computed tomography, and magnetic resonance. Vet Radiol Ultrasound 2011; 52: 81–4.

Schwarz T, Saunders J (eds). Veterinary Computed Tomography. Ames: Wiley-Blackwell 2011.

Shamir MH, Tavor N, Aizenberg T. Radiographic findings during recovery from discospondylitis. Vet Radiol Ultrasound 2001; 42: 496–503.

Thrall DE. Textbook of Veterinary Diagnostic Radiology, 5th edn. Section II: The Axial Skeleton. Philadelphia: WB Saunders 2007.

Vandevelde M, Jaggy A, Lang J. Veterinärmedizinische Neurologie. Berlin: Parey 2001.

Widmer WR, Blevins WE. Veterinary myelography: a review of contrast media, adverse effects, and technique. J Am Anim Hosp Assoc 1991; 27: 163–77.

Wisner E, Zwingenberger A. Atlas of Small Animal CT and MRI. Ames: Wiley-Blackwell 2015.

Neck (including trachea)

8

Silke Hecht

8.1 Anatomy and indications

8.1.1 Anatomy

The **larynx and trachea** are air-filled and thus easily distinguished from surrounding soft tissues (muscles, vasculature, oesophagus, etc.) (Fig. 8.1). The trachea courses parallel to the cervical spine in the neck region and deviates ventrally within the thorax (Fig. 8.2). The degree of ventral tracheal deviation and the angle between the thoracic spine and the trachea are larger in deep-chested than shallow-chested dogs.

The position of the larynx and trachea varies with changes in head and neck position. Ventral flexion of the neck during the radiographic procedure results in caudal displacement of the larynx and rightward and dorsal displacement of the trachea (Fig. 8.3). The position of the larynx and trachea is also affected by adjacent space-occupying processes (e.g. mass lesions originating from the pharynx, oesophagus or retropharyngeal lymph nodes). Displacement by pathological processes must be distinguished from normal positional variations.

The **laryngeal cartilages and tracheal rings** mineralize with increasing age especially in dogs and are better visible than in young animals.

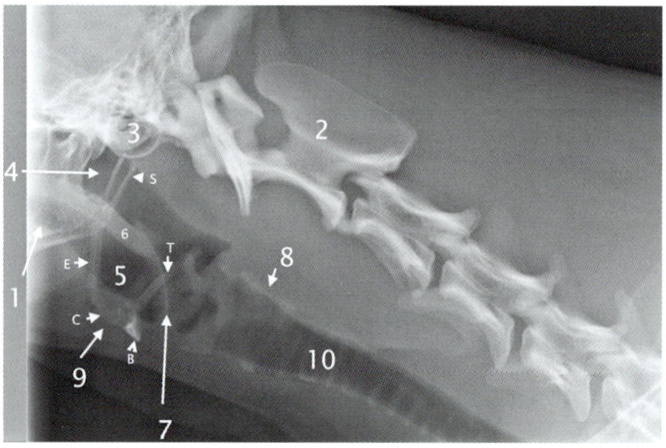

Fig. 8.1 Normal lateral radiograph of the neck in a dog. 1 Mandible, 2 Axis (second cervical vertebra), 3 Tympanic bullae (right and left side superimposed), 4 Nasopharynx, 5 Oropharynx, 6 Soft palate, 7 Epiglottis, 8 Cricoid cartilage, 9 Hyoid apparatus (right and left side superimposed; B Basihyoid, C Ceratohyoid, E Epihyoid, S Stylohyoid, T Thyrohyoid), 10 Trachea.

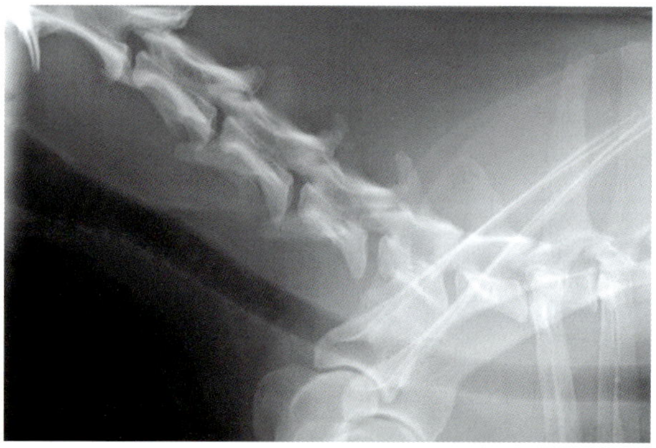

a

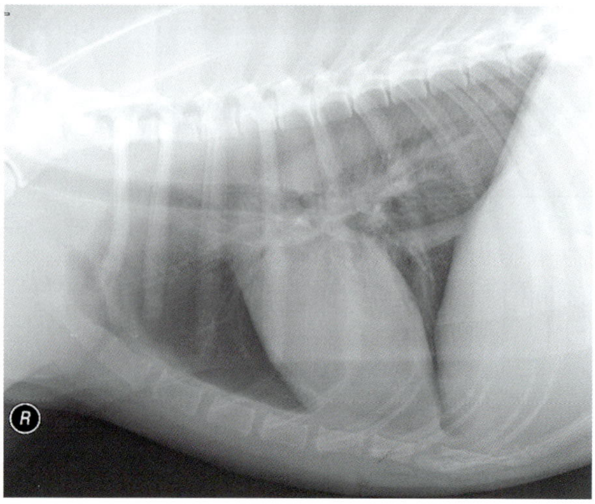

b

Fig. 8.2 Normal course of the trachea in a dog in the cervical region a and within the thorax b (R = right).

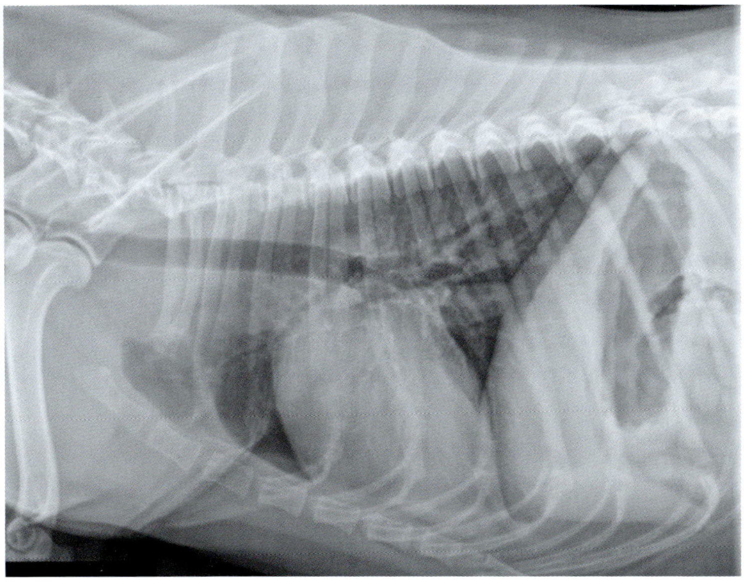

a

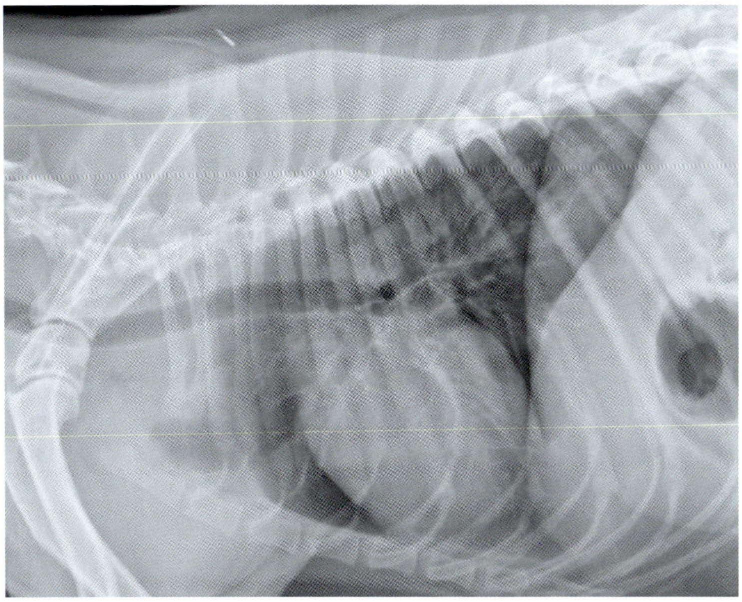

b

Fig. 8.3 Physiological variations of the appearance of the trachea with straight neck positioning a and neck flexion b.

The **oesophagus** is not normally visible on radiographs. However, a small amount of intraluminal air may be a physiological variant. The radiographic examination of the oesophagus is covered in detail in Chapter 13.

8.1.2 Indications

Indications for a radiographic examination of the cervical soft tissues include:

- respiratory difficulty
- difficulty swallowing
- palpable or visible cervical mass lesions
- neck trauma.

8.2 Radiographic technique and positioning

8.2.1 Technique

While at least two orthogonal radiographs are required for the radiographic evaluation of most regions of the body, a single lateral view of the neck may suffice depending on the indication. Ventrodorsal or dorsoventral projections are often of limited value due to superimposition of the larynx and trachea with the spine. However, ventrodorsal or oblique ventrodorsal radiographs in addition to the lateral projection may be helpful in further evaluation of, for example, a lateralized cervical soft-tissue swelling.

Radiographic evaluation of the cervical soft tissues requires the use of a different technique than a radiographic evaluation of the cervical spine, and the concurrent evaluation of the spine and cervical soft tissues including larynx and trachea may not be possible on the same radiograph. Radiography of the spine is covered in Chapter 7.

8.2.2 Positioning

Adequate cervical radiographs require straight positioning, which can often only be accomplished with the patient under heavy sedation or anaesthesia. Anatomic landmarks that can be used for assessment of patient positioning include the tympanic bullae, hyoid apparatus and transverse processes of cervical vertebrae. Depending on patient size, the radiograph may be acquired as a tabletop technique or using a grid (Fig. 8.4).

8.3 Diseases of the neck

Many diseases affecting the cervical soft tissues manifest as generalized or focal cervical swelling or a mass causing narrowing or displacement of the larynx or trachea (Fig. 8.5). Other possible radiographic findings may include gas inclusions or radiopaque foreign bodies. Compromise of the airways and dyspnoea typically result in secondary dilatation of the pharynx (Fig. 8.6).

8.3.1 Diseases of the larynx

Neoplasia

Laryngeal neoplasia is rare. Affected animals typically present with a history of change in vocalization, difficulty swallowing, exercise intolerance or progressive dyspnoea. The most common tumour types in young animals include laryngeal oncocytoma, osteosarcoma and rhabdomyoma/rhabdomyosarcoma. Tumours reported in older animals are usually of either epithelial (e.g. squamous cell carcinoma) or mesenchymal cell origin. Lymphoma is the most common laryngeal tumour in the cat. Tumours originating from adjacent tissues (e.g. thyroid gland or tonsils) may invade the larynx and may be difficult to distinguish from primary laryngeal tumours.

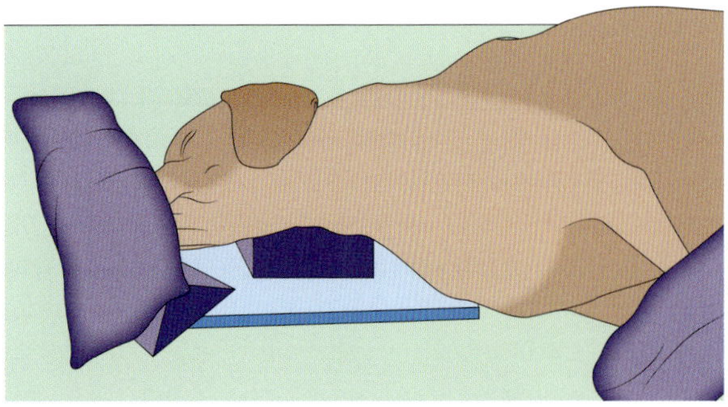

Fig. 8.4 Patient positioning for radiographic evaluation of the neck. Positioning aids must be radiolucent (e.g. foam wedges) so they do not obscure the area of interest.

Radiographic findings The most common finding with laryngeal tumours is a soft-tissue opaque and sometimes mineralized mass within the laryngeal region, possibly associated with destruction of one or more laryngeal cartilages. A presumptive diagnosis of a mass is usually straightforward, as the intraluminal component of the soft-tissue opacity lesion contrasts with surrounding gas. Affected animals typically suffer from some degree of upper airway obstruction, resulting in airway dilatation proximal to the obstructive lesion due to increased respiratory effort (Fig. 8.7).

Foreign body

Aspiration of foreign material may occur, for example during food intake or play. In contrast to animals with

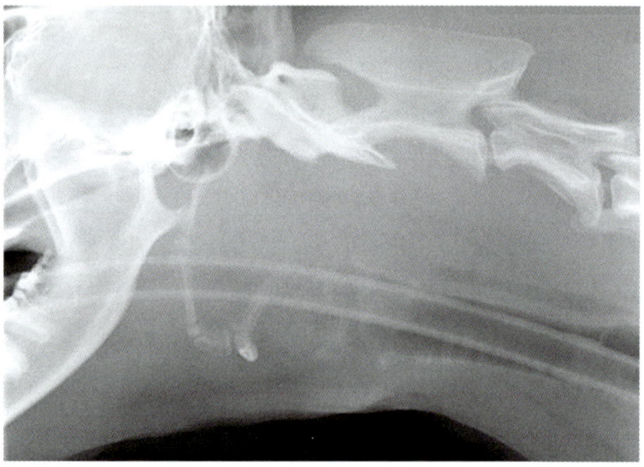

Fig. 8.5 Generalized soft-tissue swelling of the neck with obliteration of the airways and ventral displacement of the larynx and trachea due to markedly enlarged retropharyngeal lymph nodes. This radiograph was obtained under general anaesthesia as indicated by the presence of an endotracheal tube.

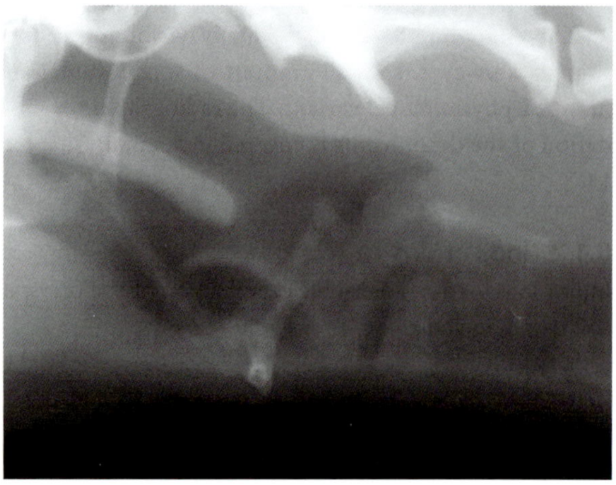

Fig. 8.6 Marked dilatation of the pharynx due to an obstruction at the level of the distal trachea.

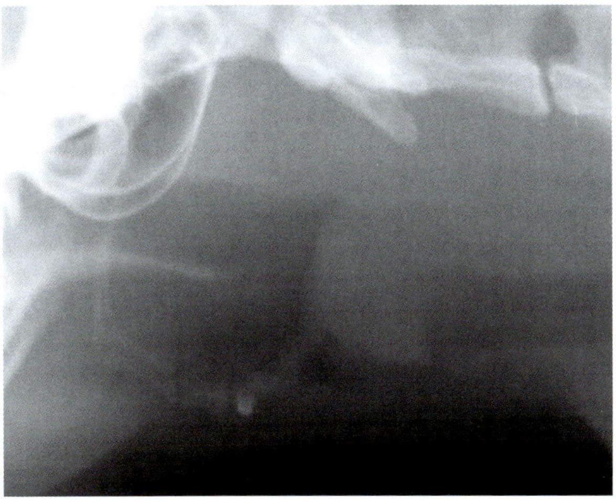

Fig. 8.7 Laryngeal mass (tumour) resulting in near-complete obstruction of the laryngeal lumen and severe secondary dilatation of the pharynx.

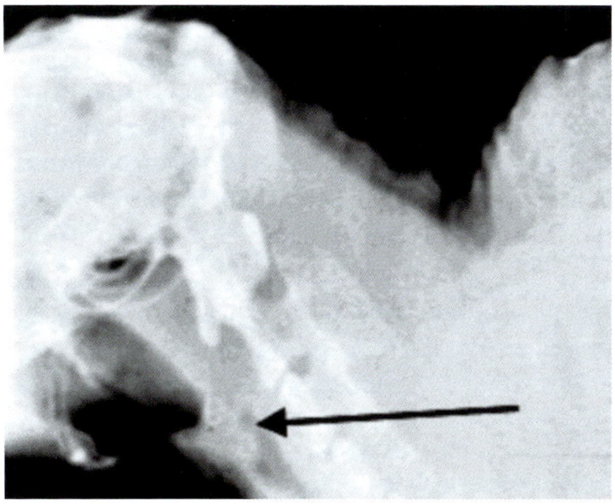

Fig. 8.8 Triangular foreign body (a piece of dry food, arrow) within the larynx of a cat.

slowly progressive upper airway obstruction (such as with tumours), animals with foreign body aspiration typically present with acute and often severe dyspnoea, retching, difficulty swallowing and salivation.

RADIOGRAPHIC FINDINGS The intraluminal foreign body is usually easily visualized even if not of bone or metal opacity, as it contrasts with adjacent air. As with other types of upper airway obstruction, secondary dilatation of the pharynx is common (Fig. 8.8).

Oedema and stenosis

Laryngeal oedema may develop, for example secondary to irritation/trauma (such as intubation) or may be secondary to an allergic reaction. True laryngeal stenosis is rare and may be congenital or acquired (secondary to trauma). Affected animals present with respiratory and/or swallowing difficulty, retching and reluctance to move.

RADIOGRAPHIC FINDINGS A radiographic diagnosis of laryngeal oedema or stenosis is not easy. Comparison of radiographs of the same animal at a different point in time or of another animal of the same or similar breed and age may be helpful. Radiographic abnormalities include diffuse narrowing or swelling of the larynx with airway compromise. Concurrent intraluminal fluid accumulation may further obscure the normally air-filled lumen. In contrast to perilaryngeal disease processes such as abscesses and tumours, which may also result in generalized laryngeal narrowing, there is no evidence of swelling or a mass associated with the adjacent soft tissues.

Laryngeal paralysis

Laryngeal paralysis is a rather common disease in older dogs which is characterized by incomplete or absent abduction of the arytenoid cartilages during inspiration. Clinical signs range from inspiratory stridor to severe dyspnoea. Possible inciting causes may include trauma, inflammation, neoplasia and diffuse neuromuscular disease; however, most cases are idiopathic. This condition is extremely rare in cats.

RADIOGRAPHIC FINDINGS The radiographic examination of patients with laryngeal paralysis is often unrewarding, as radiographs are commonly normal. A change in size and shape of the lateral ventricles may be noted in some cases. Radiographic signs of upper airway obstruction may also be present. The main role of cervical radiographs in animals presented with possible laryngeal paralysis is the exclusion of other causes of inspiratory stridor and dyspnoea such as laryngeal neoplasia or foreign body.

Fractures and neoplasia of the hyoid apparatus

These conditions are rare. Hyoid fractures may be caused by bite wounds or strangulation and are associated with acute clinical signs such as dyspnoea, difficulty swallowing and pain. Clinical signs with hyoid neoplasia are insidious in onset.

RADIOGRAPHIC FINDINGS Fractures or osseous neoplasia of the hyoid apparatus may result in loss of normal arrangement/dislocation of normally symmetric osseous structures. Concurrent soft-tissue swelling and possibly gas inclusions in the surrounding soft tissues due to connection with the laryngeal lumen are possible. Compromise of the airway is common and usually associated with radiographic indicators of upper airway obstruction.

8.3.2 Diseases of the trachea

Most tracheal diseases are associated with generalized or focal narrowing of the tracheal lumen. Familiarity with physiological tracheal diameter is important for diagnosis of abnormal tracheal size (e.g. with tracheal collapse or hypoplasia). Several different definitions of 'normal' tracheal diameter have been published. As with radiographic measurements of other organs, tracheal measurements must be weighted in light of clinical and other findings.

- The normal tracheal diameter should be similar to or only slightly smaller than the laryngeal diameter at the level of the cricoid cartilage.
- A method developed by Harvey and Fink (1982) considers differences between dogs of different breeds and body habitus. Tracheal diameter is divided by the height of the thoracic inlet. Dogs of non-brachycephalic breeds should have a mean trachea-to-thoracic inlet ratio of 0.2, brachycephalic breeds (except Bulldogs), 0.16 and Bulldogs, 0.13. In this study, all Bulldogs with a ratio <0.09 had clinical signs of tracheal hypoplasia.

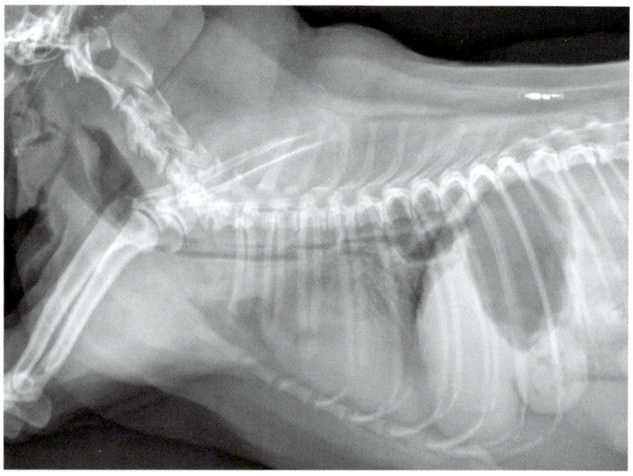

Fig. 8.9 Severe tracheal collapse in a dog. There is extensive marked narrowing of the cervical and intrathoracic trachea, and the mainstem bronchi are collapsed. Note gas dilatation of the oesophagus and the stomach due to dyspnoea and aerophagia. Multifocal intervertebral disc space collapse and ventral spondylosis deformans affecting the cervical spine in particular are incidental in this patient.

Tracheal and mainstem bronchial collapse

This is probably the most common tracheal disease in veterinary patients. It is usually an acquired condition in small- and dwarf-breed dogs. The disease is extremely rare in cats. Affected animals typically present with coughing episodes elicited by exercise, pulling on a leash or palpation of the neck.

RADIOGRAPHIC FINDINGS The disease is characterized by narrowing of the tracheal and/or bronchial lumen. It is usually a dynamic condition in which the cervical trachea, thoracic trachea and/or mainstem bronchi partially or completely collapse during respiration.

With severe tracheal collapse, a diagnosis may be possible based on a regular lateral thoracic radiograph (Fig. 8.9). However, owing to the dynamic nature of the condition, comparative radiographs during inspiration and expiration (Fig. 8.10) or an examination under fluoroscopy is needed to document tracheal or mainstem bronchial collapse in most patients. In some dogs, there is no notable change in airway diameter during regular respiration, requiring elicitation of a cough by means of tracheal or laryngeal palpation for diagnosis (Fig. 8.11).

Some clinicians prefer an endoscopic over a radiographic diagnosis of tracheal collapse. Imaging is given preference by others due to the risk of general anaesthesia and possible inability to extubate the patient following the endoscopic procedure.

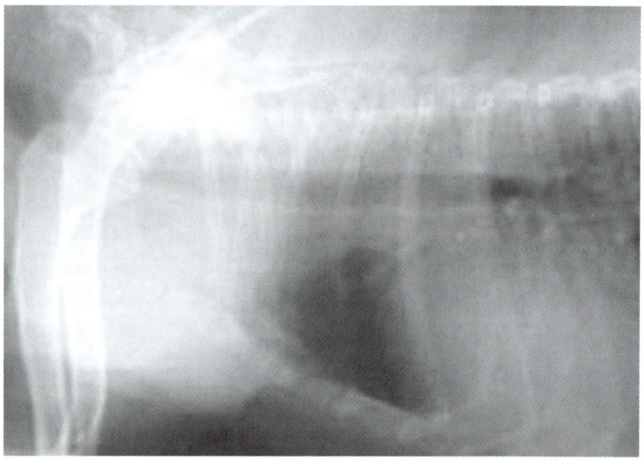

a

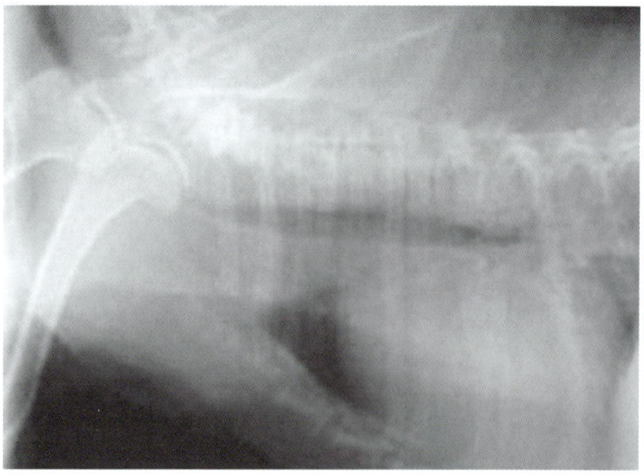

b

Fig. 8.10 Expiratory a and inspiratory b radiographs in a dog with dynamic collapse of the caudal cervical trachea. Narrowing of the tracheal lumen cranial to the thoracic inlet is worse on the inspiratory b than the expiratory a image.

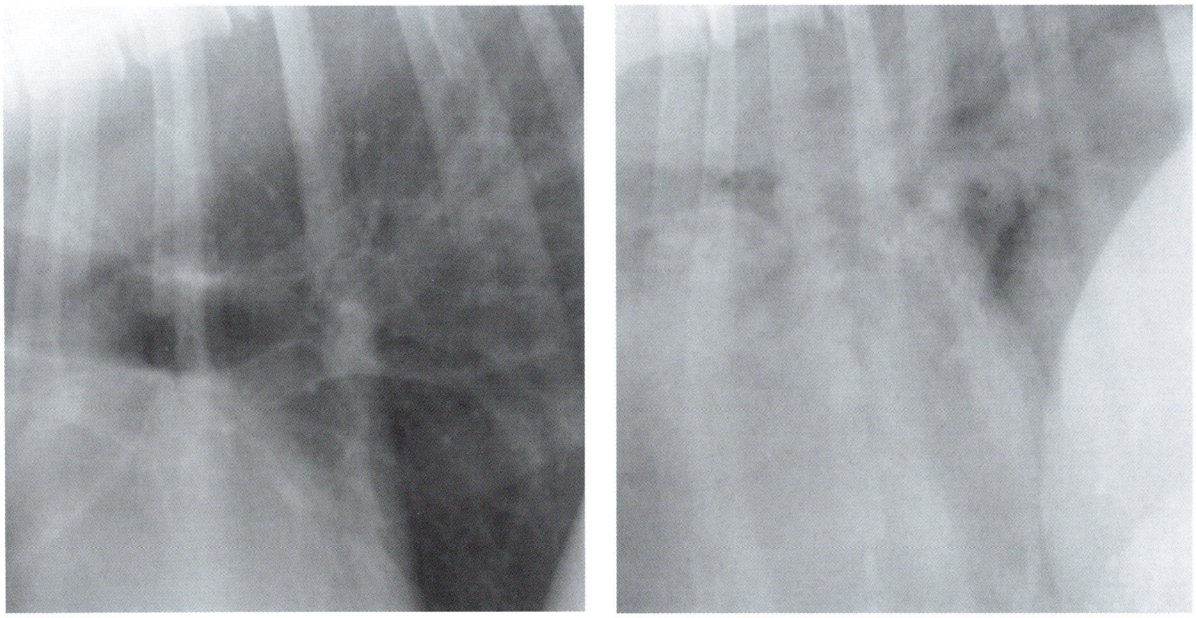

Fig. 8.11 Mainstem bronchial collapse in a dog. Radiographs obtained during inspiration a and during coughing b demonstrate complete obliteration of the bronchial lumen during the coughing episode.

Interpretation of a notable change in airway diameter with respiration and coughing, and a confident diagnosis of airway collapse, may be challenging. As a rule of thumb, tracheal or mainstem bronchial collapse is characterized by significant (more than 50%) narrowing of the airway lumen during respiration or coughing. However, minor variations in tracheal and mainstem bronchial diameter with respiration are expected in normal animals. In addition, marked airway narrowing may be seen in some animals with a severe cough but no underlying tracheal or bronchial malacia.

The most common locations for tracheal collapse are the caudal neck during inspiration and the caudal intrathoracic trachea/mainstem bronchi during expiration. This is related to intrathoracic pressure changes during respiration. The intrathoracic trachea dilates during inspiration and collapses during expiration. The cervical trachea is not affected by intrathoracic pressure changes and behaves in the opposite way (Fig. 8.12). With advanced tracheal collapse, the cervical and/or thoracic trachea may be damaged to a degree that collapse is permanent. Documentation of a dynamic component is not necessary in these cases (see Fig. 8.9).

A redundant dorsal tracheal membrane associated with the cervical trachea is a common incidental finding in dogs. In contrast to tracheal collapse, animals are asymptomatic. Radiographic differentiation from true tracheal collapse is possible as the actual dorsal wall of the trachea (i.e. the dorsal aspect of the tracheal cartilages) is visible dorsal to the soft-tissue band overlying the tracheal lumen (Fig. 8.13 and 8.14).

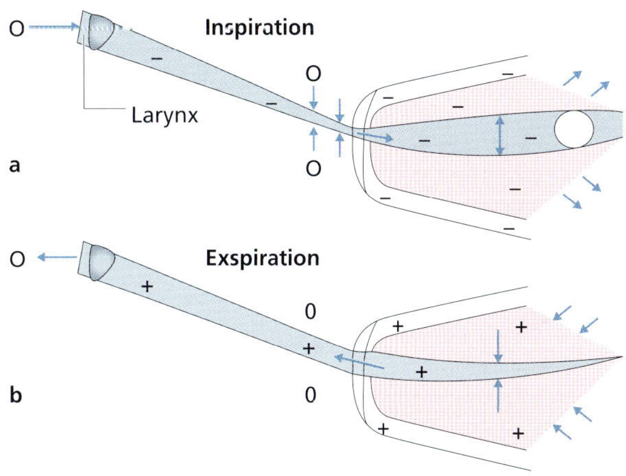

Fig. 8.12 Schematic illustration of dynamic changes in tracheal diameter during inspiration and expiration in cases of a cervical and b intrathoracic tracheal collapse.

With chronic tracheal collapse, secondary pulmonary and cardiac changes including cor pulmonale may develop.

Hypoplasia

This is a congenital condition characterized by generalized static (i.e. non-dynamic) narrowing of the tracheal lumen (Fig. 8.15). Brachycephalic dog breeds (e.g. Bulldog, Boston Terrier) are predisposed. Affected animals present at a young age with respiratory difficulty, failure to thrive and reluctance to move. Therapy-resistant and recurrent airway infection is also a common presenting complaint.

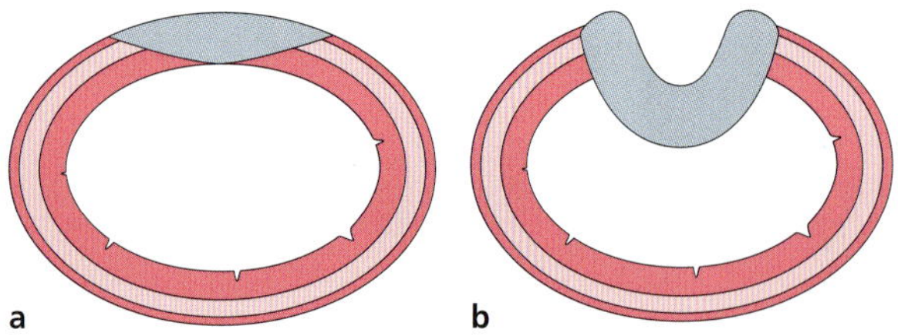

Fig. 8.13 Schematic illustration of a normal trachea a compared with a case of redundant tracheal membrane b in cross-section.

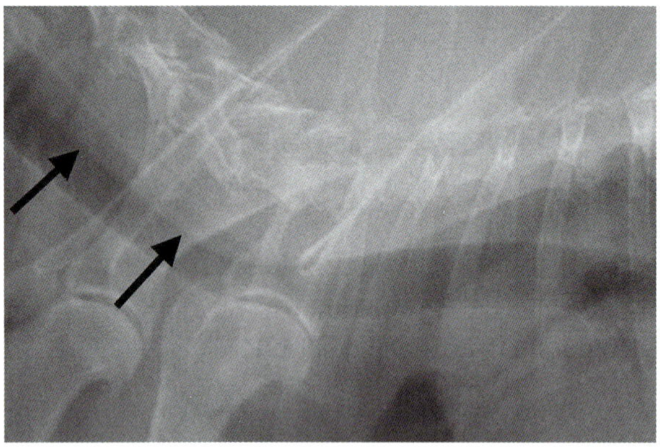

Fig. 8.14 Lateral radiograph of the caudal neck and cranial thorax in a dog with a redundant dorsal tracheal membrane. There is a tubular structure of soft-tissue opacity superimposed with the dorsal lumen of the trachea (arrows). The actual dorsal tracheal wall is visible dorsal to this line. This is commonly an incidental finding and should not be confused with tracheal collapse.

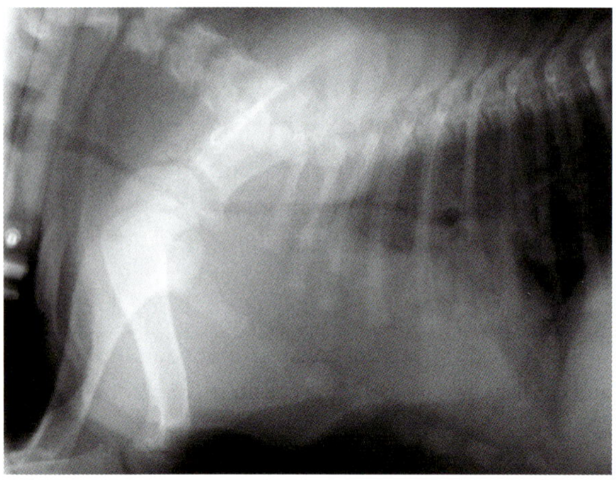

Fig. 8.15 Tracheal hypoplasia in a Bulldog puppy. The lumen of the trachea is generally narrowed, and tracheal diameter is significantly smaller than the diameter of the larynx. An alveolar pattern is associated with the cranioventral lung fields, consistent with aspiration/bronchopneumonia.

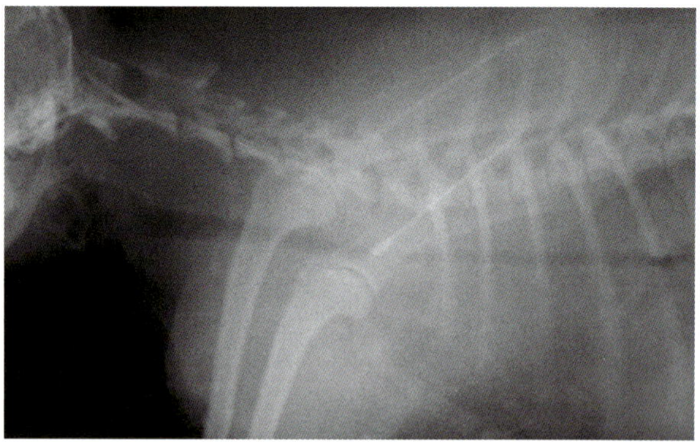

Fig. 8.16 Radiograph of the neck and thorax in a dog with rodenticide toxicity. There is marked generalized narrowing of the tracheal lumen due to haemorrhage into the tracheal wall.

Generalized wall thickening of the trachea (e.g. secondary to haemorrhage with rodenticide toxicity, Fig. 8.16; or due to inflammation or neoplastic infiltration) may also result in generalized luminal narrowing and be mistaken for tracheal hypoplasia. However, a distinction can usually be made taking into account the patient's breed, age and clinical history.

Tracheitis/tracheobronchitis

'Kennel cough' and other inflammatory / infectious (viral and bacterial) diseases of the trachea and bronchi are very common, especially in young dogs. Affected animals typically present with a cough of varying severity. Superinfection with bacteria following a primary viral infection may result in additional symptoms such as fever, lethargy or anorexia.

Radiographic findings Cervical and thoracic radiographs in animals with acute and uncomplicated tracheitis / tracheobronchitis are typically normal. In severe cases and when there is superinfection with bacteria, tracheal oedema may result in luminal narrowing. Intraluminal accumulation of secretions may result in increased soft-tissue / fluid opacity in the tracheal lumen. Severe or chronic bronchitis is characterized by a bronchial lung pattern. With bronchopneumonia, an alveolar lung pattern is identified in the cranioventral lung fields. These abnormalities are covered in Chapter 9.

Stenosis

With tracheal stenosis there is a focal, segmental narrowing of the trachea. While the congenital form is rare in small animals, acquired stenoses secondary to tracheal inflammation or fibrosis due to trauma (e.g. bite wounds or overinflation of an endotracheal tube cuff) are relatively common. Like all diseases resulting in narrowing of the tracheal lumen, affected animals present with dyspnoea of variable severity.

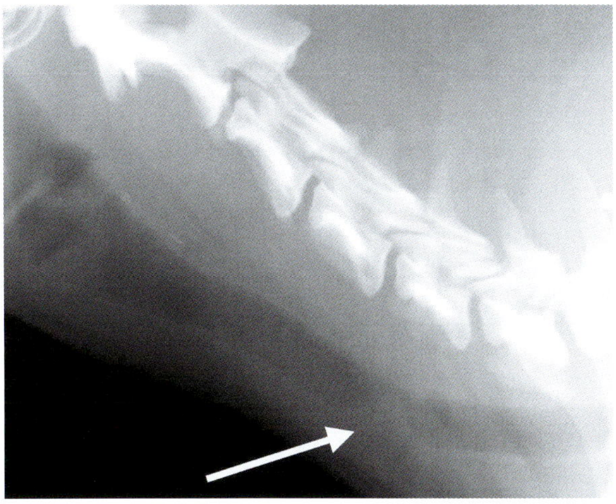

Fig. 8.17 Radiograph of the neck in a dog with tracheal stenosis. Focal circumferential narrowing of the trachea is noted at the level of the fifth cervical vertebra (arrow).

Radiographic findings The predominant radiographic finding is a focal and often circumferential narrowing of the trachea (Fig. 8.17). Regional deformity of the tracheal cartilages is possible. Tracheal stenosis may mimic a wall-associated tracheal mass (tumour or granuloma), and care must be taken to distinguish these entities.

Tracheal mass lesion(s)

Differential diagnoses for mass lesions originating from the tracheal wall include granulomas, polyps and tumours. A granuloma may develop secondary to a tracheal foreign body, surgical procedure (tracheostomy), or parasite infection (e.g. *Filaroides*). Like laryngeal neoplasia, tumours of the trachea are rare. Possible primary tumour types include lymphoma, squamous cell carcinoma, chondroma/chondrosarcoma, leiomyoma, osteoma and adenocarcinoma. As described for laryngeal tumours, invasion of the trachea by tumours originating from adjacent soft tissues is possible.

Radiographic findings Intraluminal extension of a wall-associated mass results in narrowing of the tracheal lumen (Fig. 8.18). Depending on the tumour type, location and chronicity of the process, the lesion may range in size from a few millimetres to several centimetres, may result in circumferential narrowing of the trachea as with tracheal stenosis, may result in destruction of tracheal cartilages, or may mineralize. Secondary findings may include pharyngeal and/or tracheal dilatation, pulmonary hyperinflation and metastatic disease to regional lymph nodes or lung.

Tracheal injury and rupture

Tracheal injury or rupture is typically caused by external (e.g. bite wound) or internal trauma (overinflated cuff of an endotracheal tube). As the intrathoracic trachea is fairly protected from injuries, the cervical trachea is much more commonly affected. Perforation of the trachea results in gas leakage into the surrounding soft tissues (Fig. 8.19). Depending on aetiology, location and severity of the injury, this may result in subcutaneous emphysema, gas accumulation within the soft tissues of the neck, pneumomediastinum, and possibly pneumothorax and pneumoretroperitoneum. Clinical signs in affected animals may range from none through subcutaneous emphysema to severe dyspnoea if tracheal patency is compromised.

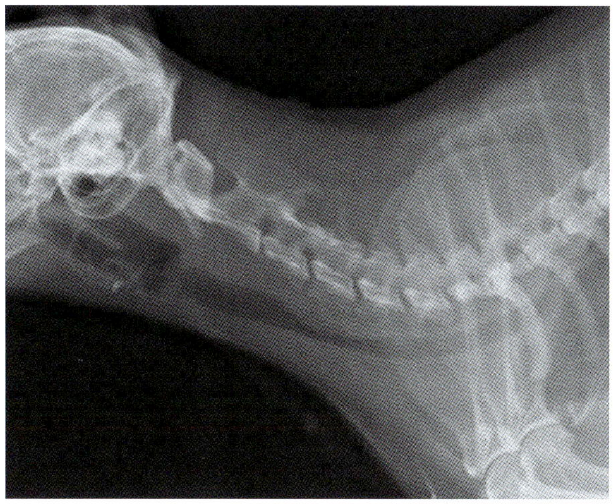

Fig. 8.18 Tracheal neoplasia (lymphoma) in a cat. A mass is associated with the dorsal wall of the trachea, extending from the level of the third through sixth cervical vertebrae. Note marked dilatation of the pharynx secondary to partial tracheal obstruction. The diagnosis was made based on endoscopic biopsies.

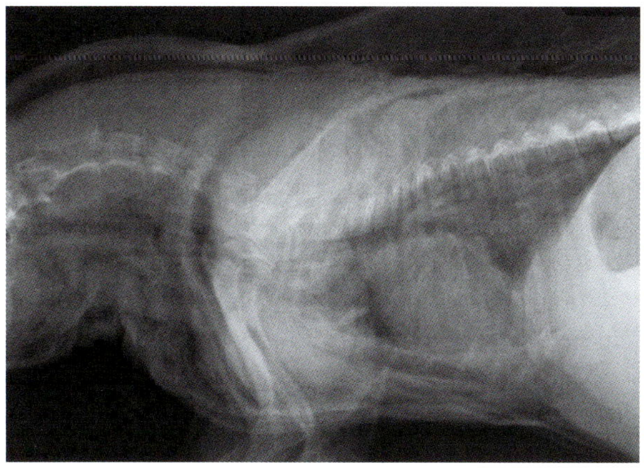

Fig. 8.19 Tracheal rupture in a dog following bite wounds to the neck. There is disruption of the cervical trachea, and extensive gas accumulations are present within the soft tissues of the neck, the mediastinum and the subcutaneous tissues.

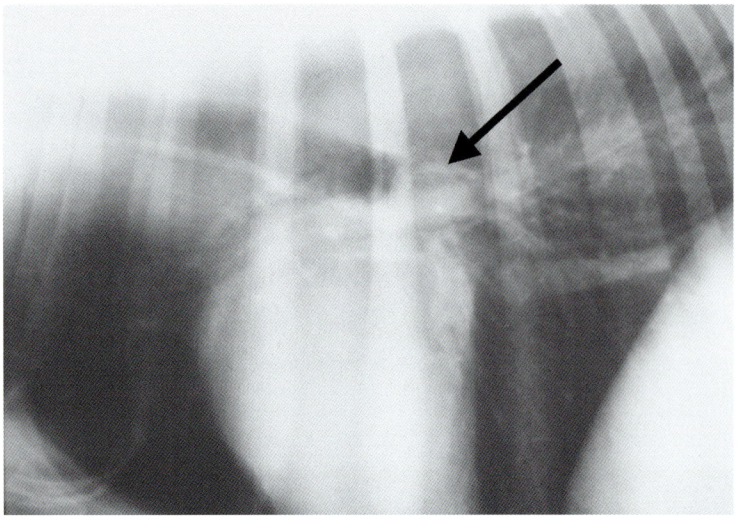

Fig. 8.20 Round, thin-walled intraluminal tracheal foreign body (acorn; arrow) at the level of the tracheal bifurcation. Note the abrupt end of the air-filled lumen of the trachea at the cranial margin of the foreign body.

RADIOGRAPHIC FINDINGS The severity of radiographic abnormalities varies with the severity of the injury. In most severe cases of tracheal rupture, discontinuity of the trachea and separation between individual tracheal cartilages may be seen. However, this may be difficult to identify due to concurrent soft-tissue swelling and superimposition of gas within surrounding tissues. Additional findings include extensive gas inclusions within the soft tissues of the head and neck, within the subcutaneous tissues, along the trachea and other mediastinal structures (pneumomediastinum), and in severe cases pneumothorax and pneumoretroperitoneum due to extension of mediastinal gas.

Foreign body

Patients with tracheal foreign bodies present with similar history and clinical signs to patients with laryngeal foreign bodies. Foreign material may be aspirated, for example during eating or play. Depending on the size and location of the foreign body, affected animals typically present with acute and severe dyspnoea and cough.

RADIOGRAPHIC FINDINGS Even foreign bodies of low radiographic opacity are usually clearly visible as they contrast with adjacent intraluminal air (Fig. 8.20). Findings secondary to partial or near-complete airway obstruction include dilatation of the pharynx, larynx and trachea proximal to the obstructive lesion. Depending on the position of the foreign body, a (partial) collapse of the airway distal to the obstructive lesion may be seen. The diagnosis of a tracheal foreign body is best made on a lateral view due to superimposition of the trachea over the spine on ventrodorsal or dorsoventral projections.

References and further reading

Berry CR, Gallaway A, Thrall DE, Carlisle C. Thoracic radiographic features of anticoagulant rodenticide toxicity in 14 dogs. Vet Radiol Ultrasound 1993; 34: 391–6.

Hammer AS, Kessler M. Tumoren des Larynx und der Trachea. In: Kessler M (ed.). Kleintieronkologie, 2nd edn. Stuttgart: Parey MVS 2005; 305–7.

Harvey CE, Fink EA. Tracheal diameter: analysis of radiographic measurements in brachycephalic and non-brachycephalic dogs. J Am Anim Hosp Assoc 1982; 18: 570.

Kneller SK. Larynx, pharynx, and trachea. In: Thrall DE (ed.). Textbook of Veterinary Diagnostic Radiology, 5th edn. St. Louis: Saunders Elsevier 2007; 489–94.

Macready DM, Johnson LR, Pollard RE. Fluoroscopic and radiographic evaluation of tracheal collapse in dogs: 62 cases (2001–2006). J Am Vet Med Assoc 2007; 230: 1870–6.

Owens JM, Biery DN. Thorax (noncardiac). In: Owens JM, Biery DN (eds). Radiographic Interpretation for the Small Animal Clinician. Baltimore: Williams & Wilkins 1999; 147–84.

Thorax (excluding the heart)

9

Silke Hecht

9.1 Anatomy and indications

9.1.1 Anatomy

Radiographs of the thorax allow evaluation of the thoracic wall, diaphragm, mediastinal structures, pleural space, cardiovascular structures, lung, and any extrathoracic structures included in the collimation (caudal neck, cranial abdomen, proximal forelimbs) (Fig. 9.1 and 9.2).

Thoracic wall

Structures of the thoracic wall include the skin, subcutaneous soft tissues and fat, sternum, thoracic vertebrae, ribs, intercostal muscles and parietal pleura.

RADIOGRAPHIC FINDINGS There are major differences in the appearance of the thoracic cavity in dogs of different sizes and breeds (Fig. 9.3). The appearance of the thorax in cats is less variable. Certain normal anatomic structures of the thoracic wall (nipples, mineralized costal cartilages, fat, and skin folds) may mimic but should not be confused with pathological changes. These 'pitfalls' will be covered in more detail in the discussion of individual disease processes.

Diaphragm

The diaphragm separates the thoracic from the abdominal cavity. It consists of two anatomic components. The **diaphragmatic crura** consist of striated musculature and are important for respiratory motion. They originate from the thoracic wall (specifically, ribs, sternum and vertebrae) and insert on the passive compartment of the diaphragm, the tendinous **cupula**. There are three openings within the diaphragm, connecting the thoracic cavity with the peritoneal cavity and retroperitoneal space, respectively, and providing passage for organs, vessels and nerves. The aorta, azygous vein and thoracic duct pass through the

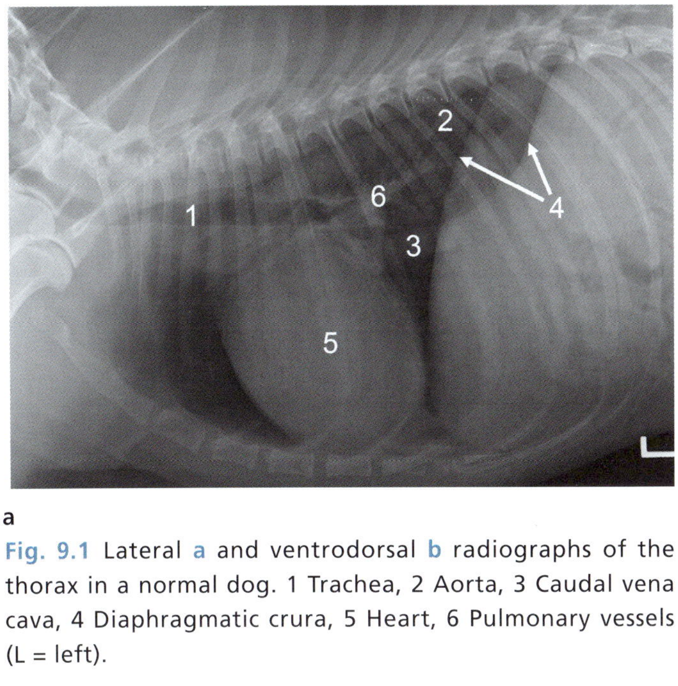

a

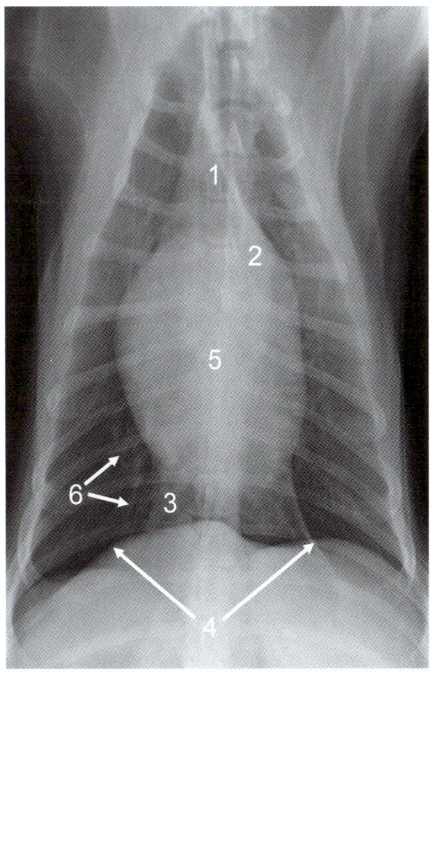

b

Fig. 9.1 Lateral a and ventrodorsal b radiographs of the thorax in a normal dog. 1 Trachea, 2 Aorta, 3 Caudal vena cava, 4 Diaphragmatic crura, 5 Heart, 6 Pulmonary vessels (L = left).

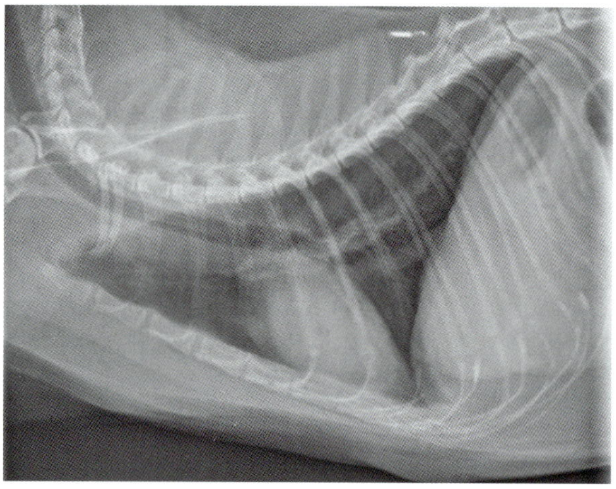

a

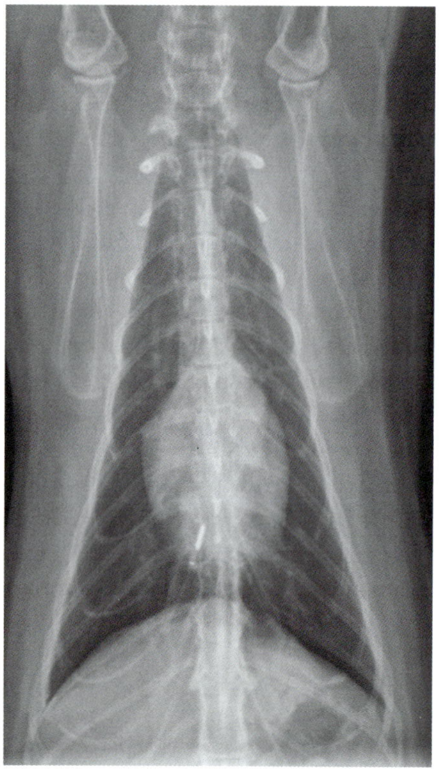

b

Fig. 9.2 Lateral a and ventrodorsal b radiographs of the thorax in a normal cat.

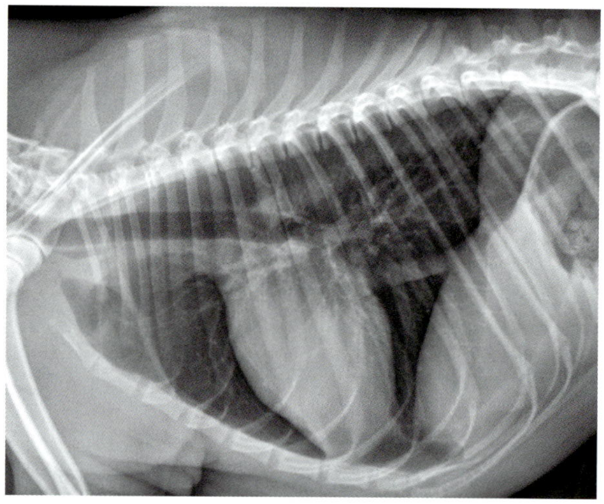

a

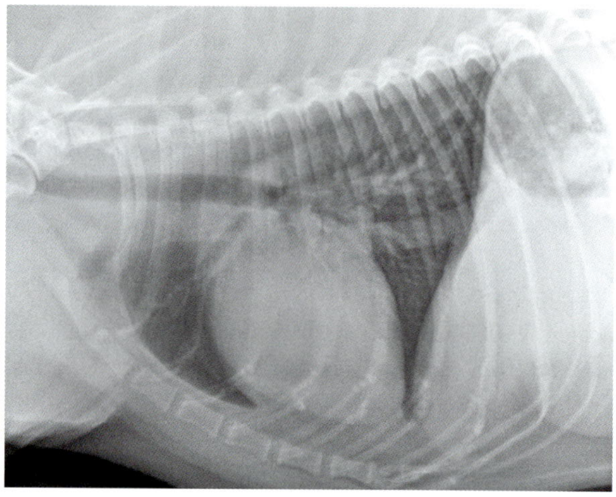

b

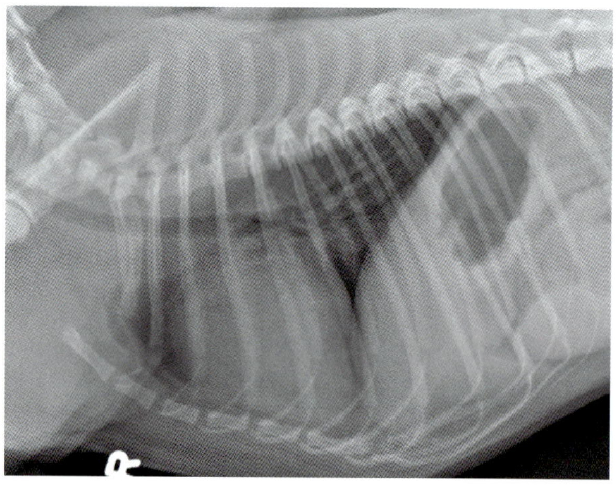

c

Fig. 9.3 Variations in thoracic conformation in dogs of different breeds. Note differences in radiographic appearance of the thoracic wall, mediastinal structures, cardiac silhouette and intrathoracic fat (R = right).

a Deep-chested dog (e.g. Collie, Irish Setter).

b Average dog (e.g. Golden Retriever, Labrador Retriever).

c Barrel-chested dog (e.g. Boston Terrier, Bulldog).

aortic hiatus, the oesophagus and vagus nerves traverse through the **oesophageal hiatus**, and the caudal vena cava passes through the **caudal vena cava foramen**.

RADIOGRAPHIC FINDINGS The cranial surface of the soft-tissue opaque diaphragm is delineated by its interface with air-filled lung. A large part of the caudal margin of the diaphragm silhouettes with the liver and is not recognized as a separate structure. The ventral aspect of the caudal margin of the diaphragm may be visible due to adjacent falciform fat, especially in obese animals. The radiographic appearance of the diaphragm depends on several factors.

- Species and breed.
- Body condition.
- Respiratory phase.
- Intra-abdominal conditions (degree of gastric distention, intra-abdominal space-occupying lesions).
- Thoracic diseases.
- Radiographic projection: On a lateral thoracic radiograph, the dependent diaphragmatic crus (i.e. the crus closer to the film) is pushed cranially. In combination with other findings, this indicator can be used to distinguish a right lateral from a left lateral thoracic radiograph (see section 9.2). The diaphragmatic crura and cupula may form three distinct bulges on a ventrodorsal (VD) view (especially evident in large-breed and deep-chested dogs), while the diaphragm usually appears as a single dome on a dorsoventral (DV) view. However, this is inconsistent and not a very reliable indicator of the radiographic projection.

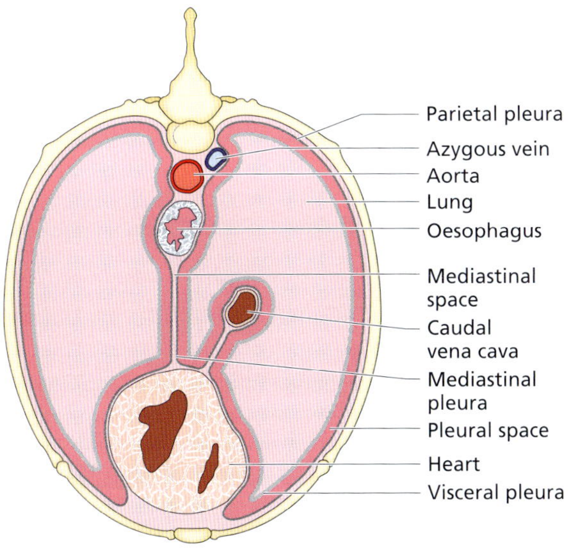

Fig. 9.4 Schematic anatomic drawing of the pleural and mediastinal space at the level of the middle mediastinum. The parietal pleura covers the inner thoracic wall and reflects in the ventral and central aspect of the thorax to become the mediastinal pleura, which borders the mediastinal space. The lung is covered by visceral pleura.

Pleural space

The thorax has a **right and a left pleural cavity**, which are separated by the mediastinum and mediastinal structures (Fig. 9.4). The **parietal pleura** (covering the inside of thoracic wall) and the **visceral pleura** (covering the lung) form the border of the pleural space. In the ventral aspect of the thorax near the midline, the parietal pleura of both pleural cavities reflects dorsally and becomes the **mediastinal pleura**.

RADIOGRAPHIC FINDINGS Pleura and pleural space are not visible on radiographs in normal animals. However, it is important to be familiar with the location of the pleural fissures between individual lung lobes to be able to identify pleural pathology (e.g. pleural effusion) (Fig. 9.5).

Mediastinum

The mediastinal space is contained within two layers of mediastinal pleura. **Mediastinal structures** include the heart, large vessels, nerves, lymph nodes, trachea, thymus, fat and oesophagus. The mediastinal space communicates cranially with the deep fascial planes of the neck, caudally with the retroperitoneal space via the aortic hiatus, and with the pleural space. The mediastinum is subdivided into a dorsal and ventral part, and into three craniocaudal compartments (cranial, middle and caudal mediastinum) for descriptive purposes (Fig. 9.6).

RADIOGRAPHIC FINDINGS Mediastinal structures visible on radiographs in normal animals include the **heart, caudal vena cava, aorta, trachea, mediastinal fat and thymus** (in young dogs). A small amount of gas may be seen within the lumen of the **oesophagus**. The oesophagus is otherwise not visible but can be further evaluated by oral administration of contrast medium (oesophagography). This technique is covered in detail in Chapter 13. The **cranial mediastinum** extends from the thoracic inlet to the heart. On the lateral view, it is dominated by the air-filled trachea and adjacent soft tissues (oesophagus and vessels). On a VD view, it appears as a soft-tissue opacity band that does not extend beyond the width of the vertebral column in most cats, and does not exceed twice the width of the vertebral column in most dogs. The thymus appears as a triangular soft-tissue opacity structure (resembling a 'sail') within the left cranial thorax in young dogs (<1 year) (Fig. 9.7). A large portion of the **middle mediastinum** is occupied by the heart. The

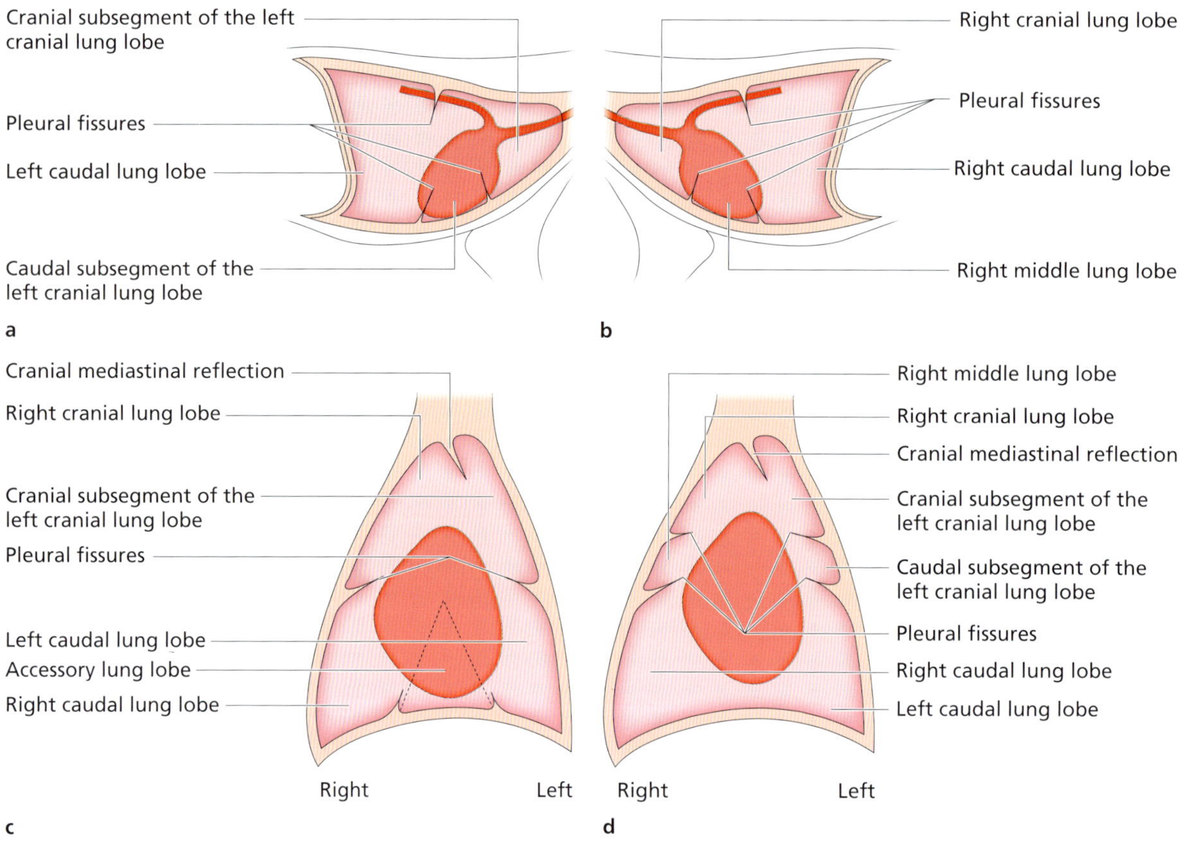

Fig. 9.5 Schematic illustration of the location of pleural fissures and lung lobes in the left half **a**, the right half **b**, the dorsal part **c** and the ventral part **d** of the thorax.

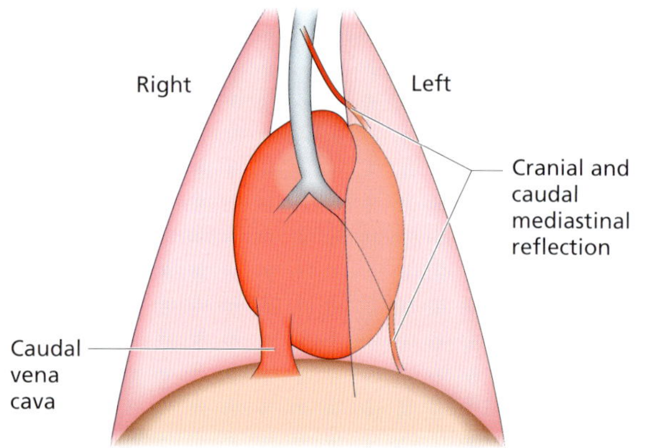

Fig. 9.6 Illustration of mediastinal subdivision into three compartments for descriptive purposes. The cranial mediastinum extends from the thoracic inlet to the heart, the middle mediastinum contains the heart, and the caudal mediastinum extends from the heart to the diaphragm.

caudal mediastinum extends from the heart to the diaphragm. Two **mediastinal reflections** are visible radiographically: The **cranial reflection** is seen on a lateral view and separates the cranial margin of the right cranial lung lobe from the tip of the cranial subsegment of the left cranial lung lobe, which extends further cranially. The **caudal mediastinal reflection** is seen on a VD view and separates the accessory from the left caudal lung lobe. Normal **mediastinal lymph nodes** are not visible radiographically. However, it is important to be familiar with their location to be able to recognize lymph node enlargement (Fig. 9.8). The radiographic anatomy of the trachea, heart and great vessels is covered in Chapters 8 and 10, respectively.

Lung

The lung consists of **air-filled components** (bronchi and their smaller branches, alveoli), **vessels and interstitial tissue**.

Radiographic findings Thoracic radiographs are characterized by **inherent high contrast** due to the differences in radiographic density between structures that are air-filled and soft-tissue opaque (e.g. vessels). **Pulmonary arteries and veins** appear as tubular soft-tissue opacities that course along and branch with air-filled bronchi. On a lateral view, arteries, bronchi and veins of a lung lobe are oriented from dorsal to ventral, on a DV or VD view from lateral to medial ('Veins are ventral and central'; see Chapter 10). **Bronchial walls** especially in young and healthy animals are normal or barely visible. They increase in prominence with thickening or calcification. The **pulmonary interstitium** represents the perivascular, peribronchial, perilymphatic and perialveolar tissues. It is not visible on thoracic radiographs in normal animals. Progressive thickening/fibrosis of these structures with age leads to a gradual increase in generalized opacity of pulmonary parenchyma.

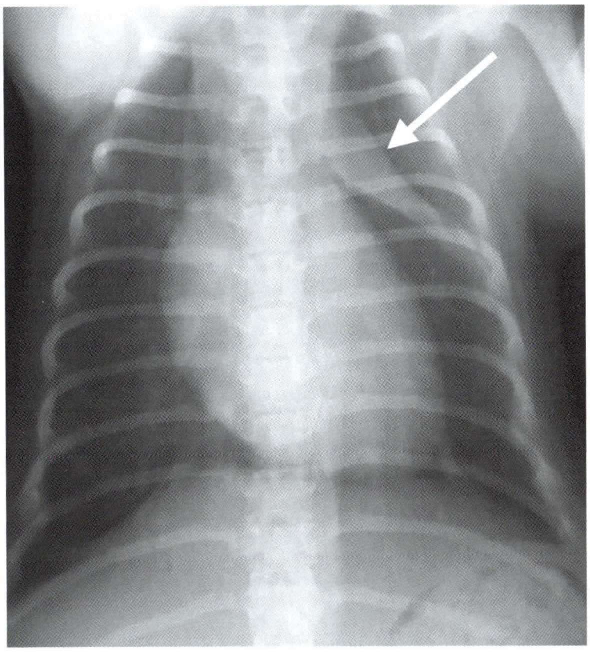

Fig. 9.7 Ventrodorsal thoracic radiograph in a young dog. The thymus is seen as a triangular soft-tissue opacity structure in the left cranial thorax (arrow). (Courtesy of Dr Amy Sato, Tufts Cummings School of Veterinary Medicine, North Grafton, USA)

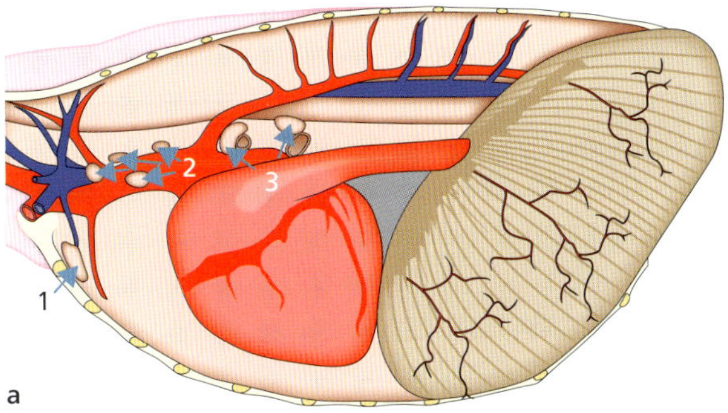

a

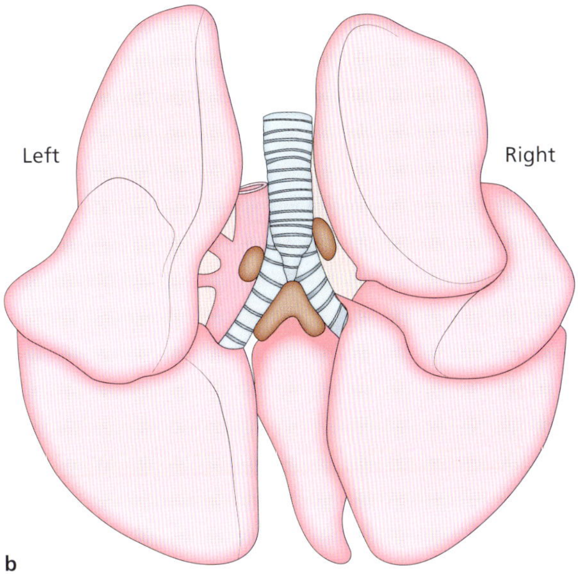

b

Fig. 9.8 Schematic illustration of the location of mediastinal lymph nodes. These are not visible in normal animals but appear as soft-tissue opacity masses in these locations when enlarged.
a View from lateral. **1** Sternal, **2** Cranial mediastinal and **3** Tracheobronchial lymph nodes.
b View from dorsal. Note location of the right, middle and left tracheobronchial lymph nodes surrounding the tracheal bifurcation.

The **right lung** in dogs and cats consists of **four** (cranial, middle, caudal and accessory) and the **left lung** of **two** lung lobes (subdivided cranial, and caudal). Lung lobe margins are marked by **pleural fissures** (see Fig. 9.5). It is important to be familiar with the location of individual lung lobes from both a diagnostic and a therapeutic standpoint. Some lung diseases occur in specific locations, and exact lesion localization is important, for planning of lung biopsy or lobectomy, for example.

9.1.2 Indications

Indications for radiographic examination of the thorax include but are not limited to:

- suspected respiratory diseases
- suspected heart disease
- staging in oncology patients
- evaluation for any thoracic anomalies prior to general anaesthesia especially in older patients
- thoracic trauma
- mass lesions, wounds and anomalies of the thoracic wall.

9.2 Radiographic technique and positioning

In most cases, a routine radiographic examination of the thorax includes at least one lateral (typically right lateral) and a ventrodorsal or dorsoventral view. If full evaluation of the lung is desired, an opposite lateral view should also be acquired. Additional radiographs and special views (horizontal beam views, oblique views, dynamic radiographs) may be appropriate depending on the indication. Especially uncooperative patients should be sedated to **minimize motion artefacts and radiation exposure** of radiology personnel. However, thoracic radiographs under general anaesthesia should be avoided, as pulmonary atelectasis develops rapidly in these animals, limiting the diagnostic value of the images.

The evaluation of **image quality** of thoracic radiographs includes assessment of **technique, positioning and phase of respiration**.

9.2.1 Technique

For most body regions, a radiograph high in contrast is desirable to accentuate subtle differences in opacity between adjacent tissues. The radiographic examination of the thorax is an exception due to the inherently high contrast of thoracic structures (air-filled lung compared with bony ribs and soft tissues). Use of a high-contrast technique for thoracic radiography would make concurrent evaluation of soft tissues, bone and lung difficult (Fig. 9.9).

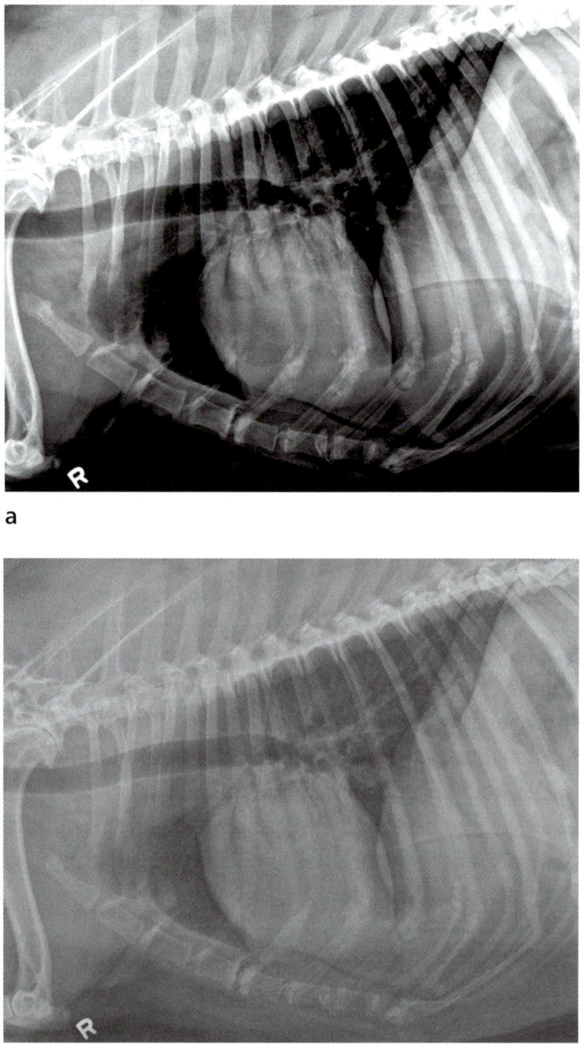

Fig. 9.9 Examples of differences in contrast with thoracic radiographs.

a High contrast radiograph. Air-filled tissues such as the trachea and lung are black, and bony structures are white. There are few intermediate shades of grey. The pulmonary parenchyma and pulmonary vessels cannot be adequately evaluated on this radiograph. A limited evaluation of the cardiac silhouette is possible.

b Low contrast radiograph. All tissues are displayed in varying shades of grey. This radiograph is of good diagnostic quality and allows evaluation of cardiovascular, pulmonary and mediastinal structures.

Image contrast is determined by exposure factors (specifically, kVp) and the type of radiographic film (conventional radiology) or reconstruction algorithm (digital radiology). **kVp** determines beam hardness, i.e. the ability of photons to penetrate tissues. An increase in kVp results in **increased transmission of photons** not only through low attenuating structures (air, fat) but also through soft tissues and bone. More photons reach the film/imaging plate, resulting in **low image contrast**. This is desirable for thoracic radiographs. Depending on the equipment and patient size, kVp values may range from 70–150.

The quality of a radiograph is also affected by **mA** and **exposure time (s)**. Exposure time should be kept as short as possible to **minimize motion artefacts**. As for other areas of the body, a **grid** should be used if the region of interest exceeds 10 cm in thickness.

9.2.2 Positioning

As with all radiographs, patient positioning should be **as straight as possible**. The X-ray field is centred on the caudal margin of the scapula and collimated from the caudal cervical region to the caudal aspect of the costal arch (Fig. 9.10).

On a well-positioned lateral view, the heads of opposite ribs are superimposed. On a well-positioned ventrodorsal or dorsoventral view, the spinous processes of the thoracic spine are superimposed with the vertebral bodies and have an oval/teardrop shape.

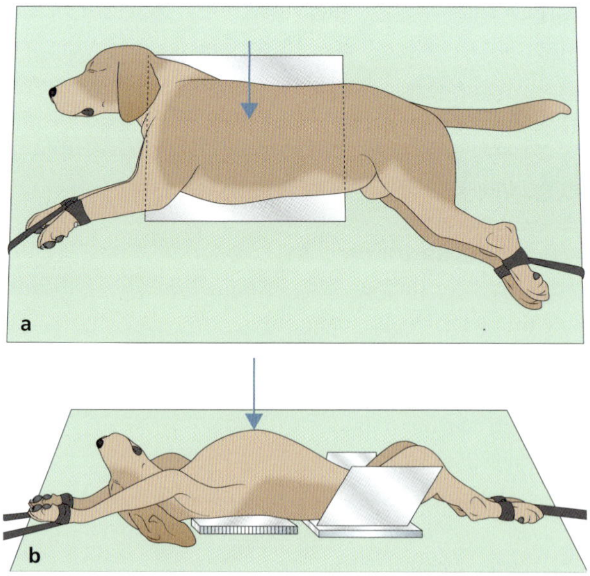

Fig. 9.10 Schematic illustration of patient positioning for a right lateral a and a ventrodorsal b thoracic radiograph. The X-ray beam is centred on the caudal margin of the scapula and extends from the caudal neck to the caudal costal arch. As with other body regions, patient positioning should be as straight as possible.

Particularly in deep-chested dogs (and to a lesser degree in small dogs and cats), the appearance of the thorax varies with positioning (Fig. 9.11):

- **Right lateral versus left lateral view:** On the right lateral view, the heart is egg-shaped, the diaphragmatic crura are parallel, and the right diaphragmatic crus (recognized by its juncture with the caudal vena cava) is positioned further cranially than the left. On a left lateral view, the cardiac silhouette often has a rounded apex and appears slightly separate from the sternum. The diaphragmatic crura diverge in the dorsal thorax, and the left diaphragmatic crus is positioned further cranially and summates with the caudal vena cava. These differences usually permit differentiation between a right and left lateral view.
- **Ventrodorsal versus dorsoventral view:** Differences between these projections are most evident in large and deep-chested dogs, and may not be apparent in small, shallow-chested dogs and cats. On a ventrodorsal view, the cardiac silhouette is elongated, and the diaphragm has three bulges representing the left and right diaphragmatic crus and the central cupula. The heart appears rounded on a dorsoventral view, and the diaphragm has a single dome. The decision to obtain a ventrodorsal versus a dorsoventral view depends on personal preference, indication for the radiographic examination and patient status. Severely dyspnoeic animals may tolerate sternal positioning better than dorsal positioning, in which case a dorsoventral view is preferable. Many examiners prefer a ventrodorsal view for evaluation of the cardiac silhouette. On the other hand, the caudal lobar pulmonary vessels are better evaluated on a dorsoventral view due to improved inflation of surrounding lung parenchyma. Mild pleural effusion may be more conspicuous on a ventrodorsal view, mild pneumothorax on a dorsoventral view.

If the cranial abdomen is included in the collimation, distribution of gas within the stomach can also aid in identification of the radiographic projection (see Chapter 13).

Many diagnoses (e.g. heart disease, thoracic trauma, pleural effusion or pneumothorax) can be made based on a single lateral view in combination with a ventrodorsal or dorsoventral radiograph. Many investigators prefer a right lateral over a left lateral view due to a more consistent appearance of the cardiac silhouette. The examiner has to be aware that the lung fields closer to the radiographic film / plate (i.e. the dependent lung) quickly become atelectatic and assume soft-tissue opacity. Pathological changes within the dependent lung (such as pulmonary metastasis or alveolar infiltrates as seen with aspiration pneumonia) silhouette with the collapsed lung, and may not be visible on the resultant radiograph (Fig. 9.12).

Special thoracic radiographic techniques include oblique views, dynamic radiographs and horizontal beam views. These techniques will be further discussed with the descriptions of specific thoracic diseases.

A right lateral radiograph allows evaluation of the left lung, a left lateral view evaluation of the right lung. In cases of suspected lung disease, or for staging in oncology patients ('met check'), opposite lateral views should always be acquired.

9.2.3 Phase of respiration (inspiration – expiration)

Thoracic radiographs should generally be acquired under maximum inspiration to ascertain optimal inflation of the lungs. Exceptions are dynamic thoracic radiographs (e.g. for a diagnosis of tracheal collapse) and radiographs acquired to rule out pulmonary emphysema.

- An **inspiratory radiograph** (Fig. 9.13a, b) is characterized by low pulmonary opacity and good contrast between the pulmonary parenchyma and soft tissues (especially the heart and pulmonary vessels). The heart and diaphragm have minimal or no contact. The diaphragm is mildly flattened and located further caudally than on an expiratory radiograph.
- On an **expiratory radiograph** (Fig. 9.13c, d) there is increased opacity to the pulmonary parenchyma, hampering evaluation of pulmonary vessels. The diaphragm is displaced cranially and in broad contact with the cardiac silhouette.

Increased pulmonary opacity on an expiratory radiograph can mimic pulmonary diseases. In addition, the decreased thoracic volume may yield the erroneous impression of cardiomegaly.

9.3 Diseases of the thorax

The radiographic evaluation of the small animal thorax may be challenging. Multiple thoracic diseases may affect more than one anatomic compartment (e.g. concurrent thoracic wall, pleural space and pulmonary lesions in a trauma case). Additionally, both significant and nonsignificant lesions may be present concurrently. It is important to evaluate all thoracic structures even if a lesion has already been identified.

9.4 Diseases of the thoracic wall

9.4.1 Extrapleural lesions

Lesions associated with the thoracic wall may be superimposed with intrathoracic structures and may on occasion be difficult to distinguish from mediastinal or pulmonary pathology.

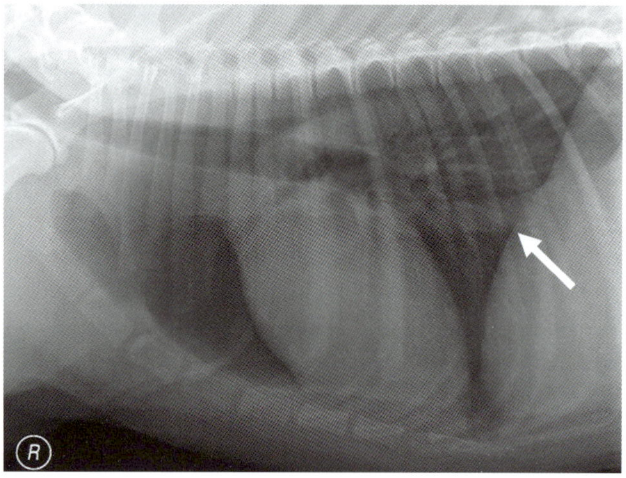

a

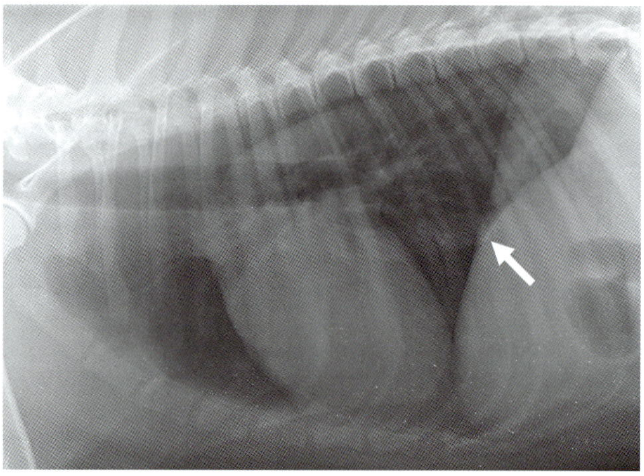

b

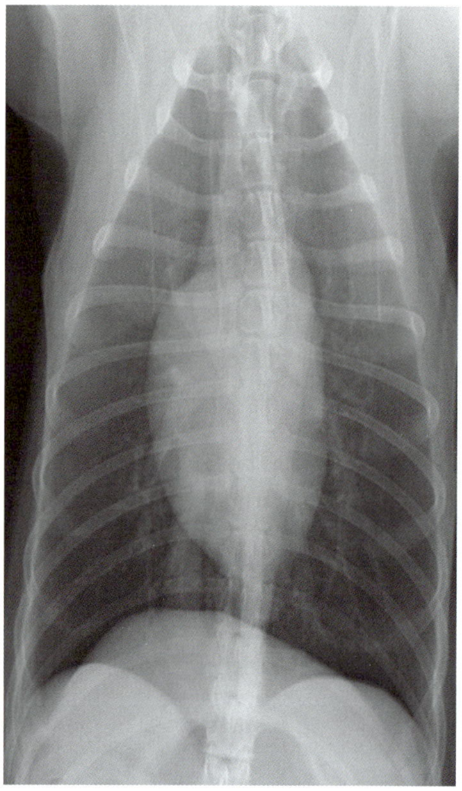

c

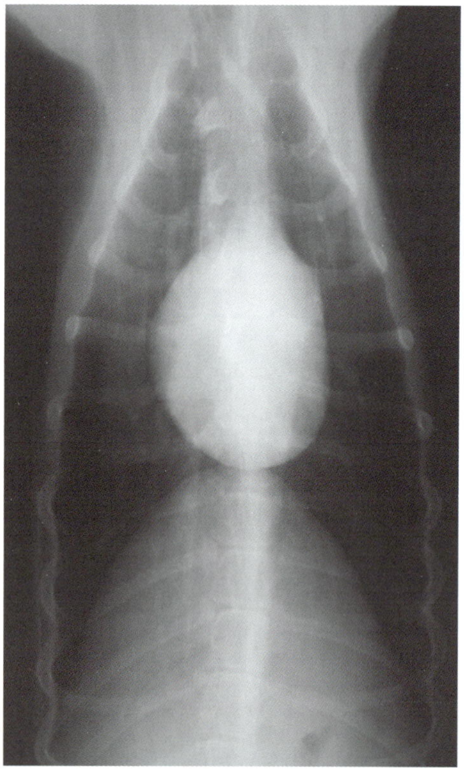

d

Fig. 9.11 Variations in appearance of the thorax depending on patient positioning.
a Right lateral radiograph. The diaphragmatic crura are parallel. The dependent (right) diaphragmatic crus is displaced cranially and can be identified based on its juncture with the caudal vena cava (arrow).
b Left lateral radiograph. The diaphragmatic crura diverge in the dorsal aspect of the thorax (appearing almost like an L). The dependent (left) diaphragmatic crus is displaced cranially. The caudal vena cava connects to the right diaphragmatic crus and is superimposed with the left diaphragmatic crus over a short distance (arrow).
c Ventrodorsal radiograph. The cardiac silhouette is elongated, and the diaphragm has three distinct domes.
d Dorsoventral radiograph. The heart is more rounded than on the ventrodorsal view, and the diaphragm only has one dome.

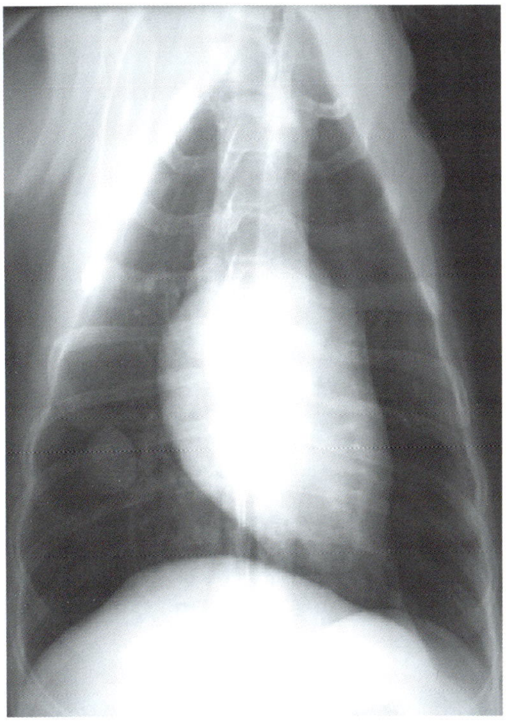

a

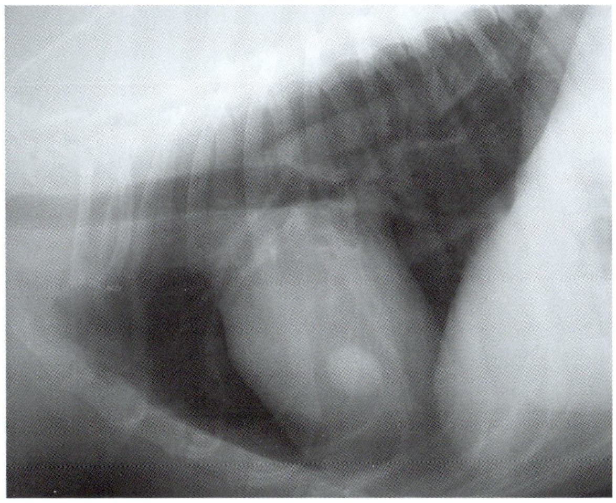

b

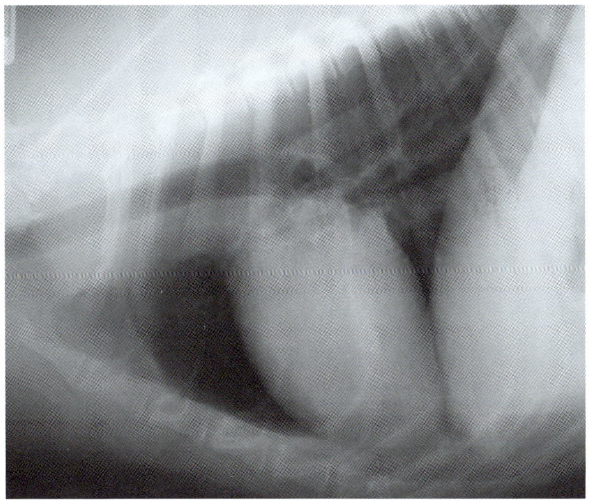

c

Fig. 9.12 Thoracic radiographs in a dog with a solitary soft tissue opacity mass (primary lung tumour) in the right middle lung lobe.

a On this ventrodorsal view, the soft-tissue opacity mass within the right middle lung lobe is visible in the plane of the sixth and seventh right intercostal spaces.

b On this left lateral view, the soft-tissue opacity mass is clearly seen and summates with the cardiac silhouette.

c On this right lateral view, the tumour is not visible due to silhouetting with adjacent atelectatic lung parenchyma.

(Courtesy of Dr Amy Sato, Tufts Cummings School of Veterinary Medicine, North Grafton, USA)

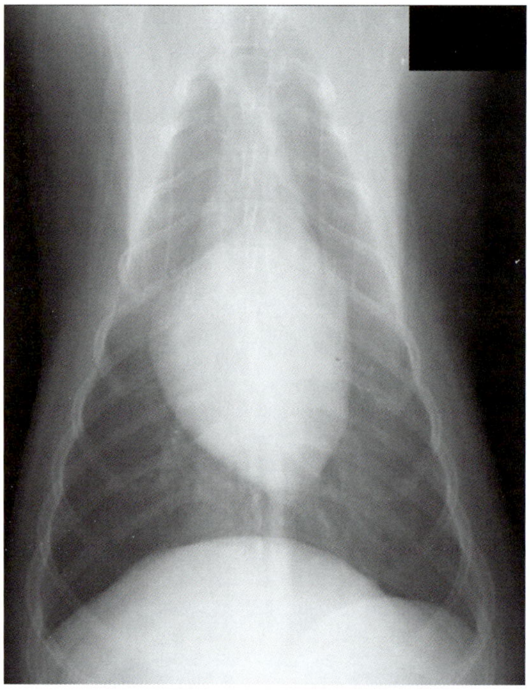

a

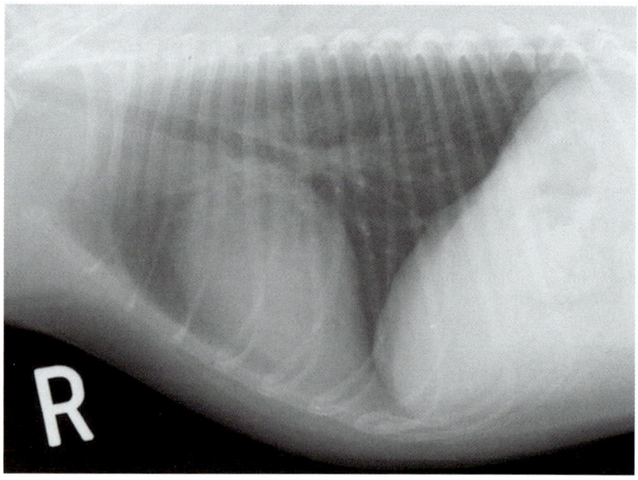

b

Fig. 9.13 a, b Ventrodorsal a and lateral b thoracic radiographs in inspiration. The lung is of low opacity, and pulmonary vessels are clearly visible. The diaphragm is mildly flattened and separate from the cardiac silhouette. (R = right).

c, d Ventrodorsal c and lateral d thoracic radiographs in expiration. Pulmonary opacity is artificially increased, which may mimic pulmonary disease and hampers evaluation of pulmonary vessels. The diaphragm is displaced cranially into the thoracic cavity and is in contact with the cardiac silhouette. The thoracic cavity appears smaller than on the inspiratory radiographs and is dominated by the cardiac silhouette, which may result in the erroneous diagnosis of cardiomegaly.

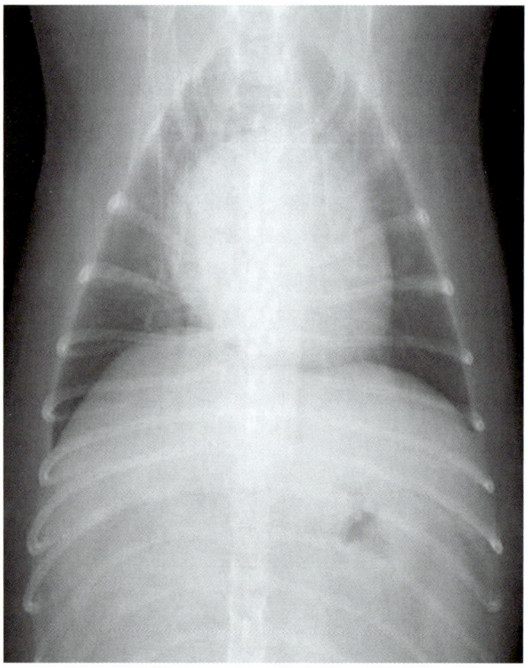

c

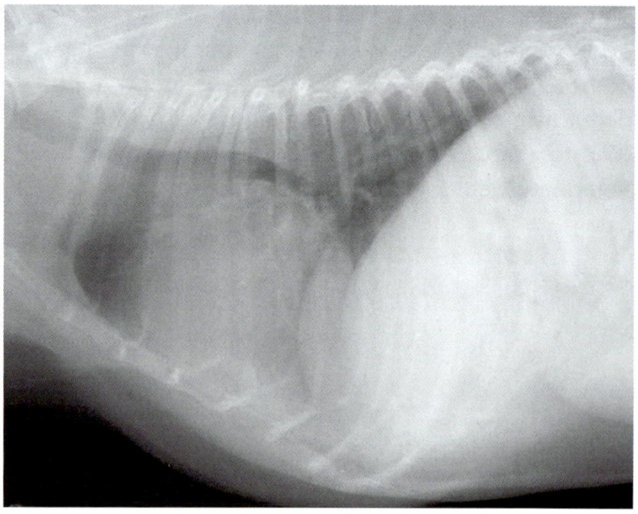

d

RADIOGRAPHIC FINDINGS The diagnosis of an extrapleural lesion (Fig. 9.14) is possible based on the following.

- Broad-based contact with the thoracic wall in at least one view and convex extension into the thoracic cavity ('extrapleural sign').
- Extension into the tissues outside the thoracic cavity.
- Associated bone abnormalities (e.g. periosteal reaction or lysis of ribs).

Oblique views or fluoroscopy may be helpful in demonstrating the extrapleural nature of a lesion in some cases.

Rib fractures

Rib fractures may be easy or difficult to identify depending on location, degree of dislocation and chronicity. Healed rib fractures are a common incidental finding on thoracic radiographs and may or may not be associated with a history of trauma. With acute thoracic trauma, additional findings such as soft-tissue swelling of the thoracic wall, pleural effusion, pneumothorax, pulmonary contusions and subcutaneous emphysema are common (Fig. 9.15). Like other fractures, rib fractures are categorized depending on location and presence and degree of displacement. With segmental fractures of adjacent ribs, abnormal mobility of the affected portion of the thoracic wall with paradoxical respiratory motion is possible ('flail chest'). In contrast to other rib fractures, surgical intervention may be required in these cases.

Primary tumours

Primary tumours of the thoracic wall commonly originate from the ribs or costal cartilages (chondrosarcoma, osteosarcoma). Origin from soft tissues of the thoracic wall is also possible. Rib associated tumours appear as mass lesions of variable size and are often associated with extensive heterogeneous mineralization. There is often at least partial destruction of the affected rib, and the mass may result in displacement of adjacent structures such as ribs, lung and even mediastinal organs (Fig. 9.16).

Secondary tumours

Metastases to ribs (e.g. from carcinoma) typically affect more than one rib at a time. They may appear as lytic and/or periosteal lesions, are often small and may be difficult to identify.

Lipomas

Fatty thoracic wall masses are common incidental findings especially in older dogs. They are less opaque than adjacent soft tissues and typically well defined.

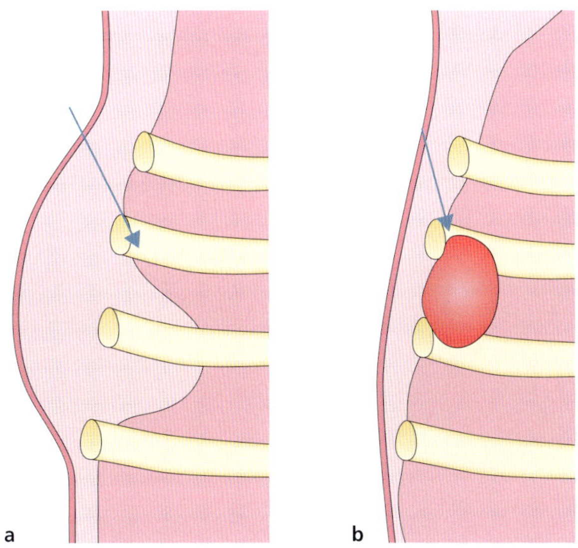

Fig. 9.14 Schematic illustration of an extrapleural a compared with a peripheral pulmonary b mass lesion.
a The extrapleural (thoracic wall) mass is in broad-based contact with the thoracic wall, has a convex margin towards the adjacent lung, and extends into the soft tissues outside the thoracic cavity. There is an obtuse angle between the mass and the adjacent normal thoracic wall (arrow).
b The pulmonary mass is limited to the lung and has an acute angle with the thoracic wall (arrow).

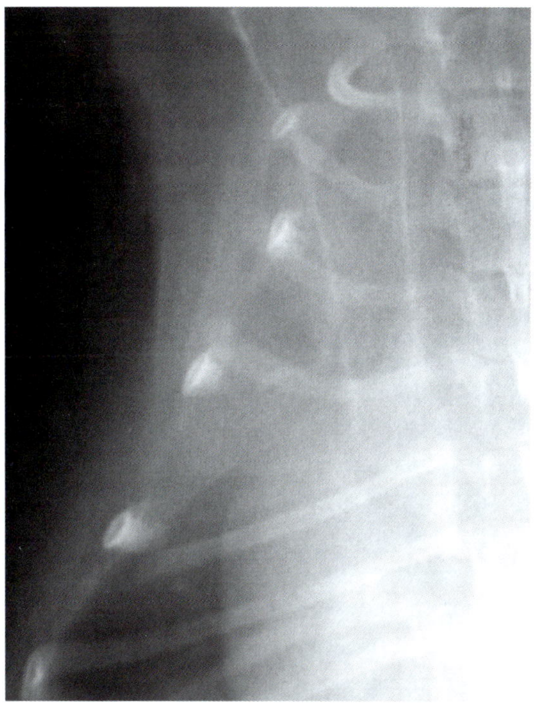

Fig. 9.15 Close-up of a ventrodorsal thoracic radiograph in a dog following thoracic trauma (bite wound). There are moderately displaced transverse fractures of the second through fifth right ribs. The adjacent right cranial lung lobe is of homogeneous increased opacity, consistent with pulmonary contusion.

Abscesses and granulomas

Inflammatory thoracic wall lesions appear as mass lesions of variable size and opacity and cannot usually be distinguished from neoplastic conditions. Depending on size, location and chronicity, concurrent rib lesions may be noted along with soft-tissue swelling. Foreign material within the lesion or gas inclusions may suggest inflammatory aetiology; however, an underlying tumour cannot usually be ruled out based on imaging findings alone.

9.4.2 Abnormal opacity of the thoracic wall

Subcutaneous emphysema

Inclusion of gas within the soft tissues of the thoracic wall is commonly seen following thoracic trauma. Air may reach the subcutaneous tissues and spread along the thoracic wall secondary to injury to intrathoracic air-filled structures (lung, trachea) or secondary to a perforating skin injury.

> RADIOGRAPHIC FINDINGS Subcutaneous gas inclusions appear as linear to irregularly marginated regions of decreased opacity between soft tissues of the thoracic wall (Fig. 9.17).

Soft-tissue mineralization

Increased radiographic opacity of the soft tissues of the thoracic wall may be focal or diffuse. Examples of underlying causes include dystrophic mineralization of soft-tissue lesions (e.g. neoplasia), metastatic mineralization and calcinosis cutis.

9.4.3 Thoracic wall anomalies

Congenital thoracic wall anomalies are not uncommon and are often incidental.

With **pectus excavatum,** the sternum is displaced dorsally, and on a lateral view projects dorsal to the costochondral junctions. This results in a decrease of the dorsoventral thoracic diameter and displacement of intrathoracic structures (Fig. 9.18). Affected animals may show signs such as exercise intolerance, respiratory difficulty or growth retardation, or may be asymptomatic.

Pectus carinatum is characterized by a ventral protuberance of the sternum and is usually an incidental finding in animals.

An **abnormal number of rib pairs and/or asymmetry of the last pair of ribs** are common and typically associated with spinal anomalies (transitional vertebrae, abnormal vertebral formula).

9.5 Diseases of the diaphragm

Evaluation of the diaphragm should include assessment of its position, contour, symmetry and continuity. Identification of a functional diaphragmatic anomaly requires inspiratory and expiratory radiographs or fluoro-

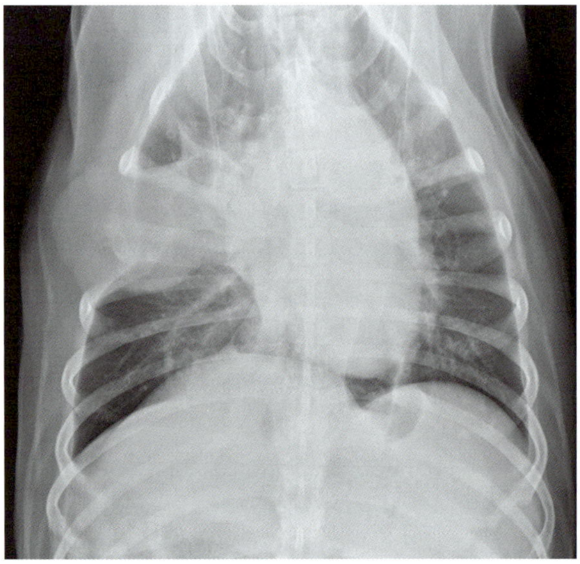

Fig. 9.16 Ventrodorsal thoracic radiograph in a 16-year-old mixed-breed dog with a primary tumour of the thoracic wall (osteosarcoma of the sixth right rib). A rounded, irregularly marginated soft-tissue opacity mass with extensive lysis of the underlying rib is associated with the right thoracic wall. The mass displaces the adjacent ribs and extends both into the thoracic cavity and subcutaneous tissues.

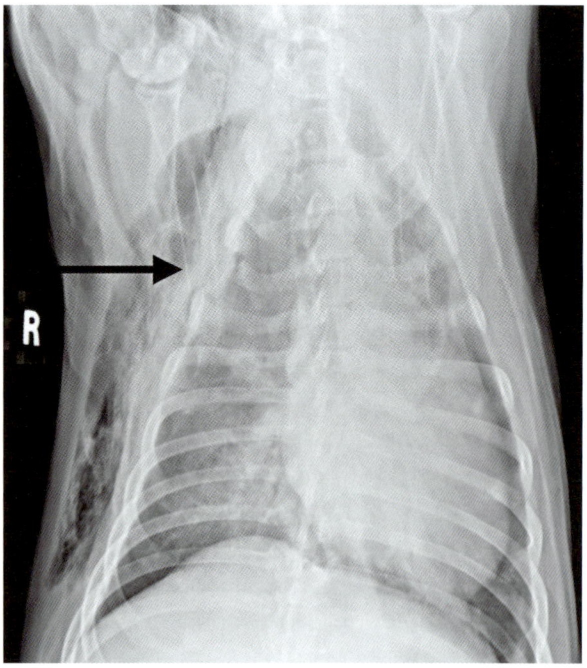

Fig. 9.17 Subcutaneous emphysema in a dog presented after being impaled on a stick. Extensive gas inclusions are associated with the soft tissues of the right thoracic wall. A fracture of the third right rib (arrow) is also noted (R = right).

scopic examination of the thorax during respiration. Multiple factors influence the radiographic appearance of the diaphragm, many of which are not associated with actual diaphragmatic diseases or anomalies.

- Cranial displacement of the diaphragm may be related to expiratory radiographs and may also be seen in adipose animals, patients with abdominal pain and patients with space-occupying intra-abdominal lesions.
- The diaphragm is displaced caudally with pulmonary emphysema and tension pneumothorax.
- Asymmetry and an abnormal contour of the diaphragm may be related to true diaphragmatic abnormalities such as hernia, paralysis or masses. However, these findings may also result from pulmonary or pleural diseases causing an increase or decrease in thoracic volume, or from adjacent space-occupying lesions associated with the thorax or cranial abdomen (Fig. 9.19).

The effect of positioning and respiratory phase on the appearance of the diaphragm is covered in section 9.2.3.

9.5.1 Diaphragmatic paralysis

Functional diaphragmatic anomalies are rarely documented in small animal practice and may be compensated for by the action of abdominal muscles.

RADIOGRAPHIC FINDINGS A diagnosis requires inspiratory and expiratory radiographs or fluoroscopy. In affected animals the entire or part of the diaphragm is hypomotile. Diaphragmatic asymmetry and paradoxical diaphragmatic motion may also be observed.

9.5.2 Diaphragmatic hernia

This is the most common diaphragmatic anomaly and is characterized by herniation of abdominal structures into the thoracic cavity.

Traumatic diaphragmatic hernia (rupture)

With a traumatic diaphragmatic rupture, there is tearing of the diaphragm or avulsion of the diaphragm from its insertion site with variable herniation of abdominal organs into the thoracic cavity. It is usually the result of recent or prior trauma. With acute diaphragmatic hernia, affected animals often present with respiratory difficulty. Animals

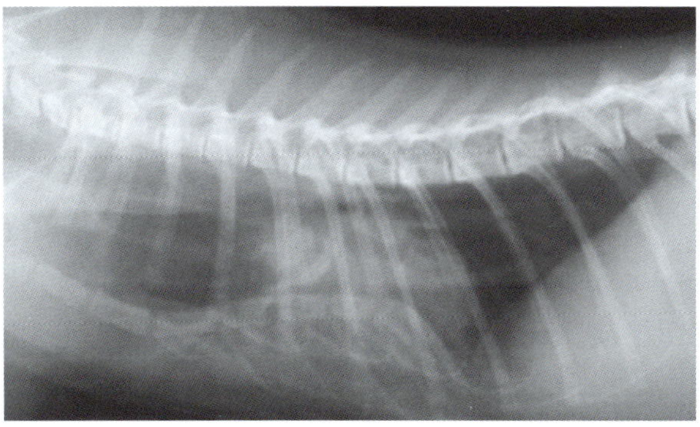

Fig. 9.18 Pectus excavatum in a 4-month-old cat. The caudal part of the sternum is displaced dorsally, resulting in marked reduction of the dorsoventral diameter of the thorax.

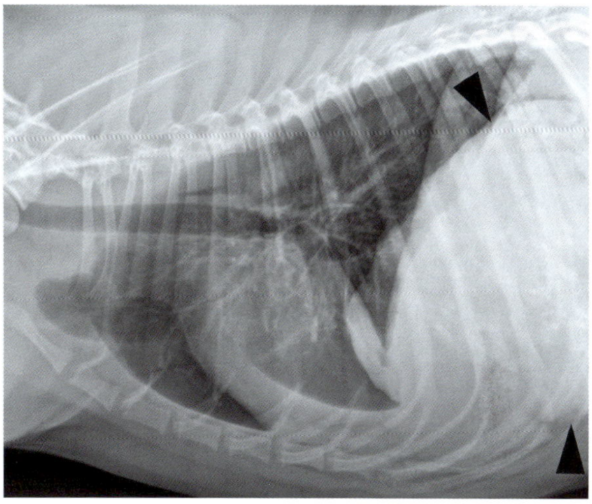

a

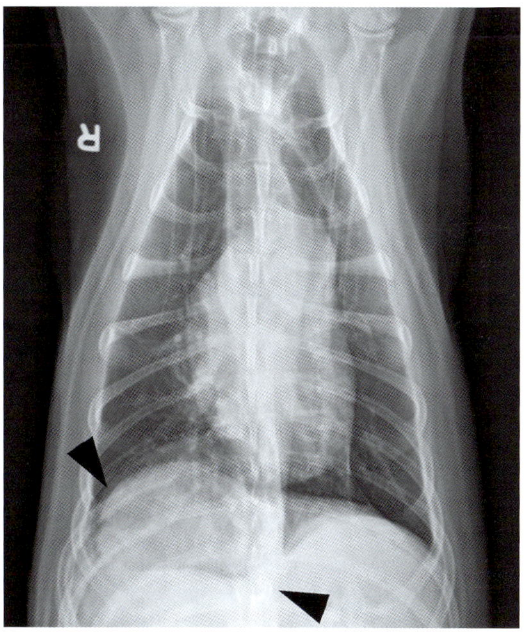

b

Fig. 9.19 Unusual contour and asymmetry of the diaphragm due to a thoracic wall mass (osteosarcoma) with intra-abdominal extension. The lateral a and ventrodorsal b radiographs show destruction of the distal part of the tenth right rib and a large mineral opacity mass within the right cranial abdominal quadrant (arrowheads). The right diaphragmatic crus is displaced cranially (R = right).

with chronic diaphragmatic hernias may or may not exhibit clinical signs, and a diagnosis may be made months or even years after trauma.

RADIOGRAPHIC FINDINGS The diaphragm is discontinuous, and various organs may be found within the thoracic cavity (Fig. 9.20). Concurrent indicators of thoracic trauma such as pleural effusion, rib fractures, pulmonary contusion or pneumothorax are common. On abdominal radiographs, unusual small size of the hepatic silhouette and absence of abdominal organs may be noted.

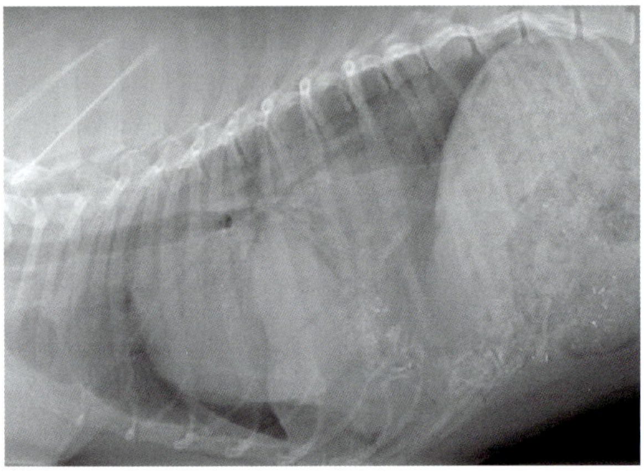

a

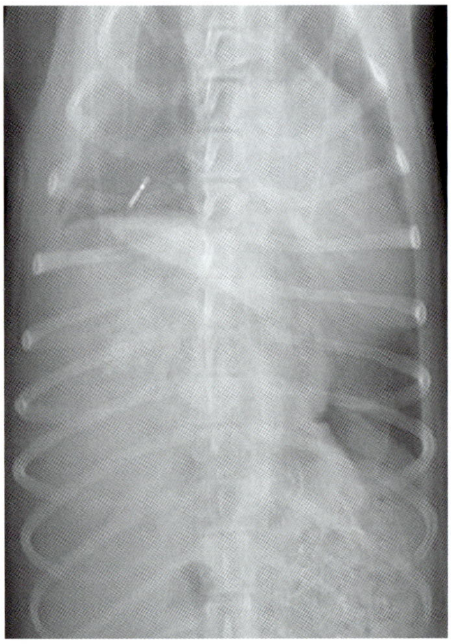

b

Fig. 9.20 Traumatic diaphragmatic hernia (rupture) in an 11-year-old dog following a road traffic accident. On the lateral a and ventrodorsal b thoracic radiographs there is discontinuity of the right diaphragmatic crus with herniation of abdominal viscera into the thoracic cavity.

Even though a radiographic diagnosis of diaphragmatic rupture sounds straightforward, concurrent abnormalities such as pleural effusion may complicate matters. In addition, intrathoracic mass lesions or focal effusion silhouetting with the diaphragm may mimic the presence of abdominal organs within the abdominal cavity. When in doubt, additional radiographs (horizontal beam views), oral contrast medium administration to demonstrate the presence of gastrointestinal segments within the thoracic cavity, or advanced diagnostic imaging such as ultrasound or computed tomography (CT) may aid in diagnosis (Fig. 9.21).

True diaphragmatic hernia (congenital)

With congenital diaphragmatic hernias there is a defect associated with the diaphragm; however, the integrity of the peritoneum and pleura is often maintained.

RADIOGRAPHIC FINDINGS Intra-abdominal fat or part of the liver focally protrudes into the caudoventral thorax (often mediastinum) (Fig. 9.22). This is usually an incidental finding and should not be confused with a tumour or abscess of the diaphragm or caudal mediastinum.

Peritoneo-pericardial diaphragmatic hernia (PPDH)

With this condition there is a congenital defect within the ventral (tendinous) part of the diaphragm, connecting the peritoneal with the pericardial space. Various abdominal organs can herniate into the pericardium. This condition is more common in cats than in dogs. Affected animals may be asymptomatic or present with problems related to herniated organs (e.g. vascular compromise of the liver or intestinal obstruction). Concurrent congenital sternal anomalies may be present.

RADIOGRAPHIC FINDINGS The cardiac silhouette is enlarged, has an abnormal contour and is in broad-based contact with the ventral diaphragm. Distinct margins of herniated organs may or may not be visible. The intra-abdominal hepatic silhouette is typically smaller than normal (Fig. 9.23).

Hiatal hernia

With this condition there is herniation of abdominal organs (typically the stomach) through the oesophageal hiatus into the caudodorsal thoracic cavity. This is covered in more detail in section 13.3.5.

9.5.3 Other diseases

Other diseases and anomalies of the diaphragm are rare. **Abscesses or tumours** appear as mass lesions of variable location and size. Confirmation of diaphragmatic origin of these lesions usually requires advanced imaging such as fluoroscopy, ultrasound or CT.

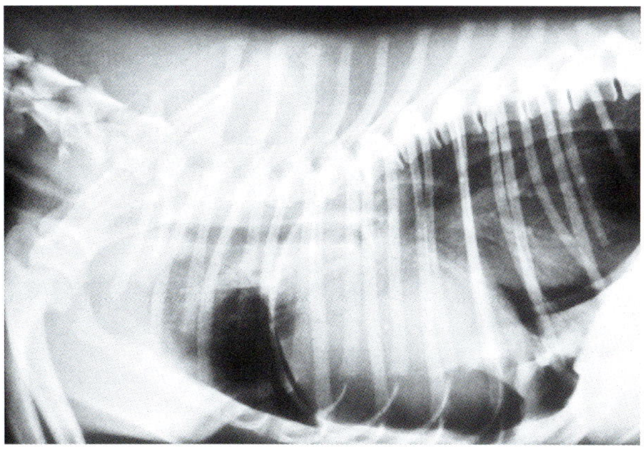

a

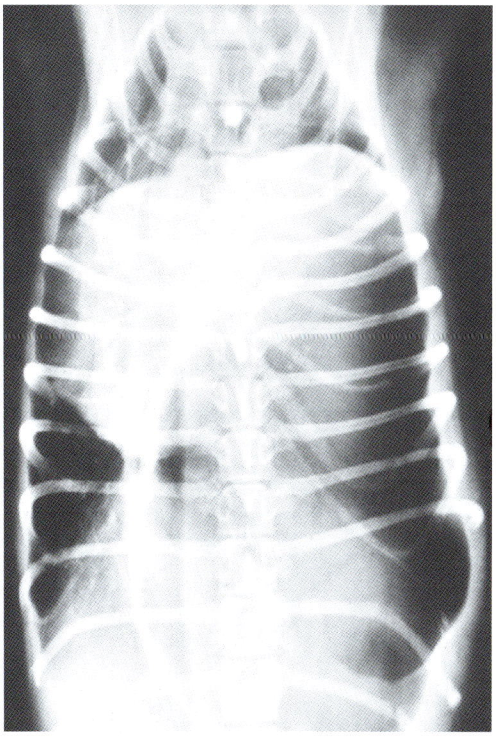

b

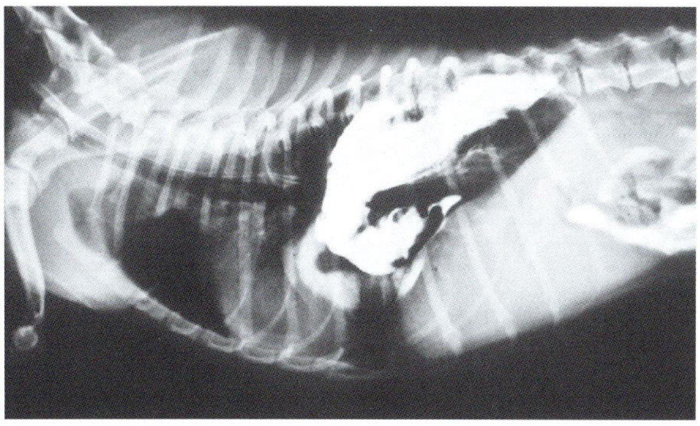

c

Fig. 9.21 Lateral a and ventrodorsal b thoracic radiographs in a 1-year-old Yorkshire Terrier presented with acute dyspnoea 10 days following a bite wound to the thorax. The entire left half of the thorax is occupied by a gas distended structure that results in rightward displacement of the cardiac silhouette. Following oral contrast medium administration c, the suspicion of diaphragmatic rupture with herniation and incarceration of the stomach is confirmed (tension gastrothorax). The stomach is less distended than on survey radiographs. Note also left-sided rib fractures best seen on the ventrodorsal view b.

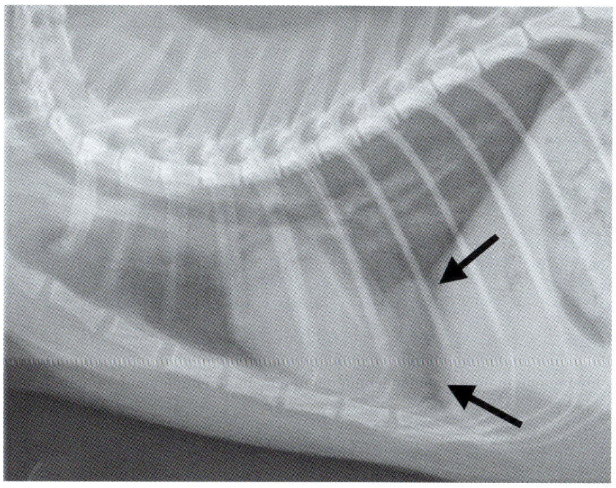

Fig. 9.22 Incidental finding of a congenital (true) diaphragmatic hernia in a 4-year-old cat. A dome-shaped fat opacity protrusion is associated with the cranioventral margin of the diaphragm (arrows).

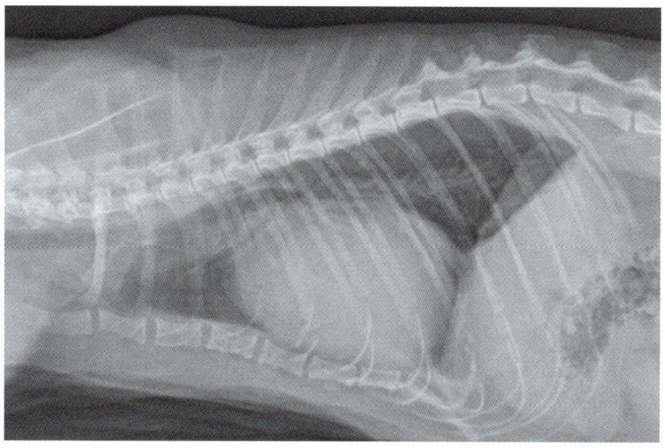

Fig. 9.23 Incidental finding of a peritoneo-pericardial diaphragmatic hernia in a 10-year-old cat. The cardiac silhouette is enlarged, has an unusual contour and silhouettes with the ventral aspect of the diaphragm. The intra-abdominal hepatic silhouette is smaller than normal.

Muscular dystrophy is a rare condition in dogs and cats which on radiographs results in a zig-zag contour of the diaphragm.

9.6 Diseases of the pleura and pleural space

As mentioned above, the pleural space is a potential space between the parietal and visceral pleura and separating adjacent lung lobes (see section 9.1.1). The normal pleura is not visible on radiographs apart from the mediastinal reflections. With thickening of the pleura or accumulation of material in the pleural space (cellular infiltrates, fluid, gas), radiographic identification becomes possible. Pleural abnormalities may be primary but are more commonly seen secondary to or in association with other thoracic disease processes.

9.6.1 Pleural effusion

Fluid accumulation within the pleural space may be unilateral or bilateral, focal or generalized. Dogs and cats have small mediastinal fenestrations, resulting in bilateral distribution of pleural effusion in most instances except for very viscous (cellular, proteinaceous) types of fluid. Different types of pleural effusion (exudate, transudate, lymphatic effusion and haemorrhage) cannot be distinguished radiographically, and thoracocentesis with fluid analysis is typically the next step following diagnosis of pleural effusion. As a rule of thumb, approximately 100 ml of pleural effusion must be present to be visible on thoracic radiographs.

Radiographic findings With mild pleural effusion, thin pleural fissure lines become apparent between adjacent lung lobes (Fig. 9.24). With increasing severity, the following radiographic abnormalities are noted.

- Widening of the pleural fissures.
- Retraction of the lung lobes from the thoracic wall and diaphragm.
- Accumulation of fluid opacity material within the ventral thorax with a scalloped margination of the ventral lung lobes.
- Rounding of the lung lobes.
- Silhouetting of pleural fluid with the heart and diaphragm (Fig. 9.25).

Repetition of thoracic radiographs following thoracocentesis may allow identification of underlying disease processes obscured by pleural effusion on initial radiographs (e.g. mediastinal mass lesions or diaphragmatic rupture).

A small volume of pleural effusion is easier to identify on a ventrodorsal than on a dorsoventral radiograph where it may be obscured by the adjacent sternum. A larger volume of pleural effusion silhouettes with the cardiac silhouette on a DV view, hampering evaluation of the cardiovascular structures. On the other hand, radiographic evaluation of the cardiac silhouette remains possible on a VD view even with a larger volume of effusion, as the heart remains located in the nondependent portion of the thorax and is surrounded by air-filled lung rather than fluid (Fig. 9.26).

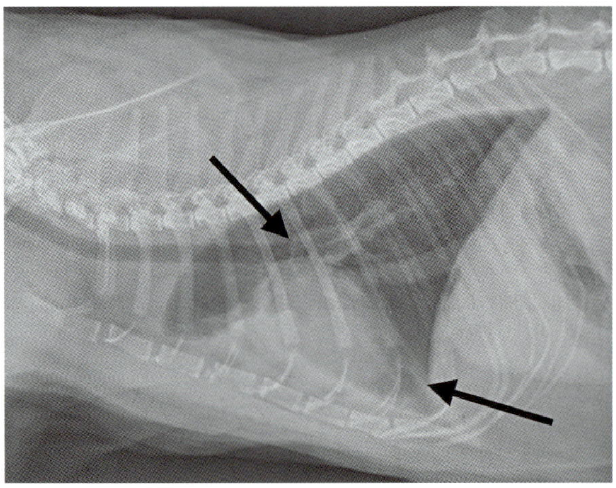

Fig. 9.24 Mild pleural effusion in a cat. Pleural fissures appear as approximately 2 mm wide soft-tissue opacity lines (arrows), and a small amount of soft-tissue opaque material silhouettes with the ventral aspect of the heart.

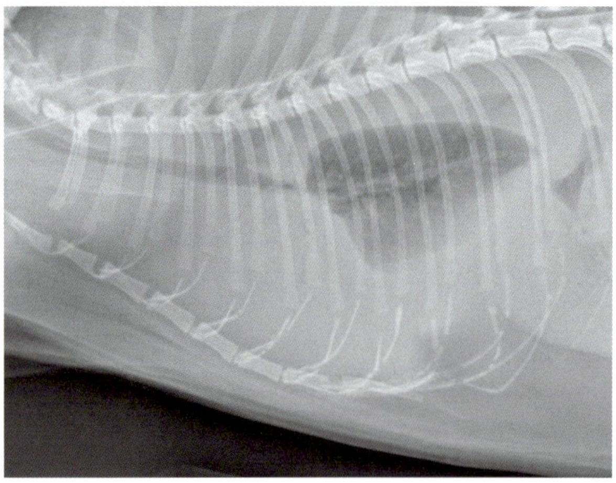

Fig. 9.25 Severe pleural effusion in a cat with cranial mediastinal lymphoma. A large amount of soft-tissue opaque material silhouettes with the heart and diaphragm. The lung lobes are rounded, surrounded by fluid and retracted from the thoracic wall. A mass within the cranial mediastinum was confirmed with ultrasound.

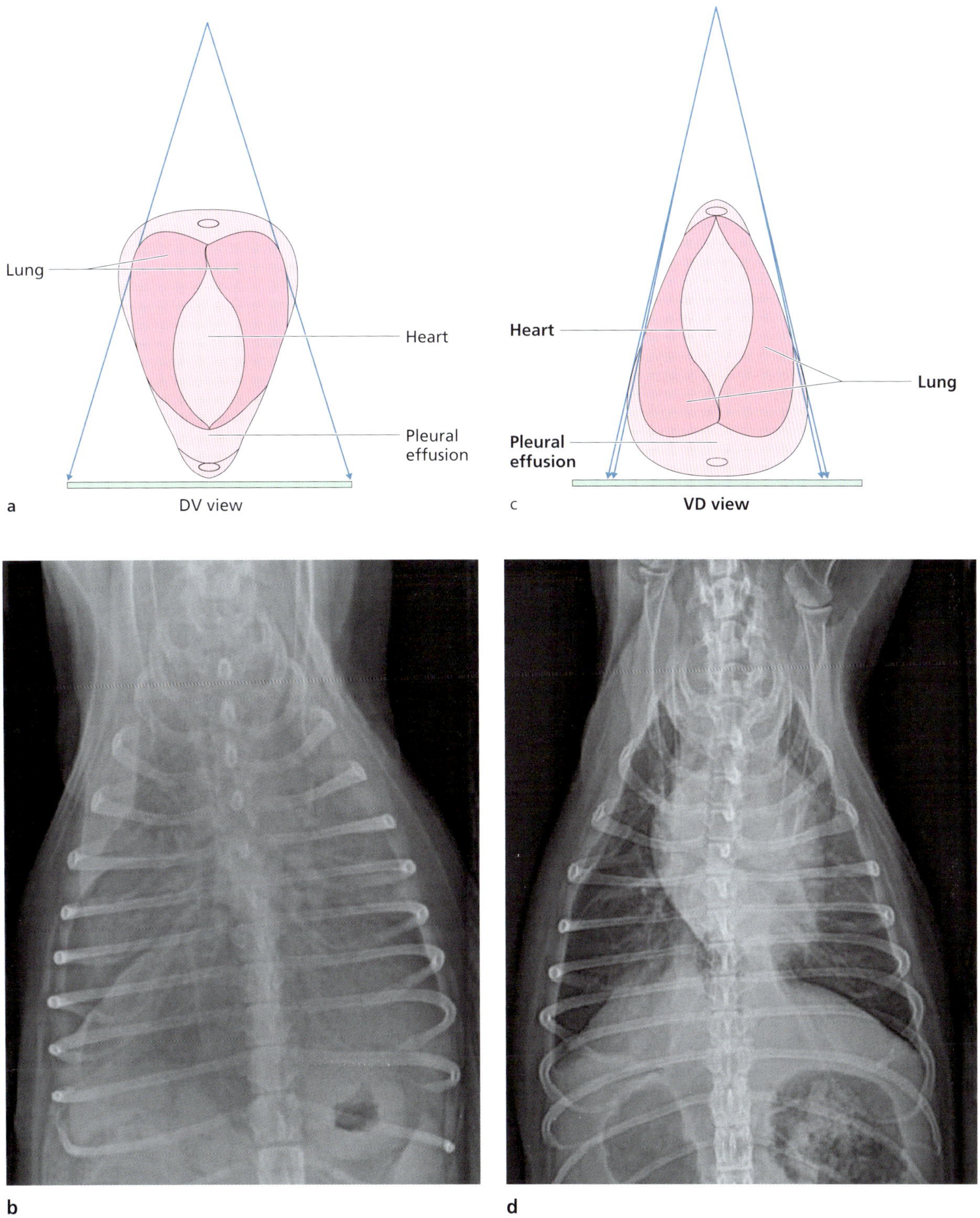

Fig. 9.26 Effect of patient positioning on thoracic radiographs in animals with pleural effusion.

a, b Schematic cross-sectional image of the thorax in a patient positioned in sternal recumbency a and corresponding dorsoventral radiograph of the thorax b. On this DV view, fluid accumulates dorsal to the sternum which may go unnoticed in cases of mild pleural effusion. However, the presence of a larger volume of pleural fluid results in silhouetting of pleural effusion with the cardiac silhouette and diaphragm, hampering evaluation.

c, d Schematic cross-sectional image of the thorax in a patient positioned in dorsal recumbency c and corresponding ventrodorsal radiograph of the thorax d. On the VD view, pleural effusion accumulates in the dorsal part of the thorax and surrounds the caudodorsal lung lobes, allowing diagnosis even in mild cases. Even with severe pleural effusion, limited assessment of the size and shape of the heart is possible as it is surrounded by pulmonary parenchyma rather than fluid.

Superimposition of pleural effusion and pulmonary parenchyma often results in the impression of increased radiographic pulmonary opacity. This may lead to an erroneous diagnosis of pulmonary disease. In addition, severe pleural effusion may hamper visualization and evaluation of the heart, mediastinal structures and diaphragm.

Pitfalls

Obesity: Suprasternal fat accumulation in obese animals (especially dogs) may result in a region of increased opacity in the ventral thorax and mimic pleural effusion. Unlike with true pleural effusion, the cardiac silhouette is delineated by surrounding fat and has clearly visible margins. Widened pleural fissure lines are absent (Fig. 9.27).

Pleural thickening: Pleural thickening is to some degree a normal ageing change, and thin, soft-tissue opaque pleural fissure lines are commonly seen as an incidental finding in older animals (especially dogs). These may be difficult to distinguish from mild pleural effusion; however, pleural fissure lines are typically very thin and sharply delineated, and other indicators of pleural effusion are lacking (Fig. 9.28).

Chest wall conformation: The conformation of the costochondral junctions as well as excessive skin folds may mimic pleural effusion especially in chondrodystrophic dogs (Fig. 9.29).

9.6.2 Pneumothorax

The most common reason for gas accumulation within the pleural space is thoracic trauma, either associated with a penetrating thoracic wound and subsequent entry of air into the pleural space, or due to air leaking from damaged lung parenchyma. Other possible aetiologies of pneumothorax include rupture of a cavitary lung lesion (bulla, cavitary lung tumour, abscess), infection of the pleural space with gas-producing bacteria or interventional procedures (thoracocentesis, lung biopsy, etc.). A thorough history and evaluation of the radiographs for any concurrent findings are needed for full patient assessment. A pneumothorax may be unilateral or bilateral, symmetric or asymmetric. As described for pleural effusion, mediastinal fenestrations usually result in the distribution of air in both pleural cavities.

RADIOGRAPHIC FINDINGS With pneumothorax, gas opacity is identified in the periphery of the thorax, with retraction and well-defined outer margins of the lung lobes. In contrast to regions of normal pulmonary parenchyma, pulmonary vessels and bronchi are lacking in regions of free pleural air (Fig. 9.30). The retracted lung is of increased opacity compared to normal pulmonary parenchyma due to decreased air content (atelectasis).

On lateral radiographs, there is apparent separation of the heart from the sternum. This is caused by accumulation of free air in the nondependent part of the thorax, collapse of the dependent lung, and displacement of the heart into the dependent part of the thorax with gravity (Fig. 9.31).

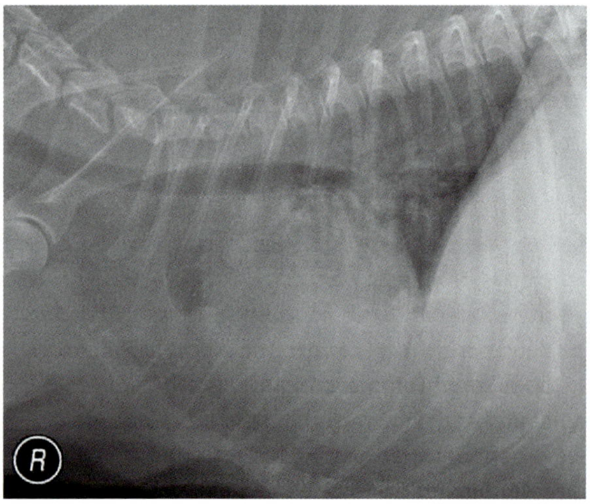

Fig. 9.27 Suprasternal accumulation of fat can mimic pleural effusion. Note that the cardiac silhouette is clearly delineated by surrounding fat, and pleural fissure lines are absent (R = right).

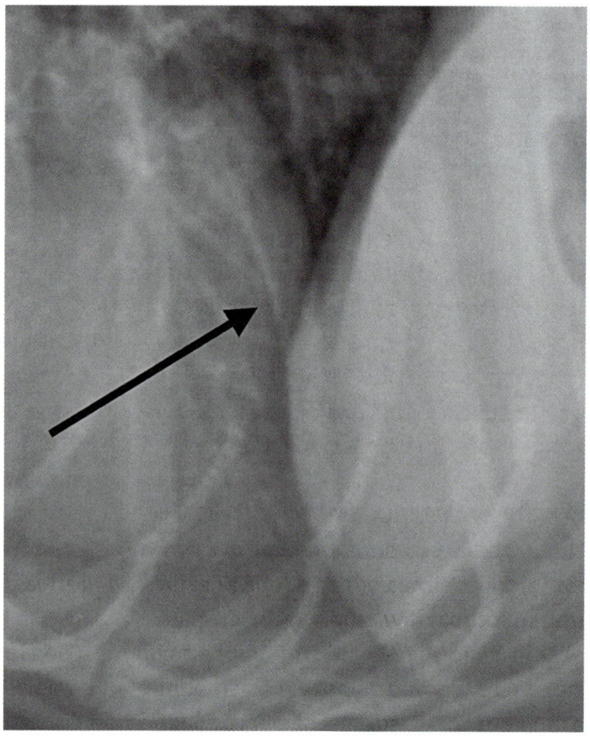

Fig. 9.28 Incidental finding of a thin pleural fissure line (arrow) between the middle and caudal lung lobes in an older dog due to pleural thickening.

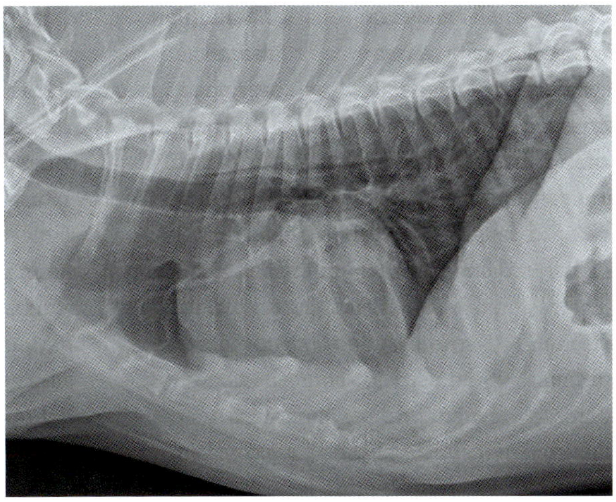

Fig. 9.29 Chondrodystrophic chest wall conformation. A scalloped region of soft-tissue opacity is noted along the costochondral junctions and may result in an erroneous diagnosis of pleural effusion. Note that margins of the cardiac silhouette remain clearly visible, pleural fissure lines are absent and the caudodorsal lung lobes extend to the thoracic wall and diaphragm.

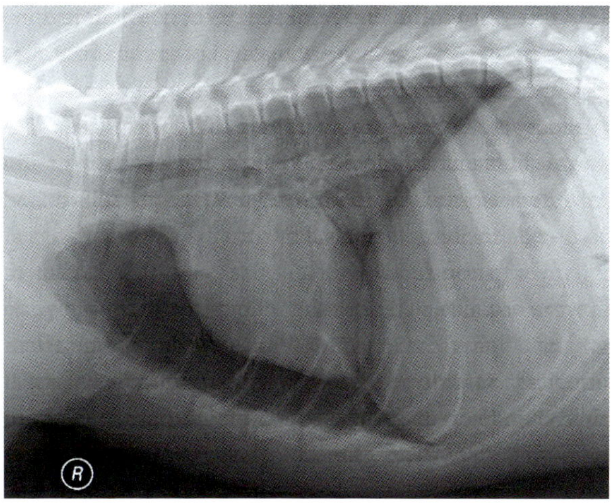

a

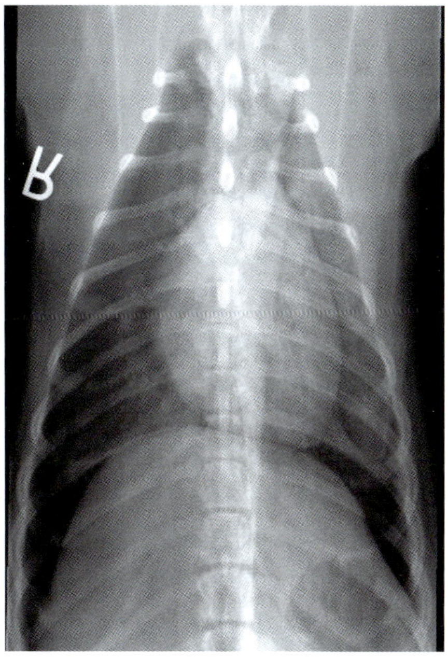

b

Fig. 9.30 Pneumothorax in a dog. There is separation of the lung lobes from the thoracic wall and sternum on the lateral a and ventrodorsal b thoracic radiographs. The lung margins are clearly delineated. Note generalized diffuse increase in pulmonary opacity due to atelectasis (R = right).

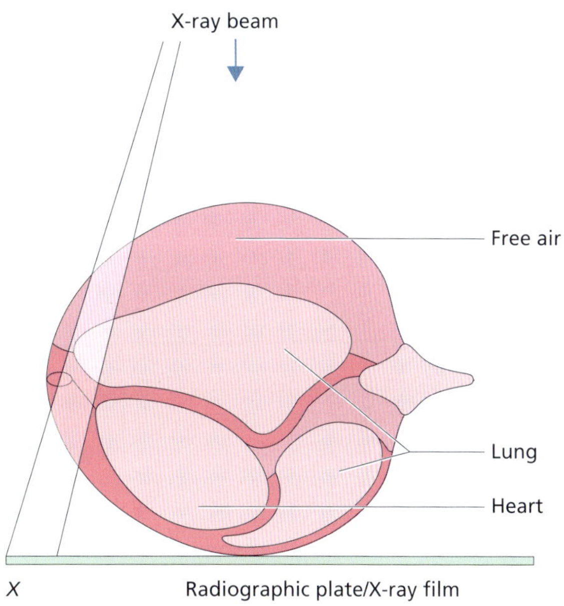

Fig. 9.31 Schematic illustration of the distribution of free air within the pleural space and intrathoracic structures in a patient with pneumothorax and in lateral recumbency. Free air ascends to the nondependent part of the thorax. The dependent lung collapses, and the heart 'falls' into the dependent part of the thorax. Radiographically, this appears as separation of heart and sternum (**X**).

A pneumothorax is more easily recognized on a dorsoventral than a ventrodorsal radiograph. Free air ascends into the nondependent part of the thorax and accumulates adjacent to the sternum on a VD view. On a DV view, free air surrounds and results in retraction of the caudodorsal lung lobes (Fig. 9.32).

Tension pneumothorax is defined as a situation where air progressively accumulates within the pleural space due to a one-way valve effect (such as seen with a perforating thoracic wound). The pressure within the pleural space exceeds atmospheric pressure, hampering pulmonary inflation during inspiration. Radiographic indicators include severe pneumothorax with extreme pulmonary collapse and marked caudal displacement and tenting of the diaphragm.

Pitfalls

Chest wall conformation: Physiological separation of the heart from the sternum on lateral thoracic radiographs is a common finding in deep-chested dogs and may mimic a pneumothorax. Upon close inspection, pulmonary vessels and bronchial structures can be traced into the region between the heart and sternum (Fig. 9.33).

Skin folds projected over the thorax may result in regions of increased and decreased opacity and result in an erroneous impression of pneumothorax. Pulmonary vessels are typically visible within the questionable region. Additionally, skin folds often extend beyond the margins of the thorax (Fig. 9.34).

Microcardia: Small size of the cardiac silhouette (e.g. in cases of hypovolaemia, shock or hypoadrenocorticism) may result in separation of the heart from the sternum on lateral views and mimic a pneumothorax. This is further discussed in Chapter 10.

Overexposure: On overexposed radiographs, lung parenchyma is figuratively 'burned out'. This problem most commonly occurs in the periphery of the thorax on VD or DV views. Especially in deep-chested dogs, there is marked discrepancy in the degree of X-ray attenuation between the largest thoracic diameter (at the level of the mediastinum, spine and sternum) and the smallest thoracic diameter (peripherally along the ribs). A large part of the X-ray beam is attenuated in the central region of the thorax, while most X-rays easily penetrate the peripheral lung fields, resulting in extreme exposure of the X-ray film or plate at this level. Differentiation between overexposure and pneumothorax requires evaluation of adjacent structures (ribs and soft tissues of the thoracic wall) for indicators of overexposure, and thorough assessment of corresponding lateral radiographs for any indicators of pneumothorax.

9.6.3 Infiltrative diseases of the pleura

Inflammatory or neoplastic infiltrative pleural diseases may be seen in association with other intrathoracic disease processes or may be an isolated problem. Primary pleuritis in small animals is rare. Primary (mesothelioma) or secondary (metastatic) neoplastic infiltration of the pleura is also uncommon.

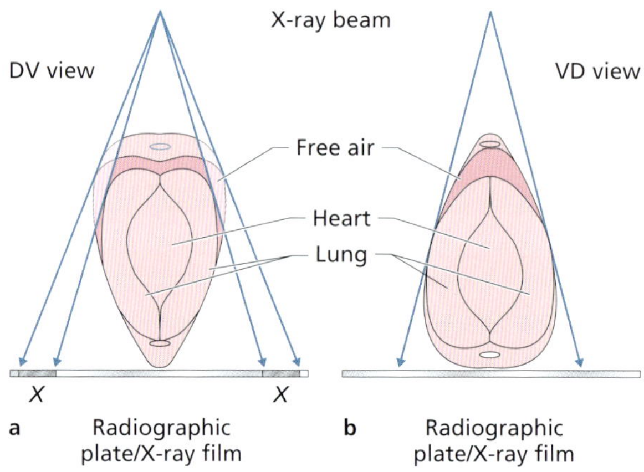

Fig. 9.32 Schematic illustration of distribution of free air in the pleural space on a dorsoventral a and ventrodorsal b view. On the DV view, air accumulates in the dorsal part of the thorax and surrounds the caudodorsal lung lobes. Even a small volume pneumothorax is easily recognized due to good contrast between pulmonary parenchyma and surrounding air (X). On the VD view, air accumulates adjacent to the sternum and may not be noted in mild cases.

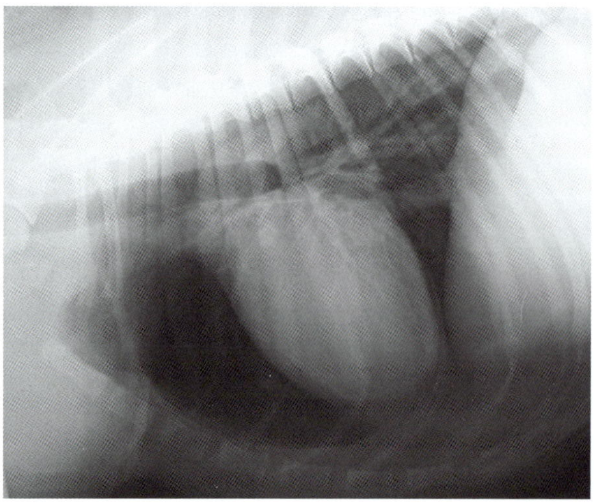

Fig. 9.33 False impression of pneumothorax in a deep-chested dog. The heart is separate from the sternum. However, on close inspection, pulmonary vessels and bronchial structures are identified between the heart and the sternum, which would not be the case with pneumothorax.

RADIOGRAPHIC FINDINGS With most infiltrative pleural diseases, concurrent pleural effusion is present which may be the predominant radiographic abnormality. Other possible radiographic findings include pleural masses or pleural thickening which may be difficult to distinguish from pulmonary or extrapleural lesions. Chronic disease processes result in rounding of the retracted lung margins ('restrictive pleuritis').

9.7 Diseases of the mediastinum

The mediastinum is formed by folding of the parietal pleura in the dorsal and ventral thorax. It is located on the midline, separates the left and right pleural space, and contains the heart, vessels, nerves, lymph nodes, trachea, thymus, fat and the oesophagus. Mediastinal abnormalities and disease processes can be subdivided into diseases of the mediastinal space (pneumomediastinum, mediastinal fluid accumulation), and diseases of specific mediastinal organs. Diseases of the trachea, heart and oesophagus are covered in Chapters 8, 10 and 13, respectively.

Mediastinal masses may originate from mediastinal organs such as the oesophagus or thymus, or may not be organ associated. This chapter will cover the radiographic diagnosis of mediastinal mass lesions and possible differential diagnoses. As discussed for the pleural space, mediastinal disorders often do not occur in isolation but are found in association with other abnormalities. For example, patients with tumours of the cranial mediastinum often have a concurrent pleural effusion due to impaired venous or lymphatic return to the heart. In patients with pneumomediastinum other signs of thoracic trauma such as pneumothorax or fractures may be present.

A **mediastinal shift** into the left or right pleural space is very common and does not necessarily indicate a pathological process. The most common reason for shifting of the mediastinum and mediastinal organs is (temporary) loss of lung volume due to lateral recumbency (positional atelectasis). The dependent lung collapses within a few minutes, more so in patients under general anaesthesia than in awake animals.

RADIOGRAPHIC FINDINGS A decrease in lung volume results in a shift of the cardiac silhouette from the midline on a VD or DV view. The collapsed (atelectatic) lung is diffusely increased in opacity (Fig. 9.35). The degree and duration of these abnormalities depend on individual

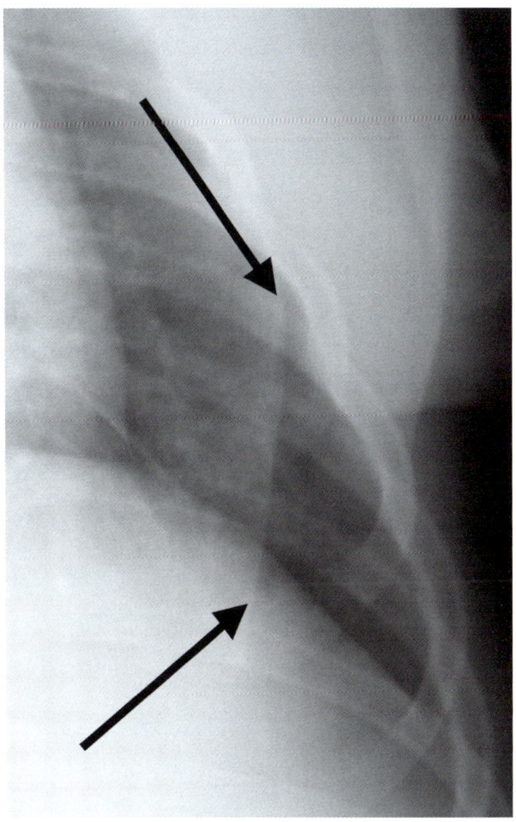

Fig. 9.34 'Pseudopneumothorax' in a dog due to superimposition of a skin fold over the left caudal thorax (arrows) and resultant artificially decreased opacity of the periphery of the left caudal lung lobe. Pulmonary vessels are associated with the region of decreased opacity, which would not be the case with true pneumothorax. Additionally, the skin fold extends beyond the thoracic margins and is also superimposed with the cranial abdomen.

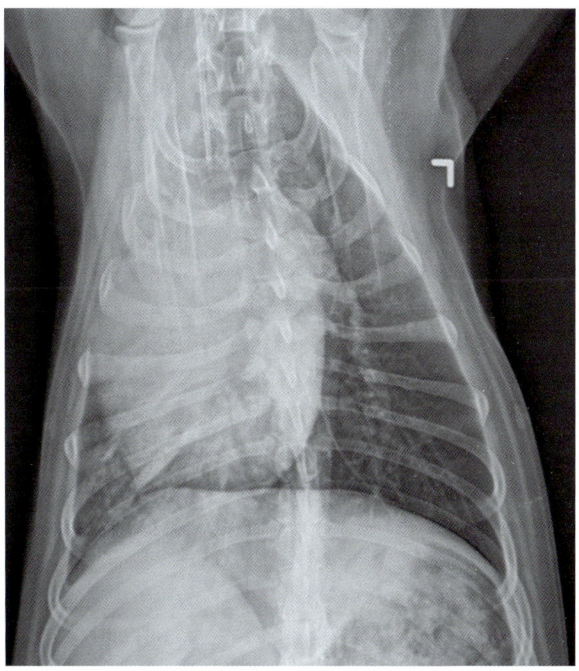

Fig. 9.35 Positional atelectasis and mediastinal shift to the right due to prior right lateral recumbency under general anaesthesia. The right lung is collapsed and of increased opacity. The cardiac silhouette is entirely located within the right half of the thorax (L = left).

factors, duration of prior lateral recumbency, respiratory capabilities of the patient, and patient status (under anaesthesia versus awake).

Positional atelectasis and mediastinal shift significantly interfere with evaluation of thoracic structures. Thoracic radiographs under general anaesthesia are generally discouraged for this reason. If thoracic radiographs under anaesthesia are unavoidable (e.g. in highly aggressive animals), the patient should be positioned in sternal recumbency and be ventilated with positive pressure ventilation.

Other factors that may affect the position of the mediastinum include abnormal conformation of the thoracic wall (e.g. pectus excavatum), space-occupying intrathoracic processes such as lung tumours, diaphragmatic rupture with organ displacement into the thorax, or overinflated (emphysematous) lung. Displacement of the cardiac silhouette and mediastinum and compromise of pulmonary parenchyma by these processes is referred to as 'push atelectasis'. Conversely, pulmonary volume loss (e.g. following lung lobe resection or bronchial obstruction) or pleural adhesions may result in mediastinal shift into the ipsilateral hemithorax ('pull atelectasis'). In cases where a reason for abnormal mediastinal position cannot be identified, repeat radiographs at a later point in time are indicated.

If the quality of thoracic radiographs is limited by positional atelectasis and mediastinal shift to a degree that evaluation of pulmonary parenchyma is not possible, radiographs should be repeated at a later point in time. Repeat radiographs are also indicated if an abnormal mediastinal position is noted and a cause other than anaesthesia or lateral recumbency is suspected.

Obliquely positioned ventrodorsal or dorsoventral views may result in the erroneous impression of mediastinal shift. Adequate evaluation of mediastinal position requires straight positioning.

9.7.1 Mediastinal mass lesions and generalized mediastinal widening

Mediastinal mass lesions

Tumours within the mediastinum and mediastinal mass lesions of other aetiologies are relatively common. Mediastinal masses may originate from mediastinal structures or may

Table 9.1 Differential diagnoses for mediastinal mass lesions depending on location.

Location	Differential diagnoses
Cranioventral	Lymphoma Thymoma Enlarged sternal and/or cranial mediastinal lymph nodes (in typical location) Mediastinal cyst (cats) Others
Craniodorsal (ventral to the trachea)	Heart base tumour Focal megaoesophagus (vascular ring anomaly) Others
Caudoventral	Special types of diaphragmatic hernia (e.g. peritoneo-pericardial diaphragmatic hernia) Others
Caudodorsal	Hiatal hernia Parasitic oesophageal granuloma (Spirocerca lupi) Others
Hilar region	Enlarged tracheobronchial lymph nodes Heart base tumour Others
Dorsal	(Generalized) megaoesophagus, oesophageal foreign bodies, oesophageal tumours and oesophageal/paraoesophageal abscesses Paraspinal tumours Others
Variable	Abscess or granuloma Haematoma Other tumours

not be organ associated. Common differential diagnoses for lesions in certain locations are listed in Table 9.1. However, the finding of a mediastinal mass lesion is often nonspecific, requiring further diagnostic steps such as contrast studies (oesophagography), ultrasound, CT (± angiography), endoscopy, fine-needle aspiration or biopsy for a definitive diagnosis.

RADIOGRAPHIC FINDINGS Mediastinal mass lesions typically appear as soft-tissue opacities of variable shape and size that result in abnormal increased opacity of the mediastinum on lateral views and mediastinal widening on ventrodorsal or dorsoventral views. Small masses may appear separate from the cardiac silhouette (Fig. 9.36 and 9.37). Larger masses silhouette with the heart and result in displacement of the trachea (Fig. 9.38). Concurrent pleural effusion is common especially with cranial mediastinal masses due to impaired venous and lymphatic return to the heart.

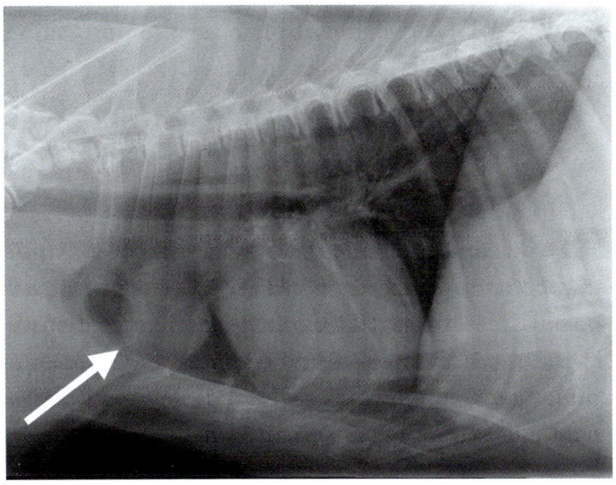

a

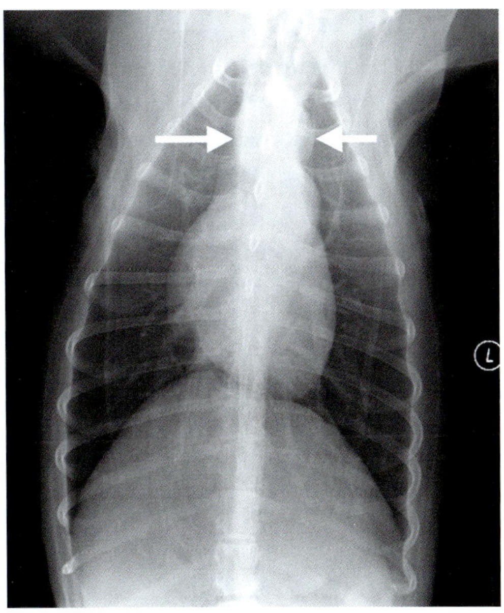

b

Fig. 9.36 Cranial (cranioventral) mediastinal mass in a 12-year-old dog.
a On the lateral view, a well-circumscribed, round, soft-tissue opacity mass is present cranial to the cardiac silhouette (arrow).
b On the ventrodorsal view, the cranial mediastinum is widened and of soft-tissue opacity (arrows). Biopsy of the cranial mediastinal mass was performed under ultrasound guidance and yielded a diagnosis of thymoma (L = left).

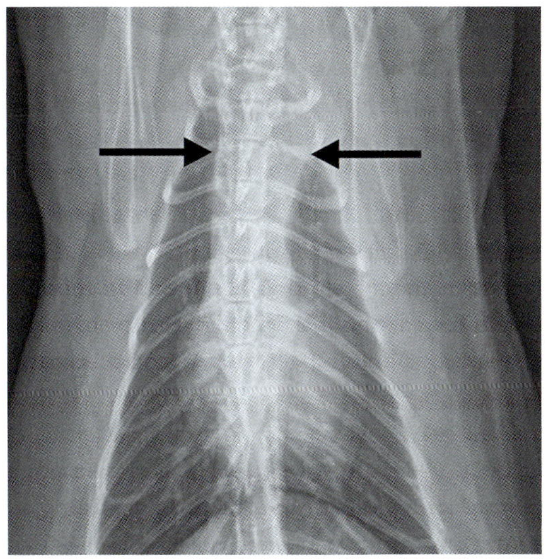

a

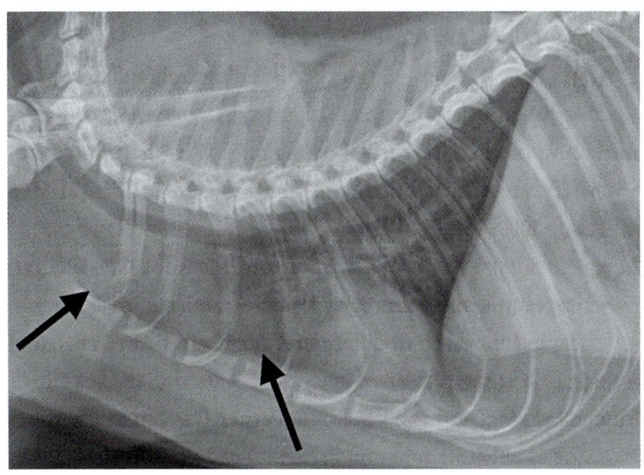

b

Fig. 9.37 Incidental finding of a cranial mediastinal cyst in a 10-year-old cat.
a On the VD view, the cranial mediastinum is widened and of soft-tissue opacity (arrows).
b On the lateral view, a rounded to elongated soft-tissue opacity mass lesion is present cranial to the cardiac silhouette (arrows). A diagnosis of a cyst rather than a solid mass was made based on ultrasound and fine-needle aspiration.

Lymphadenopathy

Mediastinal lymph node enlargement is a special type of mediastinal mass. Enlargement of only one (or one group) of lymph nodes often indicates an infectious or neoplastic process in the tributary area.

- Enlarged **sternal lymph nodes** appear as soft-tissue opacity mass lesions in the cranioventral mediastinum. They are in broad-based contact with the cranial sternum (first through third sternal segment) on lateral thoracic radiographs (Fig. 9.39 and 9.40). The tributary area includes part of the thoracic wall, the thymus, cranial mammary complexes, pleura and peritoneum. Diagnostic workup of a patient with lymphadenopathy limited to the sternal lymph nodes should always include evaluation of the peritoneal cavity.
- The **cranial mediastinal lymph nodes** are located along the cranial vena cava. When enlarged, they appear as poorly defined soft-tissue opacity masses within the cranial mediastinum resulting in dorsal displacement of the trachea (Fig. 9.40). The tributary area includes muscular and skeletal portions of the neck and thoracic wall, cranial mediastinal structures and pleura. Isolated enlargement of these lymph nodes is relatively rare.
- The **tracheobronchial lymph nodes** primarily drain the lung and bronchi but also receive tributaries from caudal mediastinal structures and the diaphragm. Enlargement of these lymph nodes results in poorly defined soft-tissue opacity mass lesion(s) around the tracheal bifurcation on radiographs (Fig. 9.40). On a lateral view, a J-shaped course of the caudal trachea and separation of the caudal lobar bronchi may be noted. Moderate or severe tracheobronchial lymph node enlargement results in lateral deviation of the mainstem bronchi on a VD or DV view. Common differential diagnoses for enlargement of this lymph node group include round cell tumours (e.g. lymphoma) and fungal infections in endemic areas. Even though mild to moderate enlargement of these lymph nodes may occur in patients with primary lung tumours, this is typically best evaluated using CT. Primary pulmonary neoplasia rarely results in radiographically visible tracheobronchial lymph node enlargement.

Enlargement of the middle tracheobronchial lymph node may result in a widened angle between the right and left caudal lobar pulmonary bronchi on a VD or DV view. This appears similar to the 'bow-legged cowboy' sign seen with left atrial enlargement. These two conditions are easily distinguished when evaluating corresponding lateral views. Enlargement of the left atrium results in dorsal displacement of the tracheal bifurcation, while enlargement of the middle tracheobronchial lymph node results in a soft-tissue opacity mass dorsal to the bifurcation with ventral displacement and a J-shaped course of the caudal trachea.

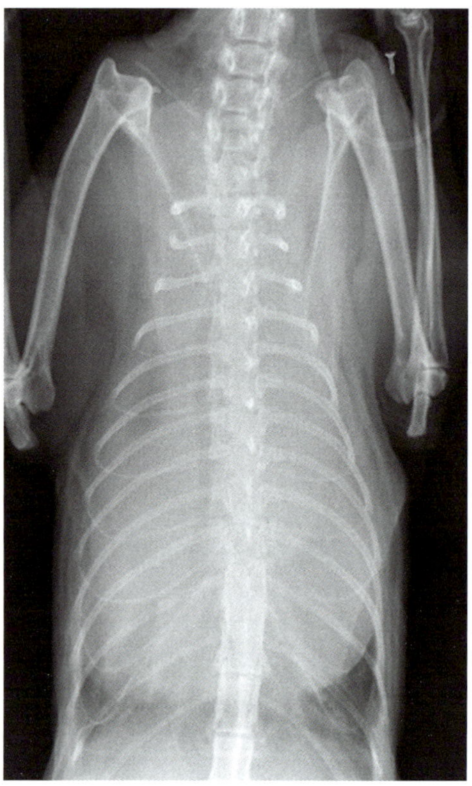

a

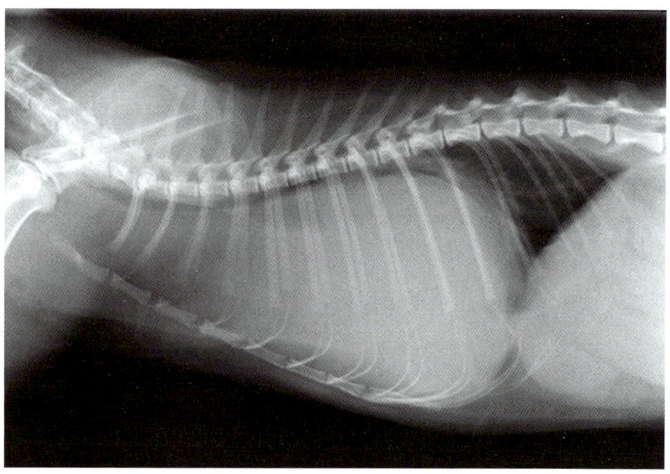

b

Fig. 9.38 a, b Orthogonal thoracic radiographs in a 1-year-old cat with a very large cranial mediastinal mass. The cranial mediastinum contains soft-tissue opaque material and is widened. The trachea is displaced dorsally, the tracheal bifurcation is displaced caudally, and the mass silhouettes obscure the cardiac silhouette. Ultrasound-guided fine-needle aspiration yielded a diagnosis of lymphoma.

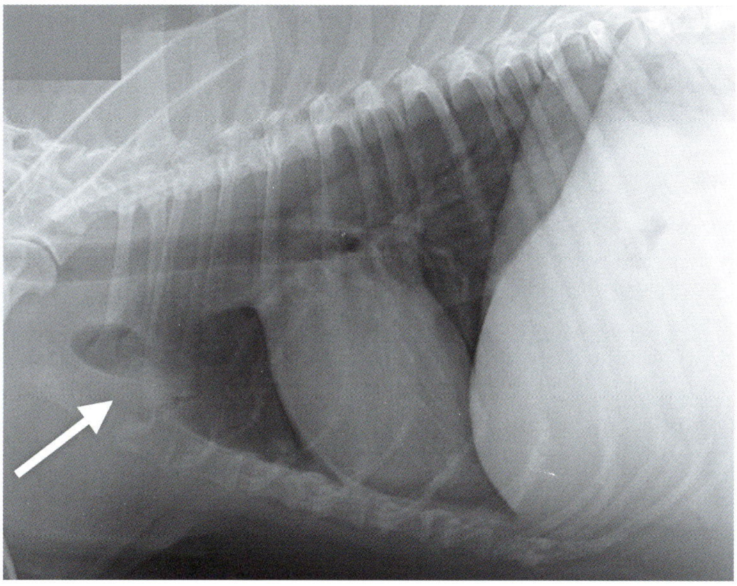

Fig. 9.39 Enlarged sternal lymph node (arrow) in a dog presented with haemoabdomen due to a ruptured splenic tumour.

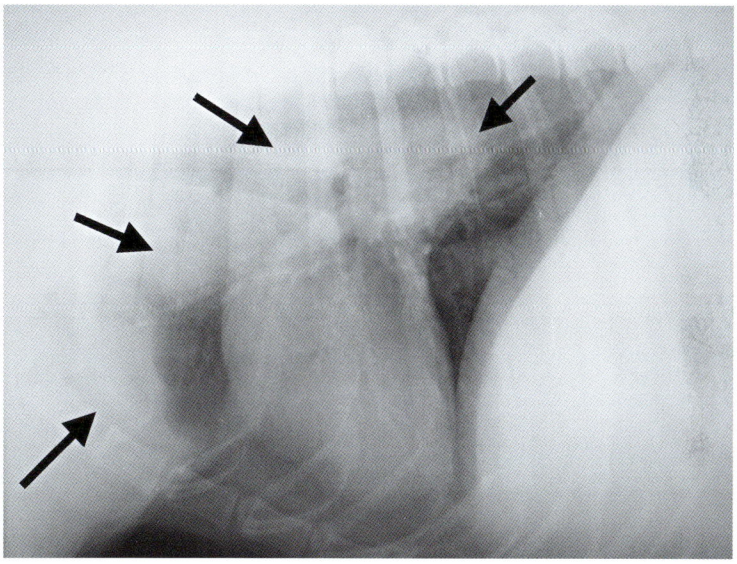

a

Fig. 9.40 Generalized thoracic lymphadenopathy in a dog with lymphoma.
a On the lateral thoracic radiograph, soft-tissue opacity mass lesions are identified in the region of the sternal, tracheobronchial and cranial mediastinal lymph nodes (arrows).
b On the less exposed ventrodorsal view, the mediastinum appears generally widened.
c On the more exposed ventrodorsal view, the course of the bronchi (marked by dotted lines) is easier to evaluate. Enlargement of the tracheobronchial lymph nodes results in lateral deviation of the caudal main stem bronchi. A soft-tissue opacity mass lesion (corresponding to the middle tracheobronchial lymph node) is located between these bronchi and results in a blunted angle (resembling a double opacity or 'bow-legged cowboy' sign also seen with left atrial enlargement).

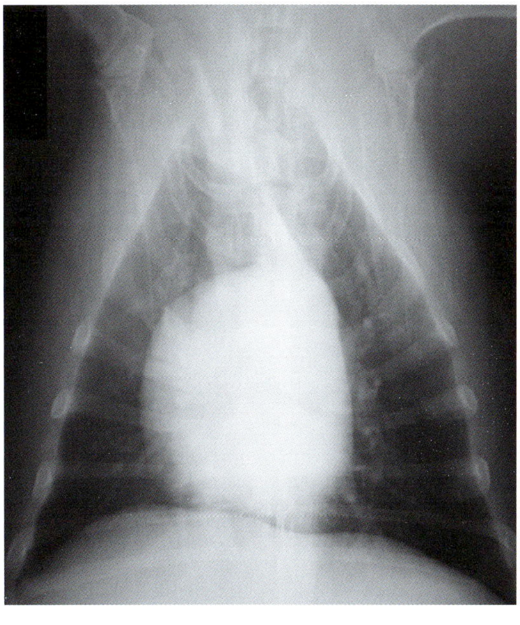

b

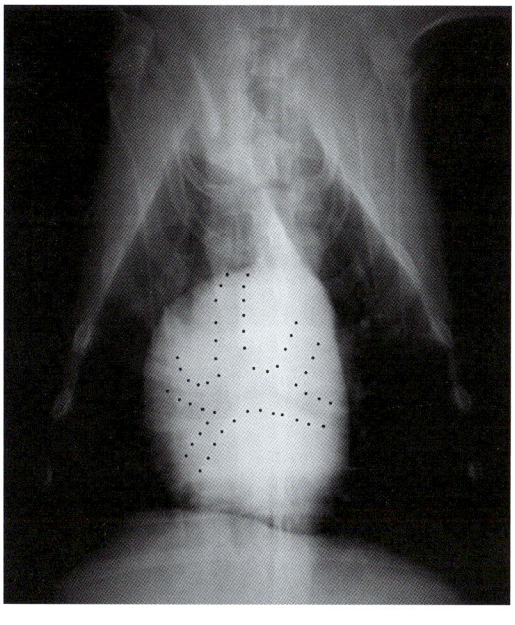

c

Generalized enlargement of the thoracic lymph nodes is most commonly seen with a generalized infiltrative neoplastic process (e.g. lymphoma, histiocytic sarcoma) and with fungal disease (animals in endemic areas or with a travel history).

Mediastinal effusion

Fluid accumulation within the mediastinal space is best identified on a VD or DV view. On a lateral view, there is a diffuse increase in radiographic opacity of the entire thorax (most notably overlying the lung), as fluid distributes over the entire height of the mediastinum and homogeneously summates with overlying structures (Fig. 9.41a). On a VD or DV view, the mediastinum appears generally widened, is of homogeneous soft-tissue opacity and silhouettes with the heart (Fig. 9.41b). A large volume of mediastinal effusion may result in tracheal compression. Due to the connection between the mediastinal space and the pleural space, concurrent pleural effusion may be present.

In theory, any kind of fluid (transudate, modified transudate, exudate) may accumulate within the mediastinum. However, in the author's experience, most cases of clinically relevant mediastinal effusion appear to be related to haemorrhage (secondary to rodenticide toxicity, neoplasia, trauma) or infection (mediastinitis, e.g. secondary to oesophageal perforation). In the latter case, the concurrent presence of mediastinal air is expected.

> **Pitfalls**
>
> **Fat deposition in the (cranial) mediastinum** may result in mediastinal widening and mimic a mediastinal mass or mediastinal effusion on VD/DV views (Fig. 9.42a). This is a common finding especially in bulldog type dogs. However, in contrast to true mediastinal masses, the cranial margin of the heart typically remains visible on lateral thoracic radiographs (Fig. 9.42b). If a distinction between mediastinal fat deposition and a mass or fluid accumulation is not possible on radiographs, advanced imaging modalities such as ultrasound or CT are helpful if accessible.

9.7.2 Pneumomediastinum

Gas accumulation within the mediastinum may be seen secondary to gas accumulation in the soft tissues of the neck (penetrating wound, tracheal injury or rupture, or iatrogenic causes such as repeat jugular venous puncture or aspiration/biopsy of cervical structures), ruptured bronchial or subpleural lesions with subsequent leakage of air, and oesophageal injuries. Most cases of pneumomediastinum result from some sort of external trauma; however, spontaneous air leakage (e.g. secondary to bronchial tears with severe cough) is possible.

The mediastinum and retroperitoneal space are connected via the aortic hiatus, and pneumoretroperitoneum is a common consequence of pneumomediastinum. Retrograde ascent of air from the retroperitoneal space

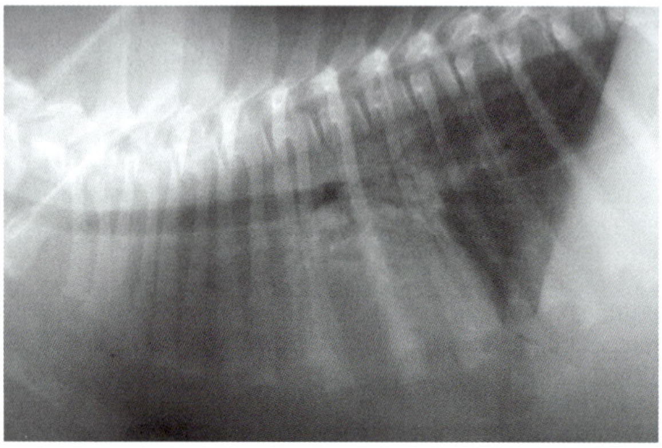

a

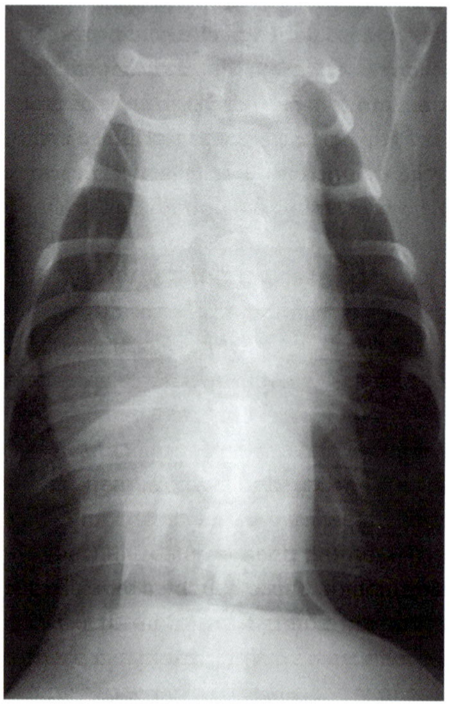

b

Fig. 9.41 Mediastinal effusion (haemorrhage) due to rodenticide toxicity in a young dog.
a On the lateral view, the entire thorax including the lung appears diffusely increased in opacity. The cranial margin of the cardiac silhouette is poorly defined due to silhouetting with mediastinal effusion.
b On the ventrodorsal view there is generalized widening of the mediastinum. Mediastinal effusion silhouettes with the heart, and the cranial and caudal margins of the cardiac silhouette are not clearly visible.
(Courtesy of Dr Amy Sato, Tufts Cummings School of Veterinary Medicine, North Grafton, USA)

is also possible but rare. Air may leak from the mediastinal into the pleural space and result in pneumothorax. Conversely, pneumothorax does not typically cause a pneumomediastinum. Finally, free mediastinal gas may escape into the fascial planes of the neck.

RADIOGRAPHIC FINDINGS Pneumomediastinum results in decreased radiographic opacity of the mediastinum and good contrast between mediastinal structures that are not normally visible (vessels and oesophagus; Fig. 9.43). This is best seen on a lateral view. Mediastinal widening may occur in severe cases and is best seen on ventrodorsal or dorsoventral views. Possible concurrent or secondary findings include pneumothorax, pneumoretroperitoneum, gas within the soft tissues of the neck and subcutaneous emphysema.

A gas-dilated oesophagus (megaoesophagus) may also result in decreased opacity of the mediastinum and mediastinal widening and should not be confused with pneumomediastinum.

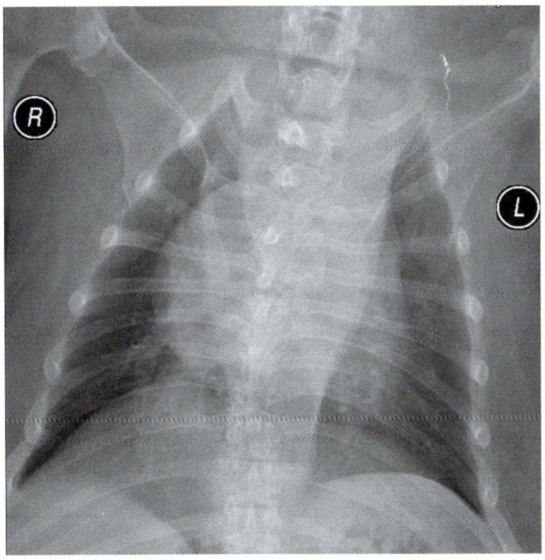

a

9.8 Diseases of the lung

The radiographic diagnosis of pulmonary diseases is difficult and probably one of the biggest challenges in small animal radiology, for the following reasons.

- Marked variability in the radiographic appearance of the normal thorax in small animals (especially dogs).
- Individual or age-related variations from normal.
- Large impact of technical and exposure factors on the appearance of thoracic structures.
- Limited ability of the pulmonary parenchyma to react to various disease processes.
- Discrepancies between radiographic findings and clinical patient presentation.

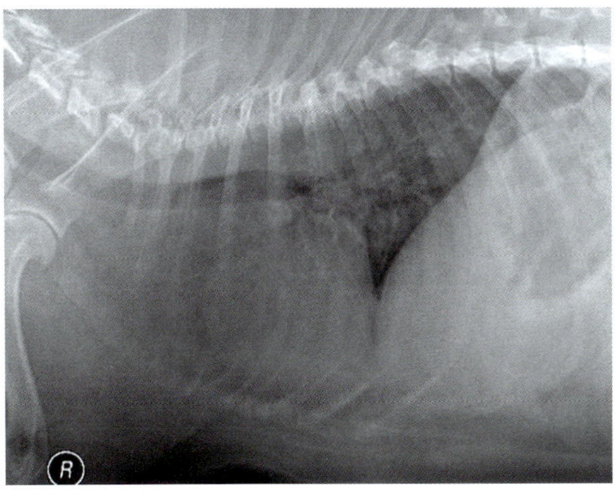

b

Fig. 9.42 Widening of the mediastinum due to fat deposition in a (normal) bulldog.

a On the ventrodorsal view there is widening of the cranial mediastinum and displacement of the trachea to the right, mimicking a cranial mediastinal mass lesion.

b The cranial contour of the heart is clearly visible on the lateral view, indicating the presence of fat rather than soft tissue or fluid in the cranial mediastinum (R = right, L = left).

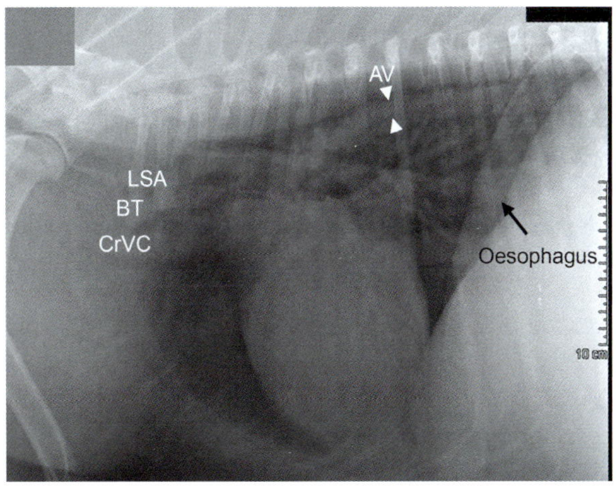

Fig. 9.43 Pneumomediastinum in a dog. Presence of gas within the mediastinum leads to improved contrast between mediastinal structures. Structures not normally visible on thoracic radiographs (cranial vena cava [CrVC], brachiocephalic trunk [BT], left subclavian artery [LSA], the outer margin of the trachea, the oesophagus, and the azygous vein [AV; arrowheads]) are visible as they are delineated by gas. Mediastinal structures that are normally recognized (heart, aorta and caudal vena cava) are also outlined by gas and are more clearly visible than normal.

Pulmonary diseases commonly have a variable radiographic appearance, and, depending on the stage and severity, may affect one or more anatomic components of the lung. Additionally, some pulmonary diseases result in only very subtle radiographic abnormalities or none at all. A normal thoracic radiograph thus does not rule out pulmonary disease.

Following identification of a pulmonary lesion, the examiner must correlate the finding with patient signalment, history and clinical signs to establish a prioritized list of differential diagnoses. Initial therapy is often based on the most likely differential diagnosis. Failure to respond to treatment may require repetition of thoracic radiographs or further diagnostic tests (ultrasound, CT, echocardiography, bronchoalveolar lavage / transtracheal wash, infectious disease testing, thoracotomy and biopsy).

A classic example is presentation of an older dog with severe dyspnoea. The patient has a history of well-controlled mitral insufficiency. Thoracic radiographs show left heart enlargement and an unstructured interstitial to alveolar pattern (see section 9.8.1) in the caudodorsal lung fields. Congestive left heart failure (cardiogenic pulmonary oedema) is the most likely differential diagnosis in this case, and therapy is instituted accordingly. However, if the patient fails to respond to treatment, other causes for a caudodorsal unstructured interstitial to alveolar pattern would have to be investigated (noncardiogenic pulmonary oedema, haematogenous pneumonia, diffuse neoplastic infiltration of the lung such as seen with lymphoma, etc.).

Pulmonary diseases can be categorized as follows.

- Distribution (generalized, multifocal, focal).
- Primary anatomic component of the lung affected (interstitium, bronchi, vessels, alveoli).
- Radiographic opacity (increased or decreased opacity of the entire lung or affected lung segment in comparison to normal).
- With (multi)focal lesion(s):
  - margination (well-circumscribed versus poorly delineated)
  - location.

Table 9.2 provides an overview of differential diagnoses for certain radiographic pulmonary abnormalities.

9.8.1 Pulmonary patterns

Depending on the part of lung affected by a certain disease process, radiographic pulmonary changes may be classified as 'pulmonary patterns' (Table 9.3 and Fig. 9.44). Identification of the predominant pulmonary pattern facilitates prioritization of differential diagnoses. However, different pulmonary patterns may occur concurrently or at different points in the course of a disease, depending on the stage, severity and chronicity, making exact classification of a lung lesion and determination of a specific diagnosis difficult. Additionally, superimposition of anomalies associated with other thoracic structures such as the thoracic wall or mediastinum with the lung may result in the impression of pulmonary abnormalities. This chapter will provide an initial overview of pulmonary patterns, followed by a discussion of specific common pulmonary diseases.

Table 9.2 Differential diagnoses for common radiographic abnormalities of the lung.

Radiographic abnormalities	Differential diagnoses	
Generalized or extensive increased pulmonary opacity	Oedema Haemorrhage Fibrosis Pneumonia (haematogenous) Diffuse infiltrative neoplasia Others	
Focal or multifocal regions of increased opacity	Focal: Primary lung tumour Granuloma Abscess Haematoma Cyst Others	Multifocal: Neoplasia (metastatic) Granulomas Others
Generalized or extensive decreased pulmonary opacity	Pulmonary hyperinflation (e.g. secondary to chronic bronchitis) Pulmonary emphysema Decreased perfusion (e.g. thromboembolic disease, right to left shunt)	
Focal region(s) of decreased opacity	Congenital or traumatic blebs and bullae Cavitary lesions (neoplasia, abscess, granuloma) Bronchiectasis	

Table 9.3 Pulmonary pattern overview and differential diagnoses.

Pulmonary pattern	Radiographic appearance	Common differential diagnoses
Normal	Pulmonary arteries and veins are of similar diameter to corresponding bronchi Bronchial walls are not or only indistinctly visible	Normal lung Early stage of many pulmonary diseases Certain pulmonary diseases not resulting in radiographic abnormalities (e.g. pulmonary thromboembolism) Non-pulmonary diseases
Bronchial	Abnormal visibility and thickening of bronchial walls ('doughnuts' or 'train tracks') Irregular margination of bronchi ± Abnormal bronchial width and shape	Allergic, parasitic and infectious lower airway diseases (e.g. bronchitis, asthma) Bronchial mineralization, e.g. with age (increased visibility but normal bronchial wall thickness and bronchial diameter)
Alveolar	Marked increase in pulmonary opacity Inability to visualize pulmonary vessels Air-filled bronchi appear as 'air bronchograms'	Pneumonia Pulmonary oedema (cardiogenic and noncardiogenic Pulmonary haemorrhage
Vascular	Abnormal size, course and/or shape of pulmonary vessels	Cardiovascular diseases (see Chapter 10)
Interstitial		
Unstructured	Increased opacity of pulmonary parenchyma (often diffuse) Poor definition of pulmonary vascular margins	Ageing change Fibrosis Infectious interstitial lung disease (e.g. viral, fungal) Pulmonary oedema (early or resolving stage) Infiltrative neoplasia (e.g. lymphoma)
Structured	Pulmonary nodule(s) or mass(es)	Primary or secondary pulmonary neoplasia Granulomatous disease Abscesses, haematomas, cysts
Miliary	Numerous small (<5 mm) nodules throughout the pulmonary parenchyma ('snowstorm')	Fungal disease Metastatic disease

Bronchial pattern

A bronchial pattern is characterized by **abnormal visibility and appearance of bronchial walls** as a result of wall thickening, fibrosis, mineralization or peribronchial infiltrates. Cellular infiltrates and oedema result in bronchial wall thickening, which occurs with many bronchial diseases. On radiographs, thickened bronchi appear as a 'doughnuts' in cross section and as 'train tracks' in longitudinal section. Age-related fibrosis and mineralization of bronchial walls is common in older dogs and may mimic bronchial disease. Common bronchial diseases in small animal patients include allergic, parasitic and infectious aetiologies. Chronic bronchial inflammation may result in irreversible bronchial dilatation (**bronchiectasis**). Another possible consequence of chronic lower airway disease is pulmonary **emphysema**, which is characterized by decreased opacity of the affected lung.

Alveolar pattern

An alveolar pattern results from **accumulation of fluid or cells in normally air-containing alveoli**, resulting in increased opacity of the affected pulmonary parenchyma. The affected lung lobes maintain their normal size and shape and are sharply delineated from adjacent normal pulmonary parenchyma. This is sometimes referred to as **'consolidation'**. Pulmonary vessels silhouette with soft-tissue opaque lung and cannot be distinguished. On the other hand, air-containing bronchi may be seen surrounded by soft-tissue opaque lung (**'air bronchograms'**). Visibility of air bronchograms is a reliable radiographic indicator of an alveolar lung pattern. However, air bronchograms may not be visible in severe cases when bronchi also contain fluid or cellular material. An alveolar lung pattern is nonspecific and may be seen with many different pulmonary diseases (e.g. bacterial pneumonia, pulmonary oedema,

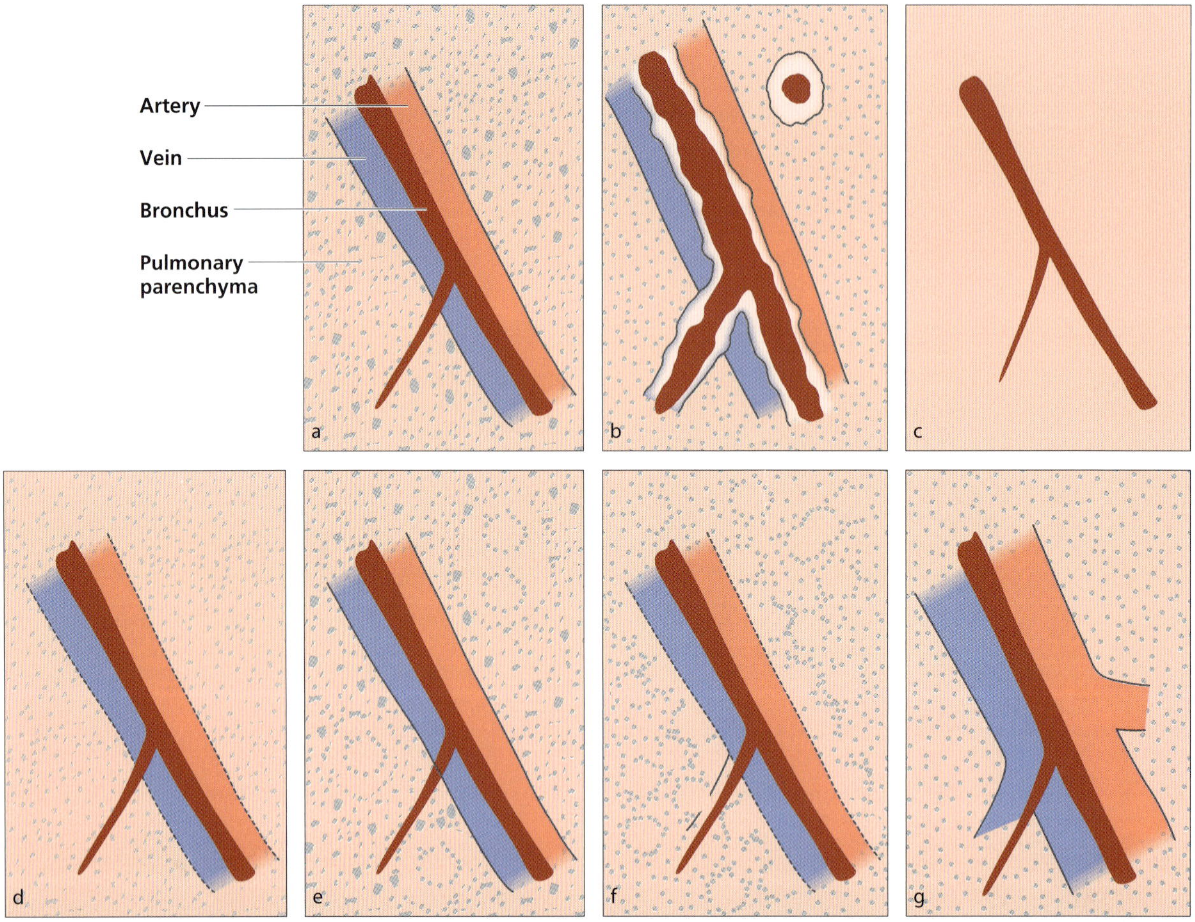

Fig. 9.44 Schematic drawings illustrating radiographic abnormalities seen with different pulmonary patterns.

a Normal lung: The pulmonary parenchyma is of low opacity. The pulmonary vessels are clearly visible as soft-tissue opacity tubular structures and have a similar diameter to the corresponding bronchus. The actual bronchial wall is not visible or only indistinctly visible.

b Bronchial lung pattern: The bronchial walls are thickened and irregularly marginated. The abnormal bronchi appear as a 'doughnuts' in cross section and as 'train tracks' between corresponding vessels in longitudinal section.

c Alveolar lung pattern: The alveoli are filled with cellular material and/or fluid. The pulmonary parenchyma has assumed soft-tissue opacity and silhouettes with pulmonary vessels which are not visible. The bronchus is air-filled and is less opaque than adjacent lung parenchyma (aka 'air bronchogram').

d Unstructured interstitial lung pattern: The interstitium contains an increased amount of cells, fluid or other material and is diffusely increased in opacity. Pulmonary opacity is lower than with an alveolar lung pattern. Pulmonary vascular margins are ill-defined but still visible.

e Structured interstitial lung pattern: One or more nodules or masses of variable size are distributed throughout the lung parenchyma.

f Miliary lung pattern: Numerous small nodules are distributed throughout the pulmonary parenchyma ('snowstorm').

g Vascular lung pattern: The pulmonary vessels are abnormal in size, course and/or shape. In this example, both the pulmonary artery and vein are enlarged compared to the corresponding bronchus.

A pathological alveolar pattern (consolidation) may sometimes be difficult to distinguish from atelectasis. If air within the alveoli has been replaced by fluid or cellular infiltrates, the lung lobe maintains its normal size and shape. With atelectasis, the lung lobe is decreased in volume, and mediastinal shift and diaphragmatic asymmetry are common concurrent findings on VD or DV views. Additionally, atelectasis often does not result in visible changes on lateral views, while radiographic abnormalities are expected with consolidation.

pulmonary haemorrhage). Some diseases predominantly affect certain areas of the lung (see section 9.8.2), which may aid in diagnosis along with patient signalment, history, clinical presentation and concurrent radiographic findings (e.g. cardiovascular or mediastinal abnormalities).

A special form of alveolar lung pattern is increased opacity of a lung lobe due to volume loss (**atelectasis**). This may result from pathological processes such as bronchial obstruction, but is more commonly the result of 'benign' factors such as lateral recumbency or general anaesthesia. In contrast to a consolidated lung lobe, an atelectatic lung lobe is smaller than normal (see Fig. 9.35).

Interstitial pattern

Pulmonary vessels, bronchi and alveoli are surrounded and supported by lung interstitium. Thickening or increased density of the interstitium due to inflammation, fibrosis, or accumulation of fluid or cellular infiltrates, results in an interstitial lung pattern. The two basic types of interstitial lung disease are the **unstructured** and the **structured interstitial pattern**.

In an unstructured interstitial pulmonary pattern, there is diffuse accumulation of cells, fluid or other material within the interstitium, resulting in an often generalized increase in pulmonary opacity. The pulmonary parenchyma is less opaque than with an alveolar pattern. The pulmonary vascular margins are ill-defined but remain visible. An unstructured interstitial pattern may progress to an alveolar pattern, when increasing severity of the disease process leads to leakage of cells or fluid from the interstitium into the alveoli. Conversely, after resolution of severe alveolar lung disease there is often a residual unstructured interstitial pattern (Fig. 9.45).

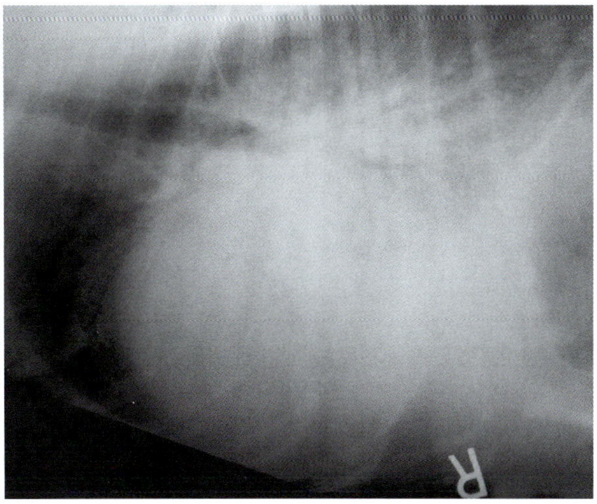

a

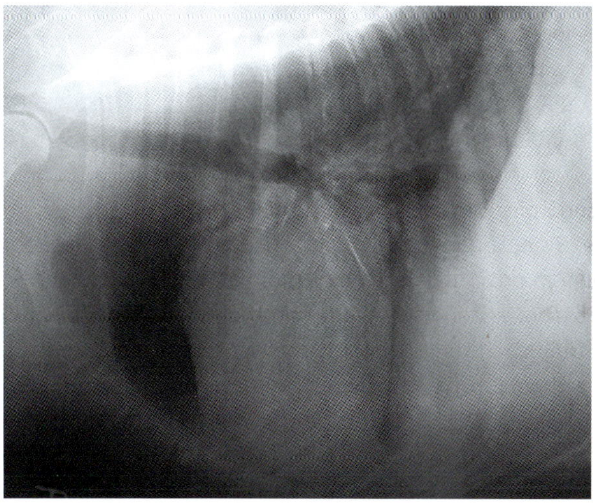

b

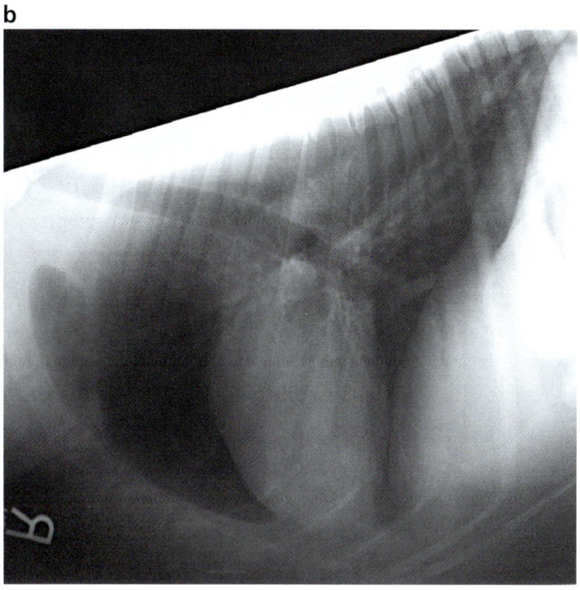

c

Fig. 9.45 Resolution of severe pulmonary oedema in a dog with congestive left heart failure (R = right).
a Alveolar lung pattern: There is diffuse increased opacity to the caudal lung fields which are of soft-tissue opacity. Neither the caudal lobar pulmonary vessels nor the caudal margin of the cardiac silhouette are visible.
b Unstructured interstitial lung pattern: There is marked improvement of pulmonary oedema. The pulmonary parenchyma remains mildly diffusely increased in opacity compared to normal (**c**). The pulmonary vessels and entire cardiac silhouette are visible.
c Normal lung: Following successful treatment of pulmonary oedema, the pulmonary parenchyma has assumed normal radiographic opacity.
(Courtesy of Dr Amy Sato, Tufts Cummings School of Veterinary Medicine, North Grafton, USA)

A diagnosis of an unstructured interstitial lung pattern is often difficult and to some degree subjective. If prior radiographs of the same patient are available, comparison of pulmonary opacity may help in identification of a change in pulmonary opacity. Alternatively, comparison to an animal of similar breed and size may be helpful.

Differential diagnoses for an unstructured interstitial pattern are similar to those listed for an alveolar pattern. Examples of possible underlying disease processes include:

- pulmonary oedema
- pneumonia
- diffuse infiltrative neoplastic processes
- pulmonary haemorrhage
- fibrosis.

A mild, diffuse, unstructured interstitial pattern is a common incidental/normal finding in older dogs.

Pitfalls

Superimposition of **subcutaneous or mediastinal fat,** especially in adipose animals, and **technical factors** (underexposure, underdevelopment, expiratory radiograph) may mimic a diffuse increase in pulmonary opacity, i.e. a diffuse unstructured interstitial pattern.

With a structured interstitial (= nodular) lung pattern, one or more nodules or mass lesions are associated with the lung. This is probably the most straightforward pulmonary pattern. Thoracic radiographs reveal one or more poorly or well-defined soft-tissue opacity nodules/masses of variable size within the pulmonary parenchyma. Differential diagnoses include:

- primary or secondary pulmonary neoplasms
- granulomas
- abscesses
- haematomas
- cysts.

A miliary pattern is a special type of a structured interstitial pattern characterized by presence of numerous small (<5 mm diameter) pulmonary nodules, giving the impression of a 'snowstorm' lung. Differential diagnoses for this finding include fungal disease and pulmonary metastases.

Vascular pattern

Pulmonary vessels are normally visible and should have a similar diameter to their corresponding bronchi. A vascular lung pattern is characterized by enlargement, small size, or abnormal course and shape of pulmonary arteries and/or veins. Different types of vascular abnormalities and their association with cardiovascular disease processes are further discussed in Chapter 10.

Pitfalls

Even though diagnosis of a structured interstitial pattern is often straightforward, there are several instances where normal or incidental findings may mimic pulmonary nodules.

End-on pulmonary vessels are round and may mimic pulmonary nodules. However, they are always superimposed with pulmonary vessels of equal or larger size, are aligned with corresponding bronchi, and are too opaque for pulmonary nodules of their size (Fig. 9.46). Additionally, they cannot be identified on orthogonal views.

Pulmonary osteomas are a common incidental finding in older dogs. They appear as small (approximately 2 mm), well-circumscribed mineral opacity nodules of variable number and distribution throughout the pulmonary parenchyma (Fig. 9.47). They are more opaque (bone or mineral opacity) than soft tissue, and despite their small size are easily seen. As a rule of thumb, true pulmonary nodules of soft-tissue opacity (e.g. metastases or granulomas) must reach approximately 5 mm in diameter (depending on position within the lung and patient size) to become visible radiographically. Pulmonary osteomas (and end-on vessels) are clearly visible despite their small size.

Skin nodules projected over pulmonary parenchyma may mimic pulmonary nodules (Fig. 9.48). When a suspicious soft-tissue opacity is identified on a radiograph, an attempt should be made to correlate it to a pulmonary nodule on the orthogonal view. If fluoroscopy is available, an attempt can also be made to visualize movement of the nodule with respiration. If confirmation of a nodule as pulmonary in origin is not possible, close inspection and palpation of the patient is indicated. Any skin nodules (including nipples) in the area of the questionable pulmonary nodule should be marked with metallic pellets or barium paste, and radiographs should be repeated. If a skin nodule was the source of the suspicious opacity in the plane of the lung fields, it will now be indicated by the metallic marker.

9.8.2 Specific lung diseases

As mentioned above, the radiographic diagnosis of specific pulmonary diseases may be difficult, as different disease processes may result in similar radiographic abnormalities. Additionally, many lung diseases are associated with concurrent abnormalities of other thoracic compartments such as the thoracic wall, pleural space or mediastinum. This chapter will cover the radiographic appearance of relatively common primary and secondary pulmonary diseases.

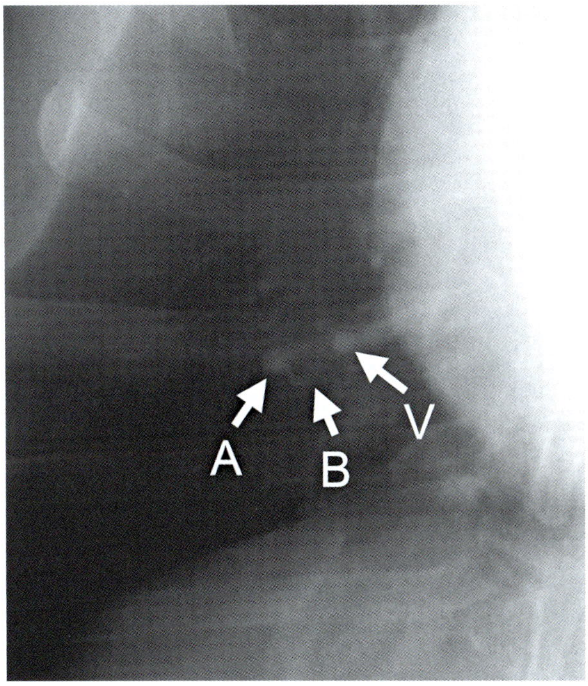

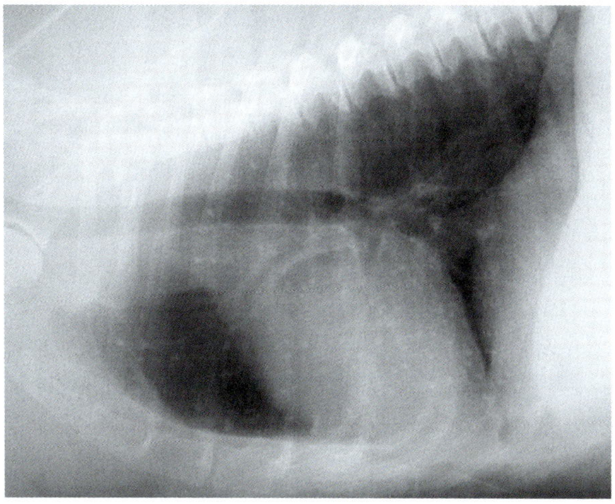

Fig. 9.47 Pulmonary osteomas in a normal older dog. There are numerous small, well-circumscribed, mineral opaque nodules throughout the pulmonary parenchyma.

Fig. 9.46 Close-up view of a ventrodorsal thoracic radiograph in a dog. Two pulmonary vessels (A = artery, V = vein) are seen in cross section (end-on) and may be confused with pulmonary nodules. However, these focal opacities are superimposed with vessels of a similar size and are in a characteristic position adjacent to a centrally located bronchus (B). They are also too radiopaque for pulmonary nodules of this size.

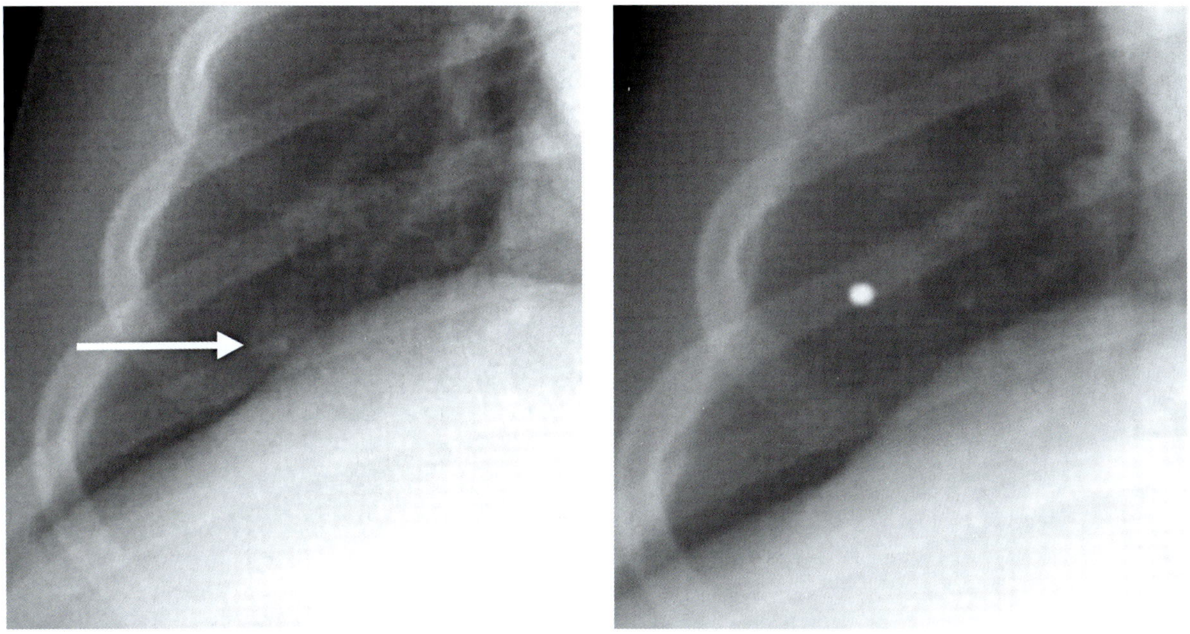

a b

Fig. 9.48 Skin nodule mimicking a pulmonary nodule.

a On this close-up ventrodorsal thoracic radiograph, a suspicious round soft-tissue opacity nodule is superimposed with the right caudal lung lobe (arrow). A palpable skin nodule was found in this location and marked with a small metallic pellet.

b The repeat radiograph shows that the metallic pellet is associated with the questionable soft-tissue opacity, confirming an artefact (skin nodule) rather than a pulmonary nodule.

(Courtesy of Dr Amy Sato, Tufts Cummings School of Veterinary Medicine, North Grafton, USA)

Pneumonia

Pneumonia is an inflammatory lung disease caused by infection with viruses, bacteria, fungi, parasites or other infectious agents. Depending on the underlying aetiological agent and the route of infection, pneumonia may result in a predominantly unstructured interstitial pattern, an alveolar pattern or a structured interstitial pattern. Concurrent bronchitis is common especially with bacterial pneumonia and results in a concurrent bronchial pattern.

Viral pneumonia is a relatively uncommon radiographic diagnosis in small animals. Thoracic radiographs may be normal or show a multifocal or generalized unstructured interstitial pattern (Fig. 9.49). Superinfection with bacteria is common and results in concurrent alveolar infiltrates.

Bacterial pneumonia is probably the most common type of inflammatory lung disease diagnosed in dogs. The diagnosis is rare in cats. Haematogenous infection (seen in puppies or immunocompromised animals) results in multifocal unstructured interstitial to alveolar patterns. Bronchopneumonia or aspiration pneumonia results in moderate to severe alveolar patterns in the cranioventral lung fields (Fig. 9.50). Concurrent bronchial and peribronchial abnormalities are common.

Mycotic pneumonia (e.g. blastomycosis, coccidioidomycosis) is common in endemic areas and may also be seen in animals with a travel history. Even though a miliary pattern is considered a classic finding with mycotic pneumonia (Fig. 9.51), fungal disease is truly the joker among lung diseases and can take on almost any pattern (unstructured interstitial and any form of structured interstitial pattern are most common). Concurrent enlargement of intrathoracic (especially tracheobronchial) lymph nodes is common.

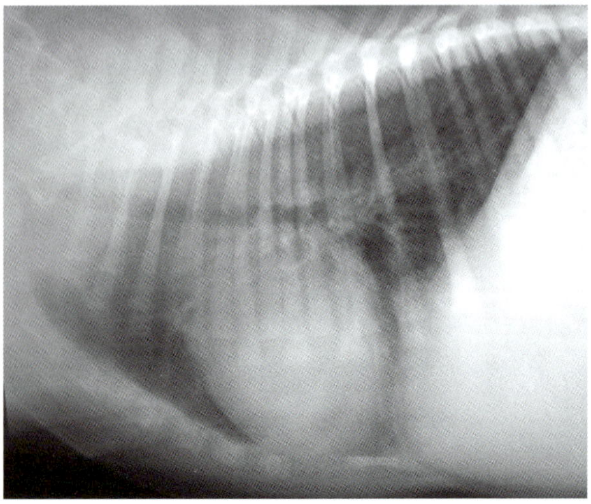

Fig. 9.49 Viral pneumonia (distemper) in a 2-month-old dog. The lung is of diffusely increased opacity, with ill-defined margination of the pulmonary vessels (unstructured interstitial lung pattern). There is a focal region of markedly increased radiographic opacity associated with the accessory lung lobe (alveolar lung pattern), which is most consistent with bacterial superinfection.

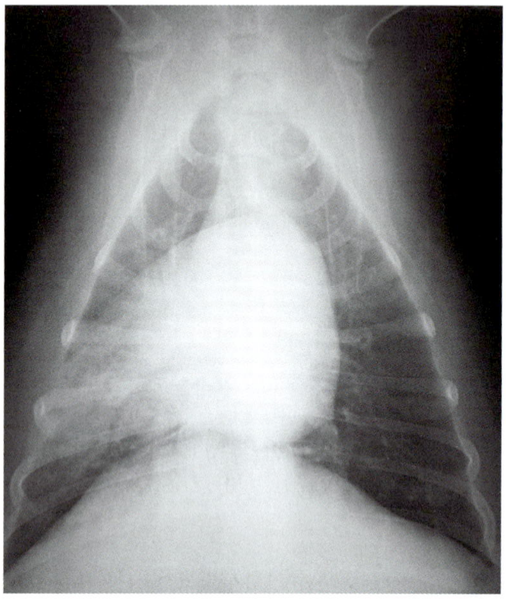

a

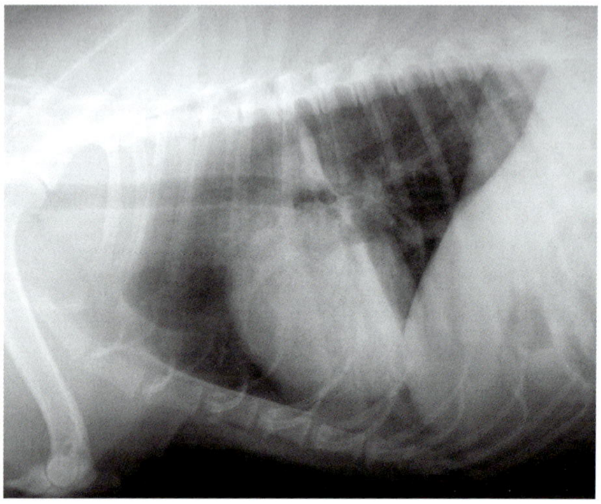

b

Fig. 9.50 a, b Bacterial pneumonia with consolidation of the right middle lung lobe in a 6-year-old dog. The affected lung lobe has an alveolar pattern characterized by homogeneous increased opacity of the entire lung lobe, loss of visualization of pulmonary vessels and tubular air bronchograms. The size and shape of the lung lobe is normal, without indication of a mediastinal shift. The remaining lung parenchyma has a diffuse unstructured interstitial pattern.

Parasitic pneumonia is rare. Infectious agents include *Toxoplasma*, *Paragonimus* and lung worms (e.g. *Aelurostrongylus*). The radiographic findings in parasitic pneumonia are variable, ranging from unstructured interstitial and bronchial lung patterns to pulmonary nodules and alveolar infiltrates.

Pulmonary oedema

Pulmonary oedema is defined as fluid accumulation within the lung. This may occur secondary to left-sided heart failure and impaired pulmonary venous return to the heart (cardiogenic pulmonary oedema) or may be unrelated to cardiovascular disease (noncardiogenic pulmonary oedema).

Cardiogenic pulmonary oedema results in a perihilar to caudodorsal unstructured interstitial to alveolar lung pattern in most dogs (see Fig. 9.45). Pulmonary infiltrates in cats are more variable and may occur in any area of the thorax. In addition to pulmonary abnormalities, enlargement of the cardiac silhouette and pulmonary vessels is often seen. Further details are discussed in Chapter 10.

Noncardiogenic pulmonary oedema can result from electric shock (e.g. biting an electrical cord), inhalation of toxic gases or smoke, strangulation, inhalation of a foreign body or asphyxia of a different aetiology, epilepsy or traumatic brain injury. The predominant radiographic finding is a fairly symmetric caudodorsal alveolar (or less commonly unstructured interstitial) lung pattern (Fig. 9.52). In contrast to cardiogenic oedema, the heart and pulmonary vessels are normal.

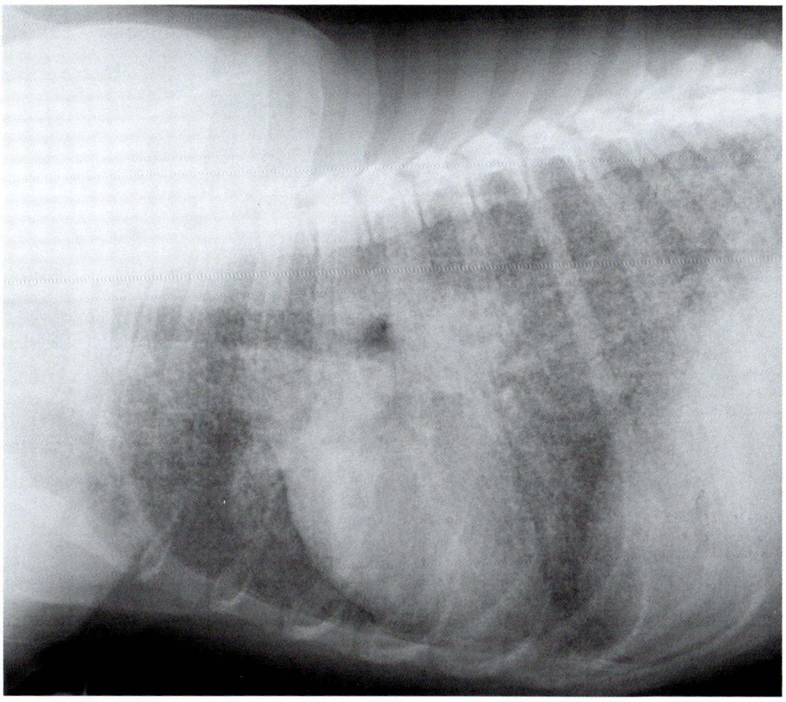

Fig. 9.51 Mycotic pneumonia in a dog. There are numerous small coalescing soft-tissue nodules throughout the entire lung, giving the impression of a 'snowstorm' (miliary lung pattern). Note also focal increased opacity dorsal to the tracheal bifurcation, indicative of enlargement of the tracheobronchial lymph nodes.

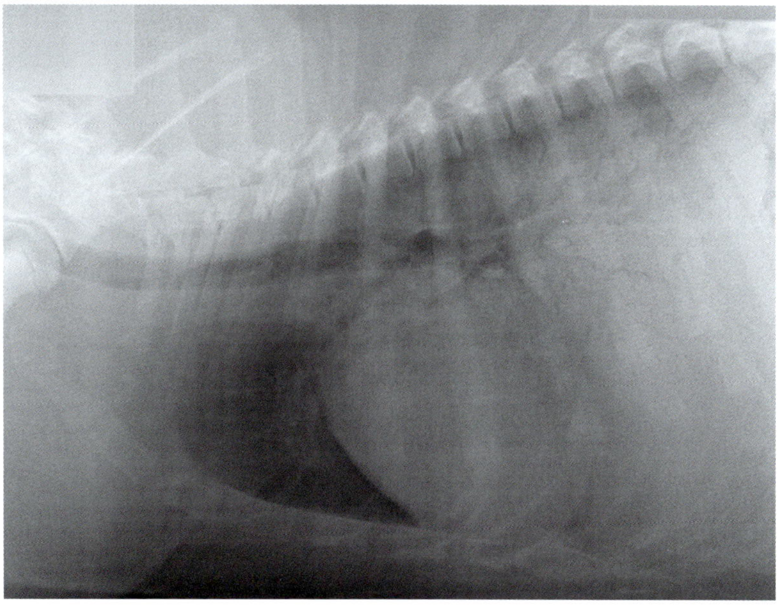

Fig. 9.52 Noncardiogenic pulmonary oedema in a dog following inhalation of toxic chemicals. A severe alveolar pattern is associated with the caudodorsal lung fields. The heart and pulmonary vessels are normal.

Even though the distribution of the pulmonary infiltrates and the appearance of the cardiovascular structures are often helpful in distinguishing cardiogenic from non-cardiogenic oedema, a radiographic diagnosis is not always possible. Patient signalment, history and clinical findings (e.g. presence of a heart murmur) are important factors to consider when making a diagnosis.

Bronchial/lower airway disease

Lower airway disease may be of **allergic** (e.g. feline asthma), **parasitic** (lungworms), or **infectious** (acute or chronic bronchitis) aetiology. Thoracic radiographs reveal a more or less pronounced bronchial (± unstructured interstitial) lung pattern (Fig. 9.53). Additional finding in chronic cases may include pulmonary emphysema or irreversible bronchial dilatation (**bronchiectasis**; Fig. 9.54).

Pulmonary neoplasia

Pulmonary neoplasia can be categorized as primary or metastatic lung disease. Diffuse infiltrative pulmonary neoplasia is also possible. Even though lung tumours are more common in older animals, they may occasionally be seen in young patients. The most common radiographic finding is a structured interstitial lung pattern (i.e. one or more nodules or masses of variable size within the pulmonary parenchyma). They may be of homogeneous soft-tissue opacity, have mineralization or be cavitary. A primary lung tumour (such as pulmonary carcinoma) typically appears as a larger solitary pulmonary mass (Fig. 9.55), while pulmonary metastases usually manifest as multiple smaller nodules (Fig. 9.56). Exceptions are certainly possible. Some pulmonary tumours (e.g. pulmonary lymphoma, miliary metastasis or bronchial carcinoma in cats) may have an atypical or unpredictable appearance and result in an unstructured interstitial, miliary or even bronchial pattern (Fig. 9.57).

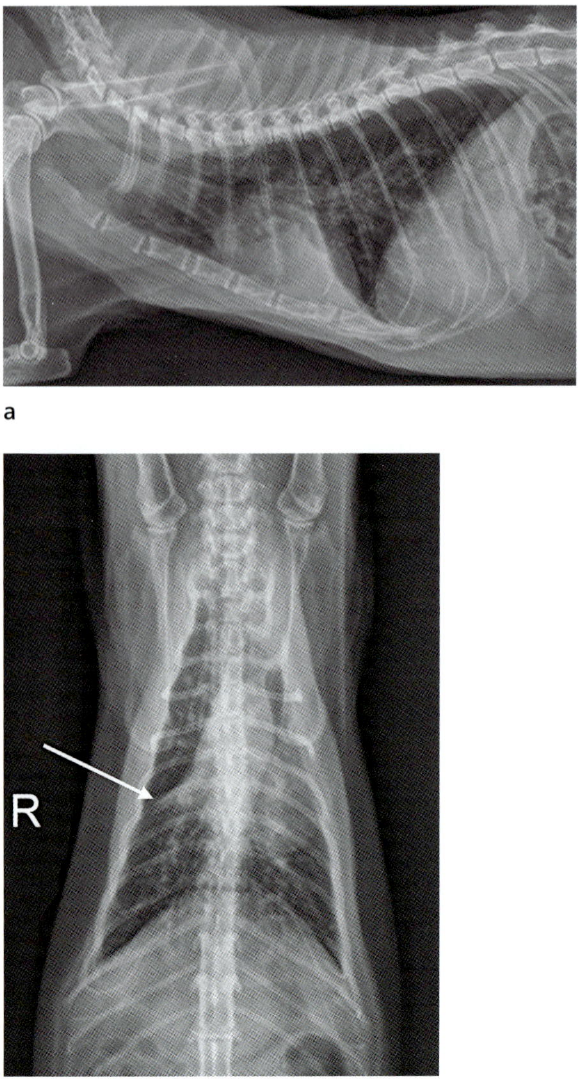

a

b

Fig. 9.53 Lateral a and ventrodorsal b thoracic radiographs in a cat with asthma. There is a generalized bronchial and unstructured interstitial lung pattern. The thickened bronchi appear as 'doughnuts' and 'train tracks'. The right middle lung lobe (arrow) is completely collapsed due to bronchial obstruction and is of homogeneous soft-tissue opacity (atelectasis). (R = right)

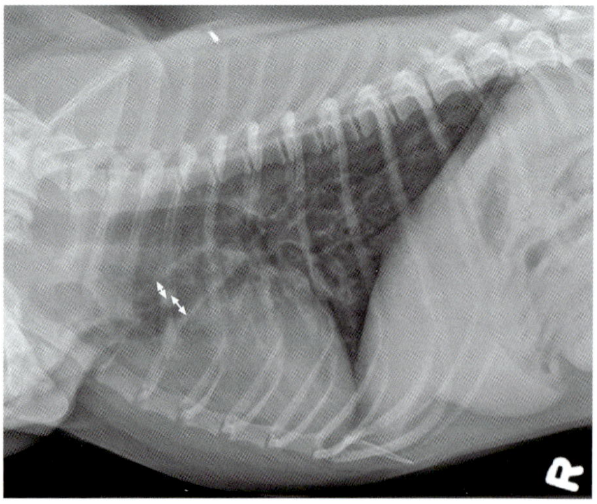

Fig. 9.54 Bronchiectasis in a 2-year-old Dachshund with chronic bronchitis. In addition to a severe generalized bronchial lung pattern, dilatation of the cranial lobar bronchi is noted (double arrows). (R = right)

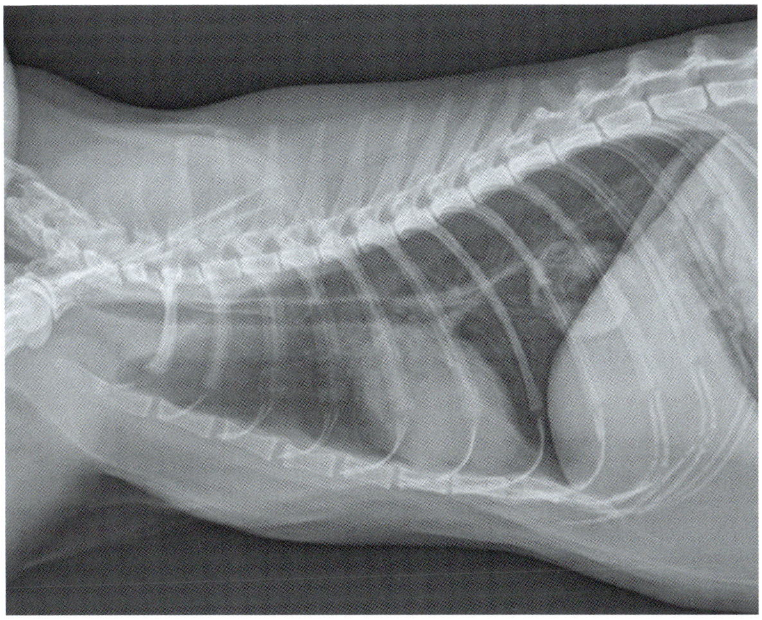

Fig. 9.55 Primary lung tumour in a cat. A solitary cavitary mass is associated with the caudal lung fields.

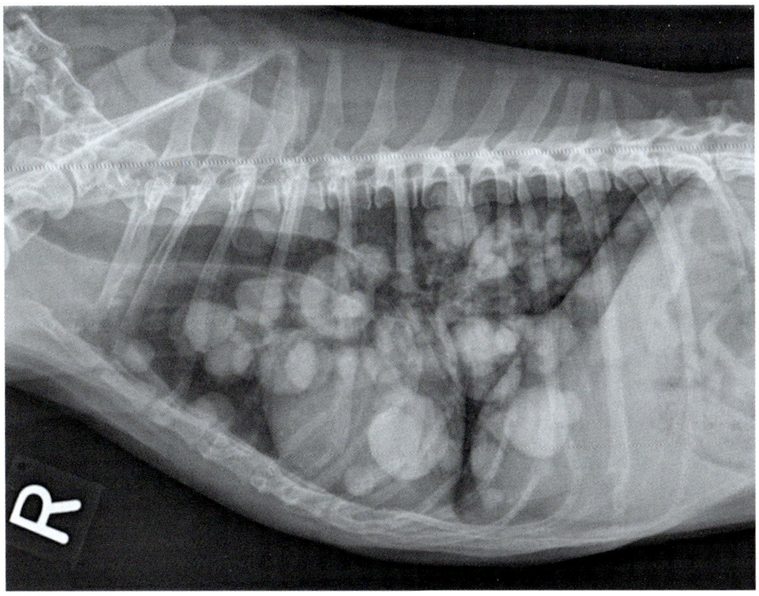

Fig. 9.56 Pulmonary metastases in a dog. There are numerous variably sized soft-tissue opacity nodules throughout the lungs (R = right).

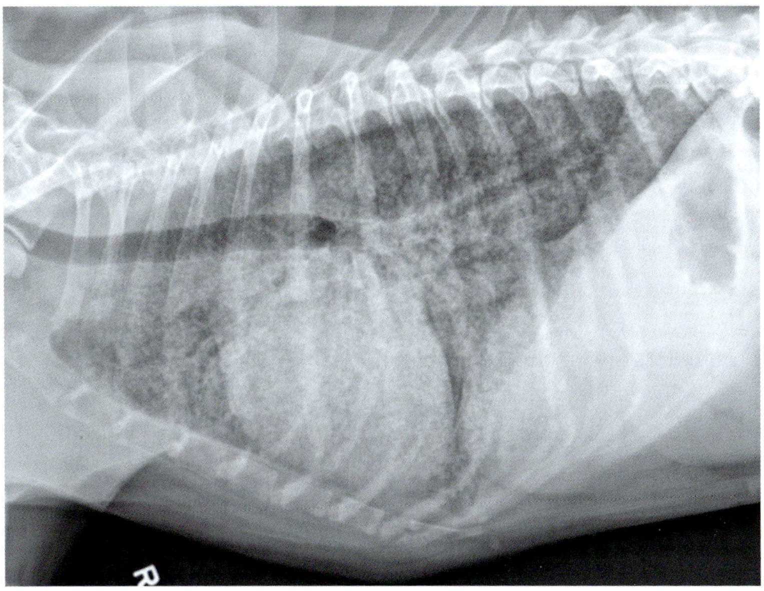

Fig. 9.57 Miliary lung pattern in a dog with metastatic pheochromocytoma (R = right).

Pulmonary haemorrhage and trauma

Pulmonary haemorrhage may occur secondary to a traumatic event (contusion) or may be related to coagulopathy (e.g. with thrombocytopenia or secondary to rodenticide toxicity). The radiographic appearance of pulmonary haemorrhage is variable and changes rapidly. Focal or generalized unstructured interstitial or alveolar pulmonary infiltrates are commonly seen and may affect any region of the lung (Fig. 9.58). Thoracic trauma may also result in cavitary pulmonary lesions (fluid-filled haematomas or air-filled bullae) which appear as well-circumscribed, round soft-tissue or air opacity regions within the pulmonary parenchyma (Fig. 9.59).

Additional findings with traumatic thoracic injuries may include subcutaneous emphysema, pleural effusion, pneumothorax and/or rib fractures (Fig. 9.60).

> Traumatic lung lesions pose a diagnostic challenge if no history or only an incomplete history is provided. As discussed above, alveolar and unstructured interstitial lung patterns are nonspecific and may have many causes other than contusion. A pulmonary haematoma may mimic a solitary lung tumour, abscess or granuloma. Additional radiographic abnormalities such as pneumothorax or rib fractures may be helpful in arriving at a diagnosis of thoracic trauma.

Lung lobe torsion

With lung lobe torsion there is rotation of one or more lung lobes around their axis. The cranial and middle lung lobes are most commonly affected. Even though a predisposition in deep-chested dog breeds is suspected, lung lobe torsions may also be seen in small-breed dogs and cats. Radiographic abnormalities include abnormal opacity of the affected lung lobe (interstitial or alveolar pattern, often associated with small diffusely distributed gas foci), segmental abnormalities of the corresponding bronchus, mediastinal shift and uni- or bilateral pleural effusion (Fig. 9.61).

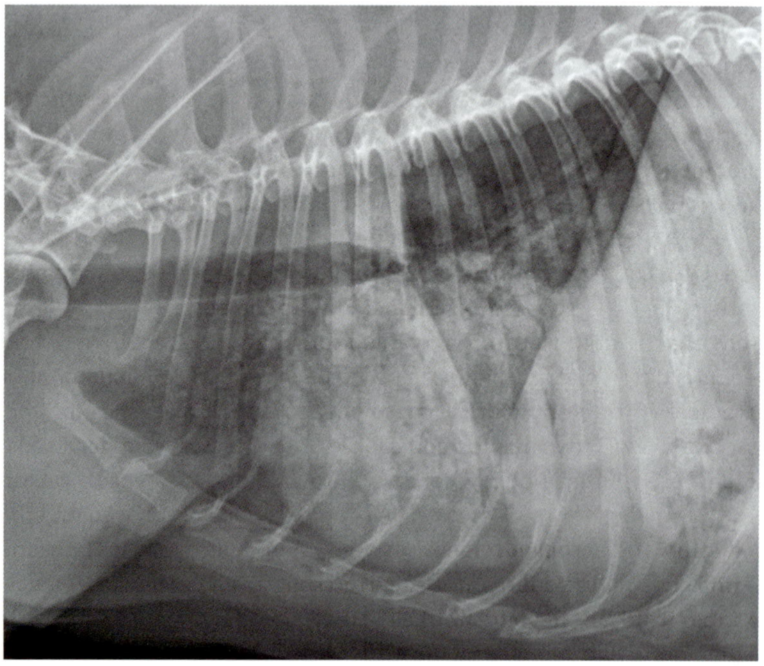

Fig. 9.58 Multifocal alveolar and unstructured interstitial pattern in a 10-year-old dog with severe thrombocytopenia. Multifocal pulmonary haemorrhage was suspected and was confirmed with necropsy and histopathology. Additional findings included interstitial pneumonia and pulmonary oedema.

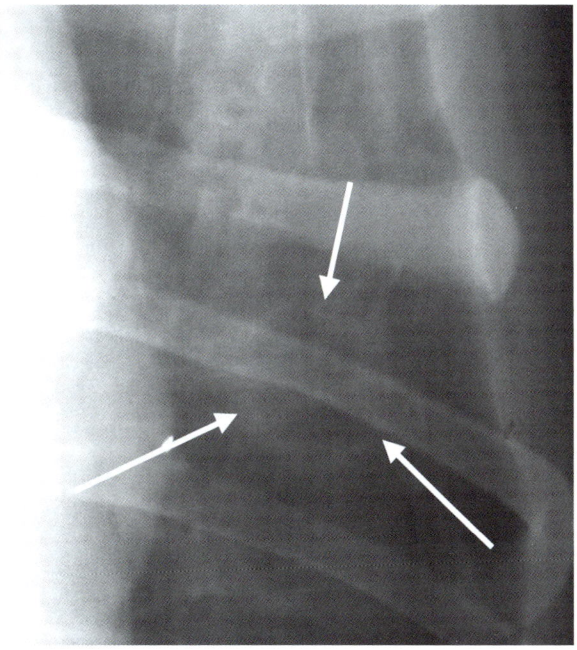

Fig. 9.59 Traumatic pulmonary bulla in a dog following a road traffic accident. The close-up view of a ventrodorsal thoracic radiograph shows a round, thin-walled gas opacity lesion within the left lung (arrows).

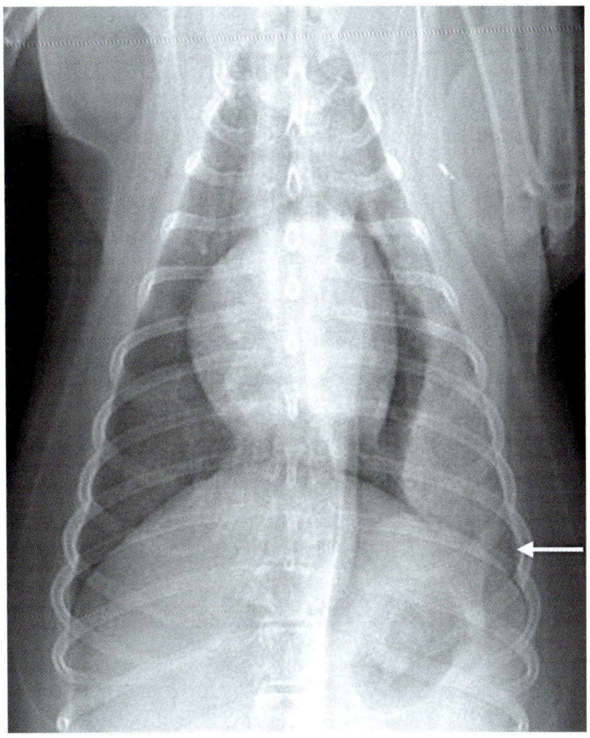

a

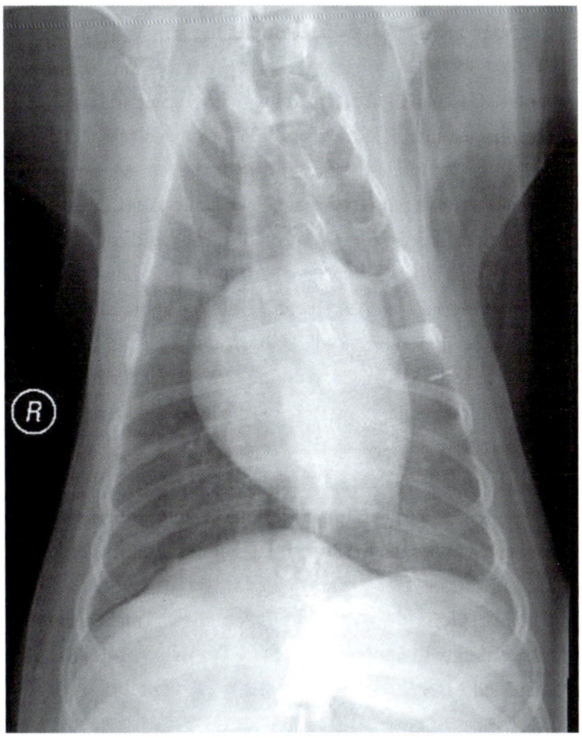

b

Fig. 9.60 Pulmonary contusion in a dog presented following a road traffic accident.

a The ventrodorsal thoracic radiograph immediately following initial presentation shows homogeneous soft-tissue opacity to the peripheral left lung fields. A mild pneumothorax (arrow) is also present.

b The (mildly oblique) repeat radiograph of the thorax two days later shows near-complete resolution of the pulmonary abnormalities (R = right).

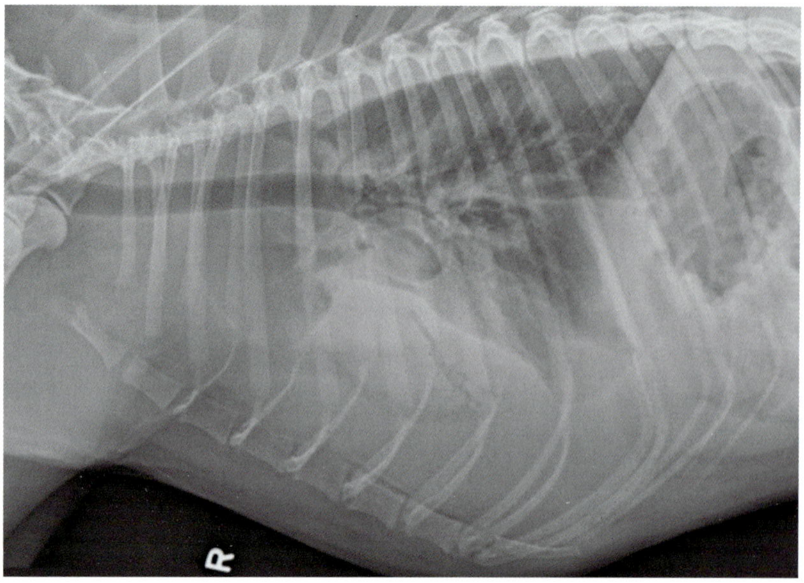

Fig. 9.61 Torsion of the caudal subsegment of the left cranial lung lobe in a dog. Findings in addition to homogeneously increased opacity of the affected lung lobe (alveolar pattern) include focal narrowing of the affected bronchus and marked pleural effusion (R = right).

References and further reading

Berry CR, Koblik PD, Ticer JW. Dorsal peritoneopericardial mesothelial remnant as an aid to the diagnosis of feline congenital peritoneopericardial diaphragmatic hernia. Vet Radiol 1990; 31: 239–45.

Berry CR, Gaschen FP, Ackerman H. Radiographic and ultrasonographic features of hypertrophic feline muscular dystrophy in two cats. Vet Radiol Ultrasound 1992; 33: 357–64.

Brinkman EL, Biller D, Armbrust L. The clinical usefulness of the ventrodorsal versus dorsoventral thoracic radiograph in dogs. J Am Anim Hosp Assoc 2006; 42: 440–9.

D'Anjou MA, Tidwell AS, Hecht S. Radiographic diagnosis of lung lobe torsion. Vet Radiol Ultrasound 2005; 46:478–84.

Little AM, Hecht S, Kirk CA, Bohling MW. What is your diagnosis? Traumatic diaphragmatic hernia in a dog. J Am Vet Med Assoc 2009; 235: 1041–2.

Lord PF, Suter PF, Chan KF, Appleford M, Root CR. Pleural, extrapleural, and pulmonary lesions in small animals: A radiographic approach to differential diagnosis. J Am Vet Radiol Soc 1972; 13:4–17.

Mitchell SL, McCarthy R, Rudloff E, Pernell RT. Tracheal rupture associated with intubation in cats: 20 cases (1996–1998). J Am Vet Med Assoc 2000; 216: 1592–5.

Ober CP, Barber D. Comparison of two- vs. three-view thoracic radiographic studies on conspicuity of structured interstitial patterns in dogs. Vet Radiol Ultrasound 2006; 47: 542–5.

Owens JM, Biery DN. Thorax (noncardiac). In: Owens JM, Biery DN (eds). Radiographic Interpretation for the Small Animal Clinician, 2nd edn. Baltimore: Williams & Wilkins 1998; 147–84.

Smith JR, LeBlanc AK, Hecht S. What is your diagnosis? Tracheal mast cell tumor in a dog. J Am Vet Med Assoc 2008; 233: 385–6.

Spencer CP, Ackerman N, Burt JK. The canine lateral thoracic radiograph. Vet Radiol 1981; 22: 262–6.

Suter PF, Lord PF. Thoracic Radiography: A Text Atlas of Thoracic Diseases of the Dog and Cat. Wettswil, Switzerland: Peter F. Suter 1984.

Suter PF, Gomez JA. Diseases of the Thorax: Radiographic Diagnosis, 2nd edn. Ames: Iowa State University Press 1987.

Thrall DE. Textbook of Veterinary Diagnostic Radiology, 4th edn. Section V: Neck and Thorax – Companion Animals. WB Saunders, Philadelphia 2002; 307–449.

Heart and great vessels

10

William H. Adams and Silke Hecht

10.1 Anatomy and indications

10.1.1 Anatomy

Heart and pericardium

The heart and surrounding pericardium are located within the middle mediastinum and surrounded by mediastinal pleura. The cardiac silhouette seen on radiographs consists of the heart itself (including blood within the cardiac chambers), origin of the large vessels (aorta and pulmonary trunk), coronary arteries and pericardium (including pericardial fat).

Individual cardiac chambers cannot be distinguished on survey radiographs. Similarly, a differentiation between heart and pericardium is not possible. A schematic illustration of cardiac anatomy including the individual cardiac chambers and the large vessels is provided in Figure 10.1. The location of the cardiac chambers and large vessels can be described using a **clock-face analogy** (Fig. 10.2). With this, a clock is mentally superimposed on the cardiac silhouette, and the cardiovascular structures are assigned specific time points. This method aids in identification of enlarged cardiovascular segments.

In **dogs** there is marked individual and breed-associated variability in the appearance of the thorax and cardiac silhouette (see also Chapter 9). Deep-chested dogs such as the Doberman or Collie have an elongated heart on the lateral view, and on a ventrodorsal (VD) view the cardiac apex is close to midline. The cardiac silhouette is more rounded in shallow-chested dogs, and the cardiac apex is pointed towards the left (Fig. 10.3).

The appearance of the cardiovascular structures in **cats** is similar across individuals and breeds. However, certain changes occur with increasing age: the long axis of the heart assumes an orientation parallel with the sternum, and a notable bulge develops associated with the aortic arch (Fig. 10.4).

The radiographic evaluation of veterinary patients for cardiovascular disease is challenging. Normal cardiac size is variable, especially in dogs, and the radiographic diagnosis of 'cardiomegaly' or 'microcardia' is to a certain degree subjective. As a rule of thumb, the cardiac silhouette should occupy approximately two-thirds of the height of the thoracic cavity on a lateral view. The width of the cardiac silhouette is approximately 2 to 2.5 intercostal spaces in cats, approximately 2.5 intercostal spaces in deep-chested dogs, and approximately 3 to 3.5 intercostal spaces in shallow-chested dogs.

To compensate for individual and breed-dependent variations, and to provide an objective assessment of normal heart size, a **'vertebral heart score'** has been developed (Fig. 10.5). The length of the heart is measured from the tracheal bifurcation to the cardiac apex, and the width of

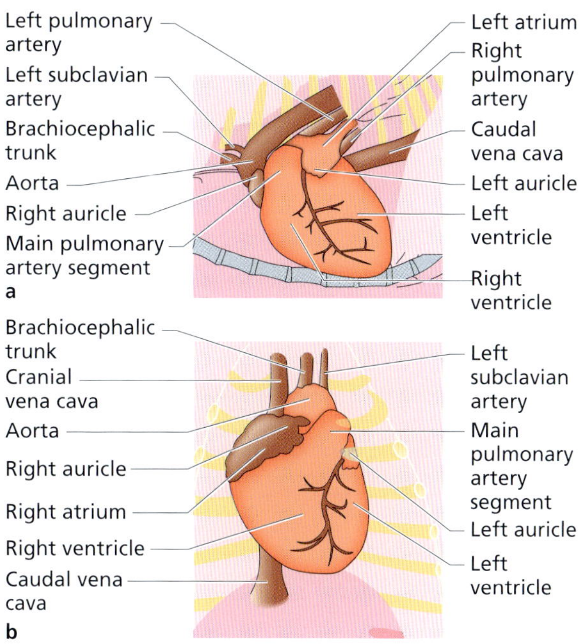

Fig. 10.1 Schematic illustration of the location of individual cardiac chambers and large vessels on a lateral a and ventrodorsal b thoracic radiograph.

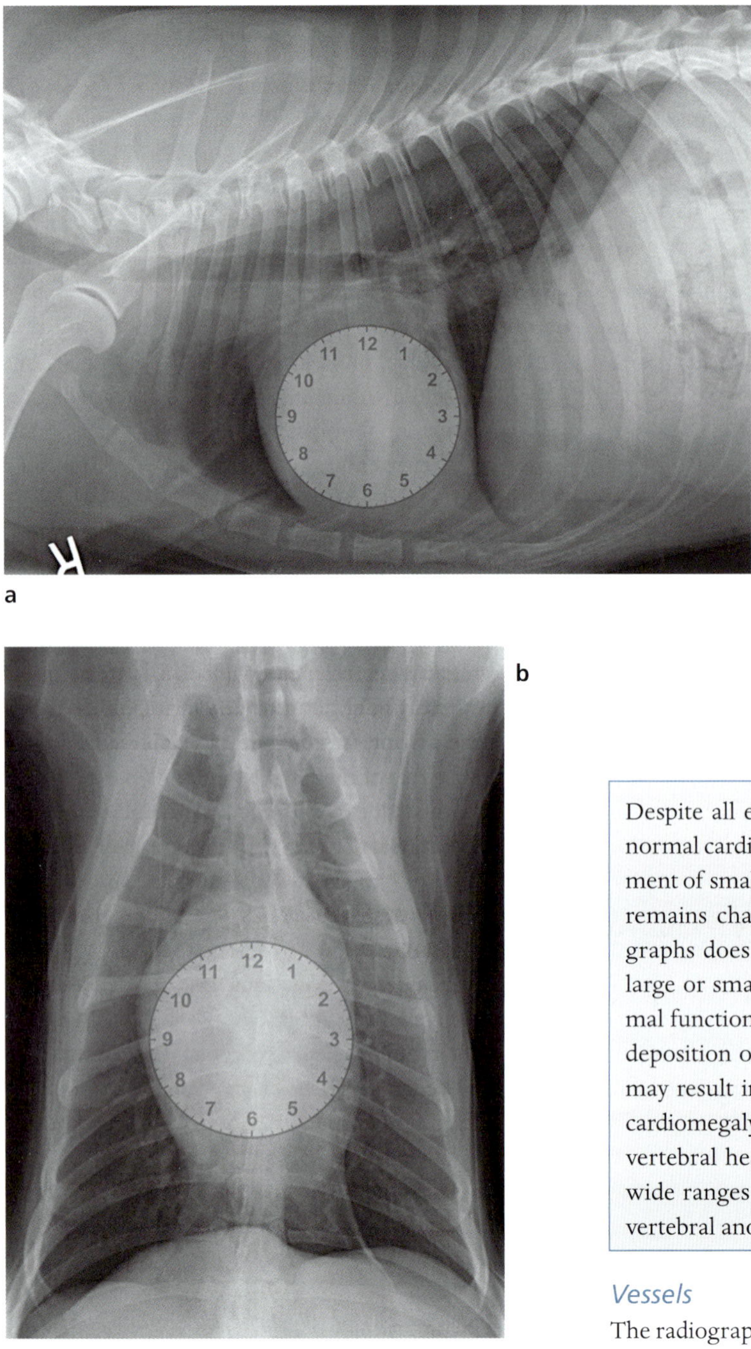

a

b

Fig. 10.2 Clock-face analogy on a lateral a and ventrodorsal b thoracic radiograph.
a Lateral view: 12 to 2 o'clock, left atrium; 2 to 5 o'clock, left ventricle; 5 o'clock, cardiac apex; 5 to 9 o'clock, right ventricle; 9 to 10 o'clock, right atrium and main pulmonary artery; 10 to 11 o'clock, aorta (R = right).
b Ventrodorsal view: 11 to 1 o'clock, aorta; 1 to 2 o'clock, main pulmonary artery; 2 to 3 o'clock, left auricle; 2 to 5 o'clock, left ventricle; 5 to 9 o'clock, right ventricle; 9 to 11 o'clock, right atrium. Note that the left atrium does not contribute to the outer margin of the cardiac silhouette but is located between the mainstem bronchi immediately caudal to the tracheal bifurcation on the VD view.

the heart is measured perpendicular to the long axis of the heart at the largest width of the cardiac silhouette. Starting at the cranial endplate of the fourth thoracic vertebra, the length and width of the cardiac silhouette are measured in terms of number of thoracic vertebrae and added together. The normal vertebral heart score in dogs has been reported as 9.7 ± 0.5 (range 8.5–10.6), and in cats as 7.5 ± 0.3.

> Despite all efforts to provide standardized values for normal cardiac size on thoracic radiographs, the assessment of small animal patients for cardiovascular disease remains challenging. Normal cardiac size on radiographs does not rule out cardiac disease, and even a large or small heart may have normal or almost normal function. Multiple variables such as pericardial fat deposition or radiographs obtained during expiration may result in the erroneous subjective impression of cardiomegaly. Even objective measurements such as the vertebral heart score remain of limited value due to wide ranges of normal and anatomic variations (e.g. vertebral anomalies).

Vessels

The radiographic anatomy of the thoracic and pulmonary vessels is relatively simple (see Fig. 10.1).

THORACIC VESSELS

The **aorta** leaves the cranial aspect of the heart and initially forms the aortic arch. The descending aorta is located within the mediastinum ventral and slightly to the left of the spine and enters the abdomen via the aortic hiatus. The **caudal vena cava** is located between the cardiac silhouette and the diaphragm, to the right of the spine on a ventrodorsal view, and in the mid thorax and superimposed with the accessory lung lobe on a lateral view.

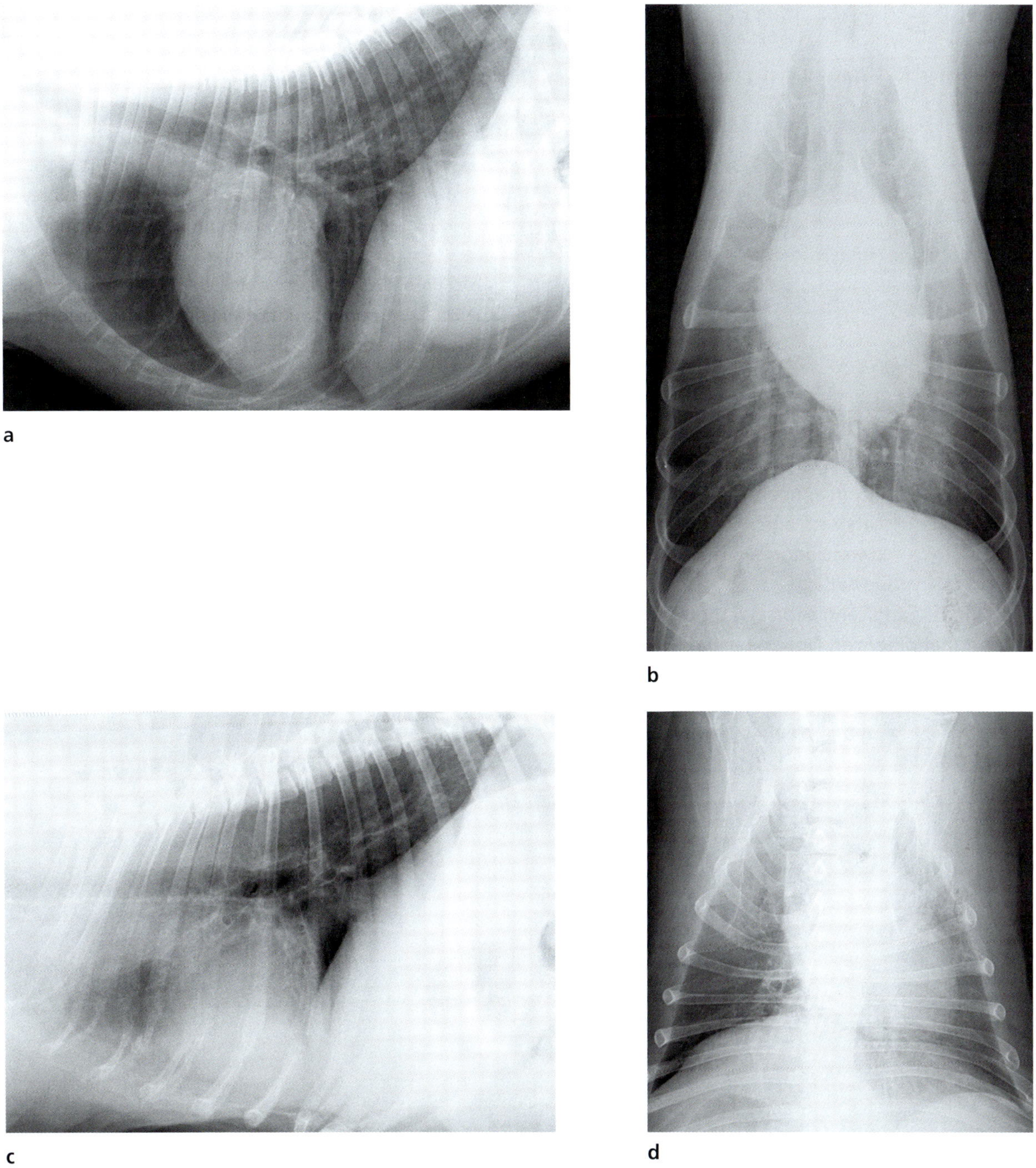

Fig. 10.3 Variations in appearance of the cardiovascular structures in dogs of different breeds.
a, b Lateral a and ventrodorsal b thoracic radiographs in a normal deep-chested dog. The cardiac silhouette is elongated, and the cardiac apex is located close to the midline.
c, d Lateral c and ventrodorsal d thoracic radiographs in a normal shallow-chested dog. The cardiac silhouette is rounded, and the cardiac apex is located within the left side of the thorax.

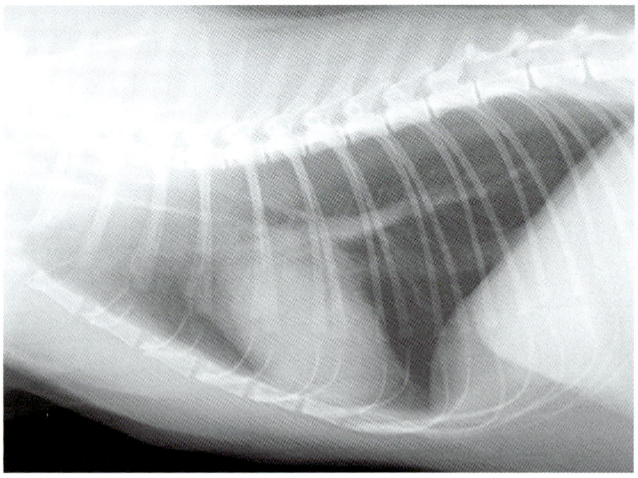

a

Fig. 10.4 Variability in appearance of the cardiovascular structures in cats with age.
a, b Lateral a and ventrodorsal b thoracic radiographs in a normal young cat.
c, d Lateral c and ventrodorsal d thoracic radiographs in a normal older cat. Note near-parallel orientation of the long axis of the heart with the sternum and the marked bulge associated with the aortic arch, particularly noticeable on the VD view (arrow). (L = left)

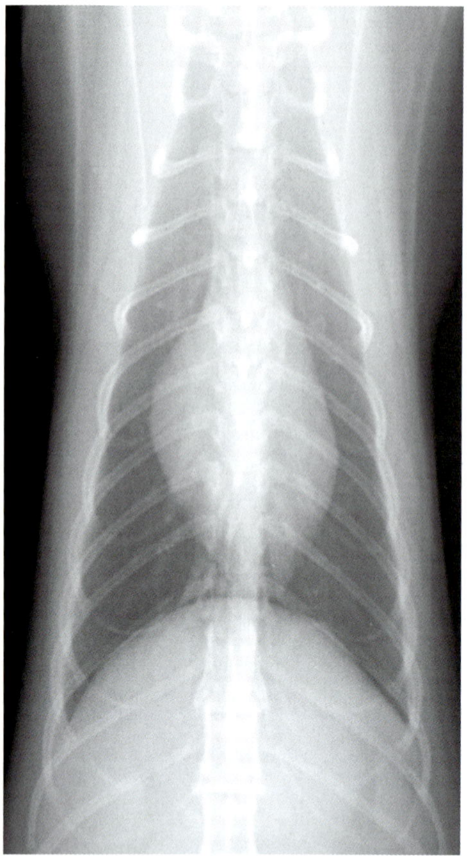

b

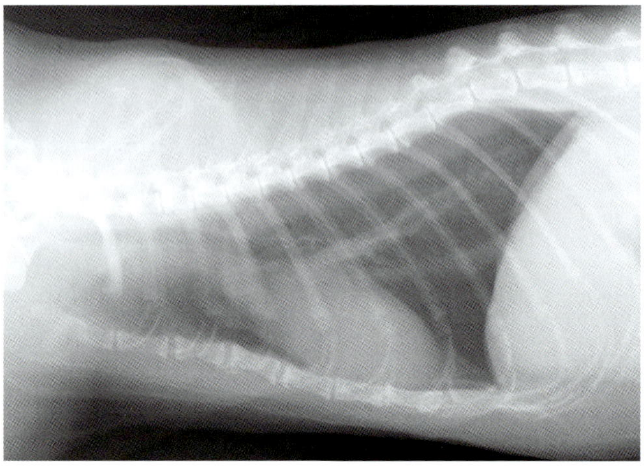

c

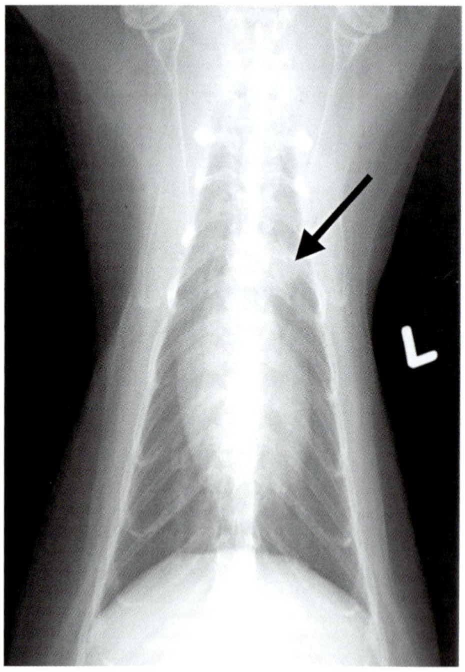

d

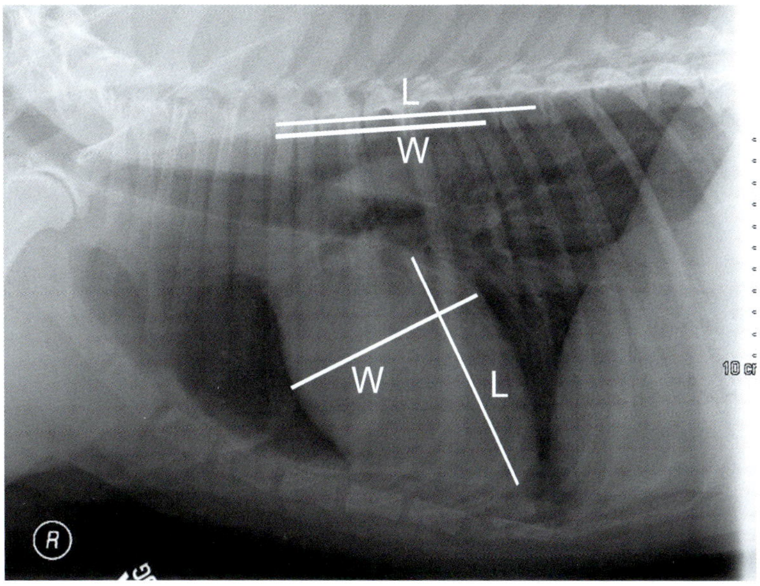

Fig. 10.5 Determination of the 'vertebral heart score'. The length (L) of the heart is measured from the tracheal bifurcation to the cardiac apex. The width (W) of the heart is measured perpendicular to the long axis at the point where the width of the cardiac silhouette is greatest. Starting at the cranial endplate of the fourth thoracic vertebra, the length and width of the cardiac silhouette are determined in terms of number of thoracic vertebrae and added together. In this example, cardiac length is 5.8 vertebrae and cardiac width is 4.7 vertebrae, resulting in a vertebral heart score of 10.5 (R = right).

> The aorta and caudal vena cava should be of similar **diameter**. However, in contrast to the aorta, the width of the caudal vena cava varies with the cardiac cycle. The size of the caudal vena cava is smaller on a radiograph obtained exactly during end-diastole than during other phases of the cardiac cycle. This should not be confused with volume depletion (dehydration, shock).

Cranial mediastinal vessels (cranial vena cava, brachiocephalic trunk, left subclavian artery) silhouette with each other and cannot be distinguished. Similarly, the azygous vein located in the dorsal mediastinum silhouettes with the aorta and is not normally visible.

PULMONARY VESSELS

The main pulmonary artery (aka pulmonary trunk) splits into the right and left caudal lobar pulmonary arteries at the level of the tracheal bifurcation. On a lateral view, the left caudal lobar pulmonary artery is located dorsal and the right caudal lobar pulmonary artery ventral to the mainstem bronchi. Pulmonary artery and vein branches course parallel with corresponding bronchi. Arteries and veins are similar in diameter at the same level and branch into smaller vessels in the periphery of the lung. Pulmonary vessels are arranged in a characteristic fashion with the accompanying bronchus (Fig. 10.6).

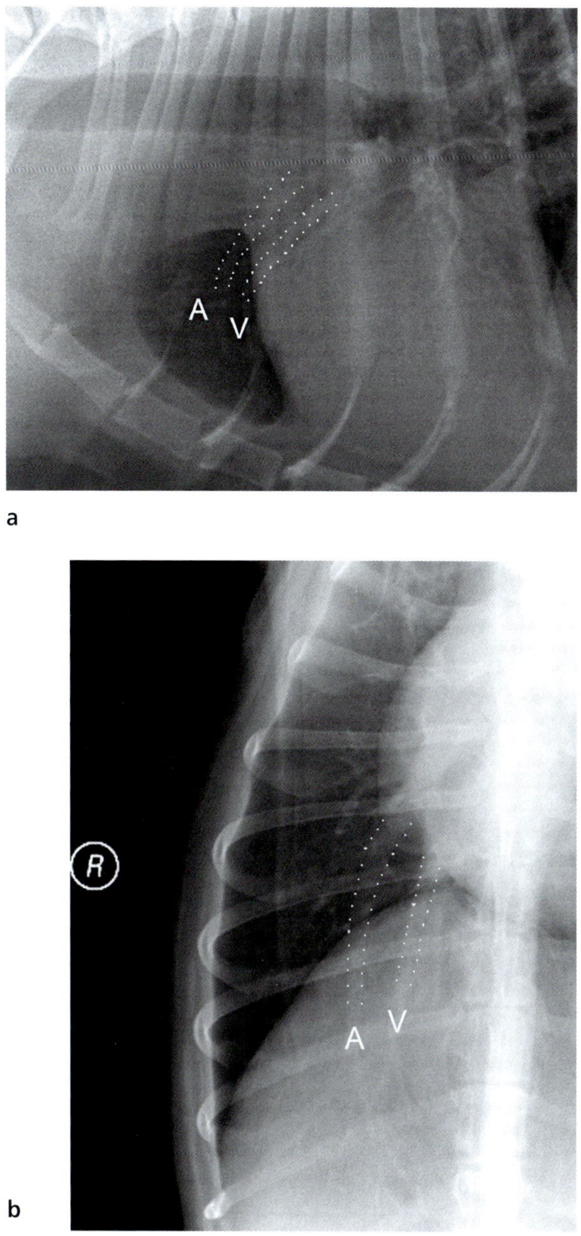

a

b

Fig. 10.6 Radiographic anatomy of the pulmonary vessels. On the lateral view a the pulmonary artery is located dorsal to the vein, and on the ventrodorsal view b the artery is located lateral to the vein (A = artery, V = vein). The bronchus located between these vessels is not clearly visible in this healthy dog (R = right).

> On a lateral view, artery, bronchus and vein are arranged from dorsal to ventral, and on a ventrodorsal view, from lateral to medial.
> **Note**: 'Veins are ventral and central'

Numerous attempts have been made to define normal pulmonary vascular diameter. In dogs, the caudal lobar pulmonary arteries and veins should not exceed the diameter of the ninth rib at their site of intersection. Another rule of thumb is that the diameter of the cranial lobar pulmonary arteries and veins should not be larger than the smallest diameter of the fourth rib. In the authors' opinion, this definition is questionable. Thus far, attempts to determine normal pulmonary vessel size in cats have failed. Like the assessment of cardiac size, the evaluation of pulmonary vessels remains to some degree subjective.

10.1.2 Indications

Indications for a radiographic examination of the cardiovascular system overlap with general indications for thoracic radiography (see Chapter 9). Specific indications include a heart murmur in symptomatic or asymptomatic patients, dyspnoea, ascites or other symptoms of congestive heart failure, and follow-up in patients medically treated for cardiac decompensation.

10.2 Radiographic technique and positioning

10.2.1 Technique

Thoracic radiographs in patients with suspected heart disease typically include a lateral and a ventrodorsal or dorsoventral view. An opposite lateral view commonly acquired for other indications may not be needed.

Depending on patient status, **sedation** should be considered, particularly in uncooperative animals. However, as discussed for other thoracic radiographs, general anaesthesia should be avoided due to the risk of pulmonary atelectasis, which may render the radiographs of limited or nondiagnostic quality.

Survey radiographs of the thorax do not provide any information about the interior of the cardiac chambers, cardiac valves, wall thickness, pressure within the heart and great vessels, or cardiac function. Additionally, the pericardium and the actual heart cannot be distinguished from each other. The role of thoracic radiographs in the evaluation of a cardiac patient is therefore limited to detection of obvious abnormalities in cardiac size and shape, appearance of the pulmonary vessels, and indicators of congestive heart failure. Advanced techniques (echocardiography [ECG] and others) are typically needed for further patient evaluation.

10.2.2 Positioning

General assessment of image quality (including evaluation of technique, positioning and respiratory phase) was discussed in section 9.2. Specific considerations in patients with suspected cardiovascular disease include the following.

- **Perfect patient positioning is mandatory**. Even minimal obliquity may mimic enlargement of cardiac chambers and interfere with adequate radiographic evaluation. The only exception is a patient with severe respiratory distress due to pulmonary oedema or pleural effusion. The diagnosis of congestive heart failure can typically be made on a limited radiographic study. In this case, immediate treatment of heart failure takes precedence over radiographic perfection. However, radiographs should be repeated following improvement of clinical signs.
- **Appearance of the cardiac silhouette differs depending on patient positioning.** The cardiac apex appears elongated on a right lateral view and somewhat rounded on a left lateral view. This difference is subtle and usually goes unnoticed during image interpretation. Differences observed on dorsoventral versus ventrodorsal views are more pronounced. On a dorsoventral view, the heart is rounded and shorter than on a ventrodorsal view, and visualization of individual chambers may be limited. On the other hand, there is improved visualization of the caudal lobar pulmonary vessels. This position is often preferred when evaluating animals in respiratory distress.

10.2.3 Contrast studies

Radiographic contrast studies of the cardiovascular system (selective and nonselective angiocardiography) have lost relevance since the introduction of safer and more accurate tests such as echocardiography, ultrasound and computed tomography (CT)/computed tomography angiography (CTA). This chapter will provide a brief explanation of these procedures. The reader is referred to specialty publications for additional information.

Nonselective angiocardiography

With this technique, a bolus of positive contrast medium is injected into a peripheral vein. Following injection, one or more static radiographs are acquired in rapid succession or fluoroscopy is used to document passage of contrast medium through the heart and great vessels. Evaluation of many cardiac structures including heart valves is generally difficult due to superimposition of contrast medium.

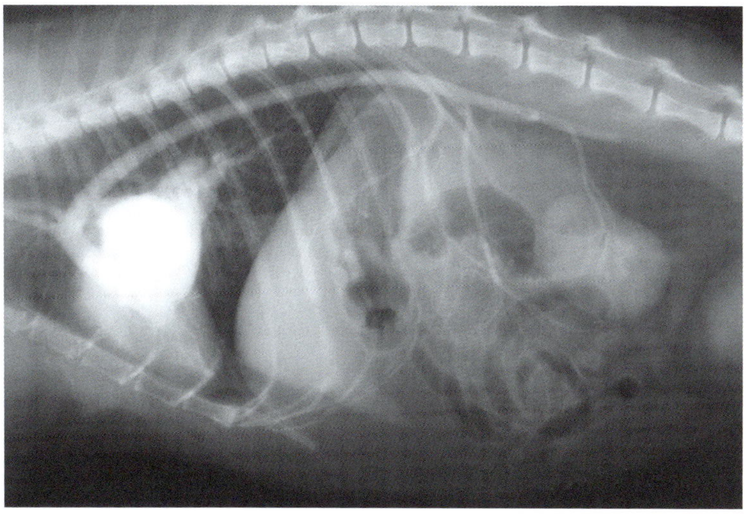

Fig. 10.7 Nonselective angiocardiography in a cat. The radiograph was obtained after the contrast bolus had passed through the right heart and lung and reached the left heart and the aorta. There is severe dilatation of the left atrium, and the lumen of the left ventricle is barely visible due to ventricular wall thickening. Note abrupt termination of contrast medium flow within the abdominal aorta caudal to the origin of the renal arteries. Diagnosis in this patient was hypertrophic cardiomyopathy with severe left atrial dilatation and aortic thromboembolism.

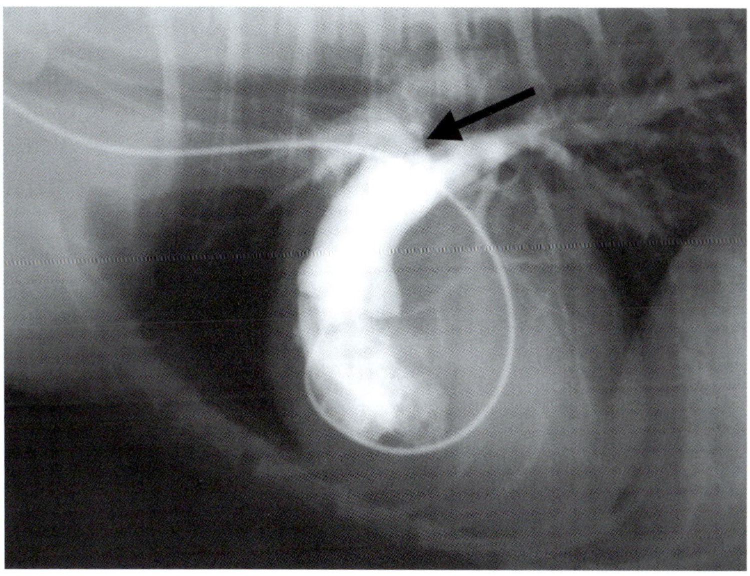

Fig. 10.8 Selective angiocardiography in a dog. The catheter passes through the jugular vein, cranial vena cava and right atrium, and the catheter tip is located in the outflow tract of the right ventricle. The right ventricle, main pulmonary artery segment and pulmonary arteries are filled with contrast medium. Even though there is no contrast medium present within the left heart, contrast medium is present within the aorta. Upon close inspection a vessel is identified connecting the main pulmonary artery and the aorta (arrow). The diagnosis in this patient was patent ductus arteriosus with a right-to-left shunt.

However, this method can provide a rough assessment of dimensions and wall thickness of cardiac chambers, passage time, cardiac or pericardial masses, as well as intracardiac or vascular obstruction (Fig. 10.7).

Selective angiocardiography

With this technique, a catheter is positioned in a specific cardiac chamber or vessel, and a directed injection of contrast medium is performed (Fig. 10.8). In addition to the information provided by nonselective angiocardiography, selective angiocardiography allows detailed assessment of valvular lesions (stenosis or insufficiency), shunts and septal defects as well as pressure measurements within different cardiovascular structures. This procedure is technically demanding and limited to specialty institutions.

10.3 Diseases of the cardiovascular system

As mentioned above, normal thoracic radiographs do not rule out heart disease, and marked breed and individual differences in the appearance of the cardiac silhouette in veterinary patients may mimic cardiovascular conditions. Nevertheless, thoracic radiographs are a useful tool in the assessment of cardiac patients. Most heart diseases result in cardiomegaly, either generalized or affecting specific chambers. This chapter will cover the radiographic changes seen with cardiomegaly, microcardia and congestive heart failure, and will discuss common congenital and acquired diseases of the cardiovascular structures.

10.3.1 Cardiomegaly and microcardia

Due to variability in normal size of the cardiac silhouette, particularly in dogs, diagnosis of cardiomegaly, especially in mild cases, is difficult and often subjective. The diagnosis is easier in severe cases and when only certain parts of the heart are affected.

Enlargement of the left atrium

- **Lateral view:** Radiographic findings include dorsal displacement of the mainstem bronchi, elongation and convex shape of the caudal margin of the cardiac silhouette, and loss of the normal caudal cardiac waist (Fig. 10.9a).
- **Ventrodorsal view:** Summation of the enlarged left atrium with the left ventricle results in a 'double opacity sign' between the caudal mainstem bronchi. The bronchi are deviated laterally and have a curved appearance, resulting in the impression of a 'bow-legged cowboy'. Enlargement of the left auricle results in a focal bulge associated with the cardiac silhouette at the 2 to 3 o'clock position (Fig. 10.9b).

Enlargement of the left ventricle

- **Lateral view:** Left ventricular enlargement results in a greater length of the cardiac silhouette, with a straight rather than curved appearance of the caudal cardiac margin. The cardiac silhouette occupies a larger percentage than normal of the dorsoventral thoracic diameter, and the trachea is displaced dorsally (Fig. 10.10a).
- **Ventrodorsal view:** The heart is longer than normal, and the cardiac apex is shifted into the left thorax. The cardiac silhouette has a bulge at the 2 to 5 o'clock position, corresponding to the location of the left ventricle (Fig. 10.10b).

Enlargement of the right atrium

- **Lateral view:** Radiographic abnormalities include a dorsal convex (J-shaped) course of the caudal trachea cranial to the tracheal bifurcation, rounding of the craniodorsal cardiac margin, and loss of the cranial cardiac waist (Fig. 10.11a).
- **Ventrodorsal view:** The cardiac silhouette has a bulge at the 9 to 11 o'clock position (Fig. 10.11b).

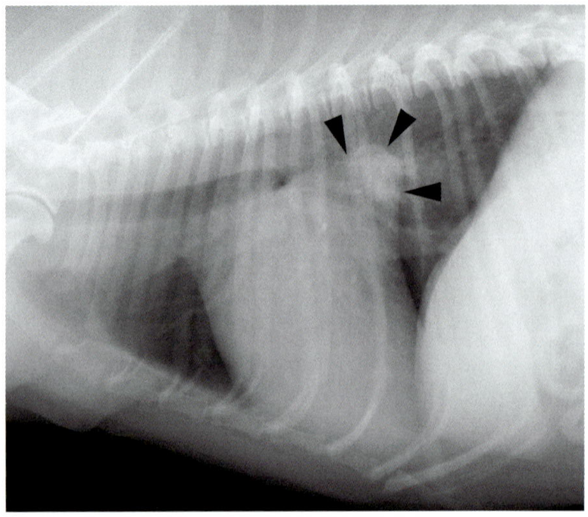

a

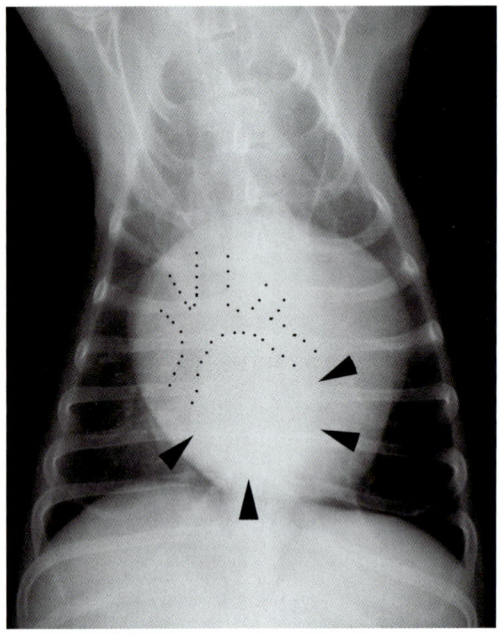

b

Fig. 10.9 Left atrial enlargement.
a On the lateral view, the caudal margin of the cardiac silhouette is elongated and has a convex shape, resulting in loss of the caudal cardiac waist. The tracheal bifurcation and mainstem bronchi are displaced dorsally by the enlarged left atrium (arrowheads).
b On the VD view, the enlarged left atrium (arrowheads) summates with the left ventricle, resulting in regional increased opacity ('double opacity sign') and widening of the angle between the caudal mainstem bronchi ('bow-legged cowboy sign'). The mainstem bronchi are indicated by the dotted lines. Note also left auricular enlargement indicated by a bulge at the 2 to 3 o'clock position.

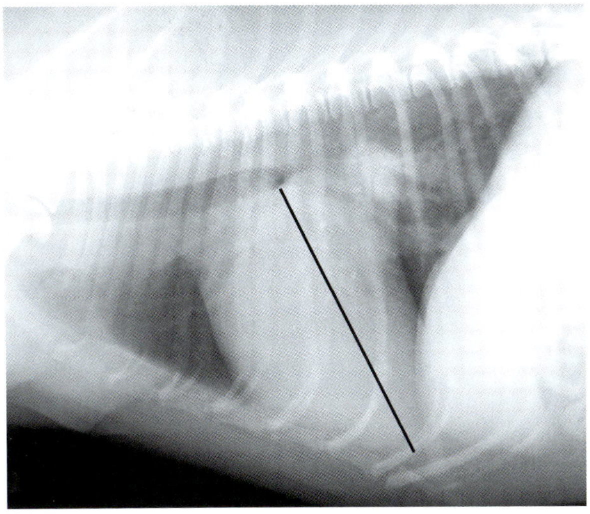

a

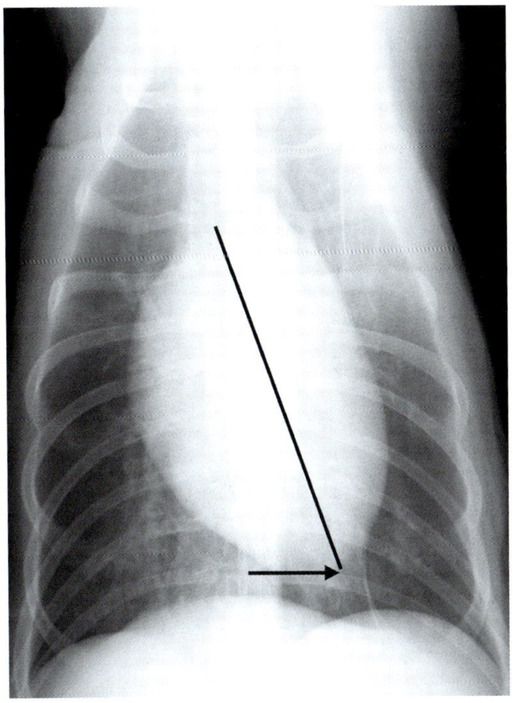

b

Fig. 10.10 Left ventricular enlargement.

a On the lateral view, the cardiac silhouette appears elongated and occupies more than two-thirds of the dorsoventral thoracic diameter. The trachea is displaced dorsally. There is also left atrial enlargement.

b On the VD view, the cardiac silhouette appears unusually long. The cardiac apex is located further to the left than normal (arrow), and there is a bulge of the cardiac silhouette at the 2 to 5 o'clock position.

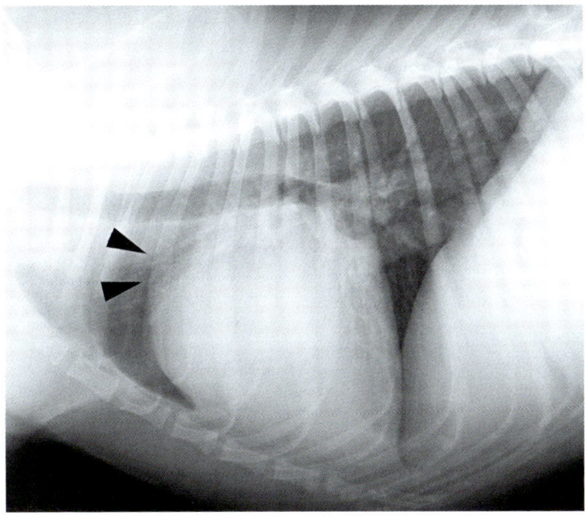

a

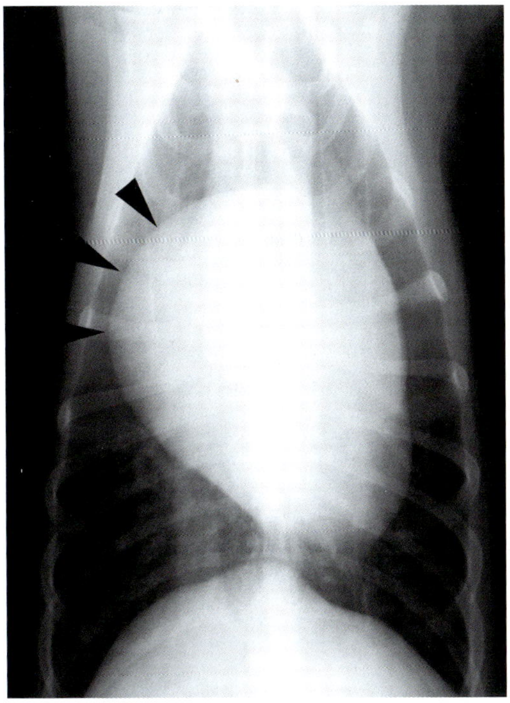

b

Fig. 10.11 Right atrial enlargement.

a On the lateral view, there is a dorsal convex (J-shaped) course of the thoracic trachea cranial to the bifurcation. Rounding of the cranial and dorsal margin of the cardiac silhouette (arrowheads) is also noted, resulting in loss of the cranial cardiac waist.

b On the VD view, there is a bulge associated with the cardiac silhouette at the 9 to 11 o'clock position (arrowheads).

Enlargement of the right ventricle

- **Lateral view:** Right ventricular enlargement results in increased width of the cardiac silhouette, increased convexity of the cranial cardiac margin, and increased contact between the heart and the sternum. The trachea often has a J-shaped course, similar to changes seen with right atrial enlargement (Fig. 10.12a).
- **Ventrodorsal view:** The heart is enlarged in the 5 to 9 o'clock position and appears rounded. These abnormalities result in the impression of a 'reverse D' shape of the cardiac silhouette (Fig. 10.12b).

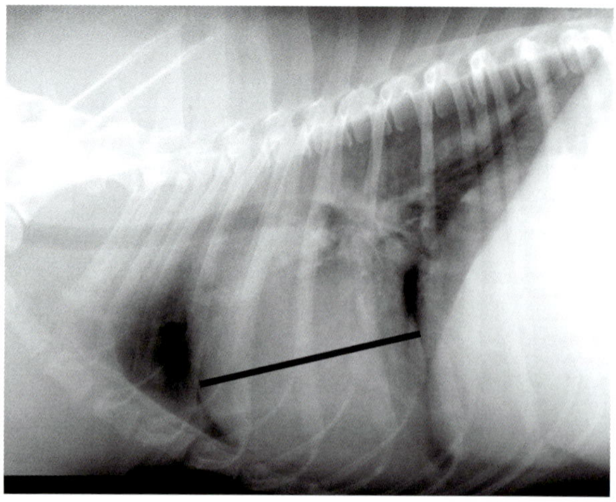

a

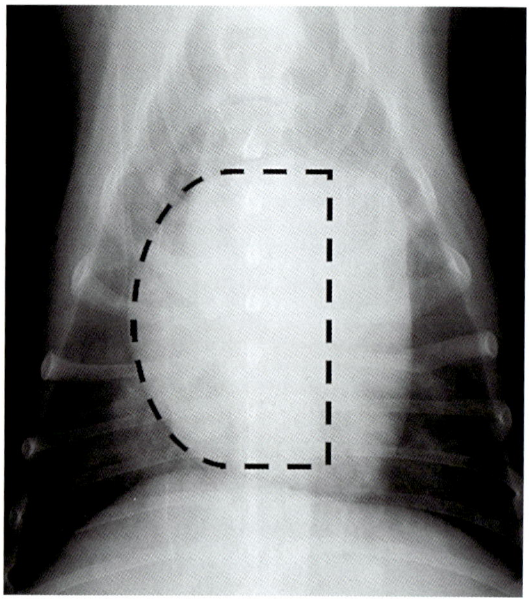

b

Fig. 10.12 Right ventricular enlargement.
a On the lateral view, the cardiac silhouette is abnormally wide, extending over approximately four intercostal spaces in width. The cranial cardiac margin is rounded, and there is increased contact between the cardiac silhouette and the sternum. A J-shaped course of the trachea is noted, suggesting concurrent right atrial enlargement.
b On the VD view, the cardiac silhouette is enlarged in the 5 to 9 o'clock position and appears rounded. This results in a 'reverse D' shape of the cardiac silhouette.

Generalized cardiomegaly

With generalized cardiomegaly, radiographic abnormalities consistent with both left and right heart enlargement are present.

Pitfalls

Technical and positioning errors, normal variations in cardiac size and shape, and non-cardiac thoracic pathology may result in the impression of generalized cardiomegaly or enlargement of specific cardiac chambers.

Examples:

- The cardiac silhouette appears disproportionately large in comparison to the underinflated lung fields on **expiratory radiographs**, resulting in the impression of generalized cardiomegaly.
- **Oblique positioning** may result in an unusual shape of the cardiac silhouette and/or may artificially decrease the distance between the cardiac silhouette and spine, giving the impression of cardiomegaly.
- **Pericardial fat deposition** results in enlargement of the cardiac silhouette and may mimic true cardiomegaly.
- **Enlargement of the tracheobronchial lymph nodes** may result in similar abnormalities to those seen with left atrial enlargement on a VD view (double opacity sign between the mainstem bronchi, and 'bow-legged cowboy' sign due to bronchial deviation). However, an enlarged left atrium will be located ventral to the tracheal bifurcation on a lateral view, while the lymph node is located dorsal to it.
- **Changes in head and neck position and mass lesions within the cranial mediastinum** may affect the course of the trachea and may give the erroneous impression of right atrial enlargement.

Microcardia

Microcardia refers to an abnormally small cardiac silhouette (i.e. less than 2.5 intercostal spaces in width), usually associated with a decrease in blood volume. Common concurrent findings include small size of the pulmonary vessels and the caudal vena cava, and hyperlucency of the pulmonary parenchyma due to underperfusion (Fig. 10.13). The most common causes of microcardia are dehydration, shock and hypoadrenocorticism (Addison's disease).

10.3.2 Congestive heart failure (cardiac insufficiency)

Cardiac insufficiency refers to an inability of the heart to handle the blood volume returning from the pulmonary and/or systemic circulation. For the purpose of this textbook chapter, 'heart failure' will be defined as changes visible on survey radiographs. Indicators of heart failure observed on echocardiography or other tests are covered in specialty textbooks.

Cardiomegaly alone is not a radiographic indicator of heart failure but may be an associated finding. Congestive heart failure may affect the left side, right side or both sides of the heart.

Left heart failure

With left heart failure, the heart is unable to efficiently pump oxygenated blood into the systemic circulation. This results in fluid backing up into the pulmonary veins and pulmonary parenchyma.

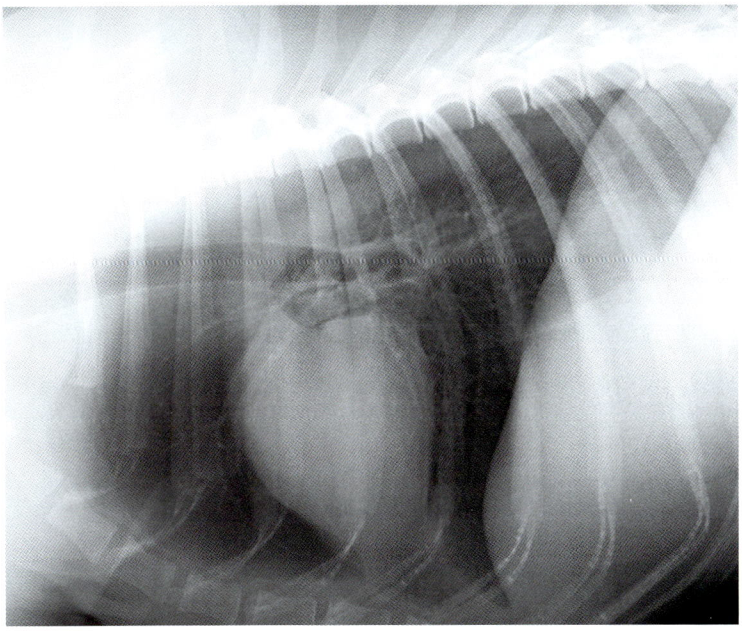

Fig. 10.13 Microcardia in a dog with shock. The cardiac silhouette measures less than 2.5 intercostal spaces in width. There is marked attenuation of the pulmonary vessels, resulting in overall decreased opacity of the pulmonary parenchyma. The caudal vena cava is also smaller than normal.

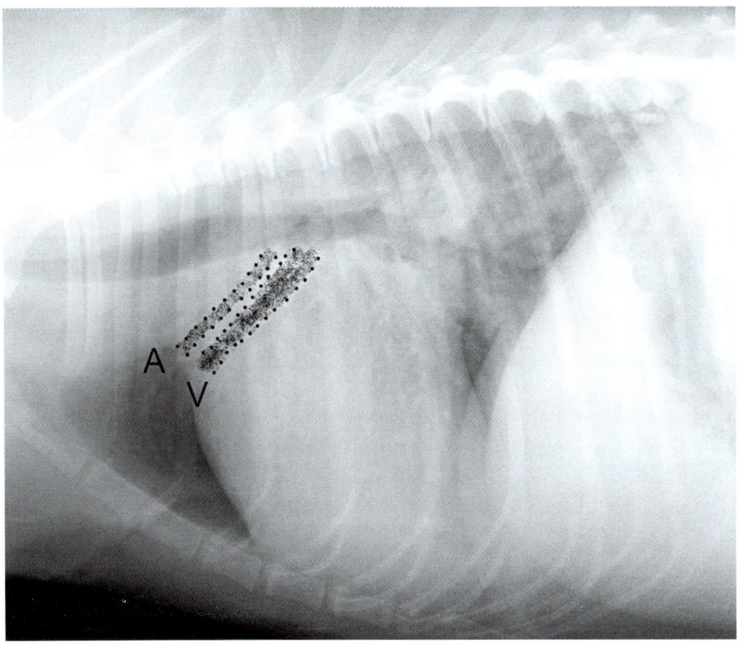

Fig. 10.14 Congestive left heart failure. The pulmonary veins (V) are larger than the corresponding arteries (A). There is increased opacity to the perihilar/caudodorsal lung fields, with poor definition of the pulmonary vascular margins. This is consistent with an unstructured interstitial to alveolar pattern and is compatible with pulmonary oedema. Note marked enlargement of the left atrium and ventricle in this patient.

Radiographic findings Left-sided congestive heart failure initially results in **enlargement of the pulmonary veins** compared to the corresponding arteries. Fluid leakage from the congested vessels subsequently results in **cardiogenic pulmonary oedema**, which, depending on severity, may appear as an unstructured interstitial to alveolar pulmonary pattern (Fig. 10.14). A bronchial pattern may also be present due to peribronchial cuffing, especially in cats. Cardiogenic pulmonary oedema predominantly affects the perihilar to caudodorsal lung fields in most dogs. The distribution of pulmonary infiltrates is more variable in cats, some dog breeds (e.g. Doberman Pinschers with dilated cardiomyopathy) and patients with acute rupture of the chordae tendineae. **Pleural effusion** is another possible consequence of left heart failure and is more commonly seen in cats than in dogs. As left heart failure results from left heart disease, enlargement of the left atrium and/or ventricle is frequently noted.

Right heart failure

With right heart failure, the heart is unable to efficiently pump blood into the lungs. This results in backup of blood into the systemic circulation and abdominal viscera, and in transudation of fluid into the peritoneal and/or pleural space.

> Pleural effusion may develop secondary to right and/or left heart failure. The veins of the parietal pleura drain into the systemic circulation. Right heart failure results in backup of blood into these vessels, which causes pleural effusion. The veins of the visceral pleura drain into the pulmonary veins. Left heart failure results in backup of blood into these vessels, also causing pleural effusion. Cats are more prone than dogs to developing pleural effusion secondary to left heart failure.

Radiographic findings Abnormalities seen with right-sided congestive heart failure include **dilatation of the caudal vena cava, hepatomegaly and ascites and/or pleural effusion** (Fig. 10.15).

10.3.3 Congenital heart diseases

Congenital heart diseases are rare, accounting for less than 10% of cardiac diseases diagnosed in dogs and cats. Overall prevalence in dogs is approximately 0.46–0.85%, in cats approximately 0.2–1.0%. An overview of the most common congenital heart diseases in dogs and cats and breed predispositions is provided in Tables 10.1 and 10.2. For information on less common congenital heart diseases the reader is referred to further literature.

By definition, congenital heart diseases are defects present at birth. Affected animals may show signs soon after birth (common, e.g. with patent ductus arteriosus), later in life (e.g. subaortic stenosis) or possibly never. A diagnosis of congenital heart disease on radiographs is very challenging due to limited ability to evaluate heart valves, pressure relationships and cardiac wall thickness. However, radiographs are valuable in the assessment of congestive heart failure, evaluation of the progress of known heart disease, and follow-up examinations in cardiac patients under therapy. They may also be helpful in initial diagnosis, especially when considering patient signalment, history and clinical examination findings (e.g. presence of cyanosis, heart murmurs, etc.). However, in most cases further imaging such as echocardiography or angiocardiography is needed for a definitive diagnosis.

Patent ductus arteriosus (PDA)

With this condition, the embryological connection between the descending aorta and the main pulmonary

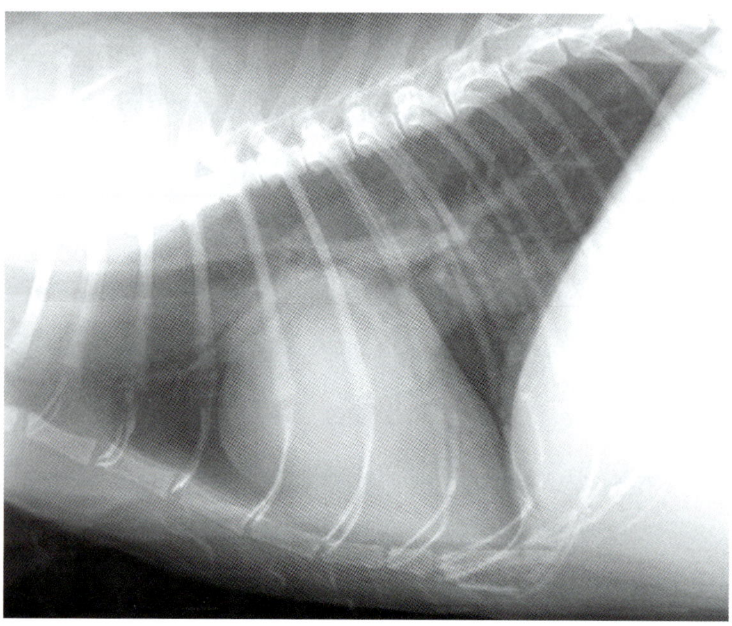

Fig. 10.15 Congestive right heart failure. The caudal vena cava is markedly dilated compared to the aorta. There is loss of serosal margin detail in the cranial abdomen, consistent with hepatomegaly and ascites. The cardiac silhouette is widened, consistent with right heart enlargement.

Table 10.1 Overview of the most common congenital cardiac diseases in dogs and breed predisposition.

Disease	Breed predisposition
Patent ductus arteriosus	Toy and Miniature Poodle, German Shepherd Dog, Collie, Pomeranian, Shetland Sheepdog, Maltese, English Springer Spaniel, Keeshond, Yorkshire Terrier, American Cocker Spaniel, Rottweiler
Pulmonic stenosis	English Bulldog, Terrier, Beagle, Mastiff, Samoyed, Miniature Schnauzer, American Cocker Spaniel, Keeshond, West Highland White Terrier
(Sub)aortic stenosis	Newfoundland, Rottweiler, Golden Retriever, Boxer
Ventricular septal defect	English Springer Spaniel
Tetralogy of Fallot	Keeshond
Mitral dysplasia	Rottweiler and other large-breed dogs
Tricuspid dysplasia	Labrador Retriever and other large-breed dogs
Persistent left cranial vena cava	
Persistent right aortic arch	German Shepherd Dog, Irish Setter
Peritoneo-pericardial diaphragmatic hernia	

Note: Modified from Kittleson and Kienle 1998; Sisson et al. 2000.

Table 10.2 Overview of the most common congenital cardiac diseases in cats.

Disease
Atrioventricular septal defect
Tricuspid dysplasia
Mitral dysplasia
Patent ductus arteriosus
Aortic stenosis
Endocardial fibroelastosis
Tetralogy of Fallot
Pulmonic stenosis
Persistent right aortic arch
Peritoneo-pericardial diaphragmatic hernia

artery segment (ductus arteriosus) remains open rather than closing normally a few days postpartum. The pressure difference between the aorta and the pulmonary vasculature results in a left-to-right shunt and pulmonary hyperperfusion. The increased volume of blood returning from the lungs to the left heart subsequently causes volume overload of the left ventricle.

Radiographic findings Radiographic abnormalities with uncomplicated PDA (i.e. left-to-right shunt) include **enlargement of the left ventricle and atrium including the auricle**, and a focal bulge associated with the cardiac silhouette at the 1 to 2 o'clock position due to **aneurysmal dilatation of the main pulmonary artery segment**. In classic cases, a **'triple bump sign'** of the cardiac silhouette will be evident on the VD view: main pulmonary artery segment (1 to 2 o'clock position), 'ductus diverticulum' (focal dilatation of the descending aorta at the level of the ductus arteriosus; 2 o'clock position), and enlargement of the left auricle (2 to 3 o'clock position) (Fig. 10.16). The **pulmonary vessels** are commonly enlarged due to hyperperfusion. Volume overload of the left ventricle may lead to **left heart failure**. The radiographic findings in patients with **atypical PDA** (right-to-left shunt, e.g. secondary to pulmonary hypertension/cor pulmonale) are variable. Indicators of pulmonary hyperperfusion are lacking.

Pulmonic stenosis

With pulmonic stenosis there is narrowing of the right ventricular outflow tract. The stenosis is typically located at the level of the pulmonary valve (valvular stenosis). Subvalvular or supravalvular location is less common. Increased resistance to right ventricular outflow results in pressure overload and hypertrophy of the right ventricle.

Radiographic findings Predominant radiographic findings include **enlargement of the right ventricle** (± atrium) and **poststenotic dilatation of the main pulmonary artery segment** appearing as a focal bulge associated with the cardiac silhouette in the 9 to 10 o'clock position on the lateral view and in the 1 to 2 o'clock position on the VD view (Fig. 10.17). The pulmonary vessels are often small. **Right heart failure** is possible due to pressure overload of the right ventricle.

(Sub)aortic stenosis (SAS)

As described for pulmonic stenosis, stenotic narrowing of the left ventricular outflow tract may be subvalvular, valvular or supravalvular. The subvalvular form (sub-

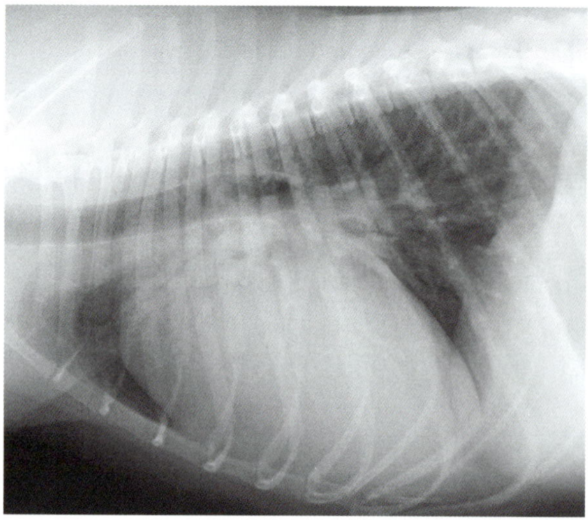

a

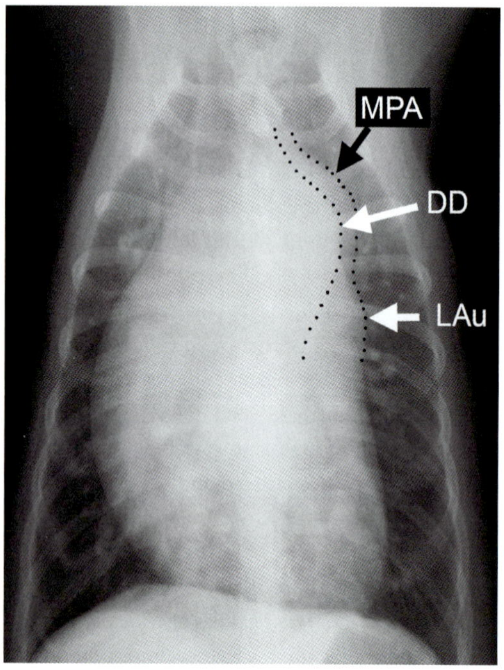

b

Fig. 10.16 Patent ductus arteriosus in a 5-month-old Pomeranian.

a On the lateral view, there is evidence of left heart enlargement and dilatation of both the pulmonary arteries and veins due to left-to-right shunting.

b The VD view reveals the classic 'triple bump sign': main pulmonary artery bulge (MPA, 1 to 2 o'clock), 'ductus diverticulum' (focal widening of the descending aorta at the level of the ductus arteriosus; DD, 2 o'clock), and enlargement of the left auricle (LAu, 2 to 3 o'clock).

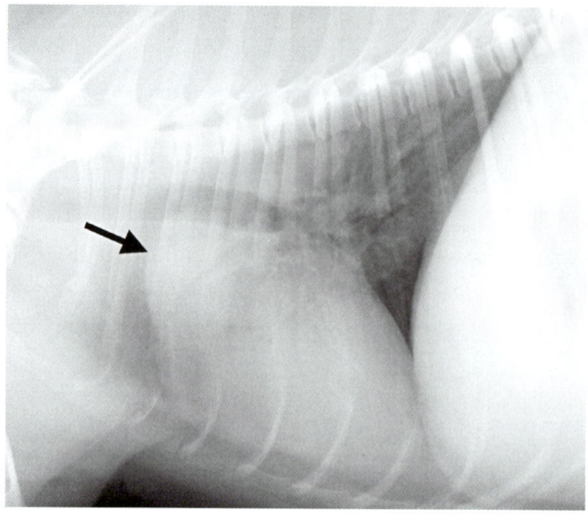

a

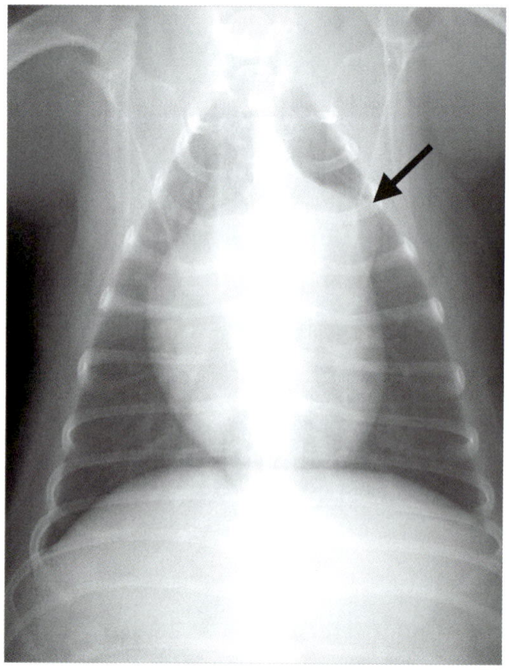

b

Fig. 10.17 Pulmonic stenosis in a 3-year-old mixed-breed dog.

a On the lateral view, the cardiac silhouette is widened (right heart enlargement), and a notable bulge is associated with the main pulmonary artery segment at the 9 to 10 o'clock position (arrow). The pulmonary vessels especially in the caudodorsal lung fields are smaller than normal.

b On the VD view, right heart enlargement indicated by increased convexity of the right atrium and ventricle is noted. There is a focal bulge at the 1 to 2 o'clock position, consistent with poststenotic dilatation of the main pulmonary artery segment (arrow).

aortic stenosis) is by far the most common. Increased resistance to left ventricular outflow results in pressure overload and hypertrophy of the left ventricle. However, left heart failure is an uncommon finding with this condition as severely affected animals typically succumb to acute death.

RADIOGRAPHIC FINDINGS Radiographic abnormalities may be **mild** or even **absent**. **Enlargement of the left ventricle** (and/or left atrium) is possible. **Poststenotic dilatation of the aortic arch** may be visible as a focal bulge associated with the cranial cardiac silhouette on a lateral view and in the 11 to 1 o'clock position on a ventrodorsal view (Fig. 10.18).

Ventricular septal defect (VSD)

With VSD the embryological connection between the left and right ventricles fails to close appropriately. This is the most common congenital heart disease in cats. Affected animals are often asymptomatic; however, with a large defect, left-to-right shunting with volume overload of the left ventricle and left heart failure may develop.

RADIOGRAPHIC FINDINGS Thoracic radiographs may be **normal** or show evidence of **left heart enlargement** ± right heart enlargement or left heart failure.

Tetralogy of Fallot

This is a complex congenital cardiac defect characterized by the presence of four concurrent abnormalities:

- pulmonic stenosis
- high ventricular septal defect
- overriding aorta
- right ventricular hypertrophy (likely to be secondary to pulmonic stenosis).

The pathophysiology of this condition is complex. Pulmonic stenosis results in pressure overload of the right ventricle. Subsequently, a right-to-left shunt develops via the ventricular septal defect.

RADIOGRAPHIC FINDINGS Predominant findings include **enlargement of the right ventricle** and an abnormal contour of the cardiac silhouette (**'boot-shaped heart'** = **'Coeur en sabot'**) (Fig. 10.19). Blood bypasses the pulmonary circulation, and the pulmonary vessels are smaller than normal.

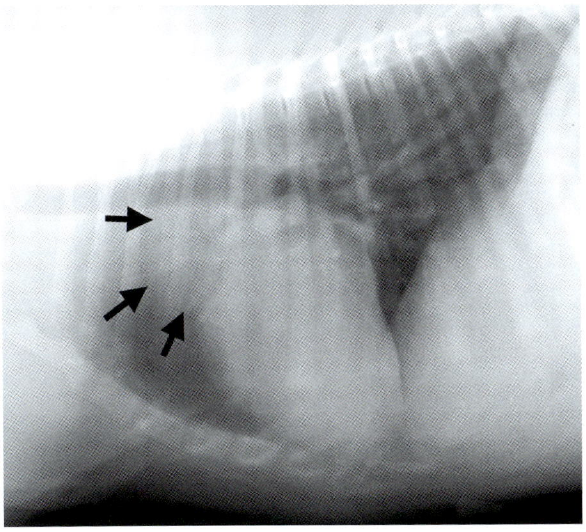

a

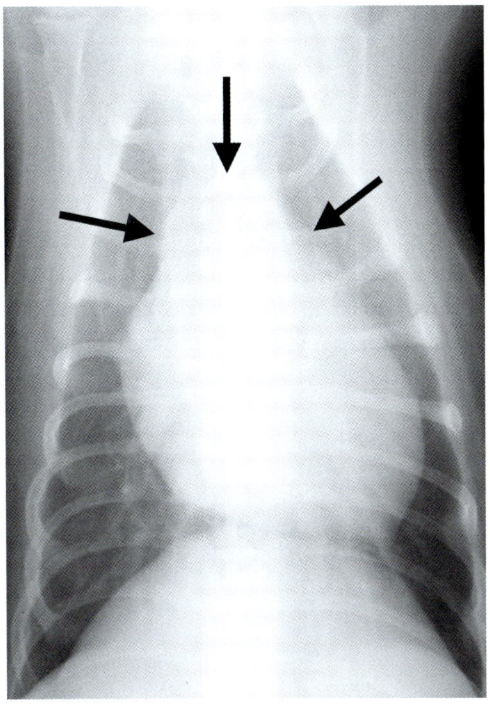

b

Fig. 10.18 (Sub)aortic stenosis in a 6-month-old Rottweiler.
a On the lateral view, there is moderate left heart enlargement. There is a large bulge of the cardiac silhouette ventral to the trachea (arrows), consistent with poststenotic dilatation of the aortic arch.
b On the VD view, there is evidence of left ventricular enlargement indicated by a bulge at the 2 to 5 o'clock position of the cardiac silhouette. The cardiac apex is displaced to the left. Enlargement of the aortic arch is evident as bulge in the 11 to 1 o'clock position (arrows).

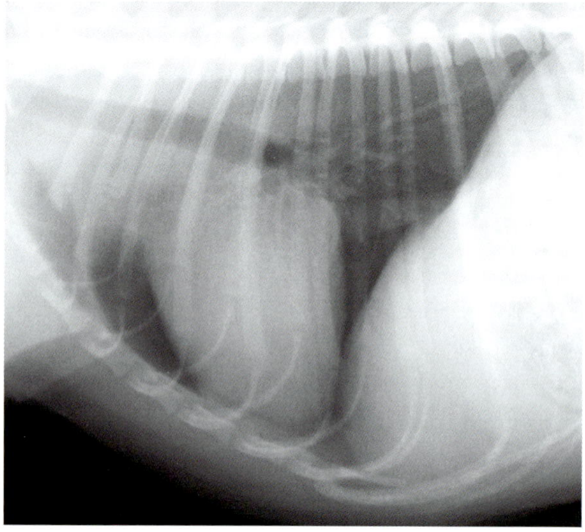
a

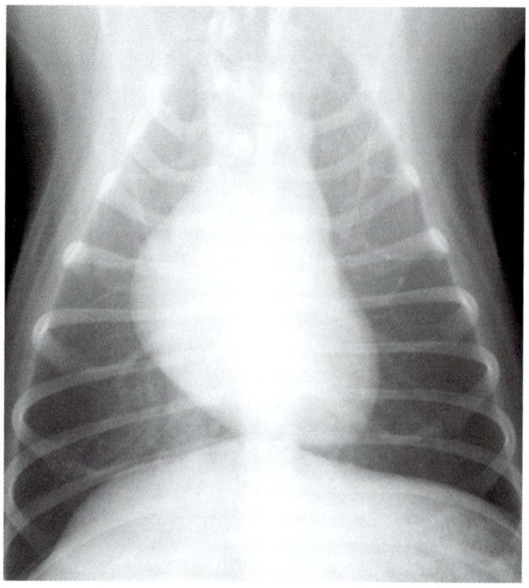
b

Fig. 10.19 Tetralogy of Fallot in a 5-month-old mixed-breed dog.

a Relatively minor abnormalities noted on the lateral view include a straight cranial cardiac contour and small size of the pulmonary vessels.

b On the VD view, there is evidence of right ventricular enlargement and an unusual 'boot-shaped' contour of the cardiac silhouette ('coeur en sabot').

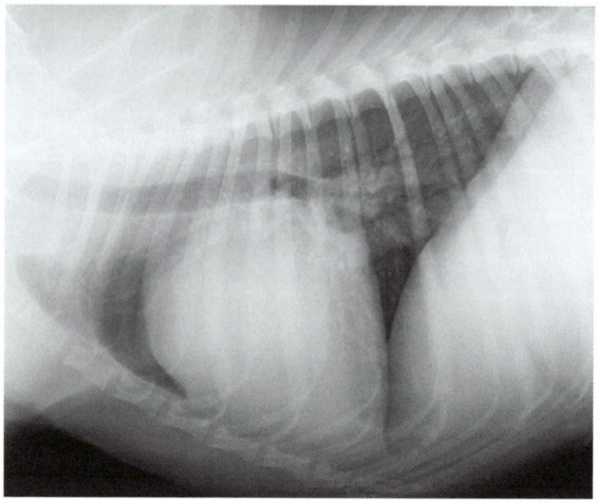
a

Fig. 10.20 Tricuspid insufficiency and right heart failure in a young Golden Retriever. Marked right heart enlargement and caudal vena cava dilatation are noted on both the lateral a and ventrodorsal b thoracic radiographs.

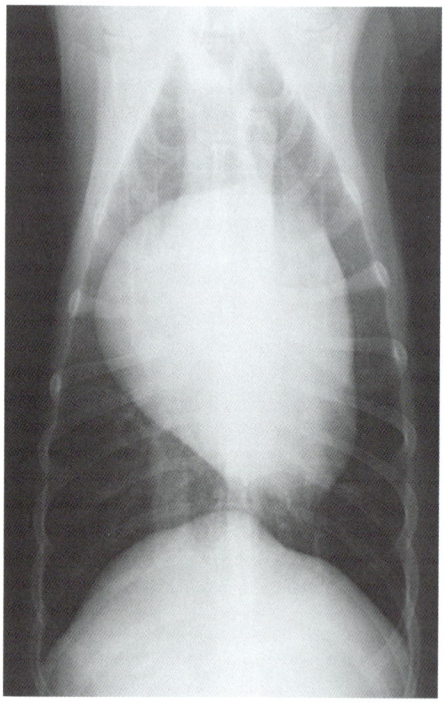
b

Mitral and tricuspid dysplasia

Mitral dysplasia is more common in cats, while tricuspid dysplasia is more common in dogs. Both conditions are characterized by abnormal conformation of the respective atrioventricular valve and resultant severe valvular insufficiency.

RADIOGRAPHIC FINDINGS The predominant radiographic finding is severe left (in case of mitral dysplasia) or severe right heart enlargement (in case of tricuspid dysplasia), respectively. Concurrent indicators of congestive heart failure are common (Fig. 10.20).

Persistent cranial vena cava

This is an occasional finding in dogs and cats, does not result in clinical signs and is thus inconsequential in otherwise heart healthy individuals. However, the abnormal anatomy may result in problems when performing a thoracotomy or procedures such as cardiac catheterization or implantation of a pacemaker. As these interventions are uncommonly performed in private practice, this condition will not be further discussed.

Persistent right aortic arch (PRAA)

This is the most common type of so-called 'vascular ring anomalies', a group of embryological abnormalities affecting intrathoracic vessels and resulting in variable oesophageal constriction. With PRAA, the right rather than the left fourth branchial arch develops to form the aorta. This has no haemodynamic consequences; however, it results in focal circumferential constriction of the oesophagus by the right aorta, heart base (including main pulmonary artery) and ligamentum arteriosum. Severe narrowing of the oesophageal lumen at the site of the vascular ring anomaly results in focal megaoesophagus. This is covered further in Chapter 13.

Peritoneo-pericardial diaphragmatic hernia (PPDH)

This is a congenital anomaly characterized by a persisting connection between the peritoneal cavity and the pericardium. This is discussed further below (see section 10. 3. 5).

10.3.4 Acquired heart diseases

Heartworm disease (dirofilariasis, angiostrongyliasis and others)

Heartworm disease may affect dogs and cats and has to be considered not only in patients from endemic areas but also in imported animals or animals with a travel history. Parasites residing within the pulmonary arteries cause endarteritis, endothelial proliferation and chronic allergic lesions. The increased afterload caused by pulmonary arterial changes results in right ventricular hypertrophy and dilatation of the main pulmonary artery segment. In addition to cardiovascular abnormalities, pulmonary changes including granulomas, infiltrates consistent with eosinophilic bronchopneumopathy, and pulmonary thromboembolism are common.

RADIOGRAPHIC FINDINGS Predominant radiographic abnormalities affect the pulmonary vessels. The **pulmonary arteries** are of increased diameter compared to the corresponding veins and have an unusual shape (tortuous course, blind and blunted endings without normal vascular branching patterns) (Fig. 10.21). In dogs, concurrent abnormalities of the cardiac silhouette (**right heart enlargement and main pulmonary artery bulge**) are common. The cardiac silhouette is often normal in cats. Allergic lung disease secondary to parasitic infestation (**eosinophilic bronchopneumopathy**) often manifests in mixed pulmonary patterns, usually with a predominant bronchial and/or unstructured interstitial component. Pulmonary granulomas may result in ill-defined pulmonary nodules. With pulmonary thromboembolism, oligaemic or alveolar regions are occasionally seen in the peripheral lung fields (Fig. 10.22). Severe heartworm disease may result in right heart failure.

Endocardiosis of the atrioventricular valves (mitral and tricuspid insufficiency)

Atrioventricular (AV) valve insufficiency secondary to degenerative valvular changes (endocardiosis) leads to the valves being unable to completely close during ventricular contraction. This results in regurgitation of blood into the atria. This condition is common and usually affects small-breed dogs. Mitral insufficiency may be an isolated condition or occur in association with tricuspid insufficiency. Isolated tricuspid insufficiency appears to be relatively rare.

RADIOGRAPHIC FINDINGS Depending on the affected valve(s), left and/or right heart enlargement with or without concurrent evidence of heart failure is noted (Fig. 10.23).

Cardiomyopathies

DILATED CARDIOMYOPATHY

This is characterized by progressive ventricular dilatation resulting in systolic dysfunction. This disease is most common in large-breed dogs, with a breed predisposition for Doberman Pinschers, Boxers and Great Danes. The disease is rare in small-breed dogs. The incidence of this condition has decreased in cats since an association with nutritional taurine deficiency has been discovered.

RADIOGRAPHIC FINDINGS With dilated cardiomyopathy there is evidence of **generalized cardiomegaly**, with or without concurrent evidence of **heart failure** (Fig. 10.24).

Radiographically, dilated cardiomyopathy and AV valve insufficiency may appear similar. However, the former predominantly affects large-breed dogs and the latter predominantly affects small-breed dogs.

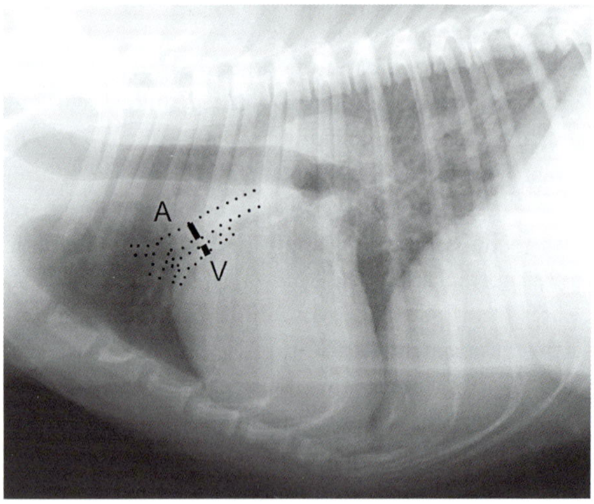

a

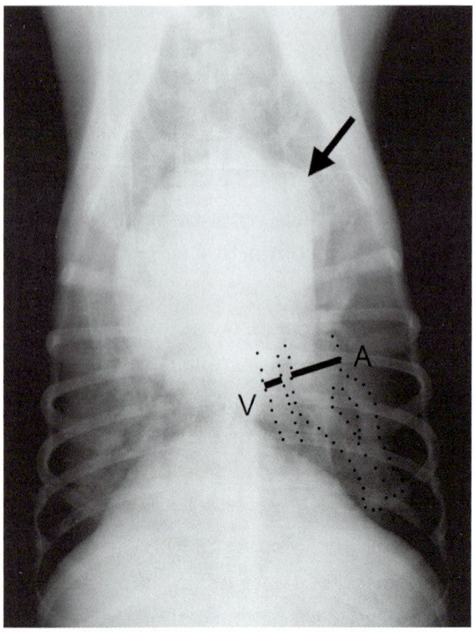

b

Fig. 10.21 Lateral a and ventrodorsal b thoracic radiographs in a dog with heartworm disease (dirofilariasis). Radiographic abnormalities include right heart enlargement and a focal bulge of the cardiac silhouette at the main pulmonary artery segment (arrow). The pulmonary arteries (A) are larger than the corresponding veins (V) and are multifocally tortuous and blunted. Throughout the lung fields, unstructured interstitial and bronchial patterns are noted, consistent with eosinophilic bronchopneumopathy.

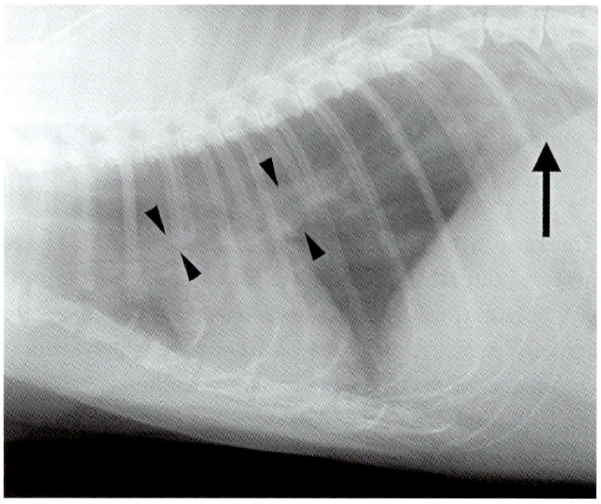

a

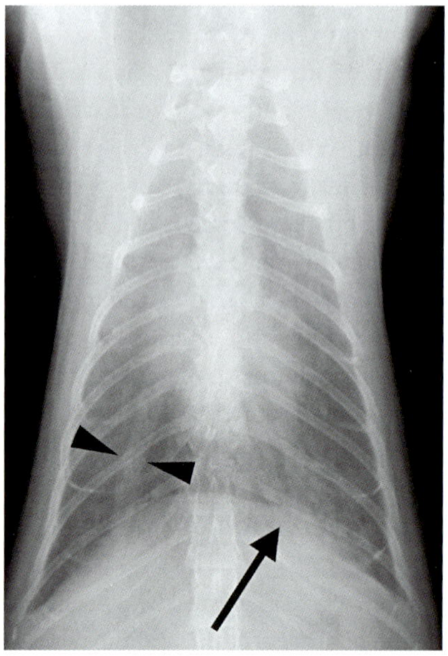

b

Fig. 10.22 Lateral a and ventrodorsal b thoracic radiographs in a cat with heartworm disease (dirofilariasis) and pulmonary thromboembolism. Several pulmonary arteries (arrowheads) are enlarged and blunted. The cardiac silhouette is only mildly enlarged. In addition to multifocal unstructured interstitial and bronchial lung patterns there is a focal fairly well-delineated alveolar pattern associated with the periphery of the left caudal lung lobe (arrow), consistent with pulmonary thromboembolism.

HYPERTROPHIC CARDIOMYOPATHY

This is characterized by progressive thickening of the myocardium, resulting in diastolic cardiac dysfunction. This disease is predominantly seen in cats. True hypertrophic cardiomyopathy is a primary disease of heart muscle, which should be distinguished from hypertrophy of heart muscle secondary to an underlying condition such as hyperthyroidism.

RADIOGRAPHIC FINDINGS Hypertrophic cardiomyopathy predominantly results in **left auricular and left atrial enlargement**, possibly associated with left ventricular and/or right heart enlargement. Severe atrial enlargement may result in a characteristic 'Valentine shape' of the cardiac silhouette on a VD view (Fig. 10.25). Evidence of (left) heart failure may or may not be present.

RESTRICTIVE CARDIOMYOPATHY

This results in decreased distensibility of heart muscle and decreased cardiac output. This condition has been described in cats.

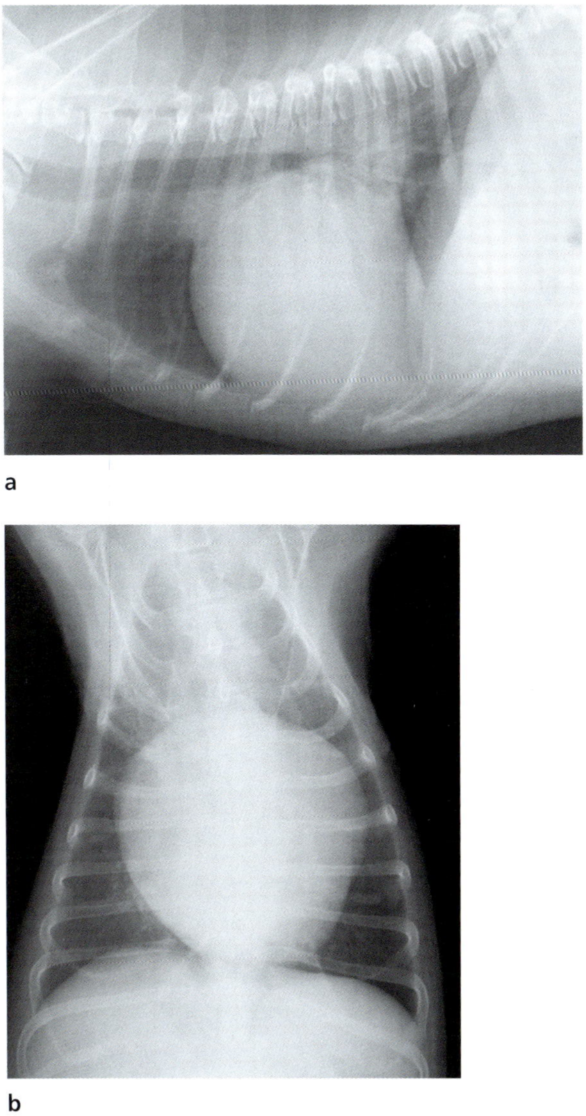

Fig. 10.23 Mitral and tricuspid insufficiency in a 10-year-old Shih Tzu. The cardiac silhouette is elongated and wide, resulting in dorsal displacement of the trachea and rounding of the cranial cardiac margin on the lateral view a as well as marked generalized cardiomegaly on the ventrodorsal view b. At this point, there is no radiographic evidence of heart failure.

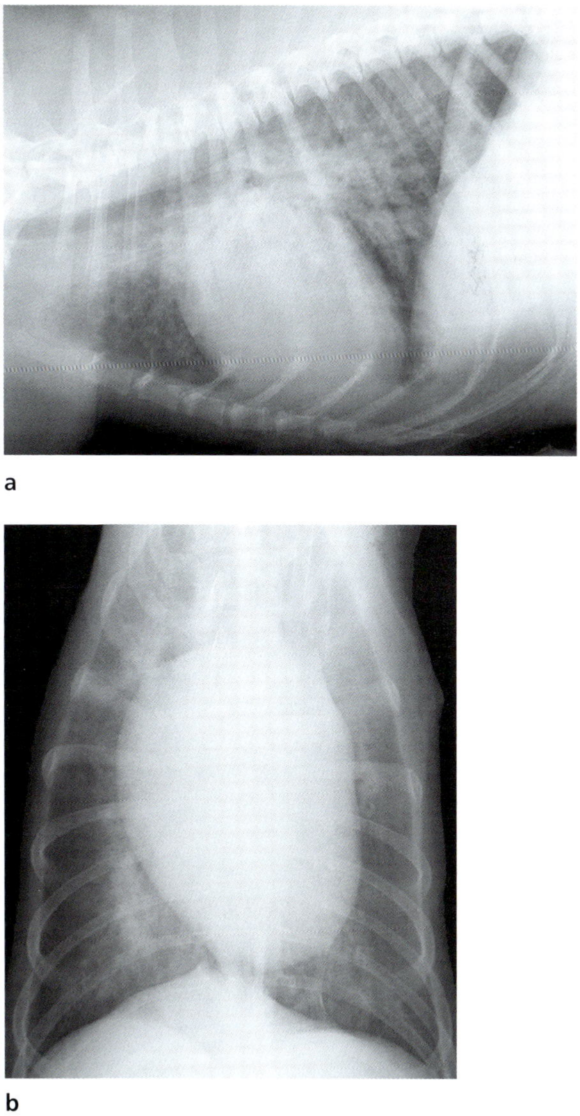

Fig. 10.24 Lateral a and ventrodorsal b thoracic radiographs in a 5-year-old Doberman Pinscher with dilated cardiomyopathy and left heart failure. Radiographic abnormalities include severe generalized cardiomegaly and a marked unstructured interstitial to alveolar pattern most notably affecting the caudodorsal lung fields, consistent with pulmonary oedema.

Radiographic findings Thoracic radiographs may be normal or show evidence of left ventricular enlargement, pericardial effusion or heart failure.

Cardiac neoplasia

Tumours of the heart are comparatively rare. Depending on the affected compartment, tumours are subcategorized as epicardial (e.g. mesothelioma, haemangiosarcoma), mural (e.g. haemangiosarcoma, lymphosarcoma) and intracavitary (e.g. haemangiosarcoma). Tumours located at the heart base (e.g. chemodectoma) are also occasionally seen.

Radiographic findings Survey radiographs may be normal or show nonspecific findings such as pericardial effusion or pulmonary metastases. Intracavitary tumours are predominantly located within the right atrium and may cause right atrial enlargement in severe cases. With heart base tumours, a mass may be evident in the cranial mediastinum, causing dorsal and rightward displacement of the intrathoracic trachea.

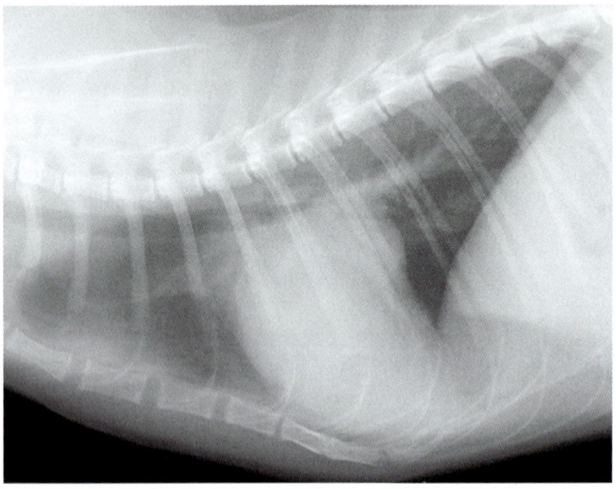

a

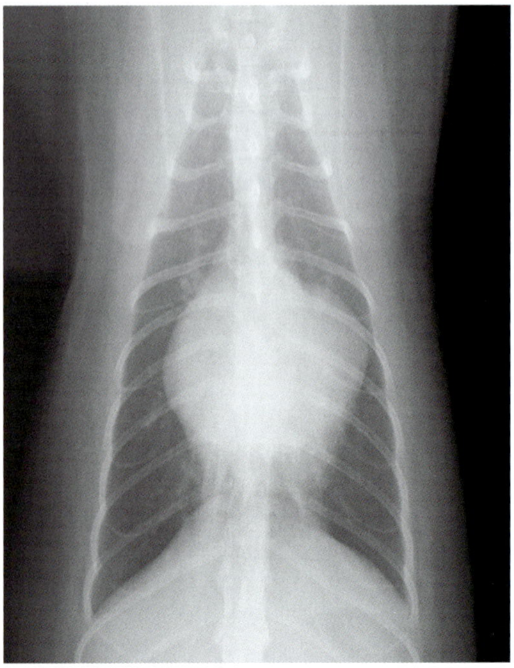

b

Fig. 10.25 Hypertrophic cardiomyopathy in a 3-year-old Oriental Shorthair cat.
a On the lateral view there is evidence of cardiomegaly, most notably affecting the left side of the heart.
b On the VD view, the cardiac silhouette has a 'Valentine shape', predominantly related to marked left auricular and atrial enlargement. The pulmonary vessels are conspicuous, suggesting early congestive heart failure.

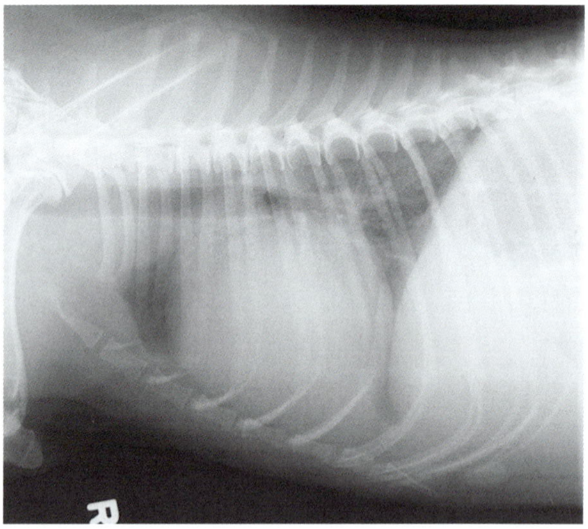

a

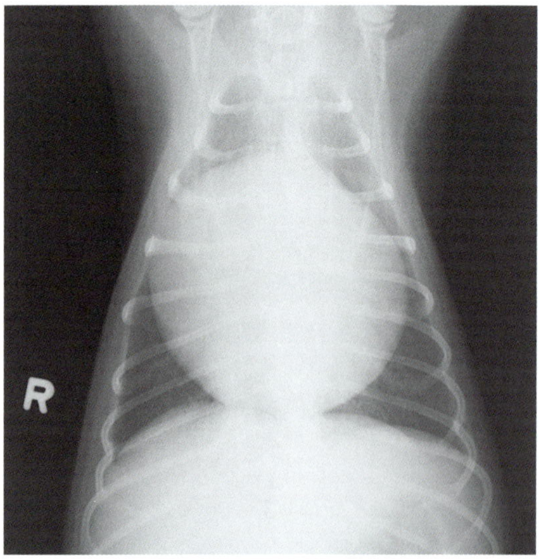

b

Fig. 10.26 Lateral a and ventrodorsal b thoracic radiographs in a 10-year-old Bichon Frise with pericardial effusion. The cardiac silhouette is markedly enlarged and globoid in shape. Marked hepatomegaly is noted, consistent with right heart failure (R = right).

10.3.5 Disorders of the pericardium

Pericardial effusion

With pericardial effusion there is fluid accumulation within the pericardial space. A large volume pericardial effusion may result in cardiac tamponade (cardiac compression) and compromised diastolic cardiac function.

RADIOGRAPHIC FINDINGS With pericardial effusion there is **generalized enlargement and globoid appearance of the entire cardiac silhouette** (Fig. 10.26). In contrast to dilated cardiomyopathy, individual chamber margins are not visible. Pericardial effusion of different aetiologies (inflammatory, infectious, traumatic, idiopathic) cannot be distinguished radiographically. With cardiac tamponade, compression of the thin-walled right heart predominates, resulting in right heart failure.

Pneumopericardium

Gas inclusions within the pericardium are a rare consequence of blunt thoracic trauma. Pneumopericardium may be an isolated finding or may be associated with pneumothorax and/or pneumomediastinum.

RADIOGRAPHIC FINDINGS Small round or linear gas opacity foci are identified adjacent to or superimposed with the cardiac silhouette.

Peritoneo-pericardial diaphragmatic hernia (PPDH)

PPDH is a congenital anomaly resulting in a persistent open connection between the peritoneal cavity and the pericardial space. This condition is often an incidental finding not associated with clinical signs.

RADIOGRAPHIC FINDINGS The radiographic appearance of PPDH varies depending on the type and degree of organ herniation. Common findings include **silhouetting of the caudoventral aspect of the cardiac silhouette and the ventral margin of the diaphragm**, and **enlargement and abnormal shape of the cardiac silhouette** (see Fig. 9.23). With herniation of intestines, tubular gas opaque structures may be present within the pericardium. Organs may be absent from the abdomen (e.g. spleen) or appear abnormally small (e.g. liver). Concurrent sternal anomalies are common.

References and further reading

Bonagura JD, Myer CW, Pensinger RR. Angiocardiography. Vet Clin North Am Small Anim Pract 1982; 12: 239–58.

Kittleson MD, Kienle RD. Small Animal Cardiovascular Medicine, 1st edn. St. Louis: Mosby 1998.

Myer CW, Bonagura JD. Survey radiography of the heart. Vet Clin North Am Small Anim Pract 1982; 12: 213–37.

Owens JM, Biery DN. Heart. In: Owens JM, Biery DN (eds). Radiographic Interpretation for the Small Animal Clinician, 2nd edn. Baltimore: Williams & Wilkins 1998; 185–216.

Sisson DD, Thomas WP, Bonagura JD. Congenital heart disease. In: Ettinger SJ, Feldman EC (eds). Textbook of Veterinary Internal Medicine, 5th edn. Philadelphia: WB Saunders 2000.

Suter PF, Lord PF. Thoracic Radiography: A Text Atlas of Thoracic Diseases of the Dog and Cat. Wettswil, Switzerland: Peter F. Suter 1984.

Thrall DE. Textbook of Veterinary Diagnostic Radiology, 4th edn. Philadelphia: WB Saunders 2002.

11 General abdomen

Tobias Schwarz

11.1 Anatomy and indications

11.1.1 Anatomy

The **abdominal cavity** is bordered by the diaphragm cranially, abdominal wall musculature ventrally and laterally, spine and lumbar musculature dorsally, and pelvic inlet caudally. It is lined by the peritoneal sac in which almost all abdominal organs are completely enveloped. The fluid-filled slit-like space between the peritoneal layers is the actual **peritoneal cavity**. The peritoneal visceral lining including the associated omentum and ligaments is of diagnostic importance and is discussed as **peritoneum** in this chapter.

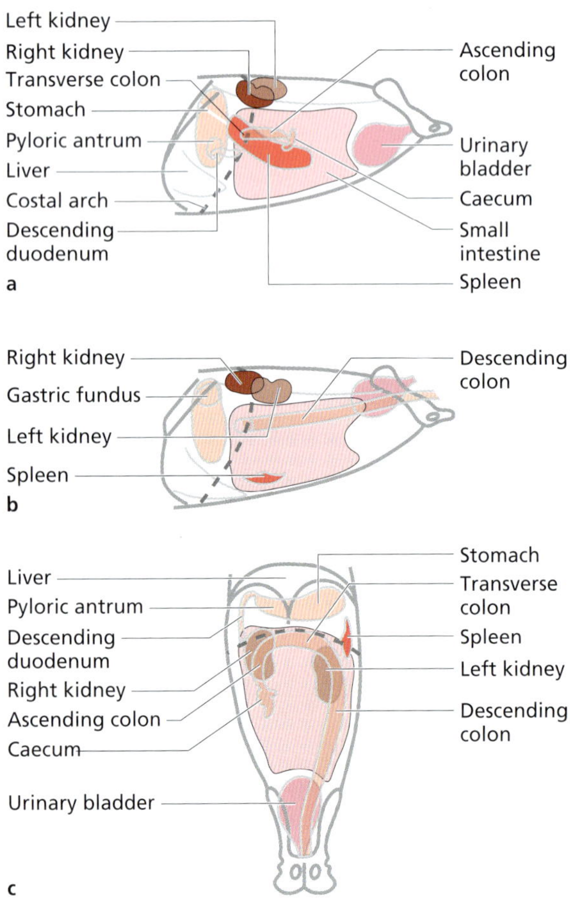

Fig. 11.1 Radiographic anatomy of the abdomen in a left lateral, b right lateral and c ventrodorsal views.

Organs not covered by peritoneum are referred to as **retroperitoneal** and include the aorta, kidneys, part of the urinary collecting system and caudal vena cava. In the context of abdominal imaging, the retroperitoneal space includes lumbar musculature, kidneys, ureters, nerves, blood and lymphatic vessels, adrenal glands and regional lymph nodes as well as the surrounding space in the dorsal abdomen.

The peritoneal cavity and retroperitoneal region are two anatomically separate spaces which do not communicate with each other (exceptions: ovary and uterine tube).

Abdominal organs that are normally visible include the stomach, small and large intestine, liver, spleen, both kidneys and the urinary bladder. However, there are differences depending on positioning (Fig. 11.1 to 11.3; Table 11.1).

- Due to direct contact with the liver, the right **kidney** in dogs is often only visible on a lateral view, while both kidneys are usually visible on both projections in cats.
- The **prostate** and **testicles** (if included in the collimation) are normally only visible in intact male dogs.
- A normal **uterus** is usually only visible in the advanced stages of pregnancy. It may occasionally be seen in nongravid small obese dogs (Fig. 11.4).
- The left lobe of the **pancreas** is often visible in well-nourished cats (Blevins and Kooreman 2003) (Fig. 11.5).
- The only part of the **small intestine** individually visible is the descending colon (to the level of the caudal duodenal flexure) if it is air-filled.
- **Adrenal glands** may on occasion be visible on radiographs if mineralized (incidental finding without clinical significance in cats; Fig. 11.6).
- The **caudal vena cava** and **abdominal aorta** are often clearly visible in small obese dogs and cats.

Table 11.1 Appearance of organ shadows in left versus right lateral recumbency.

Organ	Left lateral recumbency	Right lateral recumbency
Liver	Central location	Tendency to ventral shifting of ventral liver margin
Spleen (dog)	Often superimposed with intestinal segments and not clearly visible	Tongue-shaped soft-tissue opacity paralleling the caudal gastric wall (dependent on degree of gastric distension) Folded ventral extremity often seen as rounded soft-tissue opacity
Stomach	Soft-tissue opaque gastric content located in dependent gastric body and fundus Gas bubble in nondependent pyloric antrum	Gas bubble in nondependent gastric body and fundus Soft-tissue opaque gastric content located in dependent pyloric antrum
Gastric dilatation and volvulus (GDV; 180°)	Pyloric antrum rotated to the left, located in the dependent portion of the abdomen, often soft-tissue opaque and difficult to visualize. No obvious compartmentalization of gastric fundus	Pyloric antrum rotated to the left, located in the nondependent portion of the abdomen, contains gas and easily recognized based on compartmentalization of gastric fundus
Duodenum	Often gas filled	Often filled with soft-tissue opaque ingesta
Large intestine	Caecum (dog) and ascending colon often gas-filled Descending colon often soft-tissue opaque	Caecum and ascending colon often soft-tissue opaque Descending colon often gas-filled
Left kidney	Oval Difficult to visualize due to incomplete overlap with surrounding perinephric fat Shifted cranially due to cranial movement of the dependent left side of the diaphragm	Bean-shaped Good visibility due to surrounding perinephric fat Normal position
Right kidney	Bean-shaped Good visibility due to surrounding perinephric fat Normal position	Oval Difficult to visualize due to incomplete overlap with surrounding perinephric fat Shifted cranially due to cranial movement of the dependent right side of the diaphragm
Superimposition of kidneys	Maximal	Minimal
Free abdominal gas (VD horizontal beam view)	Gas accumulation adjacent to right abdominal wall Little risk of superimposition with gas-filled pyloric antrum and duodenum	Gas accumulation adjacent to left abdominal wall or hidden under splenic hilus Typically superimposed with gas-filled gastric fundus

Notes: Modified from Grandage 1975; Grandage 1979; Root 1974; O'Brien 1981; Love 1993; Murdoch 2001; Armbrust et al. 2000a. VD = ventrodorsal.

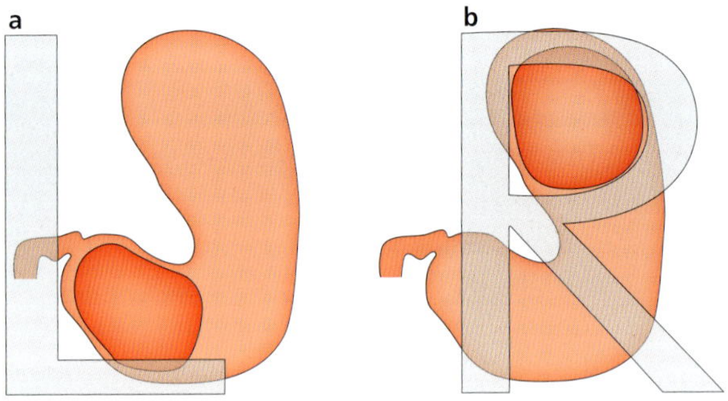

Fig. 11.2 Variations in position of the gas bubble within the stomach on lateral views dependent on recumbency.
a In left lateral recumbency, the ventrally located pyloric antrum is nondependent and gas-filled.
b In right lateral recumbency, the dorsally located gastric fundus is nondependent and gas-filled. A mental projection of the letters 'L' and 'R' over the stomach outlines the gas bubble in its respective location, which may serve as a memory aid.

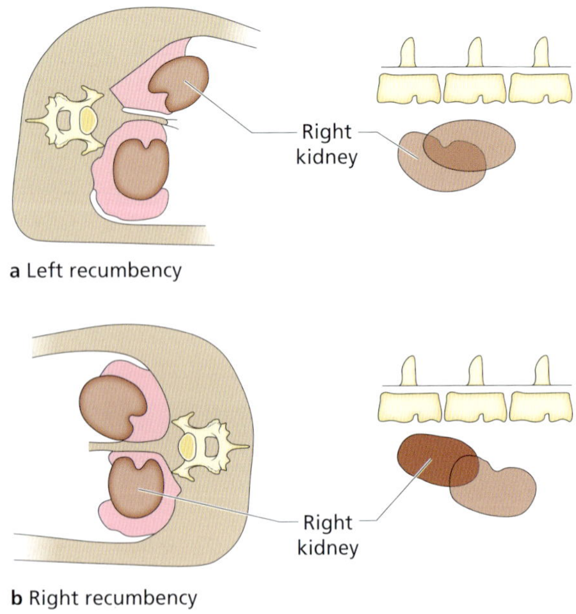

Fig. 11.3 Differences in position of the kidneys on lateral views dependent on recumbency.
a In left lateral recumbency, the nondependent right kidney falls into a horizontal position, which results in radiographic projection of the hilus and a bean shape of the renal silhouette. The renal silhouette contrasts with fat in the direction of the beam, which increases its visibility. The dependent left kidney is positioned more vertically, the hilus does not contribute to the renal silhouette, and the kidney appears oval in shape. Perinephric fat only borders the lateral aspect of the kidney, resulting in decreased visibility despite close proximity to the film. Even though the left kidney is typically located further caudally, it shifts cranially with the left part of the diaphragm, which results in marked overlap of both kidneys.
b In right lateral recumbency the situation is reversed, with one exception. The more cranially located right kidney is shifted even further, which decreases renal overlap. This recumbency is thus advantageous for evaluation of both kidneys.

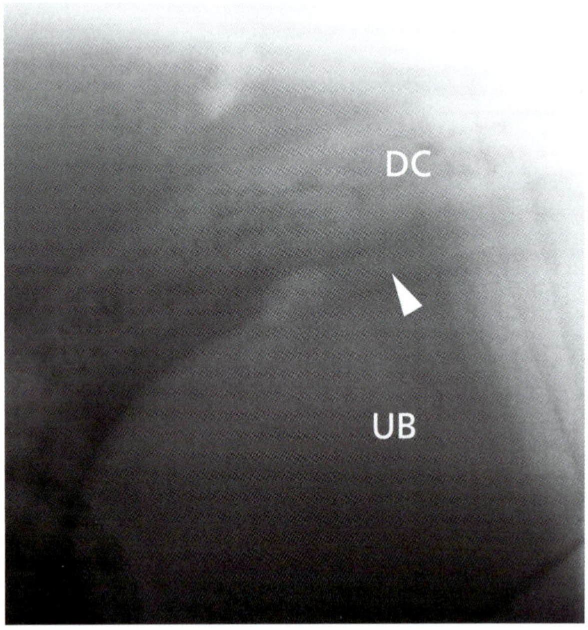

Fig. 11.4 Normal uterus (arrowhead) in a nongravid obese female dog during anoestrus. The uterus is located between the descending colon (DC) and the urinary bladder (UB) and is often not visible.

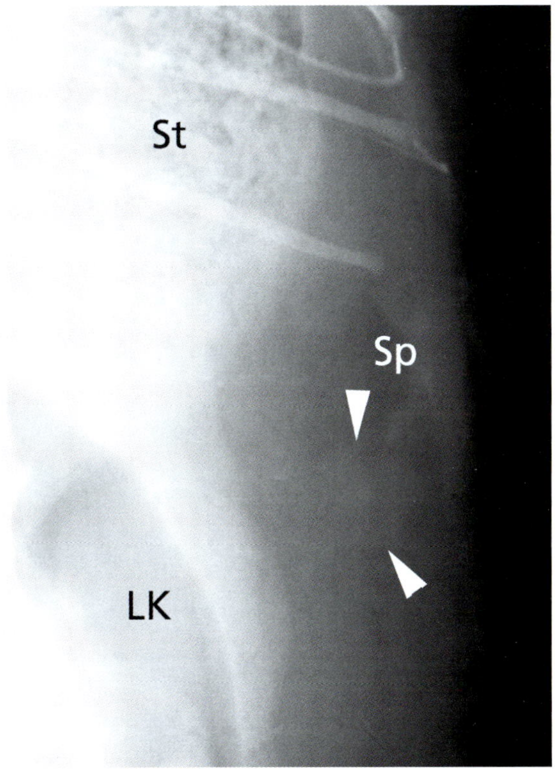

Fig. 11.5 Normal left lobe of the pancreas (arrowheads) in an 8-year-old domestic cat on a ventrodorsal view. The pancreas appears as an ill-defined soft-tissue opacity structure between spleen (Sp), stomach (St) and left kidney (LK).

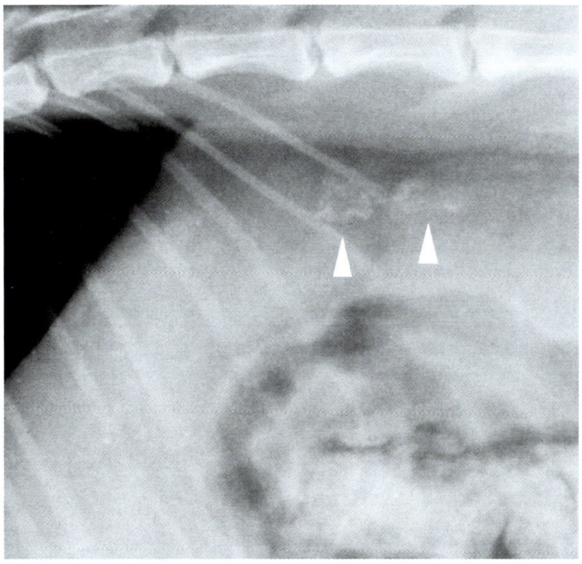

Fig. 11.6 Mineralized adrenal glands (arrowheads) in a 5-year-old domestic cat. This is an occasional incidental finding and not indicative of pathology in cats, but this is not the case in dogs!

- The branches of the **deep circumflex iliac vessels** located in the caudal lumbar region are often visible as a distinct punctate opacity (summation resulting from end-on projection of the vessel), which should not be confused with ureteral calculi (Fig. 11.7).

The adrenal glands, pancreas, gallbladder, mesentery, omentum, lymph nodes, lymphatic ducts, ovaries, uterus and prostate in neutered dogs are normally not visible except in instances listed above.

Several anatomic and positional variations of structures bordering the abdominal cavity have to be taken into consideration when evaluating abdominal radiographs.

- The appearance of the **diaphragmatic silhouette** is highly variable depending on positioning, radiographic beam centre, and respiratory phase (see Chapter 9). Increased content within the thoracic or abdominal cavity can also result in displacement of the diaphragm (Fig. 11.8).
- The **dorsal lumbar musculature** can be well developed especially in free-roaming cats and should be recognized as a physiological variant (Fig. 11.9).

- Assessment of the integrity and tension of the **ventral abdominal wall musculature** is part of the routine evaluation of the abdomen (Fig. 11.10).

As with the evaluation of other body parts, external skin structures such as the inguinal and other skin folds, nipples and prepuce are clearly visible due to adjacent contrasting air. These normal structures should not be mistaken for pathological abnormalities!

11.1.2 Indications

Indications for abdominal radiographs in small animal patients include:

- vomiting
- abdominal pain
- haematuria
- dysuria
- assessment of abnormalities noted on palpation (masses, nodules)
- abdominal distention
- tenesmus
- icterus.

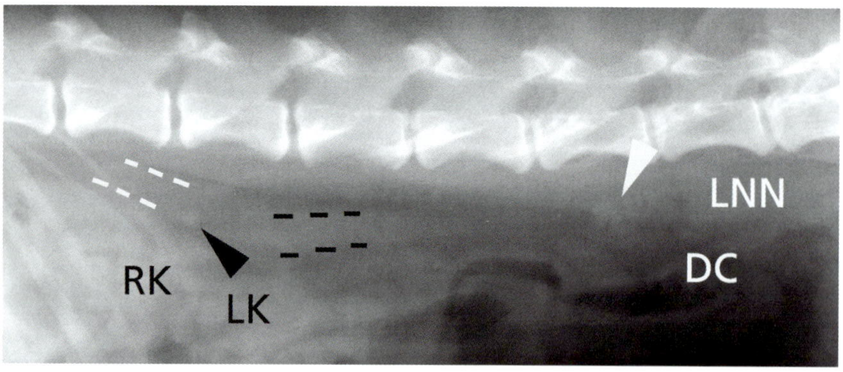

Fig. 11.7 Normal retroperitoneal space in a 1-year-old Sheltie. The aorta (white broken lines) and caudal vena cava (black open lines) are recognized as diverging tubular soft-tissue opacities dorsal to the right (RK) and left kidney (LK). Sublumbar lymph nodes (LNN) are located dorsal to the descending colon (DC) cranial to the pelvic inlet. The right renal vein (black arrowhead) and deep circumflex iliac vessels (white arrowhead) are projected end-on and appear as punctate opacities, which should not be confused with ureteral calculi.

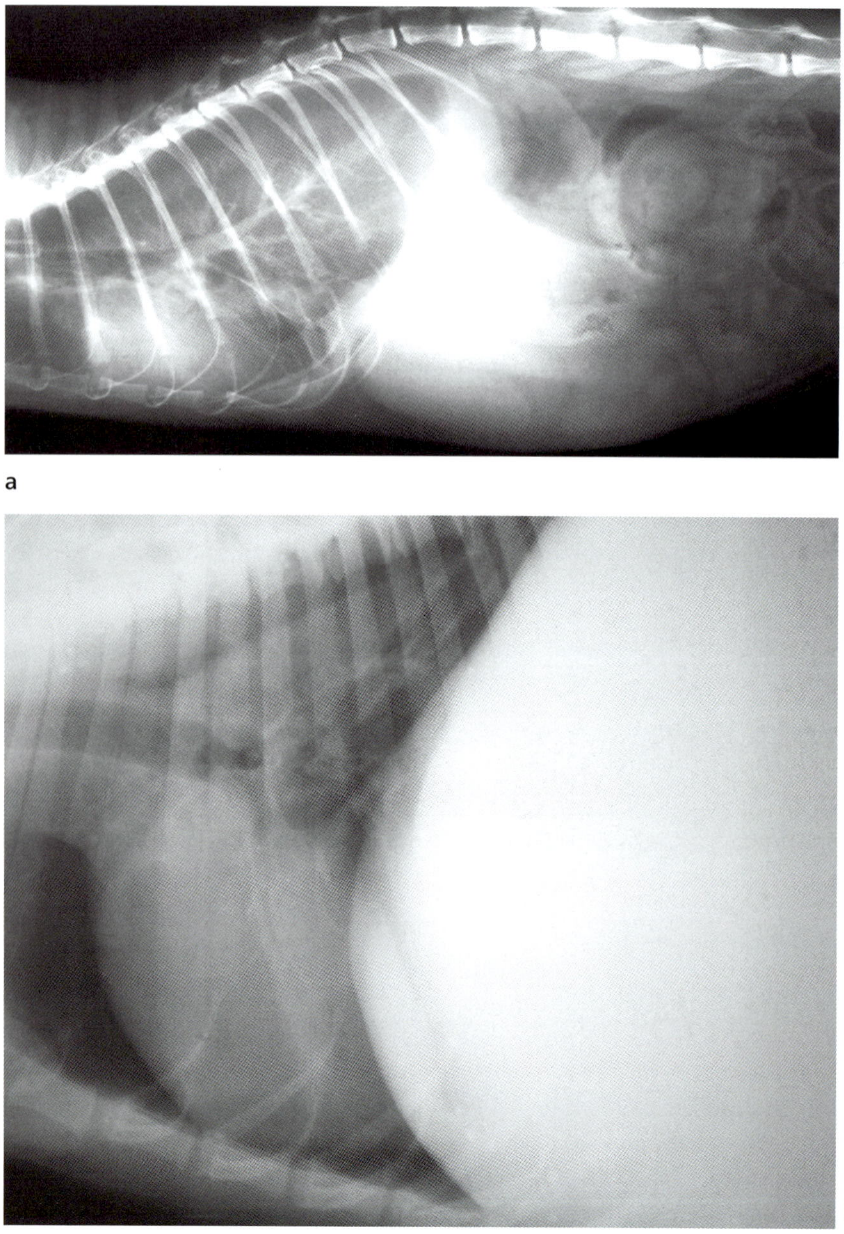

a

b

Fig. 11.8 Examples of displacement of the diaphragm due to increased filling of the thoracic and abdominal cavity, respectively.

a Caudal displacement of the diaphragm and cranial abdominal viscera in a cat with unilateral pyothorax.

b Cranial displacement of the diaphragm in a dog with severe ascites.

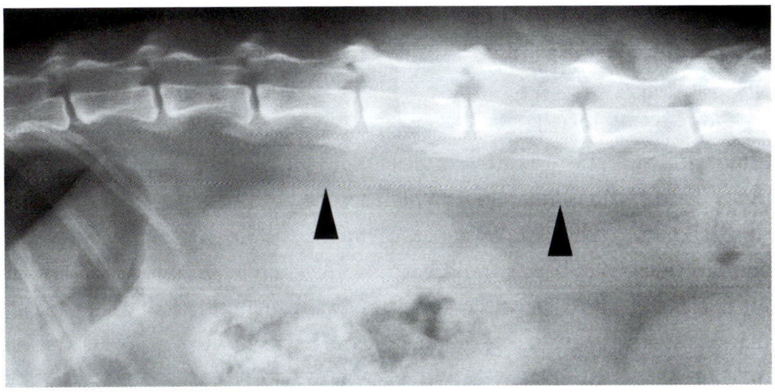

Fig. 11.9 Radiographic appearance of the lumbar musculature in an 18-year-old cat. The psoas minor muscle in cats originates from the last two thoracic vertebrae and projects as a triangular soft-tissue opacity in the caudodorsal thorax. On abdominal radiographs, the well-developed muscles are visible as a prominent soft-tissue opacity (arrowheads) superimposed with and ventral to the mid-lumbar spine.

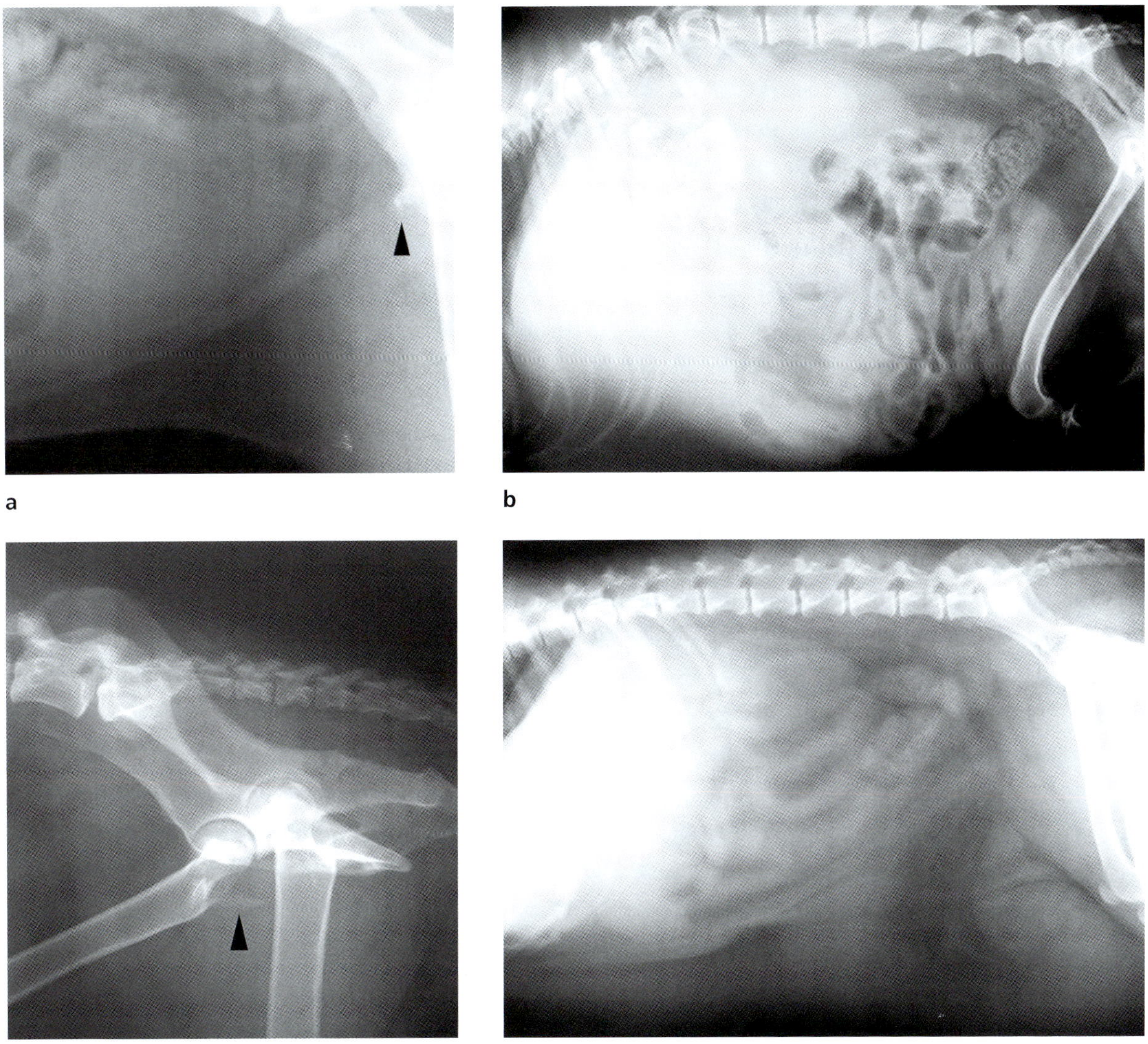

a b c d

Fig. 11.10

a Normal caudal abdominal wall musculature in a domestic cat. The insertion site of the rectus abdominis muscle on the pecten of the pubis is indicated by the arrowhead. Subfascial fat planes are indistinctly visible.

b Potbelly and hepatomegaly in a dog with Cushing's disease.

c Abdominal wall rupture and swelling with avulsion fracture of the pubis (arrowhead) in a dog following a road traffic accident.

d Inguinal hernia in a Beagle. The urinary bladder is not visible in its normal location and is displaced into the inguinal hernia sac outside the abdominal wall along with other abdominal organs.

11.2 Radiographic technique, positioning and interpretation

It is especially important for abdominal radiographs that the patient is fasted for at least 12 hours prior to the procedure if possible. For full evaluation of the urinary tract an enema may be necessary, as the colon is often superimposed with the kidneys and ureters. The hair coat should be clean and dry, especially in long-haired patients, and the patient should be brushed, as dirty or wet hair is clearly visible on a radiograph and may lead to misdiagnosis. If an abdominal ultrasound is planned, this should be performed after the radiographic examination if possible, as the contact gel causes streak artefacts.

11.2.1 Technique

For **adequate exposure,** abdominal diameter should be measured accurately at its greatest point, commonly at the level of the last pair of ribs. If there is any doubt, higher exposure parameters are given preference as overexposed radiographs are usually still diagnostic (digital radiography) or can be evaluated further using a hot lamp (conventional radiography), while underexposed radiographs are of limited or nondiagnostic quality. As there is often a marked difference in diameter between the cranial and caudal abdomen in large thin dogs, two separate acquisitions with different exposures may be necessary. Patient thickness above 10 cm requires use of a grid.

Abdominal radiographs should be taken during the **expiratory pause** in respiration. Exposure time should be kept as short as possible to minimize the risk of motion artefacts. Modern X-ray equipment automatically chooses the shortest possible exposure time to achieve the desired mAs product (**radiation quantity**). However, the investigator should be aware that a change in radiation quantity overall will affect exposure time.

The selection of **beam quality** (**energy**; kVp value) and quantity is based on established technique charts (see Chapter 2) which can be modified if needed. To optimize exposure parameters for abdominal radiographs, an attempt should be made to keep beam energy as low as possible and compensate with an increase in photon quantity. This is explained by the physical principles of radiation absorption as follows.

- A high-energy X-ray beam (i.e. high kVp value) will penetrate equally through different tissues resulting in low image contrast between abdominal soft tissues and fat.
- Increased absorption in some tissues compared to others and thus only partial transmission of the X-ray beam (i.e. low kVp value and decreased beam energy) increases image contrast.

A low-energy X-ray beam improves image contrast on abdominal radiographs: 'High kV X-ray makes the image grey.'

Following these basic principles, exposure parameters can be modified to adapt to specific situations (Fig. 11.11). To change contrast or exposure time with maintained overall exposure, one can follow the rule of thumb that an increase in beam energy by 10–15% corresponds to doubling the beam quantity.

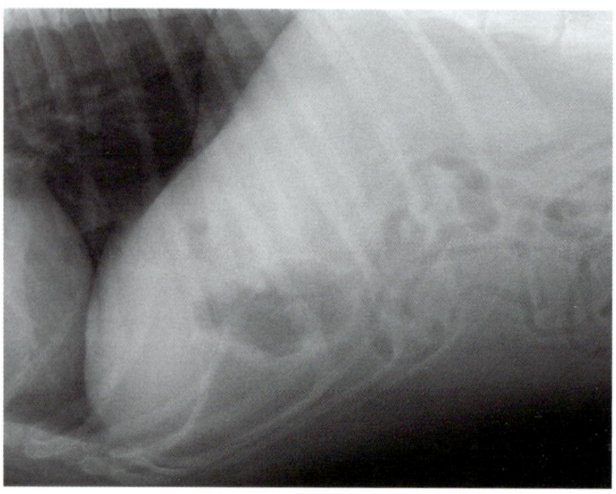

a

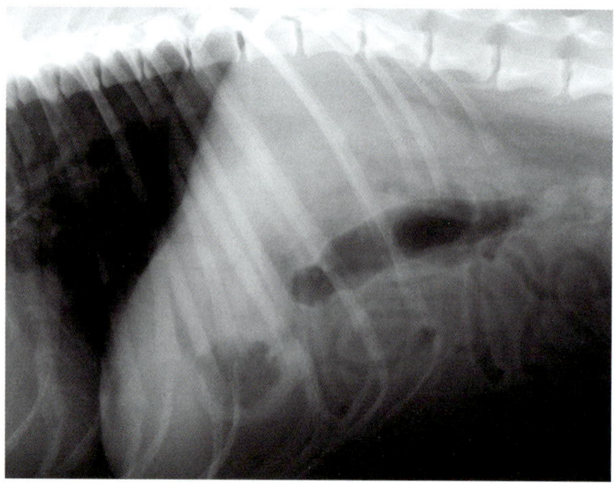

b

Fig. 11.11

a Cranial abdomen in a 2-year-old panting Boxer. To minimize motion artefacts, exposure time was kept low (5 mAs) and compensated for by increased beam energy (74 kVp). The result is a sharp but low contrast image. The kidneys are hardly visible. If rapid respiratory motion is unavoidable, this may be the best option.

b A repeat radiograph with 60 kVp and 20 mAs at normal respiration shows markedly improved image contrast. The right kidney is clearly visible.

11.2.2 Positioning

Standard projections for abdominal radiographs include lateral and ventrodorsal views. Dorsoventral views are of limited use, as the abdomen is not fully extended and the abdominal organs are compressed and displaced. Additionally, dorsal body parts are often indistinct due to the high object–film distance.

A choice of right versus left lateral recumbency is less critical; however, the examiner has to be aware of differences in abdominal organ position between these projections (see Table 11.1). Right lateral views are slightly advantageous for evaluation of the kidneys and spleen, while left lateral projections facilitate better evaluation of the pylorus and duodenum. Opposite lateral views are often helpful for complete abdominal evaluation.

As always, animals should be positioned as straight as possible for the radiographic examination. Radiographic indicators of oblique positioning in both projections are listed in Table 11.2. Positioning of **cats** is often challenging due to their natural resistance to any manipulation, especially once their initial tolerance threshold has been passed. Planning and preparation to complete the radiographic examination in the shortest possible time, possibly with the aid of instrumentation or medication (sedation), is advisable.

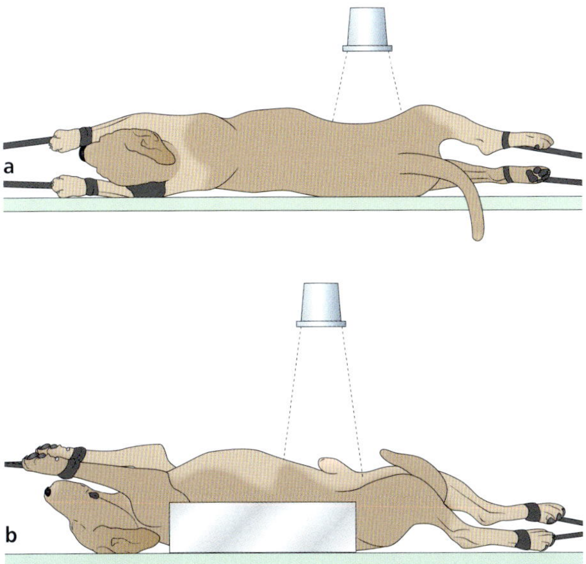

Fig. 11.12 Positioning of a dog for a lateral a and a ventrodorsal view using a fixation trough b. Depending on regional radiation safety regulations, patients can be positioned manually or using fixation devices.

> If gastric dilatation and volvulus is suspected, the lateral view should be obtained in right lateral recumbency, as dorsal displacement and dilatation of the pyloric antrum with compartmentalization of the ventral gastric fundus is best seen in this projection (see section 13.4.2)

Standard lateral views

The patient should be positioned with the legs extended (Fig. 11.12a). In deep-chested dogs, a foam wedge placed under the sternum is helpful to achieve straight positioning. This is not recommended in barrel-chested dogs, as these have a tendency to roll into a dorsal position anyway. The head and neck should be placed in a natural position without rotation. The beam collimation should not exceed the coxofemoral joints and xiphoid. In large dogs, several overlapping projections are usually necessary.

Standard ventrodorsal views

The patient is positioned with the legs extended, preferably using a V-trough (Fig. 11.12b). The xiphoid should be palpable on the midline. Alternatively, the hind legs can be angled cranially ('frog position'). This has the advantage that the inguinal folds are less conspicuous on the resultant radiograph. However, the disadvantage is a mild increase in scatter radiation, which is problematic with regard to both image quality and radiation safety considerations. The head and neck should be positioned symmetrically, as obliquity or rotation affects symmetry of the torso. The beam is collimated so it does not extend beyond the xiphoid and coxofemoral joints, and the central beam is aimed at the level of the umbilicus. In very large dogs, two overlapping views may be necessary to cover the entire abdomen.

Table 11.2 Radiographic indicators of oblique positioning on abdominal radiographs.

Ventrodorsal view	Lateral view
Laterally tilted spinous processes Incomplete superimposition of sternum and spine Asymmetric thorax	Incomplete superimposition of contralateral rib heads and bodies in dorsoventral (DV) direction Incomplete superimposition of lumbar transverse processes Incomplete superimposition of coxofemoral joints in DV direction

Modified from Love and Berry (2002).

Oblique projections

These are only used in select cases, for example when a peripheral foreign body (such as a fishing hook) has to be definitively localized within the gastric wall or peritoneal cavity.

Horizontal beam views

These are helpful for a diagnosis of free abdominal gas. The patient is positioned in left lateral recumbency, and a ventrodorsal projection is obtained (Fig. 11.13). If large animal radiographic equipment is available, standing lateral views may be considered in very large dogs (Great Dane, Irish Wolfhound) to protect both the animal and personnel during patient positioning. However, gravitational shift of organs and resultant alterations in radiographic anatomy have to be taken into consideration. For all horizontal beam views, specific radiation safety guidelines apply to ensure that the radiation dose to examiners is within acceptable limits.

'Catogram'

In general it is suboptimal to obtain whole body radiographs in small animals, as optimized imaging of different body regions requires adjustment of exposure parameters. However, the values for thoracic and abdominal radiographs are similar in cats, and whole body radiographs may be advantageous under the following circumstances:

- availability of a large cassette
- uncooperative patient with limited tolerance for repeat radiographs
- primary abdominal or systemic clinical indication (Fig. 11.14).

If the patient is evaluated primarily for respiratory disease, a 'catogram' is not advised as scatter radiation will negatively affect the ability to evaluate lung detail, and the higher beam energy used for thoracic radiographs will result in decreased abdominal contrast.

Compression radiographs

These techniques utilize radiolucent aids (wooden spoon, compression band, Plexiglas spatula) to separate superimposed abdominal organs, decrease patient diameter in large dogs, or increase back pressure from the urinary collecting system (Table 11.3). However, there is a marked risk of rupture of distended thin-walled structures such as an enlarged uterus (pyometra) or splenic and hepatic tumours, with potentially catastrophic outcome. This technique is also contraindicated if a diaphragmatic hernia is suspected.

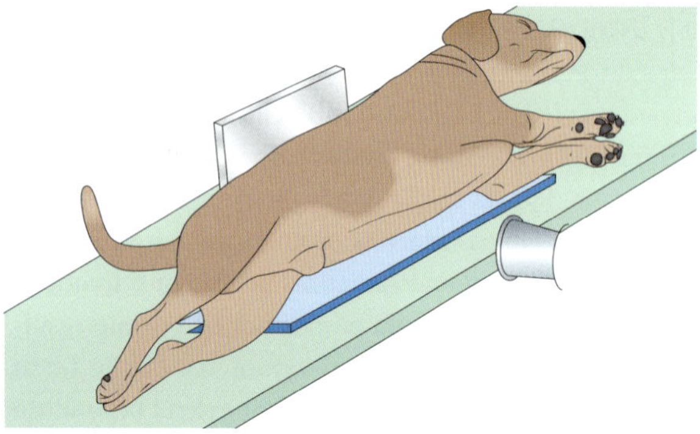

Fig. 11.13 Positioning of a dog in left lateral recumbency for a horizontal beam ventrodorsal view to demonstrate free abdominal gas.

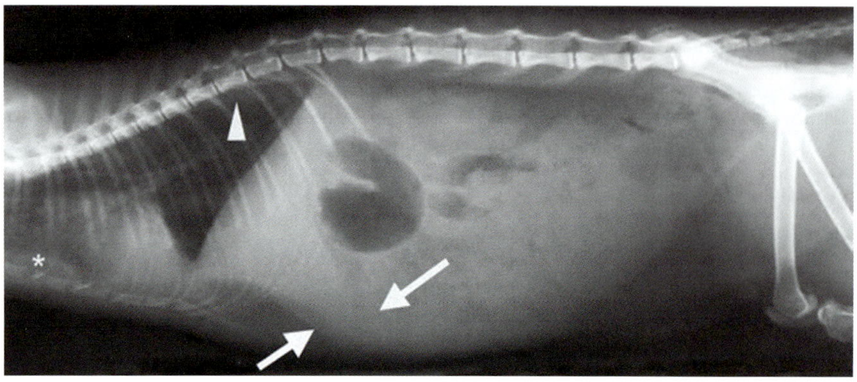

Fig. 11.14 Lateral whole body radiograph ('catogram') of a 2-year-old domestic cat presented for abdominal distention. Hepatomegaly (arrows) and an irregular loss of abdominal serosal margin detail are noted. Increasing the size of the collimated field to include the thorax allows concurrent diagnosis of unilateral pleural effusion (retraction of one caudodorsal lung lobe, arrowhead) and an enlarged sternal lymph node (*). These bicavitary changes in a young cat allow a presumptive imaging diagnosis of feline infectious peritonitis (confirmed).

Table 11.3 Examples of possible applications of abdominal compression radiography.

Potential use	Disadvantage
Differentiate ventral liver and spleen on lateral view	Often more easily accomplished with contralateral view Notable risk of rupture and (fatal) haemorrhage in case of hepatic or splenic tumour!
Evaluate equivocal small intestinal abnormality (foreign body, mass, superimposition)	Often more easily accomplished with contralateral view
Identify uroliths (kidney, ureter, urinary bladder) in case of superimposition of intestine	Displacement of overlying intestine often insufficient
Maximize filling of renal pelvis during excretory urography	Dilatation of renal pelvis secondary to compression difficult to distinguish from pathological processes
Improve radiographic image contrast in overweight large-breed dogs (e.g. Rottweilers)	Compressive band needs to be available
Distinguish an enlarged uterus from overlying intestinal segments	Notable risk of uterine perforation!

Modified from Armbrust et al. (2000b).

Table 11.4 Abdomen specific applications of basic radiation safety principles.

Basic radiation safety principles for personnel holding patients	Abdominal application
All body parts outside primary beam	Hold hind legs at level of tarsus
Adequate radiation safety clothing	Wear protective gown and gloves
Maximize distance	Patient positioning with two examiners (one at each end of the table) significantly reduces radiation dose compared to a single examiner
Minimal exposure time	Focus on minimizing unnecessary repeat radiographs; possibly consider 'catograms'
Smallest possible collimation	Use xiphoid and coxofemoral joints as markers

Modified from Hartung and Tellhelm (2000).

Radiation safety considerations

Basic principles of applied radiation safety are covered in Chapter 4. Specific considerations for abdominal radiography are listed in Table 11.4. The presence of personnel within the X-ray room during the radiographic procedure should generally be minimized. If manual positioning of the patient necessitates the presence of examiners within the room, the radiation dose can be significantly decreased by positioning one examiner at the patient's head and a second one at the feet rather than having a single individual position the animal.

11.2.3 Abdominal image contrast

Image contrast is defined as the scale of grey shades on a radiograph. A low-contrast image is characterized by numerous subtle shades of grey, resulting in a fairly homogeneous appearance of the entire image (see Fig. 11.11a). A high-contrast image has comparatively fewer shades of grey, and structures tend to appear black or white (see Fig. 11.11b). The terms **low contrast** and **high contrast** are often erroneously used to refer to the opposite meaning, which can be very confusing. Image contrast depends on technical factors as well as on physical absorption differences (**object contrast**). Only objects that differ in radiation absorption can be distinguished as lighter or darker structures on a radiograph.

The abdomen mostly consists of soft-tissue opaque organs and surrounding peritoneal and retroperitoneal fat (including the retrosternal fat pad contained within the falciform ligament). Even though these can be distinguished based on their radiographic opacity, the difference is subtle due to their comparable physical density and effective atomic numbers (Table 11.5).

The abdominal exposure technique aims at maximizing the low object contrast between fat and soft tissues by

Table 11.5 Physical absorption parameters of different substances.

Substance	Physical density (g/cm3)	Effective atomic number
Air	0.001	7.64
Fat	0.910	5.92
Water	1.000	7.42
Musculature	1.040	7.60
Bone	1.850	13.80
Lead	11.000	82.00

Expanded from Curry et al. (1990).

minimizing beam energy (see section 11.2.1). The lower the amount of intra-abdominal fat, the less likely the success of this strategy.

Fat located above or below organs rather than in between does not contribute to object contrast. Thus, extensive subcutaneous fat deposits in large-breed dogs only increase overall object thickness, which requires an increase in beam energy for sufficient penetration and results in marked loss of contrast (Schwarz et al. 2000b). This explains the often poor image quality in obese Rottweilers, for example. On the other hand, image contrast in fat cats is often good due to their overall size.

More fat does not always improve image contrast.

11.2.4 Basic principles of contrast procedures

Radiographic contrast studies improve insufficient object contrast by administering substances with increased (**positive contrast media**) or decreased (**negative contrast media**) opacity into hollow organs (viscera, vessels) or between soft-tissue organs. Positive contrast media used for abdominal imaging include iodine solutions and barium sulphate suspensions; air and carbon dioxide are used as negative contrast media (Fig. 11.15).

Among other factors, the degree of contrast depends on the organ specific contrast medium concentration. **Iodinated contrast media** progressively accumulate within the kidneys following intravenous administration, while they become increasingly dilute in the intestinal tract following oral application, due to their high osmolarity and the subsequent intraluminal accumulation of fluid. Several different ionic and nonionic iodinated contrast agents are available. The latter have a lower osmolarity; however, they are still hypertonic in most cases.

Osmolarity, pharmacological neutrality and resorption are important considerations for compatibility and thus applicability of contrast media. The applications of common abdominal contrast agents are summarized in Table 11.6.

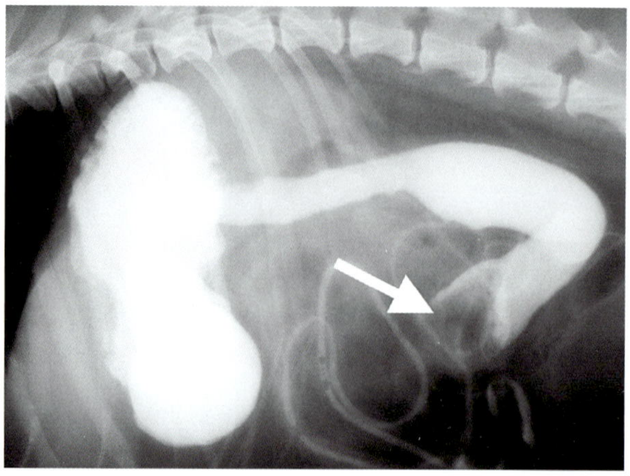

a

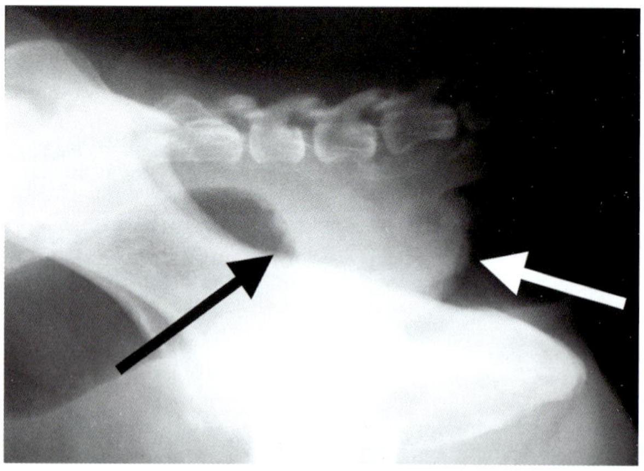

b

Fig. 11.15

a Upper gastrointestinal contrast study using iodinated contrast medium in a dog. There is only moderate mucosal detail, but the study is diagnostic for a duodenal foreign body (arrow).

b Injection of air into the large intestine in a dog (pneumocolon) outlines an intestinal tumour (arrows) felt on rectal examination.

For so-called **double contrast studies,** positive and negative contrast agents are combined to provide maximum detail of small structures (mucosal folds, ureteral openings) without superimposition. These techniques are slightly more demanding, but have proven advantageous in imaging of the stomach, large intestine and urinary bladder. Radiographic contrast studies of the different organ systems are discussed in more detail in Chapters 13 and 14.

Survey radiographs are necessary prior to any contrast study.

Table 11.6 Applications of contrast media in abdominal radiography.

Contrast medium	Application	Advantage	Disadvantage
Positive contrast media			
Barium sulphate suspension	Gastrography Upper GI contrast study Large intestine barium enema (often as double contrast study)	Neutral taste Isotonic Nonreactive Not resorbable Therapeutic effects with gastrointestinal tract irritation High contrast Cheap	Not resorbable (perforation, aspiration) High contrast (may mask lesions)
Organic iodinated contrast media (ionic or nonionic)	Upper GI contrast study	Resorbable (can be used in cases of suspected perforation)	Bitter Hypertonic (dilutes intestinal content, dehydrates) Resorbable (escapes intestine) Nonionic: very expensive Ionic: relatively expensive
	Angiography Excretory urography	Only contrast media available for intravenous applications	Hypertonic and thus dehydrating (especially ionic contrast agents)
	Peritoneogram Fistulogram Cystography (often as double contrast study) Vaginography	Only contrast media available	
Negative contrast media			
Air	Gastrography Pneumocolon Cystography	Cheap Easy application	Small risk of (fatal) vascular air embolism Poor contrast with mucosa
CO_2	Gastrography Capnocolon Cystography	Cheap (increasingly available in atmosphere!) Easy application No risk of air embolism	Poor contrast with mucosa

Expanded from Hartung and Tellhelm (2000).
Note: GI = gastrointestinal.

11.2.5 Approach and interpretation

For radiographic evaluation of the abdomen, at least two orthogonal projections are typically required. Additional views may be helpful in case of specific clinical questions (see section 11.2.2). Each abdominal structure should be assessed on both views before moving on to the next, allowing spatial localization of the object. A reliable diagnosis can only be achieved following a systematic and logical diagnostic algorithm. Individual organs are evaluated according to **Roentgen signs** (number, opacity, localization and position, margination and contour, size, shape; see also Chapter 1).

Systematic evaluation of abdominal radiographs

1. Technical assessment.
2. Evaluation of extra-abdominal structures.
   - Thorax
   - Pelvis
   - Hind limbs
   - Back
   - Skin and fur coat
3. Evaluation of the abdomen as a whole.
   - Image contrast
   - Abdominal circumference
   - Bone density
4. Evaluation of abdominal organs normally visible.
5. Are any organs visible that are normally not seen?
6. Assessment of lesions of undetermined origin.
7. Listing of findings.
8. Weighted listing of differential diagnoses.
   - Assessment of probability considering other findings.
   - Listing in order of decreasing probability.
   - Limit list to three to five likely diseases or provide a generalized statement in case of a nonspecific diagnosis. Compiling a long list of differential diagnoses is counterproductive.
9. Decide if further examinations are necessary, and if yes, which ones.

11.3 Interpretation of changes in abdominal image contrast

Radiographic image contrast is affected by numerous technical, patient specific and disease related factors. When assessing abdominal radiographs with unusually high or low image contrast, location and texture of the changes have to be taken into consideration to determine the most likely underlying cause (Table 11.7).

11.3.1 Peritoneal and retroperitoneal loss of detail

Young animals

Young animals have insufficient deposits of intra-abdominal white fat to provide adequate organ contrast. Even though an increased amount of brown fat is present, it is located mostly in an extra-abdominal position and is similar to soft tissue in its radiation absorption properties. Additionally, a small amount of abdominal effusion is physiological in puppies. Radiographic evaluation may be unrewarding for these reasons (Fig. 11.16a).

Cachexia

Similarly, poor abdominal image contrast is found in adult animals with complete loss of abdominal fat reserves. Additional findings of a tucked-up ventral abdominal wall and the inability to visualize the kidneys due to loss of retroperitoneal fat are helpful criteria in distinguishing cachexia from other causes of decreased abdominal image contrast (Fig. 11.16b).

Effusion

Transudate, exudate, purulent liquid leaking from ruptured hollow viscera, urine, bile, uncoagulated blood and lymphatic fluid can accumulate within the abdominal cavity and completely obliterate normal abdominal image contrast due to extensive spread.

The degree of loss of abdominal image contrast depends partially on the amount of intra-abdominal fat. A small amount of effusion in obese animals results in a rather irregular loss of detail.

A radiographic distinction between different types of effusion is not possible. However, location of the effusion within the peritoneal or retroperitoneal space is helpful in ranking differential diagnoses for type and origin of the fluid (Thrall 1992) (Fig. 11.16c, d). Fluid accumulation in both compartments is relatively rare.

Abdominal effusion can usually be differentiated from abdominal space-occupying lesions and lack of abdominal fat. With effusion, air-filled small intestinal segments typically float within the central abdomen (highest point, no organ displacement). With peritoneal effusion, the kidneys are often still visible and the animals have a potbelly, which is in contrast to patients with cachexia.

11.3.2 Loss of contrast due to space-occupying lesions

The more space in the abdomen that is occupied by a **homogeneous soft-tissue mass**, the less organ contrast remains between the mass and adjacent compressed and displaced soft tissues. If the abdomen is homogeneously poor in contrast, an underlying mass has to be considered as a possible differential diagnosis. If the mass is large enough and results in displacement of air-filled viscera, it can be characterized based on the direction of organ displacement (Fig. 11.17a; see also section 11.4).

Lipomatous masses (lipoma, infiltrative lipoma, liposarcoma) have a special status, as they provide good object contrast. These masses can be recognized based on organ displacement without a visible soft-tissue opacity space-occupying lesion (Fig. 11.17b, c).

Table 11.7 Criteria for evaluation of abdominal image contrast on radiographs.

Factor	Image contrast	Localization	Texture
Marked over- or underexposure	Low	Generalized	Homogeneous
High kVp	Low	Generalized	Homogeneous
Large patient diameter	Low	Generalized	Homogeneous
Young animal without fat reserves	Low	Generalized	Homogeneous
Cachexia	Low	Generalized	Homogeneous
Large volume peritoneal effusion	Low	Peritoneal; kidneys often still visible	Homogeneous
Mild peritoneal effusion in obese patient	Low	Regional – generalized	Mildly heterogeneous
Retroperitoneal effusion	Low	Kidneys not visible; normal peritoneal space	Homogeneous or streaky
Space-occupying soft-tissue mass	Low	Peritoneal or retroperitoneal	Homogeneous with organ displacement
Space-occupying lipoma or liposarcoma	High	Peritoneal or retroperitoneal	Homogeneous with organ displacement
Peritonitis and carcinomatosis	Low	Peritoneal or retroperitoneal, initially regional	Heterogeneous
Steatitis and fat necrosis	Low	Generalized; not limited to abdomen	Heterogeneous; in cats often mineralized
Visceral rupture with small volume free peritoneal gas accumulation	Low	Peritoneal	Heterogeneous with gas bubbles
Post laparotomy, pregnancy, puerperium	Low	Peritoneal	Homogeneous or irregular
Pneumoperitoneum	High	Peritoneal	Homogeneous
Pneumoretroperitoneum	High	Retroperitoneal	Homogeneous
Skin diseases, subcutaneous emphysema	Low	Generalized; not limited to abdomen	Heterogeneous
Wet or dirty hair coat	Low	Generalized; not limited to abdomen	Streaky

11.3.3 Irregular loss of (retro)peritoneal contrast

Peritonitis

Peritoneal inflammation may result from rupture of abdominal hollow viscera, abscesses, perforating abdominal wounds, leakage from gastric or intestinal fistulas, complications following laparotomy, or specific diseases such as feline infectious peritonitis (FIP).

Peritonitis results in very heterogeneous peritoneal loss of serosal margin detail, which differs significantly from most homogeneous effusions. Tributary lymph nodes including sternal lymph nodes are often enlarged (see Fig. 11.14).

Carcinomatosis

Peritoneal spread of tumour metastases is a common complication of intestinal, pancreatic, ovarian and prostatic carcinomas, and manifests as irregular loss of detail in the peritoneal and/or retroperitoneal space. In the initial stages the loss of contrast is often focal, serving as an indicator of lesion origin (Fig. 11.18a).

Pancreatitis

In advanced stages, pancreatitis results in a combination of inflammation, necrosis and saponification of peripancreatic fat due to enzymatic tissue damage (Fig. 11.18b).

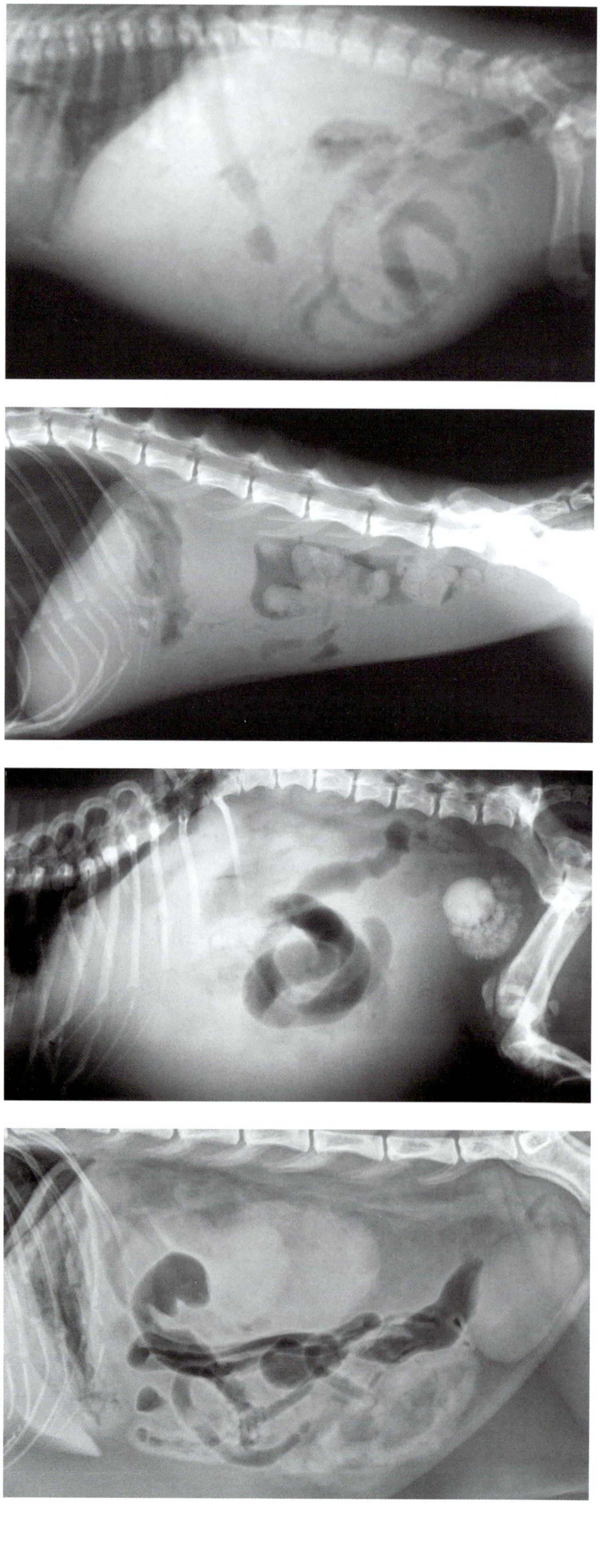

a

b

c

d

Fig. 11.16

a Normal abdomen in an 8-year-old West Highland White Terrier with a pendulous abdomen and very poor serosal margin detail. Young animals physiologically have insufficient deposits of white fat and an increased amount of peritoneal fluid. A radiographic examination is often unrewarding in the evaluation of abdominal disorders.

b Cachexia in a domestic cat characterized by generalized homogeneous loss of detail and inability to distinguish any abdominal organs, including the kidneys. The ventral abdominal wall is tucked up.

c Lateral radiograph of a dog with peritoneal effusion and bladder calculi. Gas-filled intestinal segments are floating at the highest point (central abdomen) and are not displaced by a mass. The kidneys are visible as the retroperitoneal space is not affected.

d Retroperitoneal loss of detail secondary to neoplastic renal infiltration (carcinoma) in a cat. There is irregular streaky loss of contrast dorsal and caudal to the kidneys, while the peritoneal organs are well contrasted.

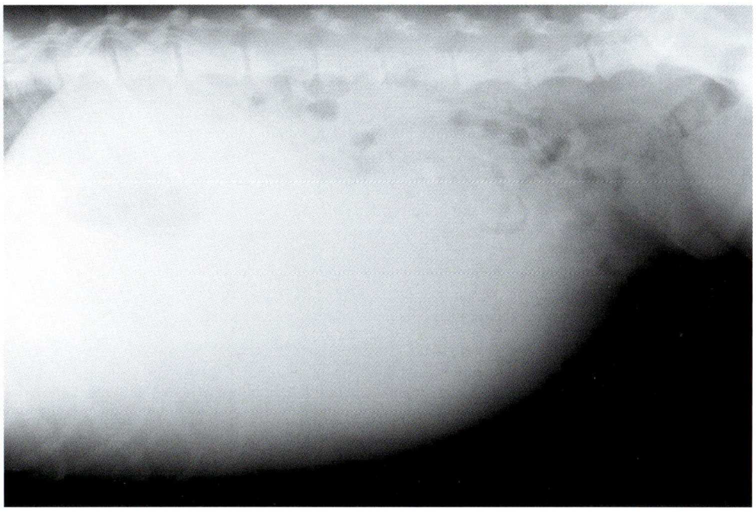

a

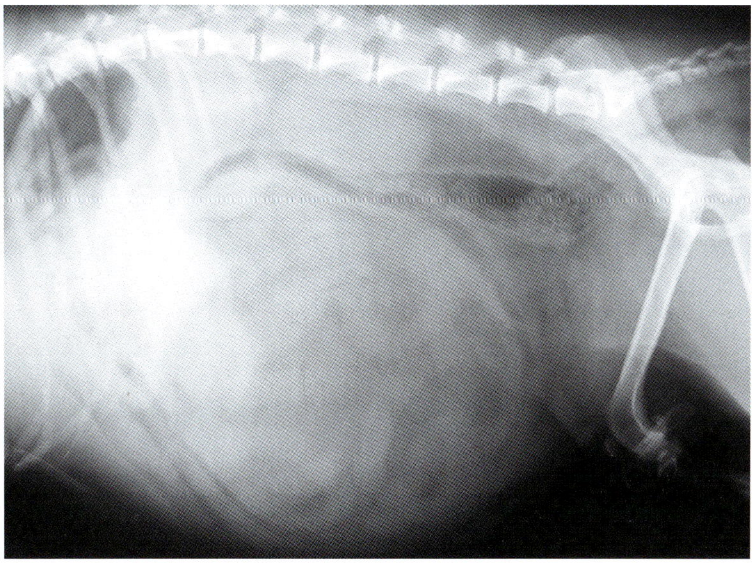

b

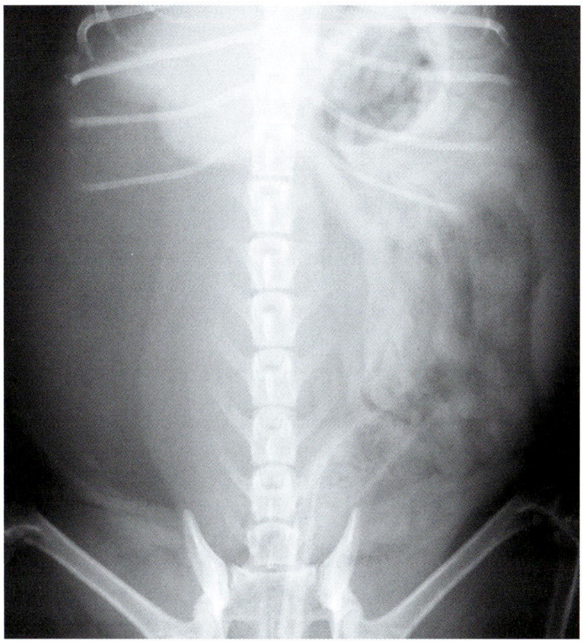

c

Fig. 11.17

a Homogeneous loss of peritoneal detail in an 8-year-old Labrador Retriever with dorsal and caudal displacement of gas-filled intestinal segments. This finding indicates a ventral or cranial mass. (Exploratory laparotomy found a cystic abdominal wall tumour without evidence of effusion.)

b Lateral view of a distended canine abdomen with peripheral organ displacement (intestines, kidneys) despite excellent soft-tissue contrast.

c The ventrodorsal view reveals the solution to the puzzle. Abdominal viscera are displaced by a fat opaque mass occupying the entire right abdominal cavity (peritoneal lipoma).

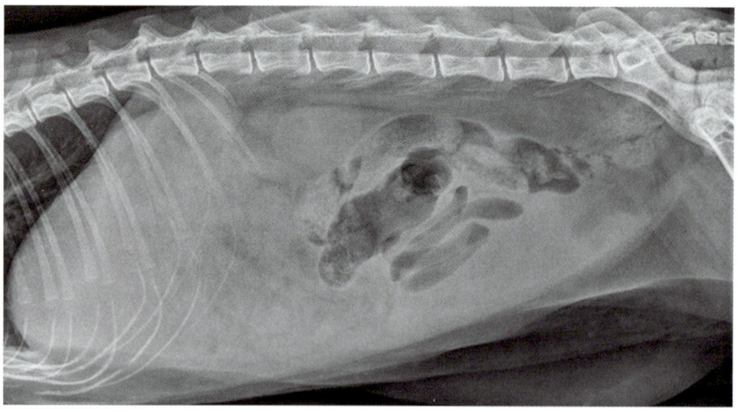

a

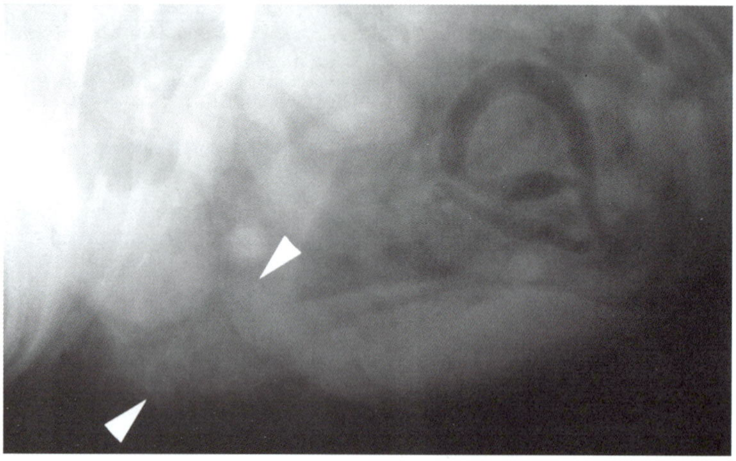

b

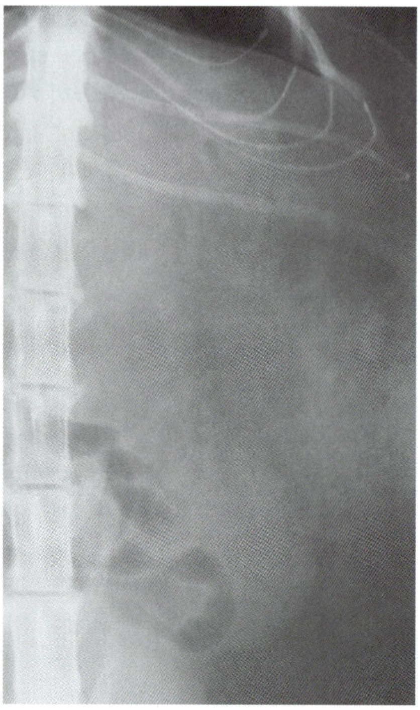

c

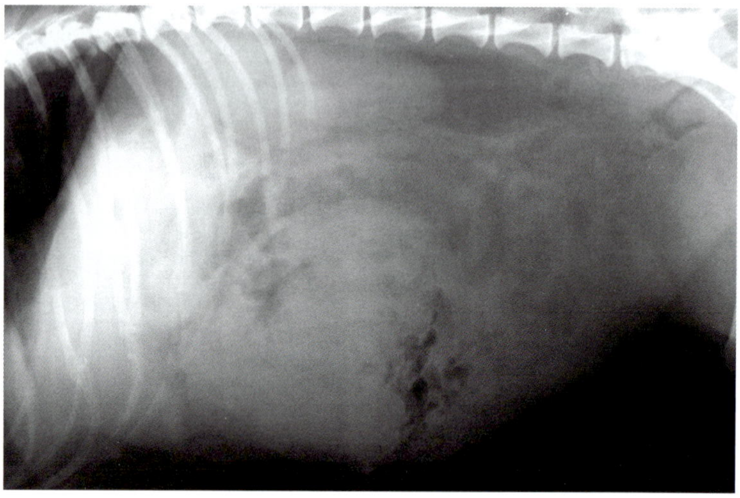

d

Fig. 11.18

a Extensive heterogeneous loss of detail in the cranioventral abdomen of a 10-year-old cat with pancreatic carcinoma. Fine-needle aspiration cytology yielded a diagnosis of carcinomatosis.

b Focal regional irregular lack of detail (arrowheads) in the cranioventral abdomen of a dog with pancreatitis.

c Ventrodorsal view of the left cranial abdomen in a 12-year-old domestic shorthair cat with steatitis. There is heterogeneous loss of intra-abdominal detail. Inflammation and necrosis of fat due to malnutrition often results in heterogeneous loss of contrast outside the abdominal cavity as well; however, this is not seen in this case.

d Rupture of a duodenal tumour with abscessation in a 5-year-old dog. There is caudal displacement of abdominal viscera and irregular loss of detail with free abdominal gas.

Other types of fat necrosis and inflammation (steatitis, pansteatitis)

These have been reported in cats fed an exclusive fish diet in the past but are very rare today (Komori et al. 2002, Root 1971). Systemic steatitis differs from peritonitis radiographically, as heterogeneous loss of detail is also present outside the abdominal cavity (Fig. 11.18c). Idiopathic nodular fat necrosis is occasionally seen in dogs and cats, and eggshell-like calcification of these lesions is common in cats (see section 11.3.6 and Fig. 11.20a). These are an incidental finding without clinical significance (Schwarz et al. 2000a).

Rupture of the gastrointestinal tract

Gastrointestinal tract rupture is always associated with peritonitis. Admixture of air with ingesta results in a mottled appearance (Fig. 11.18d). Peritoneal gas accumulations are best seen between the liver and dorsal diaphragmatic crura on a lateral view (see section 11.3.5).

Special situations

Mild homogeneous or heterogeneous peritoneal loss of detail is often seen following **laparotomy**, during **pregnancy** and during **puerperium**. If changes are mild, it is not possible to distinguish physiological from pathological processes, and a radiographic examination is often unrewarding.

11.3.4 Extra-abdominal changes with loss of contrast

Skin diseases, subcutaneous **emphysema** and a **wet or dirty hair coat** result in mild irregular loss of abdominal image contrast, which should not be confused with intra-abdominal diseases. It is key to recognize that these abnormalities extend beyond the boundaries of the abdominal cavity.

11.3.5 Abdominal accumulations of gas

Intra-abdominal gas increases abdominal contrast due to its low radiographic opacity, and abdominal viscera are often more easily visible. Possible reasons for free abdominal gas and their significance are listed in Table 11.8. To

Table 11.8 Differential diagnoses for intra-abdominal gas accumulations.

Localization	Appearance	Meaning
Parenchymal		
Liver, spleen, prostate, uterus	Disseminated gas bubbles Branching in ductal structures	Liver or splenic torsion Abscess Cholangiohepatitis Prostatic disease Fetal death (fetal vessels)
Gastric and intestinal wall	Linear gas opacities	Pneumatosis in wall necrosis, injury, sepsis, infarcts and others Not prognostic!
Urinary and gallbladder wall	Irregular gas bubbles	Infection Often concurrent diabetes mellitus
Peritoneal		
Between diaphragm and liver, wide-ranging gas bubbles	Dorsal diaphragmatic and hepatic silhouette can be differentiated Irregular gas bubbles Linear gas interface with horizontal beam views	Traumatic abdominal wall or visceral rupture Diaphragmatic hernia with pneumothorax Perforating foreign body Ruptured ulcer or tumour Following laparotomy Leakage from percutaneous gastric tube
Retroperitoneal		
Gas within retroperitoneal space	Kidneys and other retroperitoneal organs easily seen Often free gas in thorax (mediastinum)	Gas diffusion through aortic hiatus with pneumomediastinum (harmless) Abdominal wall rupture Visceral rupture

Expanded from Fischetti et al. (2004) and Morris (1992).

demonstrate a small amount of free abdominal gas, a horizontal beam ventrodorsal view in left lateral recumbency is recommended (see section 11.2.2 and Fig. 11.13).

> The presence of free abdominal gas requires immediate and thorough workup as this may indicate a life-threatening situation!

Gas accumulations within organ parenchyma

These can result from infection with gas-producing bacteria with or without abscess formation, torsion or necrosis, and often require surgical intervention (Fig. 11.19a). Gas accumulation within the wall of hollow viscera can result from ulcers, necrosis, infection and other causes (Fig. 11.19b). Intramural gas cannot be used as a prognostic indicator in cases of gastric dilatation and volvulus. Emphysematous cholecystitis and cystitis require medical management.

Pneumoperitoneum

Free gas within the peritoneal cavity is a surgical emergency if it cannot be readily explained (Fig. 11.19c). A complete resorption of air following laparotomy can take up to four weeks (Fig. 11.19d).

A diaphragmatic rupture alone cannot cause a pneumoperitoneum, as the pleural space does not physiologically contain air. However, pneumoretroperitoneum is a common consequence of pneumomediastinum (rarely pneumoperitoneum), as the aortic hiatus only has a loose covering of connective tissue and allows transition of air into the abdomen (Fig. 11.19e). A finding of free abdominal gas in this case is of no clinical significance.

11.3.6 Abdominal calcifications

Due to their high radiographic opacity, mineral opaque structures are clearly seen on abdominal radiographs even if image contrast is relatively low. Most mineralized

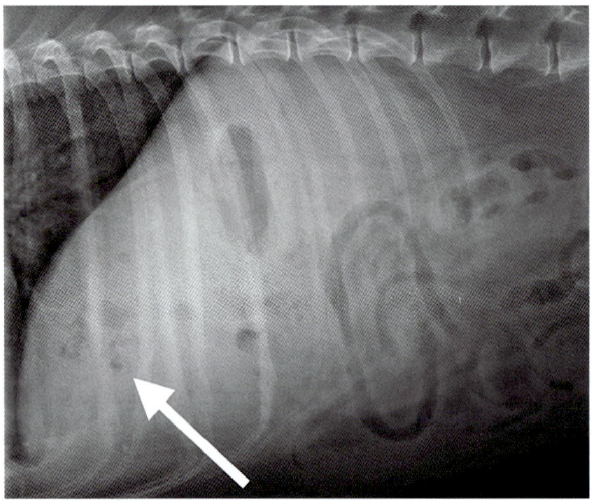

a

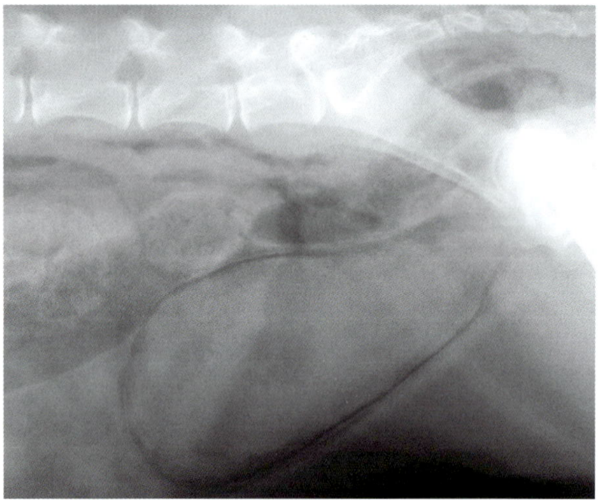

b

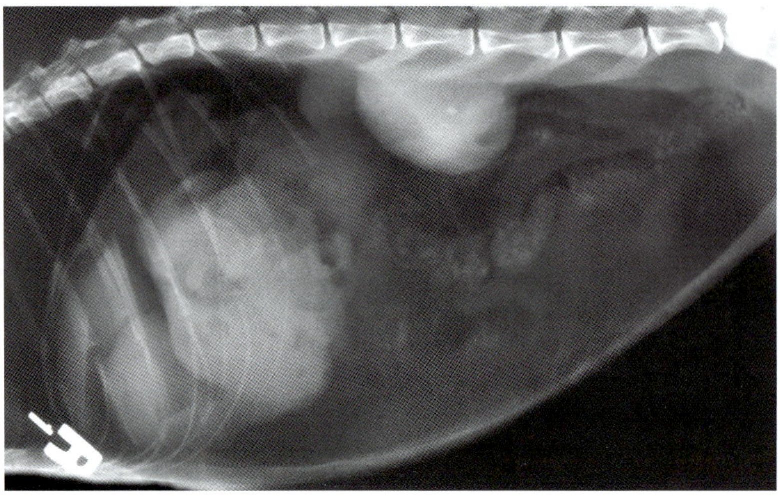

c

Fig. 11.19
a Emphysematous cholecystitis versus hepatic abscess in a dog. Multiple gas opaque bubbles are associated with the liver (arrow).
b Emphysematous cystitis in a female dog. Gas is present within the urinary bladder wall and retroperitoneal space. No reason to panic; however, diabetes mellitus should be ruled out.
c Spontaneous pneumoperitoneum in a 7-year-old cat. If there is no known reason for such gas accumulation, emergency surgery is indicated. The ultimate diagnosis in this patient was a perforating gastric lymphoma (R = right).

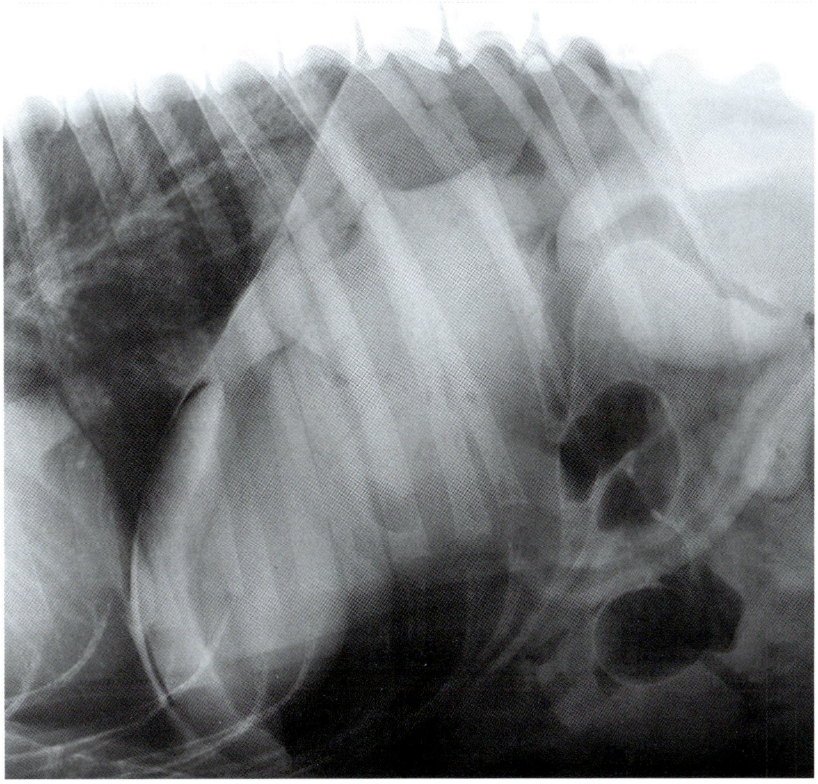

d

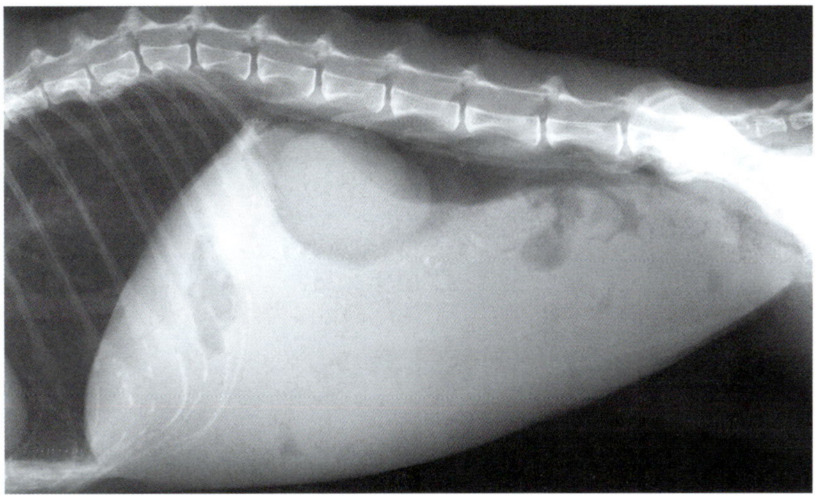

e

Fig. 11.19
d Pneumoperitoneum following laparotomy in a 9-year-old German Shepherd Dog. The diaphragm, liver, gallbladder and kidneys are well visualized due to contrasting air. An assessment of suture patency following surgical closure of hollow viscera can usually not be answered radiographically.
e Pneumoretroperitoneum in a 12-year-old cat. The gas accumulation occurred secondary to a pneumomediastinum (note distinct visibility of the thoracic aorta!) and escape of gas through the aortic hiatus. The finding of gas within the retroperitoneal space is harmless; however, the findings of pneumomediastinum and generalized loss of serosal margin detail in the peritoneal cavity require further workup.

Table 11.9 Position, appearance and meaning of common abdominal calcifications

Localization	Appearance	Meaning
Liver, spleen	Irregularly disseminated	Tumour, abscess, granuloma or haematoma with central necrosis
	Branching in ductal structures (liver)	Chronic cholangiohepatitis
Gallbladder and common bile duct	Rounded intraluminal calculi	Cholelithiasis In common bile duct may be obstructive
	Homogeneous in bladder wall	Chronic cholecystitis Neoplasia ('porcelain bladder')
Gastrointestinal tract	Rugal folds	Chronic renal insufficiency
	Ingesta, disseminated	Part of diet Upper GI contrast study
	Ingesta, local	Foreign bodies Partial obstruction Medication Enterolith
Pancreas	Irregular	Chronic pancreatitis with fat necrosis Tumour Pseudocyst
Kidneys	Bilaterally homogeneous	Nephrocalcinosis
	Focal parenchymal	Chronic infarct, abscess, granuloma or tumour with necrosis
	Renal pelvis, staghorn shape	Urolithiasis
Ureter and urethra	Focal, often rounded	Urolithiasis Separate ossification centre of os penis
Urinary bladder	Focal, often rounded	Urolithiasis
	Focal, irregular	Tumour
	Generalized, irregular	Chronic cystitis
Prostatic gland	Central, often rounded	Urolithiasis
	Generalized irregular	Intact dog: prostatitis, abscess, tumour with necrosis Neutered dog: tumour
	Eggshell-like mass dorsal to urinary bladder	Paraprostatic cysts
Uterus	Normal fetus	From day 38 (cat) /46 (dog) of pregnancy
	Abnormal fetus	Fetal death Mummification
Large vessels	Aortic wall	Chronic renal insufficiency Hypervitaminosis D Hypercalcaemia Hypothyroidism
	Aortic lumen	Calcified thrombus
Lymph nodes	Central, irregular	Feline tuberculosis Tumour Chronic infection Prior resorption of barium
Ovaries	Irregular mineralization in a large mass	Teratoma
Adrenal glands	Irregular	Cat (bilateral): incidental finding Unilateral: cortical or medullary tumour
Peritoneum	Eggshell-like	Fat necrosis (cat)
	Disseminated, irregular	Prior leakage of barium
	Localized within a mass	Tumour, abscess or granuloma with central necrosis
Skin and muscles	Streaky	Calcinosis cutis with Cushing's disease

Modified from Lamb et al. (1991). **Note:** GI = gastrointestinal.

structures seen radiographically contain calcium and are therefore often referred to as calcifications. As these are easily visible, clinicians often wonder about their importance. An overview of the most common intra-abdominal calcifications can be found in Table 11.9.

Dystrophic calcifications occur secondary to necrosis, while **metastatic calcifications** represent deposits in living tissues due to metabolic causes. **Calculi** in bodily fluids (urine, bile), **heterotopic ossification** and **tumoural calcification** are other possible causes of mineralized abdominal lesions.

Idiopathic **nodular fat necrosis** (covered in section 11.3.3) often has an eggshell-like calcification in cats (Fig. 11.20a). This is an incidental radiographic finding and should not be confused with an opaque foreign body.

Adrenal mineralization

Enlargement and calcification are the only abnormalities of the normally relatively small adrenal glands which can be visualized radiographically. If these abnormalities occur concurrently, they are almost always caused by a primary tumour of the adrenal cortex (adenoma, adenocarcinoma) or medulla (pheochromocytoma) (Fig. 11.20b, c). While adrenal mineralization in dogs is essentially pathognomonic for neoplasia, it is a common incidental finding in normal older cats (see Fig. 11.6).

Vascular mineralization

The abdominal aorta and caudal vena cava are largely inaccessible for radiographic evaluation on survey radiographs, with the exception of metastatic or dystrophic calcifications. Especially in cats with chronic renal insufficiency, the aorta is often easily recognized due to mineralization of the vessel wall (Fig. 11.20d). Ultrasound, computed tomography and possibly selective angiography are the diagnostic modalities of choice for an evaluation of vascular diseases.

11.4 Classification of abdominal masses

11.4.1 Terminology and definitions

The term 'mass' in this chapter is used to encompass both **space-occupying mass lesions** and **organomegaly,** without any implication of a specific disease process. This allows a radiographic description in situations where the origin of an increased amount of soft tissue is not immediately evident. If the organ of origin is definitively identified (e.g. in case of simple hepatomegaly), this classification may be unnecessary. However, it may still be helpful for two reasons: with increasing size, all abdominal masses have a tendency to extend into the mid abdomen, and concurrent effusion is common. The key in mass classification is recognition of displacement of other abdominal organs. This distinguishes abdominal masses from simple effusions (see Fig. 11.16 and 11.17).

Organs that are easily displaced include the small intestinal tract, colon and left kidney. However, it is important to consider that the colon and left kidney are flexible in their position even without displacement by adjacent structures. Some pairs of organs, including the spleen (dorsal) and stomach, right kidney and liver, pancreas and duodenum, prostate and urinary bladder, are closely anatomically connected, and enlargement of one organ will always result in displacement of the other.

Classification of abdominal masses is not 100% accurate and is meant as a general guideline.

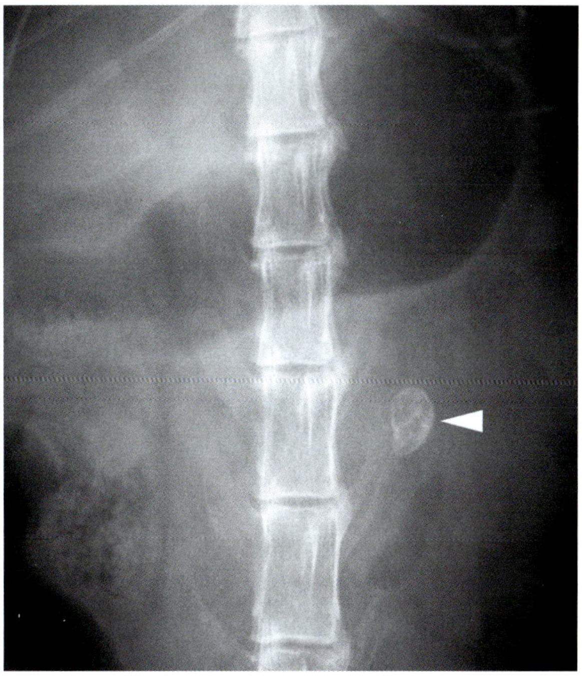

a

Fig. 11.20

a Nodular fat necrosis with eggshell-like mineralization (arrowhead) in a 16-year-old domestic cat on the ventrodorsal view. This is a common incidental finding in older well-nourished cats and of no clinical significance.

(b, c and d overleaf)

b Calcified tumour of the adrenal medulla (pheochromocytoma) in a 10-year-old (!) Boxer. The tumour results in caudoventral displacement of the left kidney.

c Calcified tumour of the adrenal cortex (adenocarcinoma, arrowhead) in an 11-year-old Yorkshire Terrier. Adrenocortical tumours are often smaller and only mildly mineralized and thus difficult to recognize. However, calcification is one of the few pathognomonic findings with adrenal neoplasms in dogs.

d Mineralization of the aorta and gastric wall in a 5-year-old domestic cat with chronic renal insufficiency. With this kind of metastatic mineralization, the aorta is more visible than usual. Following successful renal transplant, vascular mineralization often resolves.

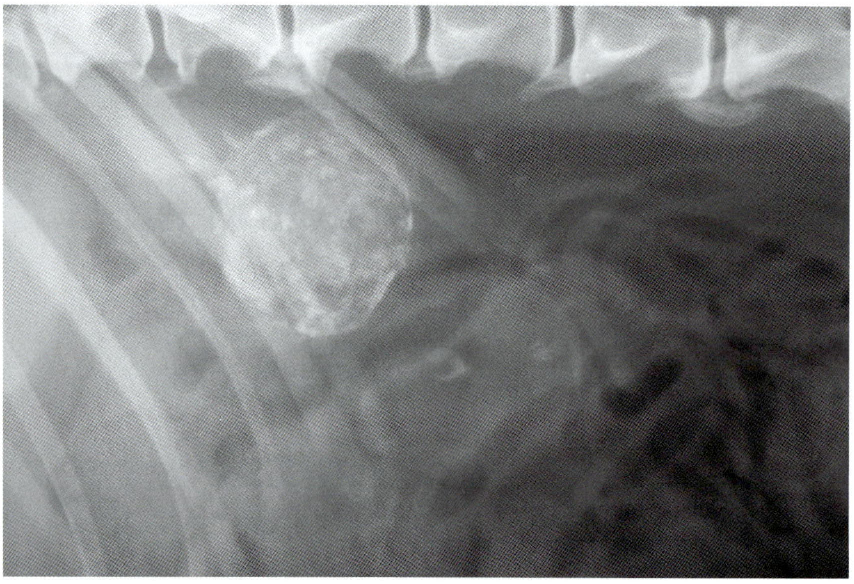

Fig. 11.20b

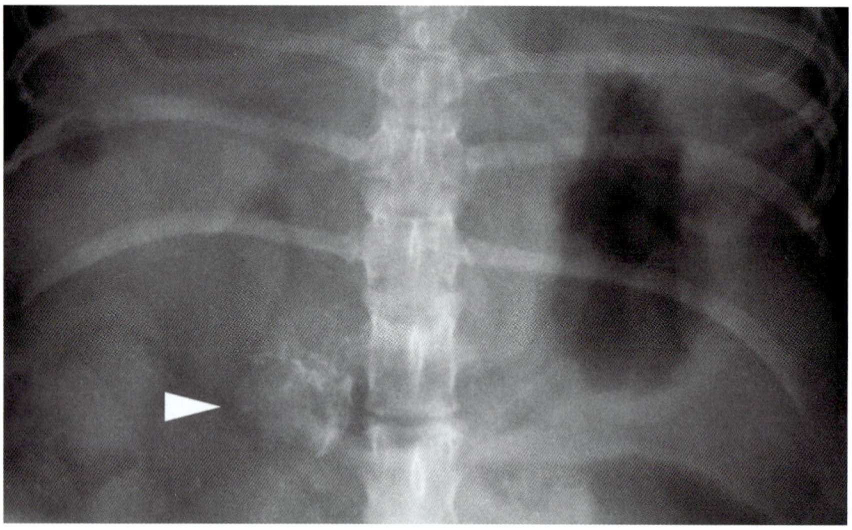

Fig. 11.20c

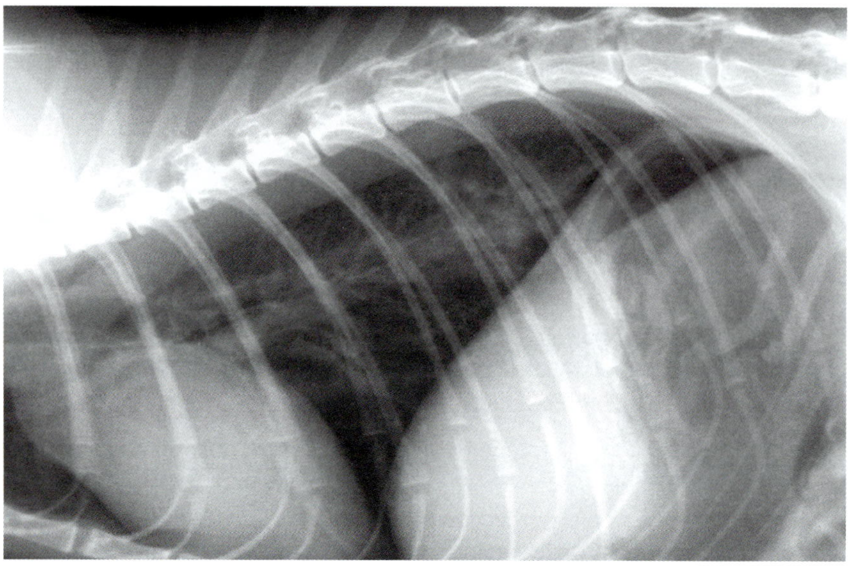

Fig. 11.20d

11.4.2 Cranial masses

These masses result in caudal and often also mild dorsal displacement of intestine (Fig. 11.21). **Liver** with **gallbladder**, **spleen**, **pancreas** and **stomach** fall into this category. Splenic masses do not affect the position of the gastric axis on lateral views, while hepatic masses often result in its counterclockwise rotation. Right-sided hepatic masses result in caudal displacement of the right kidney, while pancreatic enlargement often results in displacement of the duodenum and transverse colon within the right cranial abdomen (Fig. 11.22).

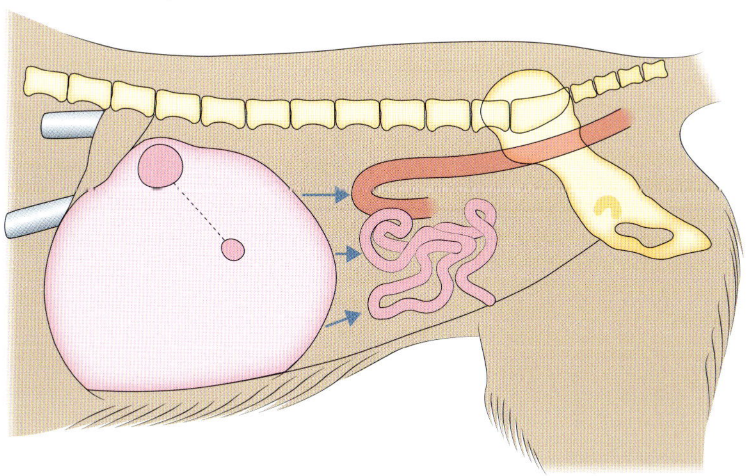

Fig. 11.21 Cranial mass. The transverse colon and small intestine are displaced caudally (arrows). Counterclockwise rotation of the gastric axis (dashed line) indicates hepatic origin.

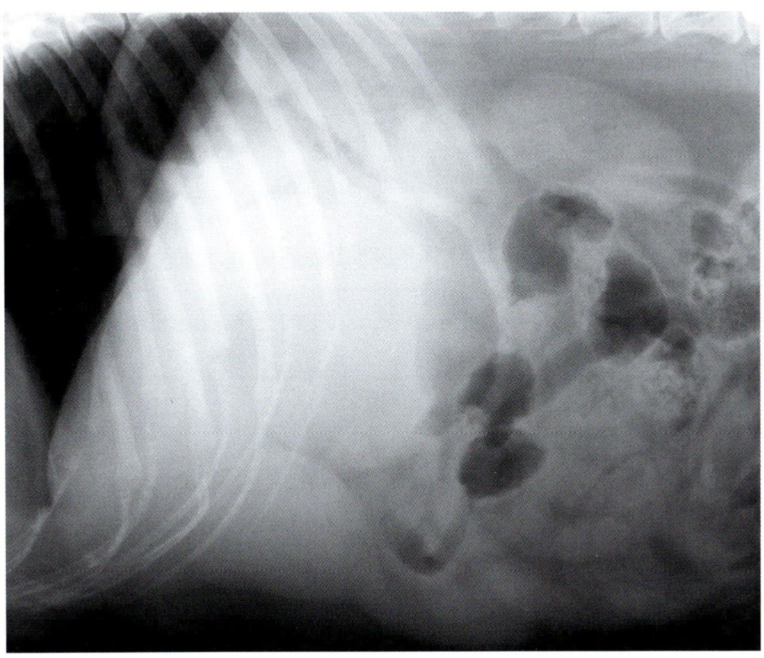

Fig. 11.22 A 12-year-old mixed-breed dog with a mass in the cranial abdomen which displaces the small and large intestine caudally. The gastric axis is markedly rotated, while the right kidney is in a normal position. These findings indicate a left-sided liver mass. The final diagnosis was hepatic carcinoma.

11.4.3 Dorsal masses

Dorsal masses mostly displace the intestine ventrally and usually also mildly cranially and caudally (Fig. 11.23).

Right-sided masses may displace the descending colon ventrally, while left-sided masses usually result in distinct ventral displacement of the descending colon. The **kidneys**, **ovaries** and **retroperitoneal lymph nodes**, potentially the **adrenal glands** (usually too small), as well as nonspecific **retroperitoneal masses** fall into this category. Differential diagnoses for renal masses are discussed further in Chapter 14.

Ovaries

These only become radiographically visible if significantly enlarged. Ovarian cysts and cystic ovarian tumours can reach considerable size, occupy most of the abdominal cavity, and may occur bilaterally (Fig. 11.24). Teratomas are a rare type of ovarian mass and are often characterized by bizarre calcifications.

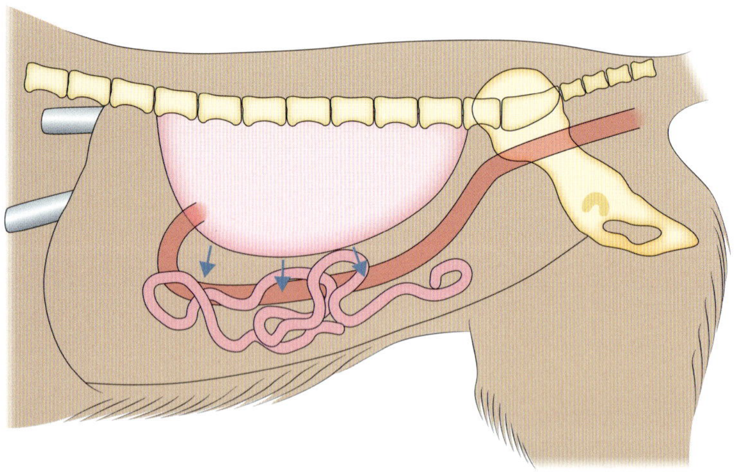

Fig. 11.23 Dorsal mass. The descending colon and small intestine are displaced ventrally (arrows). With right-sided masses the descending colon may remain in a normal position.

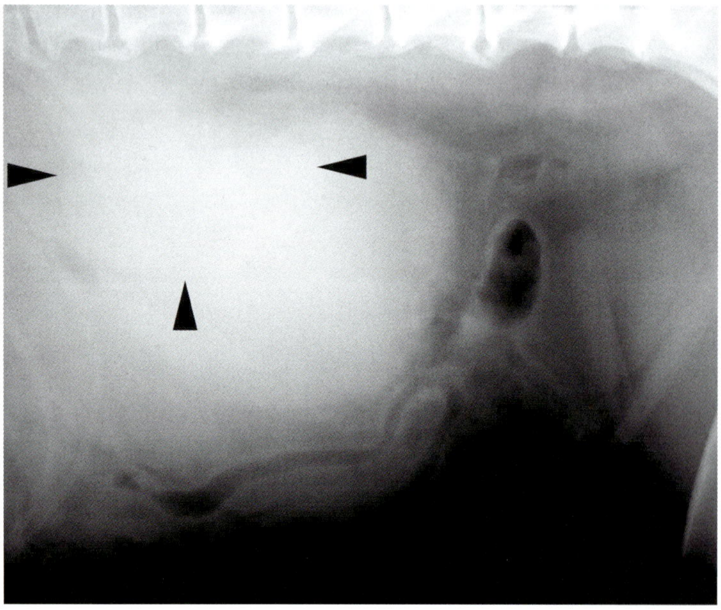

Fig. 11.24 Ovarian tumour in a 5-year-old female Labrador. The ovoid soft-tissue opacity mass displaces the small and large intestine ventrally, consistent with classification as a dorsal mass. The left kidney (arrowheads) is separate from the mass.

Aortic and sublumbar lymph nodes

Normal retroperitoneal lymph nodes are not visible. A soft-tissue opacity mass resulting in ventral displacement or compression of the descending colon cranial to the pelvic inlet is usually caused by enlargement of the sublumbar lymph nodes (Fig. 11.25).

Adrenal tumours

As discussed in section 11.3.6, these may become radiographically visible if large enough and/or associated with mineralization (see Fig. 11.20b, c). Medullary tumours in particular can become very large and result in caudal displacement of the kidneys. The examiner has to be aware that a radiographic evaluation for diagnostic workup of hyperadrenocorticism in dogs is unrewarding, as radiographically visible enlargement or tumoural calcification of adrenal glands is uncommon with this disease and difficult to recognize. Abdominal ultrasound or computed tomography are preferable in the diagnosis and evaluation of adrenal tumours.

Infiltrative tumours

Histiocytic tumours, haemangiosarcomas and liposarcomas can spread in the retroperitoneal space and cause dorsal masses. These are often difficult to distinguish from other retroperitoneal structures (Fig. 11.26).

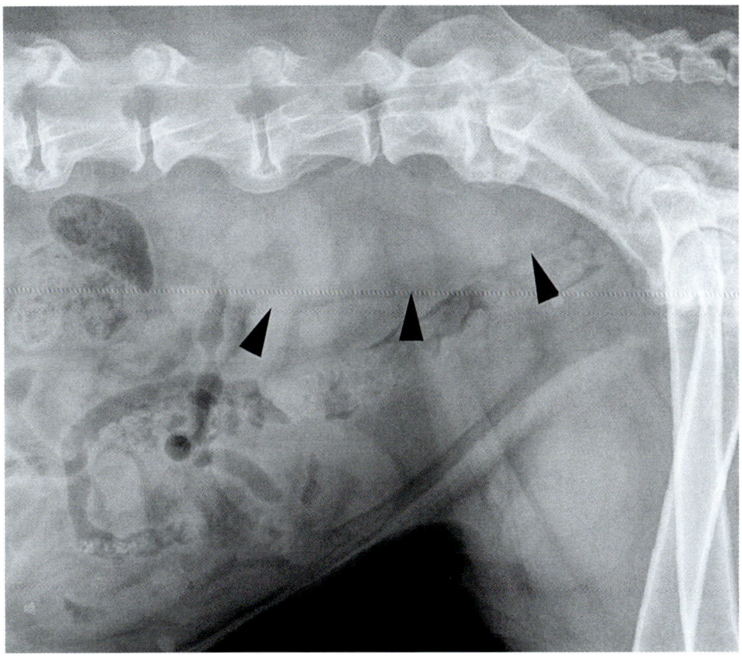

Fig. 11.25 Enlargement of the sublumbar lymph nodes (arrowheads) in a Small Munsterlander with multicentric lymphoma. The colon is displaced ventrally by the caudodorsally located mass. Small intestinal segments are superimposed with the lymph nodes.

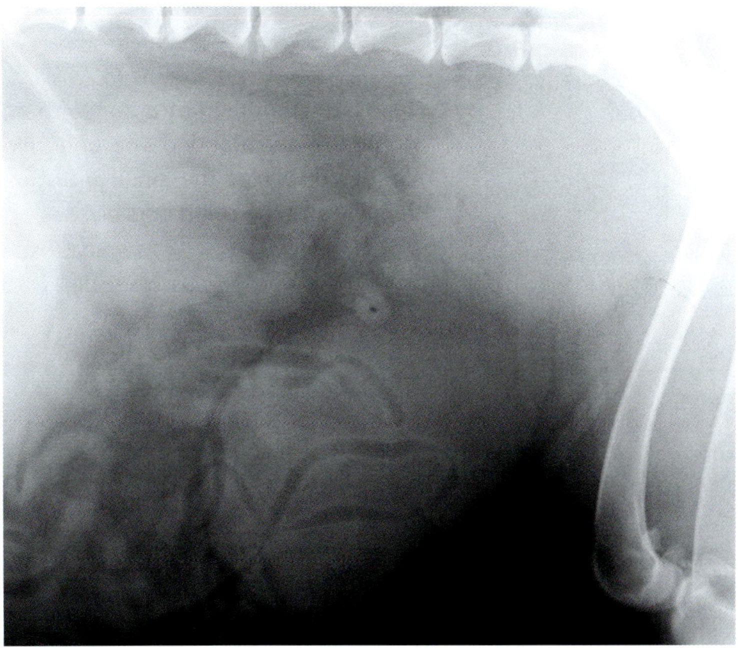

Fig. 11.26 Histiocytoma of the caudal retroperitoneal space in a 9-year-old female Golden Retriever. Radiographically, this mass cannot be distinguished from other possible organ associated masses (lymph nodes, large intestine, uterus, vagina).

Traumatic mass lesions

Hunting dogs, in particular, can present with marked retroperitoneal soft-tissue swelling and lumbar vertebral periosteal reaction when inhaled grass awns migrate into the lumbar musculature or the retroperitoneal space.

In free-roaming cats, bite wounds and secondary **abscess** formation is common in this region.

11.4.4 Caudal masses

Caudal masses displace the small intestine cranially and sometimes the descending colon dorsally (Fig. 11.27). These include the **urinary bladder**, **prostate**, **paraprostatic cysts**, **intra-abdominal testicles** and **uterus** (Fig. 11.28; see also Chapter 14).

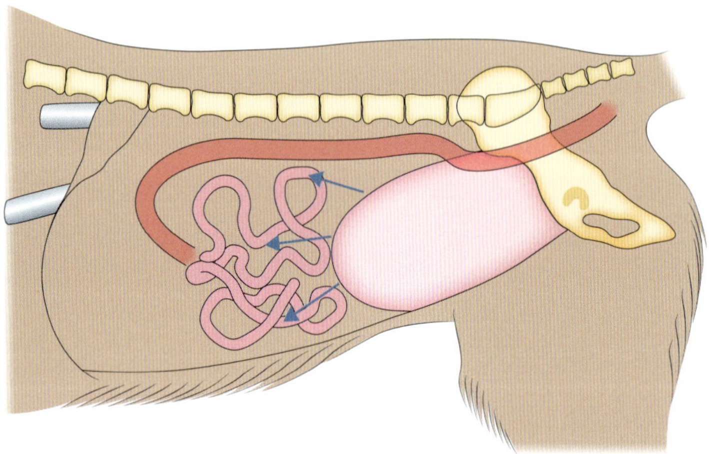

Fig. 11.27 Caudal mass. The small intestine is displaced cranially and the descending colon dorsally (arrows).

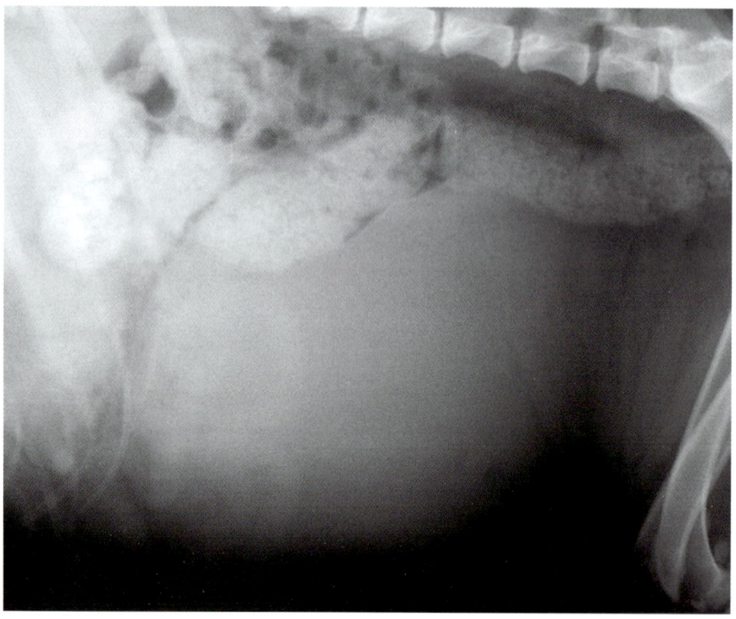

Fig. 11.28 Abdomen of a dog with an atonic urinary bladder. The enlarged bladder displaces the small intestine cranially and the colon dorsally.

Two oval soft-tissue opacities in the caudal abdomen in male dogs do not always represent the urinary bladder and prostate, as paraprostatic cysts and intra-abdominal retained testicles may appear very similar.

11.4.5 Ventral masses

Ventral masses are rare and result in dorsal displacement of intestine (Fig. 11.29). These include abdominal wall abscesses and tumours (see Fig. 11.17a), umbilical abscesses, and intra-abdominal retained testicles.

11.4.6 Central masses

Central masses displace the small intestine peripherally in all directions and the large intestine dorsally (Fig. 11.30). These include enlarged mesenteric lymph nodes, omental cysts and lipomas (see Fig. 11.17b), as well as enlarged small intestinal segments (mass, dilatation).

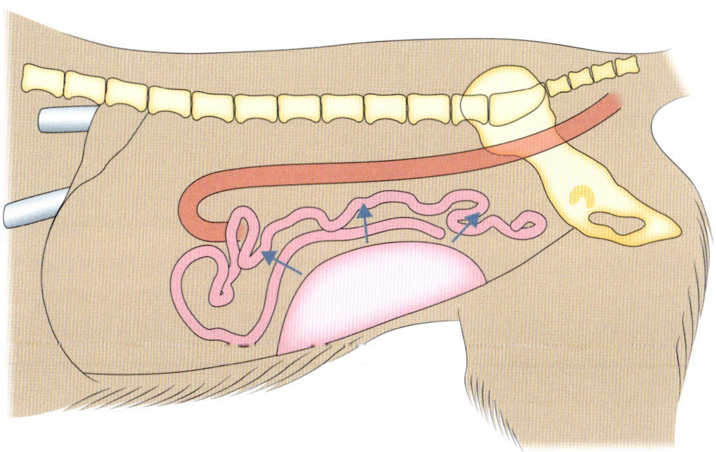

Fig. 11.29 Ventral mass resulting in dorsal displacement of the small intestine (arrows).

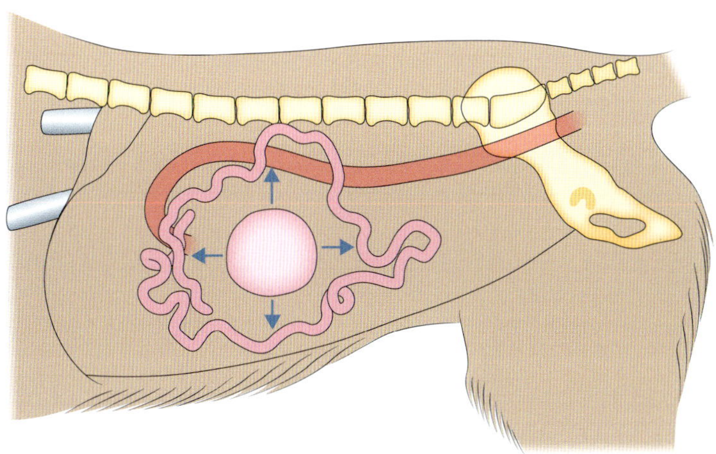

Fig. 11.30 Central mass. Small intestinal segments are displaced peripherally in all directions. The descending colon is displaced dorsally (arrows).

References and further reading

Armbrust LJ, Biller DS, Hoskinson JJ. Case examples demonstrating the clinical utility of obtaining both right and left lateral abdominal radiographs in small animals. J Am Anim Hosp Assoc 2000a; 36: 531–6.

Armbrust LJ, Biller DS, Hoskinson JJ. Compression radiography: an old technique revived. J Am Anim Hosp Assoc 2000b; 36: 531–6.

Blevins WE, Kooreman KM. The normal left limb of the pancreas is visible on survey radiographs of fat cats [Abstract]. 2002 ACVR Annual Scientific Meeting, Chicago, IL, USA. Vet Radiol Ultrasound 2003; 44: 106.

Curry TS, Dowdey JE, Murry RC. Christensen's Physics of Diagnostic Radiology, 4th edn. Philadelphia: Lippincott Williams & Wilkins 1990.

Fischetti A, Saunders HM, Drobatz KJ. Pneumatosis in gastric dilatation-volvulus syndrome. Vet Radiol Ultrasound 2004; 45: 205–9.

Grandage J. Some effects of posture on the radiographic appearance of the kidneys of the dog. J Am Vet Med Assoc 1975; 166: 165–6.

Grandage J. Posture, gravity, and radiological interpretation. J Am Vet Rad Assoc 1979; 20: 80–1.

Hartung K, Tellhelm B. Der Weg zum guten Röntgenbild. Stuttgart: Enke 2000.

Komori S, Nakagaki K, Koyama H, Yamagami T. Idiopathic mesenteric and omental steatitis in a dog. J Am Vet Med Assoc 2002; 221: 1591–3.

Lamb CR, Kleine LJ, McMillan MC. Diagnosis of calcification on abdominal radiographs. Vet Radiol 1991; 32: 211–20.

Love NE. The appearance of the canine pyloric region in right versus left lateral recumbent radiographs. Vet Radiol 1993; 34: 169–70.

Love NE, Berry CR. Interpretation paradigms for the abdomen – canine and feline. In: Thrall D (ed.). Textbook of Veterinary Diagnostic Imaging, 4th edn. Philadelphia: WB Saunders 2002, 483–92.

Morris EL. Pneumatosis coli in a dog. Vet Radiol Ultrasound 1992; 33: 154–7.

Murdoch DB. The abdomen. In: Lee R (ed.). BSAVA Manual of Small Animal Diagnostic Imaging. Gloucester: BSAVA 2001; 68–94.

O'Brien TR. Radiographic Diagnosis of Abdominal Disorders in the Dog and Cat. Davis, CA: Covell Park Vet Company 1981.

Root CR. Steatitis in cats: its radiographic appearance. J Am Vet Rad Assoc 1971; 12: 60–4.

Root CR. Interpretation of abdominal survey radiographs. Vet Clin North Am 1974; 4: 763–803.

Schwarz T, Morandi F, Gnudi G, Wisner E, Paterson C, Sullivan M, Johnston P. Nodular fat necrosis in the feline and canine abdomen. Vet Radiol Ultrasound 2000a; 41: 335–9.

Schwarz T, Störk CK, Mellor D, Sullivan M. Osteopenia and other radiographic signs in canine hyperadrenocorticism. J Small Anim Pract 2000b; 41: 491–5.

Thrall DE. Intraperitoneal vs. extraperitoneal fluid. Vet Radiol Ultrasound 1992; 33: 138–40.

12 Liver, spleen, lymph nodes and pancreas

Dagmar Nitzl and Stefanie Ohlerth

12.1 Anatomy and indications

12.1.1 Anatomy

Liver and gallbladder

Radiographic evaluation of the liver includes assessment of size, position, shape, contour and radiographic opacity. The normal organ appears as a homogeneous soft-tissue opaque structure in the cranial abdomen and contained within the costal arch. On a lateral view, the liver is located caudal to the diaphragm and lung field and cranial to the stomach. On a ventrodorsal view, the liver is located cranial to the spleen on the left side and cranial to the kidney, duodenum and pylorus on the right side (Moon Larson 2007; Owens and Biery 1999).

The liver in dogs and cats consists of a **right and left medial** and a **right and left lateral liver lobe**, a dorsal and median **caudate lobe** (with a right-sided **caudate** and a left-sided **papillary process**), and a ventral and median **quadrate lobe** (Vollmerhaus and Roos 2004a). These different lobes cannot generally be distinguished radiographically. The caudate process of the caudate lobe typically forms the caudodorsal margin of the hepatic silhouette on a lateral view and is located cranial to the right kidney. The ventral and caudoventral margins of the liver are bordered by falciform fat and are well recognized in animals with good abdominal detail (see section 11.1.1). On a left lateral view, this margin usually corresponds to the right medial liver lobe, and on the right lateral view to the left lateral liver lobe, respectively.

On a lateral view, hepatic size can be evaluated based on the position of the gastric axis, which courses through the fundus, body and pylorus of the stomach. With normal hepatic size, the gastric axis should be located between an imaginary line parallel to the ribs and a second line perpendicular to the spine (Fig. 12.1; Graham et al. 2007)

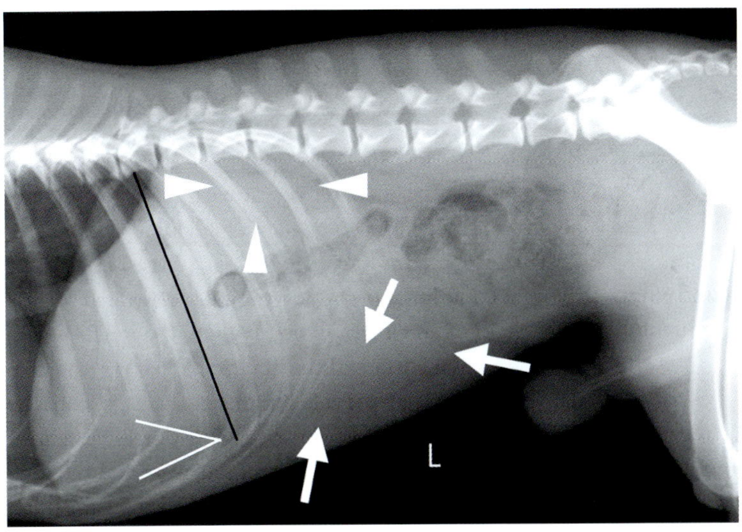

Fig. 12.1 Normal left lateral view of the abdomen in a dog. The black line indicates the gastric axis through the fundus (dorsal), corpus and pylorus (ventral). The white angle indicates the caudoventral liver margin. Arrowheads indicate the splenic head and arrows the splenic tail (L = left).

Depending on the shape of the thorax, age, phase of respiration and patient positioning, minor variations in radiographic hepatic size are possible. The caudoventral liver margin usually appears as a triangular, sharply marginated structure within or extending slightly beyond the costal arch.

Young animals physiologically have larger livers with respect to their body mass than adults, which may mimic mild to moderate diffuse hepatomegaly but should be considered normal. The liver also has a tendency to appear larger on right lateral than on left lateral views.

On a ventrodorsal view, a similar amount of normal hepatic parenchyma is present to the left and right of the spine in **dogs** (Fig. 12.2), while the liver is mostly located within the right abdomen in **cats**.

The pear-shaped **gallbladder** is located between the quadrate and the right medial liver lobes in the right abdomen. This fluid-filled structure is soft-tissue opaque and thus indistinguishable from surrounding soft-tissue opaque hepatic parenchyma.

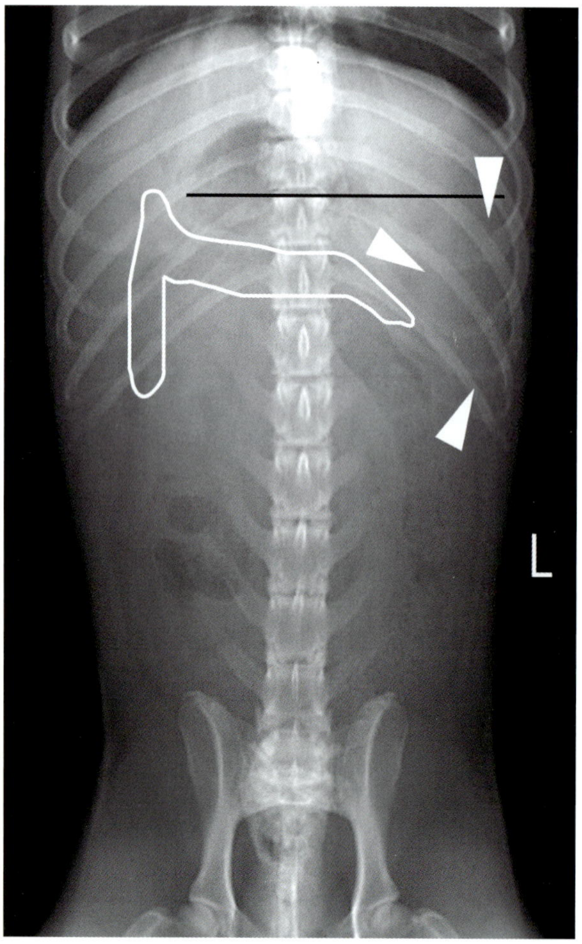

Fig. 12.2 Normal ventrodorsal view of the abdomen in a dog. The black line marks the gastric axis through the fundus (left), corpus and pylorus (right side at the level of the 10th/11th intercostal space). Arrowheads mark the splenic head adjacent to the left abdominal wall. The white line drawing outlines the expected position of the pancreas (L = left).

A markedly distended gallbladder may extend beyond the cranial ventral liver margin in **cats** and appears as a rounded soft-tissue opaque structure (best seen on lateral views). Duplication of the gallbladder in cats is a rare incidental variant.

Spleen

The spleen is a flat, elongated, smoothly marginated, homogeneous soft-tissue opaque structure located in the left cranial and mid abdomen caudal to the stomach. Its normal size is very variable in dogs. Cats generally have a smaller spleen (Graham et al. 2007; Moon Larson 2007).

The **head of the spleen** is connected to the greater curvature of the stomach in the region of the fundus via the gastrosplenic ligament. Its position is therefore relatively consistent and only varies with the degree of gastric filling. On the ventrodorsal view, it appears as a triangular structure between the gastric fundus and the cranial pole of the left kidney (Fig. 12.2). On a lateral radiograph it may also be visible craniodorsally, caudal to the gastric fundus and partially superimposed with the kidneys (Fig. 12.1).

The **body and tail of the spleen** are freely mobile in the mid abdomen. In cats they are typically visible along the left abdominal wall on a ventrodorsal view. In dogs, the splenic tail is often also visible along the ventral abdominal wall on a lateral view (Fig. 12.1) and may overlap with the caudoventral margin of the liver (Owens and Biery 1999; Vollmerhaus and Roos 2004b).

Lymph nodes

Abdominal lymph nodes are categorized into **visceral** and **parietal lymph nodes** (Vollmerhaus and Roos 2005; Bezuidenhout 2013).

> Normal abdominal lymph nodes are not visible radiographically due to their small size and soft-tissue opacity (Fig. 12.3). They become visible with significant enlargement (Frank and Mahaffey 2007; Graham et al. 2007; Owens and Biery 1999).

PARIETAL LYMPH NODES

These are located in the retroperitoneal space and are subdivided into the lumbar and iliosacral lymph centres.

The **lumbar lymph centre** in dogs and cats consists of the renal and lumbar aortic lymph nodes, which form a long chain of small lymph nodes along the renal vessels, the abdominal aorta and the abdominal part of the caudal vena cava. They provide lymphatic drainage from the kidneys, the last thoracic vertebrae, the lumbar vertebrae, the osseous pelvis, the lumbar musculature and the long paraspinal muscles, the costal pleura and the urogenital tract. Lymphatic drainage occurs via the lumbar trunks into the cisterna chyli.

The **iliosacral lymph centre** consists of the medial iliac, internal iliac (formerly hypogastric) and the sacral lymph nodes.

The **medial iliac lymph nodes** are located immediately cranial to the aortic trifurcation at the origin of the right and left external iliac arteries and ventral to the fifth and sixth lumbar vertebrae. Dogs usually have one lymph node on each side (sometimes two to three), while two to four and rarely more lymph nodes are found in cats. These lymph nodes directly drain the pelvic tissues, pelvic organs and proximal portions of the hind limbs but also receive efferent vessels from deep and superficial inguinal, ischiatic (in cats) and popliteal lymph nodes. Lymphatic drainage occurs via the lumbar trunks, the lumbar aortic lymph nodes or directly into the cisterna chyli.

The **internal iliac lymph nodes** (formerly called hypogastric) reside in the region ventral to the sixth and seventh lumbar vertebrae adjacent to the medial sacral artery, and can be located as far caudal as the lumbosacral intervertebral disc space. The variably present medial and lateral **sacral lymph nodes** lie ventral to the sacrum and caudal vertebrae. These lymph nodes drain the musculature of the pelvis, perineum and tail as well as part of the lumbar musculature, the lumbar, sacral and caudal vertebrae, pelvic bones, femora and caudal abdominal and pelvic organs. They also receive efferent vessels from the deep inguinal lymph nodes and are connected to the medial iliac lymph nodes.

VISCERAL LYMPH NODES

These include the coeliac lymph centre (splenic, gastric, hepatic and pancreaticoduodenal lymph nodes), cranial mesenteric lymph centre and caudal mesenteric lymph centre (Bezuidenhout 2013).

From a radiographic standpoint, the **cranial mesenteric lymph centre** is the most important of these lymph centres. In dogs it consists of the jejunal and colic lymph nodes, while cats have an additional one to three caecal lymph nodes. There are some species-specific differences regarding the number of lymph nodes and the tributary areas.

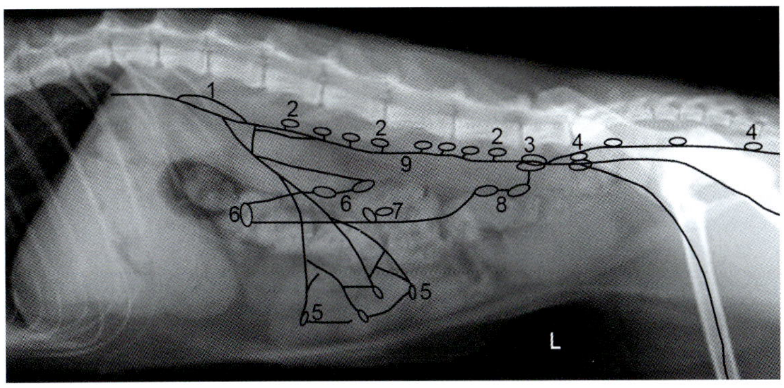

a

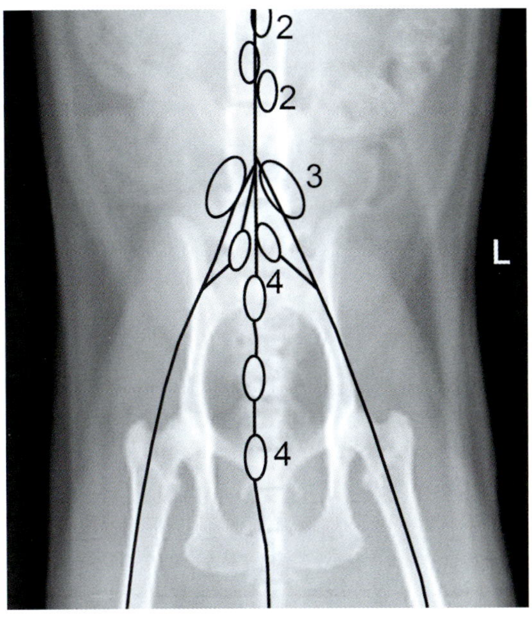

b

Fig. 12.3 Schematic drawing of the cranial mesenteric lymph centre, iliosacral lymph centre and caudal mesenteric lymph centre in a cat on a lateral a and ventrodorsal b view of the abdomen and pelvis, respectively. 1 Cisterna chyli, 2 Lumbar aortic lymph nodes, 3 Medial iliac lymph nodes, 4 Internal iliac and sacral lymph nodes, 5 Jejunal lymph nodes, 6 Colic lymph nodes, 7 Caecal lymph nodes, 8 Caudal mesenteric lymph nodes, 9 Lumbar trunk. These lymph nodes and lymphatic structures are physiologically not visible but may appear as soft-tissue opaque mass lesions in case of significant enlargement.

The **jejunal lymph nodes** in dogs predominantly drain the jejunum, ileum and pancreas, while they drain the entire small intestine and the body of the pancreas in cats. There are usually two (up to five in cats) elongated major lymph nodes and a variable number of smaller lymph nodes located along the mesojejunum and following the jejunal arteries and veins.

One to three (three to nine in cats) **colic lymph nodes** are located within the mesentery of the ascending and transverse colon, which drain the ileum, caecum and colon.

Caecal lymph nodes in cats are usually paired, located on both sides of the caecum, and are responsible for drainage of the caecum and ileum.

Drainage from the cranial mesenteric lymph centre occurs exclusively via the visceral trunk in dogs, while the caecal and colic lymph nodes drain into the lumbar trunks in cats.

Pancreas

The **right lobe** is located medial to the descending duodenum while the **left lobe** extends from the level of the gastric fundus caudally and to the left where it is located in close proximity to the spleen and cranial pole of the left kidney. The **body of the pancreas** connects both lobes in the region of the pylorus (see Fig. 12.2).

The pancreas has two ducts which connect at the level of the pancreatic body. The **pancreatic duct** empties into the descending duodenum together with the common bile duct via the major duodenal papilla, while the **accessory pancreatic duct** terminates further caudally at the minor duodenal papilla (Vollmerhaus and Roos 2004a).

In **dogs**, the pancreatic duct is smaller than the accessory pancreatic duct, or may be absent, whereas **cats** usually only have a pancreatic duct, and only occasionally is a small accessory pancreatic duct present.

> The normal pancreas is not visible radiographically. However, in obese cats, the extremity of the left pancreatic lobe is occasionally seen on ventrodorsal views as a tubular soft-tissue opaque structure in the angle between the stomach, spleen and left kidney (see Chapter 11, Fig. 11.5; Frank and Mahaffey 2007; Graham et al. 2007; Owens and Biery 1999).

12.1.2 Indications

Liver and gallbladder

Indications to acquire abdominal radiographs for evaluation of liver and gallbladder are manifold. They include palpable hepatic changes, abnormal findings on blood chemistry analysis indicating hepatic disease, and also nonspecific symptoms such as fever, vomiting, icterus, central nervous system disorders, lethargy, anorexia or abdominal pain.

Spleen

Indications for radiographic evaluation of the spleen include palpable masses in the mid abdomen, weakness, anaemia and diseases of the myeloid system.

Lymph nodes

Abdominal radiographs are obtained if there is clinical suspicion of lymph node enlargement. This may be for the purpose of tumour staging (e.g. in case of lymphoma or anal sac carcinoma) or if masses or nodules are noted on abdominal palpation.

Pancreas

As the pancreas is not normally radiographically visible and changes in the cranial abdomen cannot often be confidently attributed to pancreatic disease, a sonographic examination is preferable over abdominal radiographs if pancreatic disease is of concern. However, abdominal radiographs may be helpful in raising suspicion of pancreatic pathology in patients with clinical symptoms such as vomiting, diarrhoea, abdominal pain, lethargy and/or anorexia.

12.2 Radiographic technique and positioning

The radiographic technique and positioning of the patient for radiographic evaluation of liver, spleen, lymph nodes and pancreas is identical to those described for lateral and ventrodorsal abdominal radiographs in sections 11.2.1 and 11.2.2.

12.3 Diseases of the liver

12.3.1 Changes in hepatic size

Secondary displacement of adjacent abdominal organs (mass effect) can help in distinguishing between generalized and focal hepatomegaly. However, it is important to take into account the normal position of the stomach on ventrodorsal views, which differs between dogs (U-shaped, pylorus to the right of the spine) and cats (J-shaped, pylorus on midline) (see also section 13.1.1).

The radiographic examination may aid in identification of the underlying cause of hepatomegaly (Table 12.1). However, further diagnostic tests including ultrasound and cytological or histological examination of tissue samples are usually needed for a definitive diagnosis.

> The size of the liver on survey radiographs of the abdomen is best assessed based on the gastric axis as well as the location, shape and contour of the caudoventral liver margin (see section 12.1.1; Graham et al. 2007; Moon Larson 2007; Owens and Biery 1999).

Table 12.1 Differential diagnoses for hepatomegaly.

Generalized hepatomegaly		Focal hepatomegaly
Sharply marginated, rounded liver margins	Irregular liver margins	
Diffuse infiltrative neoplasia such as lymphoma	Multifocal or metastatic neoplasia	Neoplasia
Congestion	Cysts	Cyst
Hepatic lipidosis	Granulomas	Granuloma
Steroid hepatopathy	Abscesses	Abscess
Acute hepatitis	Nodular hyperplasia	Nodular hyperplasia
	Hepatic cirrhosis	Liver lobe torsion

Generalized hepatomegaly

With generalized hepatomegaly, the pylorus of the stomach is displaced caudodorsally and the gastric axis caudally on a lateral view (Fig. 12.4), resulting in extension of the caudoventral liver margin beyond the costal arch (Moon Larson 2007).

On a ventrodorsal view (Fig. 12.5), the gastric axis is also displaced caudally. The pylorus is shifted to the left, the gastric fundus to the right, and the right kidney, the head of the spleen, the transverse colon and the cranial duodenal flexure are displaced caudally.

The shape and contour of the liver can provide additional information about the underlying hepatic pathology (Table 12.1).

A **slightly rounded, blunt contour** in an enlarged liver may be seen with:

- hepatic lipidosis (e.g. in association with diabetes mellitus in cats)
- steroid hepatopathy (secondary to hyperadrenocorticism or iatrogenic)
- passive venous congestion of the liver (e.g. secondary to right heart failure or obstruction of the caudal vena cava)
- acute inflammation (granulomatous hepatitis such as seen with feline infectious peritonitis, cholangiohepatitis and in association with acute pancreatitis)
- diffuse neoplastic infiltration such as with lymphoma (Fig. 12.4 and 12.5).

If the **caudoventral angle** of the enlarged liver is **irregular, blunted or significantly rounded**, differential diagnoses should include:

- primary neoplasia (e.g. hepatocellular carcinoma or cholangiocarcinoma)
- secondary neoplasia (sarcoma or carcinoma metastasis or lymphoma)
- nodular hyperplasia
- hepatic abscesses
- cysts
- granulomas.

Focal hepatomegaly

Depending on the location and size of a focal hepatomegaly, displacement of the gastric axis may or may not

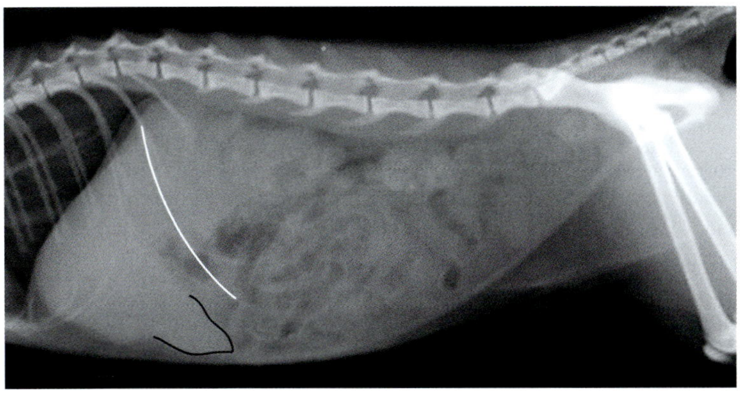

Fig. 12.4 Left lateral view of the abdomen in a cat with moderate generalized hepatomegaly. The gastric axis (marked by a white line) is caudally displaced. The caudoventral liver margin (black triangle) extends caudally beyond the costal arch and is rounded. The cytological diagnosis following ultrasound-guided fine-needle aspiration was lymphoma.

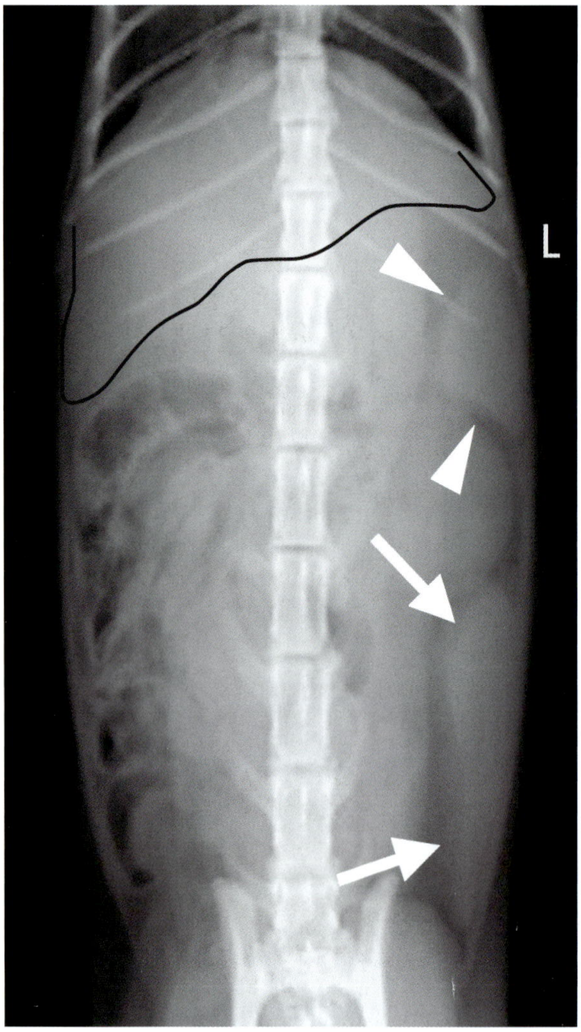

Fig. 12.5 Ventrodorsal view of the abdomen in a cat with moderate generalized hepatomegaly and splenomegaly. The caudal margin of the liver (black line) extends caudally beyond the costal arch and is rounded. The head of the spleen (arrowheads) as well as the body and tail (arrows) are larger than normal and also have rounded margins. Cytological diagnosis following ultrasound-guided fine-needle aspiration of liver and spleen was lymphoma (L = left).

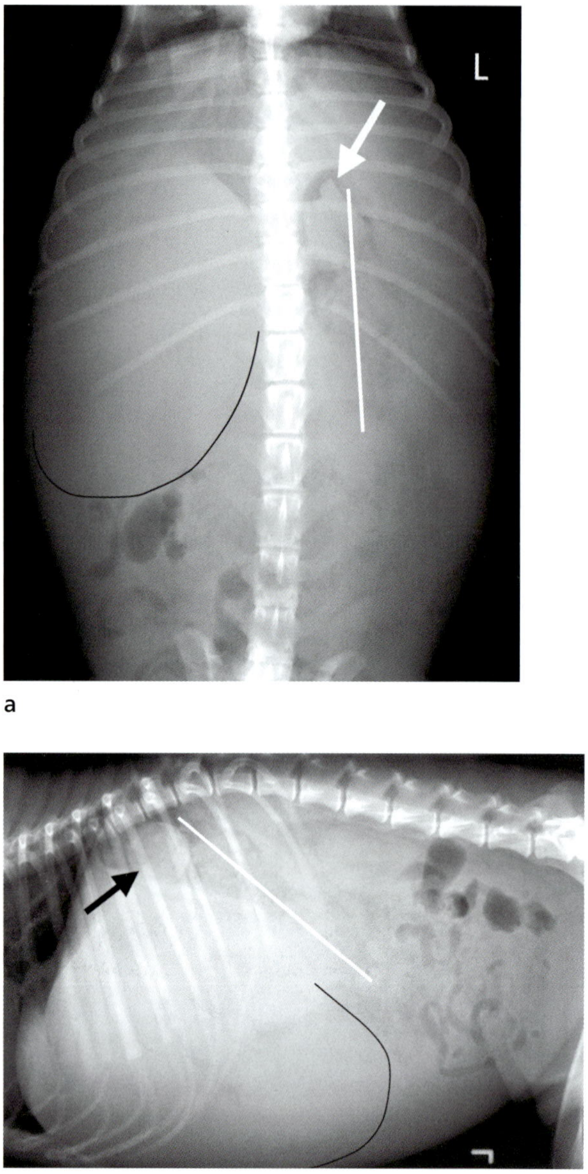

Fig. 12.6 Ventrodorsal a and left lateral b abdominal radiographs in a dog with severe focal hepatomegaly originating from the right lateral liver lobe. The caudoventral contour of the right lateral liver lobe (black line) extends far beyond the costal arch and is significantly rounded. The gastric axis (white line) is displaced caudodorsally and towards the left. The final diagnosis was echinococcosis. The gastric foreign body within the fundus (arrows) is an incidental finding at this point (L = left).

be observed. A change in position of abdominal organs bordering the liver can aid in identification of an enlarged hepatic lobe (see also section 11.4.2; Moon Larson 2007).

For example, with a mass associated with the **left lateral liver lobe**, the gastric fundus is displaced to the right on a ventrodorsal view and the stomach is displaced caudally and dorsally on a lateral view. The small intestine and spleen are located further caudal than normal in both projections.

A focal mass of the **right lateral liver lobe** (Fig. 12.6 and 12.7) is characterized by displacement of the duodenum medially (ventrodorsal view) and dorsally (lateral view).

Enlargement of the **caudate lobe**, especially the **caudate process**, is recognized by caudal displacement of the right kidney in both projections.

Differential diagnoses for focal hepatomegaly are numerous, and this radiographic finding is nonspecific (see Table 12.1). The following have to be considered:

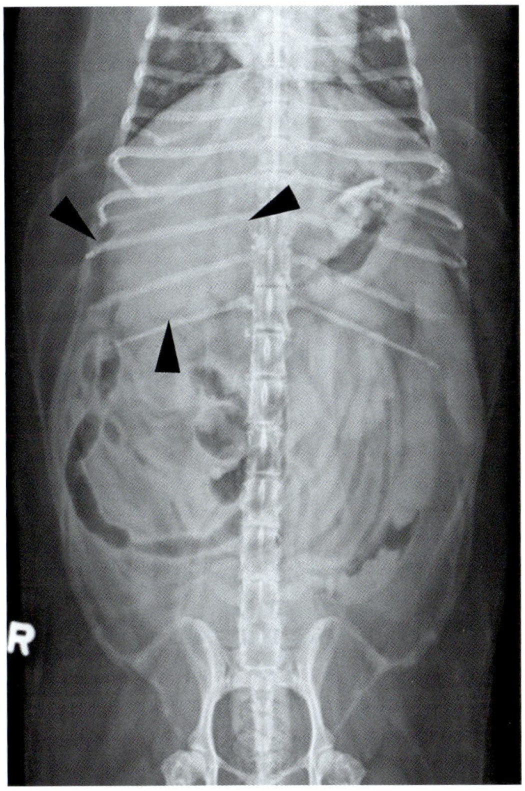

a

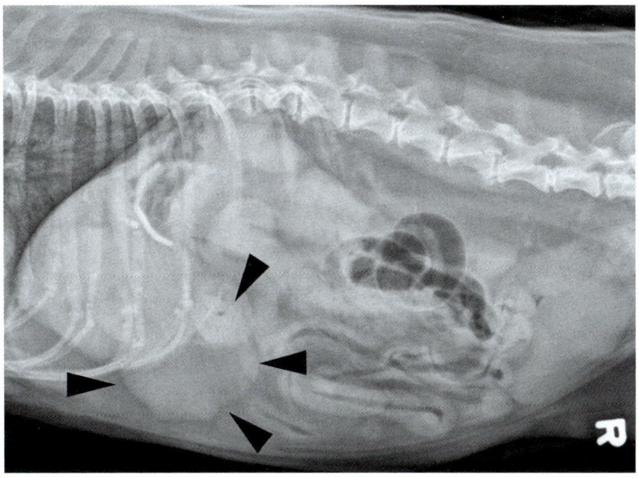

b

Fig. 12.7 Ventrodorsal a and right lateral b abdominal radiographs of the abdomen in a dog with focal enlargement of the right lateral liver lobe. The caudal and ventral contour of the right lateral liver lobe (black arrowheads) extends beyond the costal arch, is rounded and has irregular margins. The gastric axis is displaced caudodorsally and towards the left. Cytological diagnosis was undifferentiated hepatic neoplasia. The foreign body within the gastric fundus and degenerative changes of the spine are incidental findings (R = right).

- primary neoplasms such as hepatocellular carcinomas, cholangiocarcinomas, hepatomas or adenomas
- metastatic neoplasms
- abscesses
- granulomas
- hepatic or biliary cysts
- parasitic cysts
- nodular hyperplasia.

Liver lobe torsion is a rare cause for focal hepatomegaly. This may be seen secondary to trauma, gastric dilatation, hepatic masses or congenital abnormalities of hepatic ligaments; however, the exact cause is unknown. The left lateral liver lobe and the caudate process of the caudate liver lobe are most commonly affected. Concurrent abdominal effusion results in a decrease in radiographic abdominal serosal detail (Sonnenfield et al. 2001).

Microhepatia

For a diagnosis of microhepatia, the same criteria are used as for hepatomegaly (see sections 12.1.1 and 12.3.1). The gastric axis and duodenum are shifted cranially (Fig. 12.8 and 12.9; Graham et al. 2007; Moon Larson 2007), and there is the impression of not enough soft tissue between the diaphragm and gastrointestinal tract. A focal decrease in liver size is less conspicuous but may result in cranial displacement of adjacent organs. A mild cranial shift of the gastric axis is a normal variant in deep-chested dogs as the liver in these animals is located relatively far cranially and ventrally (Fig. 12.10).

A common underlying cause of small hepatic size is a portosystemic shunt. Venous blood from the gastrointestinal tract, which normally enters the liver via the portal vein or its respective branches, bypasses the liver and reaches the systemic circulation via one or more abnormal vessels. Portosystemic shunts may be extrahepatic (especially in cats, small and medium-sized dogs) or intrahepatic (especially in large-breed dogs) in location and may be congenital or acquired (Santilli and Gerboni 2003).

Microhepatia in **congenital portosystemic shunts** is caused by lack of trophic factors needed for hepatic development, which do not reach the liver in sufficient amounts due to the vascular anomaly. Additional common radiographic findings include bilateral renomegaly attributed to an increased amount of trophic factors within the blood stream, and urinary calculi (Santilli and Gerboni 2003).

Acquired shunts develop secondary to long-standing portal hypertension caused, for example, by chronic liver disease or arteriovenous fistulae. Depending on the underlying cause, the liver may be small, of normal size or enlarged. In contrast to congenital shunts, in these cases concurrent abdominal effusion is common and manifests radiographically as loss of serosal margin detail.

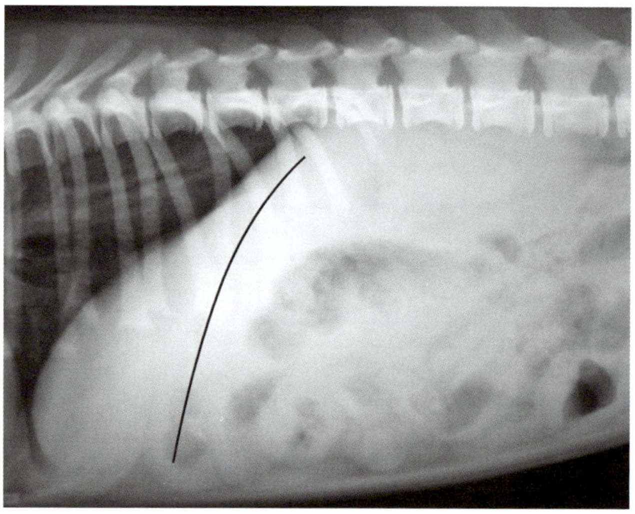

a

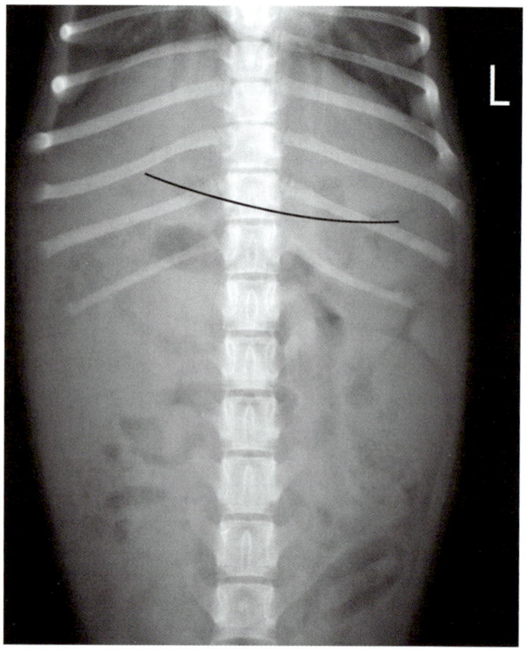

b

Fig. 12.8 Left lateral a and ventrodorsal b radiographs of the abdomen in a young dog with generalized microhepatia. The cranially displaced gastric axis is indicated by a black line. Final diagnosis was a porto-azygos shunt (L = left).

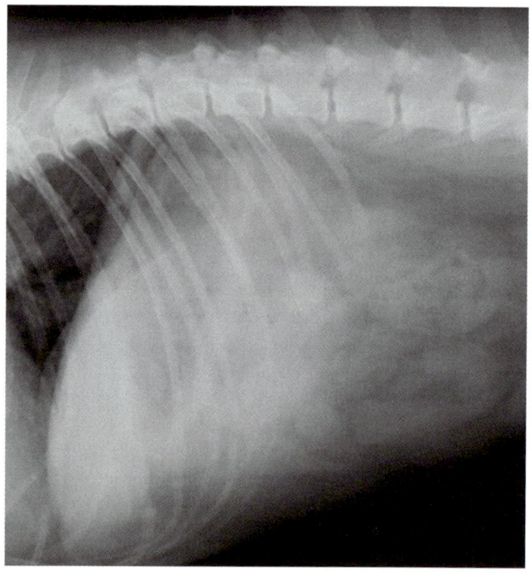

Fig. 12.9 Right lateral view of the abdomen in a dog with generalized microhepatia. The caudoventral margin of the hepatic silhouette is located cranial to the costal arch, and the gastric axis is cranially displaced. A diagnosis of a portocaval shunt was made by means of scintigraphy. (Courtesy of Dr William H. Adams, University of Tennessee)

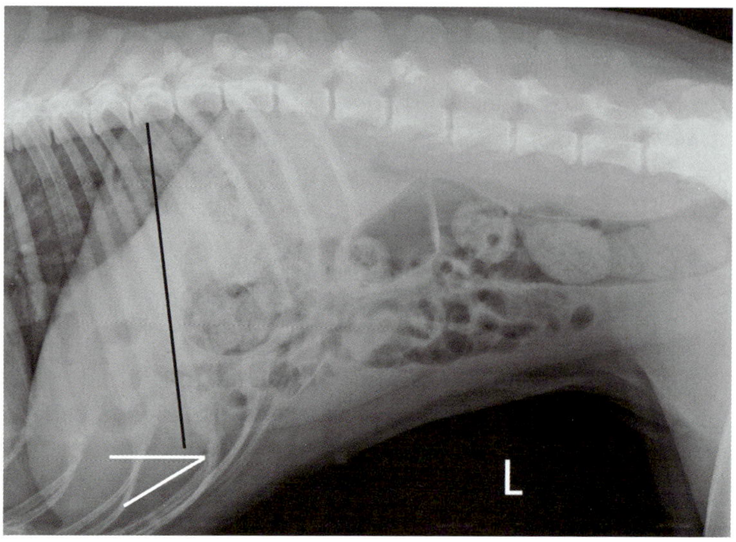

Fig. 12.10 Normal left lateral view of the abdomen in a thin, deep-chested dog. The black line marks the gastric axis, which is in perpendicular orientation to the spine. The white triangle indicates the caudoventral liver margin, which is contained within the costal arch. This can result in a subjective impression of microhepatia (L = left).

Abdominal ultrasonography is the least invasive method for direct visualization of the portosystemic shunt vessel(s) (Fig. 12.11). Alternatively, or depending on ultrasonographic findings, selective angiography (e.g. mesenteric portography; Fig. 12.12), helical computed tomography or scintigraphy can be used for definitive diagnosis and further characterization of a portosystemic shunt.

Other differential diagnoses for microhepatia include:

- congenital microvascular dysplasia which also results in insufficient portal blood supply to the liver
- hepatic cirrhosis
- chronic active hepatitis
- diaphragmatic ruptures or hernias.

The latter may result in complete or partial herniation of hepatic tissue into the pleural or pericardial space and thus in a reduction of hepatic size within the abdomen. To allow differentiation from real microhepatia, evaluation of the diaphragmatic contour and the thorax is indicated (see section 9.5.2).

12.3.2 Changes in radiographic opacity

The normal liver is radiographically of homogeneous soft-tissue opacity. Any change in opacity is pathological (Owens and Biery 1999; Moon Larson 2007).

Decreased opacity

Markedly decreased opacity in the hepatic silhouette is caused by gas inclusions (see also section 11.3.5; Table 11.8). Gas can reach the liver through the portal or systemic circulation or ascend through the biliary tract. Branching linear gas opacities within the liver resembling air bronchograms in a consolidated lung lobe (see section 9.8.1) correspond to **gas accumulations in a ductal system**. Gas inclusions within the portal venous system may occur secondary to mucosal necrosis of stomach or small intestine such as seen with gastric dilatation and volvulus.

Emphysematous cholecystitis results in a focal accumulation of gas within the gallbladder wall and/or gallbladder lumen in the right cranial ventral liver. This condition is rare and usually caused by gas-producing bacteria such as *Clostridium perfringens*. This disease is also occasionally seen in association with diabetes mellitus.

Necrotic liver tumours and **hepatic abscesses** are an important differential diagnosis for emphysematous cholecystitis. These can be focal or multifocal, occur in variable locations within the hepatic parenchyma, and usually appear radiographically as poorly or irregularly marginated gas opacity foci within the hepatic parenchyma (Fig. 12.13). Iatrogenic causes of intrahepatic or biliary gas (following surgical procedures involving incision of the common bile duct or the gallbladder) are rare.

Increased opacity

Hepatic mineralization is rare (see also section 11.3.6; Table 11.9). Radiographically, focal or multifocal regions of increased opacity are noted (Fig. 12.14). This may be an incidental finding in older animals or may be associated with chronic granulomas, abscesses, haematomas, nodular hyperplasia, neoplasia (e.g. extraskeletal osteosarcoma or cholangiocarcinoma) or parasitic cysts.

Mineralization of the biliary tree results in a branching linear mineral opaque pattern within the liver. Mineral opaque calculi within the gallbladder (**cholelithiasis**) or bile ducts are usually incidental findings (Fig. 12.15). These consist of cholesterol, bilirubin, or a mixture of both sub-

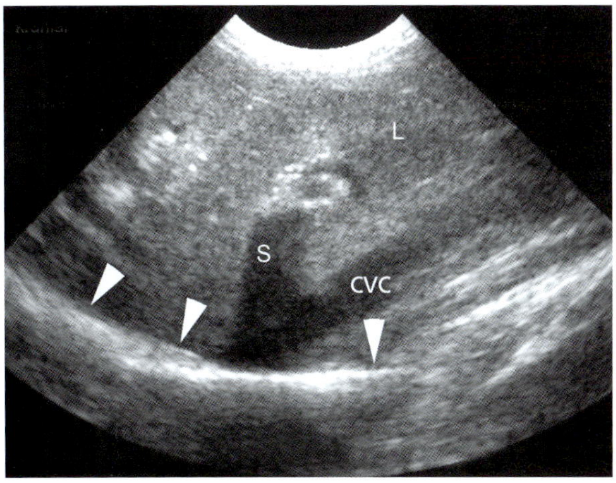

Fig. 12.11 Longitudinal B-mode ultrasound image of the liver (L) in a dog with portacaval shunt. The shunt vessel (S) terminates into the caudal vena cava (CVC) immediately caudal to the diaphragm (white arrowheads).

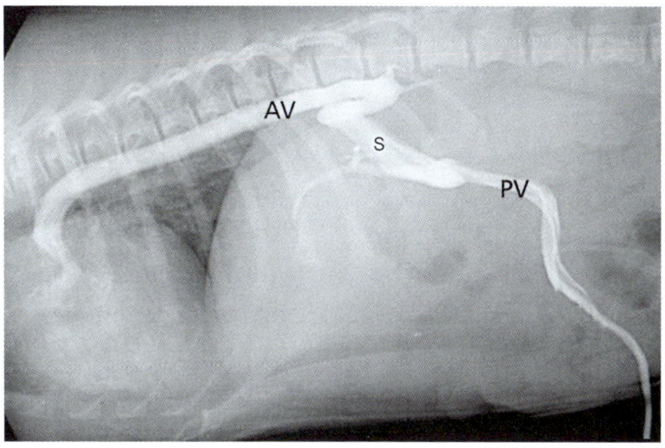

Fig. 12.12 Intraoperative mesenteric portography (lateral view) in a young dog with congenital porto-azygos shunt. Following catheterization of a mesenteric vein, positive contrast medium was injected and radiographs were obtained. A large shunt vessel (S) connects the portal vein (PV) to the azygos vein (AV), bypassing the liver.

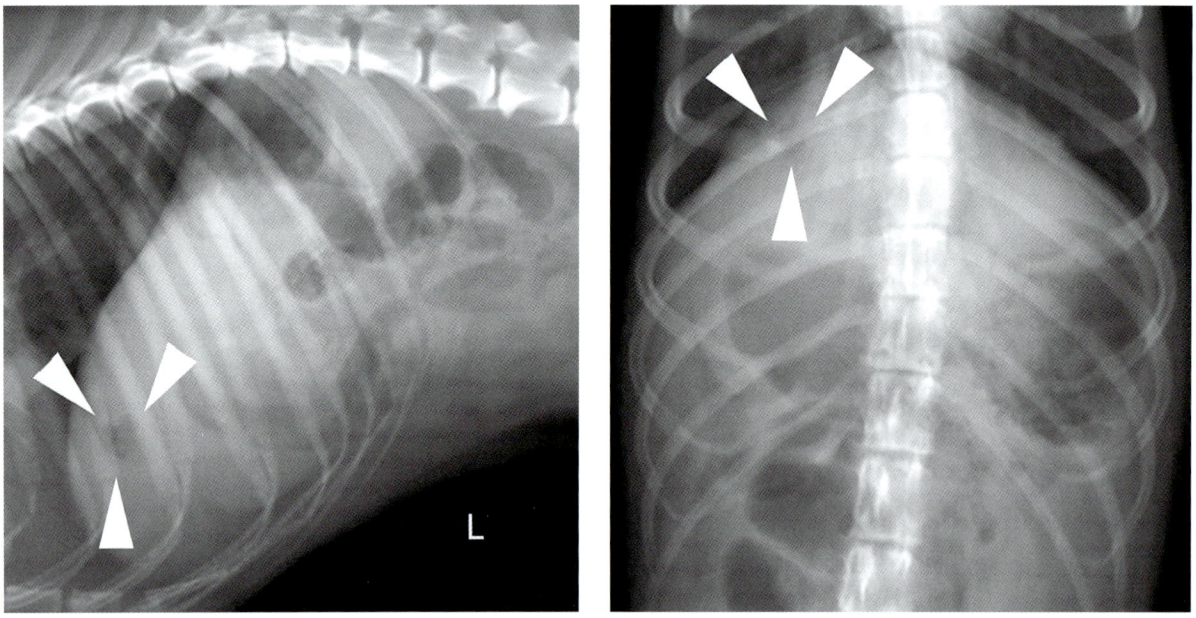

a b

Fig. 12.13 Left lateral a and ventrodorsal b radiographs of the cranial abdomen in a dog with a hepatic abscess. The focal gas accumulation in the right cranial hepatic parenchyma is marked by arrowheads (L = left).

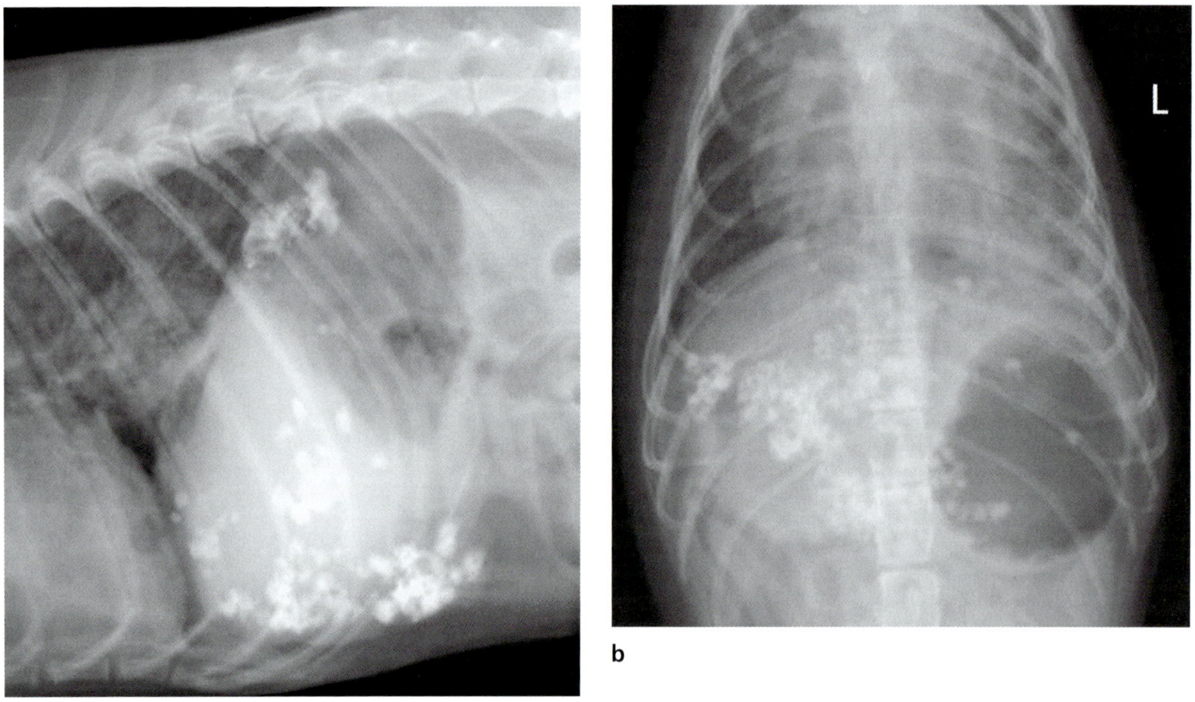

b

a

Fig. 12.14 Left lateral a and ventrodorsal b radiographs of the cranial abdomen in a dog with multiple nodular foci of hepatic mineralization of undetermined aetiology (differential diagnoses included parasitic granulomas or dystrophic mineralizations) (L = left).

stances and usually only become clinically relevant if they result in obstruction of the common bile duct. Choleliths may be associated with **cholecystitis**, which does not result in radiographic abnormalities and requires diagnosis by other means, for example ultrasonography. Necrotizing cholecystitis may cause perforation of the gallbladder wall, and the resultant peritonitis may cause loss of serosal margin detail in the cranial abdomen.

Mineralization of the gallbladder wall may be seen with cholangiocarcinomas, cholecystitis and mucinous hyperplasia.

12.4 Diseases of the spleen

12.4.1 Generalized splenomegaly

Splenic size in dogs is highly variable and dependent on age and activity level. Younger and more active dogs have larger spleens compared to quieter and older animals (Moon Larson 2007). Physiologically, German Shepherd Dogs and related breeds have larger spleens than other breeds, although this information is not readily found in the literature.

Generalized splenomegaly may be **medically induced** by administration of phenothiazine (e.g. acepromazine), barbiturates (e.g. thiopental) or propofol (Owens and Biery 1999; Baldo et al. 2012). Reasons for **pathological, generalized splenomegaly with smooth but blunted margins** (Table 12.2) include:

- diffuse infiltrative neoplasia such as lymphoma, mast cell tumour and disseminated histiocytic sarcoma (see Fig. 12.5)
- vascular congestion secondary to portal hypertension

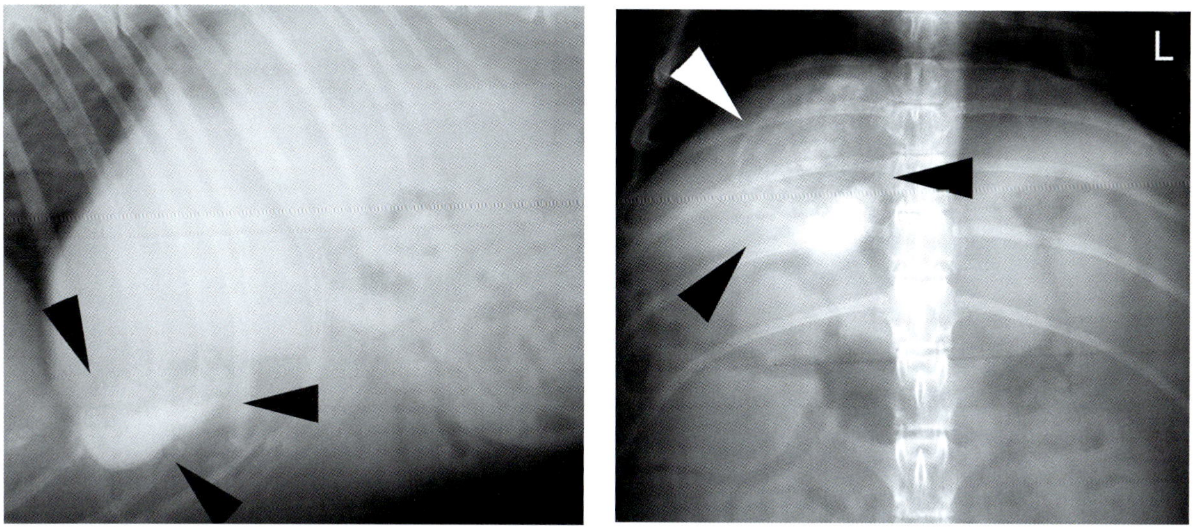

a b

Fig. 12.15 Left lateral a and ventrodorsal b radiographs of the cranial abdomen in a dog with gallbladder calculi and mineralized gallbladder sediment (arrowheads) (L = left).

Table 12.2 Differential diagnoses for splenomegaly.

Generalized splenomegaly		Focal splenomegaly
Smoothly marginated, blunted margins	Irregular margins	
Nodular hyperplasia	Nodular hyperplasia	Nodular hyperplasia
Diffuse, infiltrative neoplasia	Neoplasia	Neoplasia
Venous congestion	Abscess	Abscess
Sedation or anaesthesia	Haematoma	Haematoma
Haemolytic anaemia	Infarct	
Breed variation	Splenic torsion	
Splenitis		

- splenic torsion (see below)
- gastric dilatation and volvulus
- immune-mediated haemolytic anaemia and thrombocytopenia
- hyperplasia secondary to chronic anaemia
- bacterial or mycotic infections.

RADIOGRAPHIC FINDINGS An enlarged spleen appears wider, thicker, longer and thus bluntly marginated compared to a normal spleen. Splenic enlargement results in displacement of the small intestinal tract caudally and dorsally, which is best seen on a lateral abdominal view. On a ventrodorsal view, the enlarged splenic head displaces the small intestine and the cranial part of the descending colon to the right and caudally. The splenic tail is variable in position and can be located in the mid abdomen, along the left flank to reach the level of the urinary bladder, or within the right cranial abdomen. In that location it can result in medial displacement of the descending duodenum, the descending colon and the caecum.

Splenic size in **cats** is less variable than in dogs; however, splenomegaly results in similar displacement of adjacent organs.

Splenic torsion

This is most commonly seen in large, deep-chested dogs (commonly Great Danes and German Shepherd Dogs) and can occur alone or in association with a gastric volvulus. Splenic torsion without concurrent gastric volvulus may be chronic, and affected animals present with anorexia, vomiting, abdominal pain and anaemia. With splenic torsion the spleen rotates around its pedicle, which results in occlusion of venous drainage and potentially arterial blood supply (Weber 2000).

RADIOGRAPHIC FINDINGS Abdominal palpation and abdominal radiographs reveal moderate to severe splenomegaly resulting in a mass lesion in the mid abdomen. Additionally, the spleen may exhibit a **characteristic reverse C-shape** due to the splenic head and tail both being located in the mid abdomen. Concurrent abdominal effusion is common and results in loss of serosal margin detail. Due to the ligamentous connection between spleen and stomach the **gastric fundus may be displaced caudally and medially**, and the triangular soft-tissue opaque shadow of the splenic head is no longer visible in its typical left craniodorsal location. In some cases, splenic torsion promotes the intraparenchymal proliferation of anaerobic gas-producing bacteria, and numerous gas opacity foci are noted throughout the splenic parenchyma (Fig. 12.16).

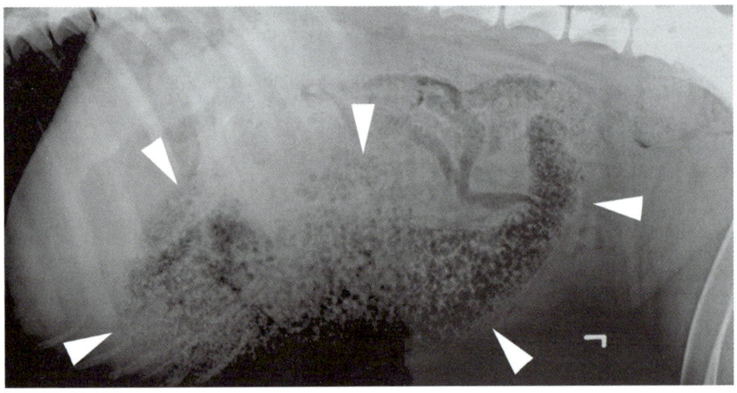

Fig. 12.16 Left lateral view of the abdomen in a dog with splenic torsion and secondary necrosis as well as infection with gas-producing bacteria. Arrowheads mark the severely enlarged spleen located in the mid ventral abdomen. Numerous gas opacity foci are noted throughout the spleen resulting in a bubbly appearance (L = left).

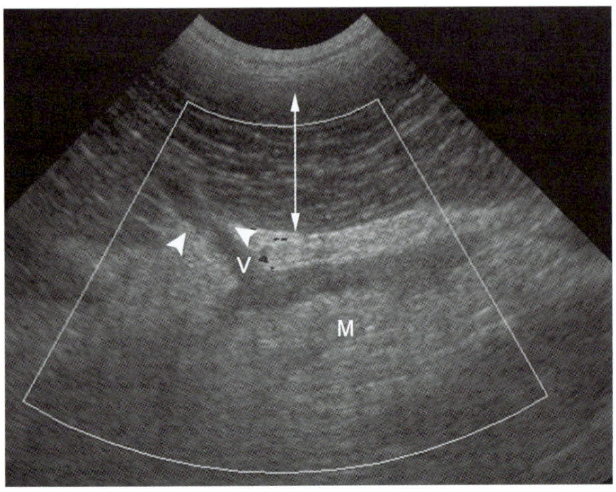

Fig. 12.17 B-Mode ultrasound image (colour Doppler) of the spleen and splenic veins in a dog with a strong suspicion of splenic torsion. There is no evidence of blood flow in the splenic veins (V), and the splenic parenchyma (double-headed arrow) appears heterogeneous and hypoechoic with anechoic foci, which is consistent with a 'lacy pattern' reported for this disease. The two arrowheads mark the perivenous hyperechoic triangle of mesenteric fat bordering the splenic hilus (M = mesentery).

A suspicion of splenic torsion based on radiographs can be confirmed by means of ultrasonographic evaluation (Fig. 12.17).

12.4.2 Focal splenomegaly

Focal splenomegaly is a common cause of a mid to cranial abdominal mass in dogs (Fig. 12.18; see also section 11.4; Moon Larson 2007; Owens and Biery 1999).

Depending on the location of the mass, adjacent organs are displaced as described for generalized splenomegaly on lateral and ventrodorsal views (see section 12.4.1). Masses are variably well circumscribed and can usually be connected to the remainder of the spleen on one or both projections (Fig. 12.18).

As the spleen is mostly located within the left abdomen in **cats**, masses originating from the splenic body or tail are typically located within the left or ventral abdomen.

Differential diagnoses for splenic masses include haematomas, abscesses, nodular hyperplasia (Fig. 12.18 and 12.19), neoplastic lesions such as haemangiosarcoma (Fig. 12.20), other sarcomas and carcinoma. These cannot be distinguished radiographically.

Haematomas and **nodular hyperplasia** of the spleen are very common findings in dogs, can reach considerable size and are often incidental findings.

Haemangiosarcomas (Fig. 12.20) are common in large-breed dogs such as German Shepherd Dogs, Golden Retrievers, Boxers and Great Danes. These tumours are prone to rupture. Animals with haemoabdomen secondary to rupture of a splenic mass commonly present with abdominal distention, weakness, anaemia and possibly a palpable abdominal mass.

RADIOGRAPHIC FINDINGS Depending on the severity of intra-abdominal haemorrhage, loss of serosal margin detail may be noted adjacent to the spleen or throughout the abdomen. A splenic mass may or may not be visible.

Abdominal ultrasound may aid in further evaluation of a patient with a splenic mass and abdominal effusion. However, only a cytological or histological examination can ultimately provide a definitive distinction between malignant and benign neoplasia, haematoma and nodular hyperplasia.

Splenic abscesses are rare in dogs and cats. These may occur in conjunction with regional or systemic infections. They may also occur in association with a splenic torsion or gastric volvulus.

RADIOGRAPHIC FINDINGS In case of infection with gas-producing bacteria, small gas bubbles may accumulate within the spleen, and appear as small, round, radiolucent foci distributed within the soft-tissue opaque splenic parenchyma.

Fig. 12.18 Left lateral a and ventrodorsal b radiographs of the abdomen in a dog with a mass located within the mid-ventral abdomen (arrowheads), believed to originate from the splenic tail based on its position. The cytological diagnosis was splenic nodular hyperplasia (L = left).

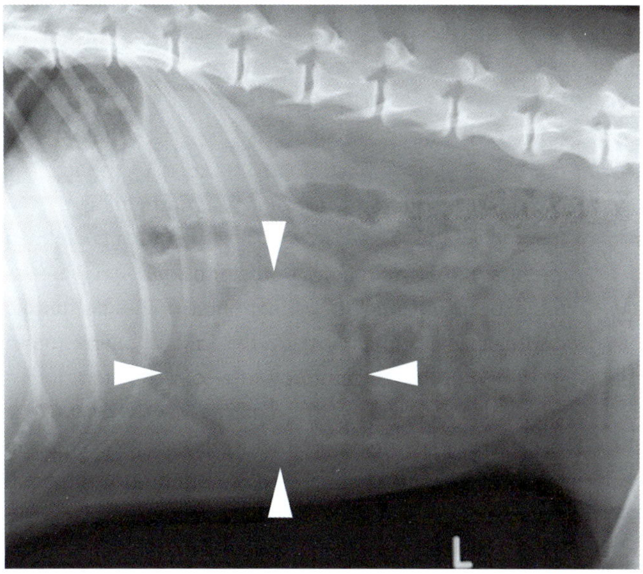

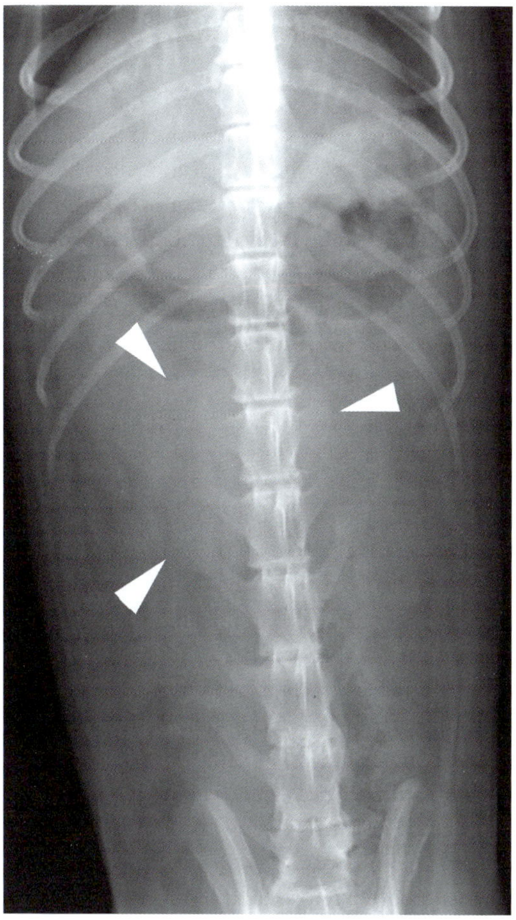

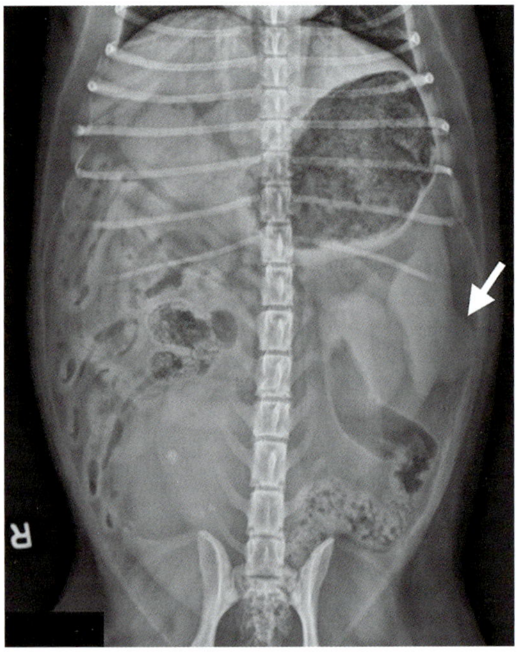

Fig. 12.19 Ventrodorsal view of the abdomen in a dog with a focal mass associated with the spleen (arrow). Cytological diagnosis was nodular hyperplasia.

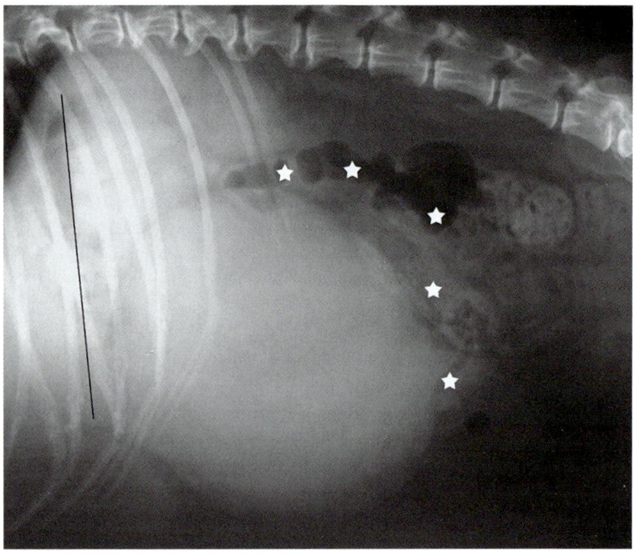

Fig. 12.20 Left lateral view of the abdomen in a dog with suspicion of a large splenic mass in the mid-ventral abdomen. The gastric axis (black line) is displaced cranially and the intestinal segments are displaced caudodorsally (stars). Histopathological diagnosis was haemangiosarcoma.

12.5 Diseases of the lymph nodes

> Abdominal lymph nodes are only visible on radiographs if they are significantly enlarged or mineralized.

Usually, the only intra-abdominal lymph nodes that are recognized as being enlarged on survey radiographs are the nodes of the **lumbar lymph centre** and **iliosacral lymph centre** ('sublumbar lymph nodes'), which are surrounded by retroperitoneal fat, and the lymph nodes of the **cranial mesenteric lymph centre** ('mesenteric lymph nodes') (Frank and Mahaffey 2007; Graham et al. 2007; Owens and Biery 1999).

SUBLUMBAR LYMPH NODES Enlargement of the sublumbar lymph nodes is recognized as a region of increased soft-tissue opacity or a soft-tissue opacity mass in the retroperitoneal space at the level of the kidneys to approximately the fourth lumbar vertebrae (lumbar lymph centre), ventral to the fifth and sixth lumbar vertebrae (medial iliac lymph nodes), ventral to the sixth and seventh lumbar vertebrae (internal iliac lymph nodes), or ventral to the sacrum and caudal vertebrae (sacral lymph nodes), respectively. In case of severe enlargement, the mass may extend further cranially and caudally and result in ventral displacement of the caudal descending colon and the rectum (Fig. 12.21; see also section 11.4). However, it is important to note that the position of the colon is flexible in many animals, and ventral displacement without associated sublumbar soft-tissue swelling may be a variation of normal.

The reason for lymph node enlargement is usually neoplastic infiltration, either primary such as seen with lymphoma or secondary as with metastases from carcinomas or other tumours in the pelvic region (urinary bladder, urethra, prostatic gland, testicles, rectum or perineum), the caudoventral abdominal wall or the hind limbs.

Lymph node enlargement secondary to inflammation is less common but may be seen, for example secondary to infection or inflammation of the perineum, caudal abdominal cavity or pelvic canal. Clinically, this may be associated with hind limb oedema caused by obstruction of lymphatic drainage or compression of the caudal vena cava or iliac veins.

MESENTERIC LYMPH NODES Severe enlargement of the mesenteric lymph nodes is recognized as a poorly defined soft-tissue opacity mass or region of increased soft-tissue opacity in the mid abdomen resulting in peripheral displacement of the intestinal tract (Fig. 12.22; see also section 11.4).

As with sublumbar lymphadenomegaly, the underlying cause is a neoplastic or inflammatory disease process of the tributary area or of the lymph node itself (e.g. lymphoma, metastatic intestinal tumours such as adenocarcinoma, leiomyosarcoma/gastrointestinal stromal tumour or

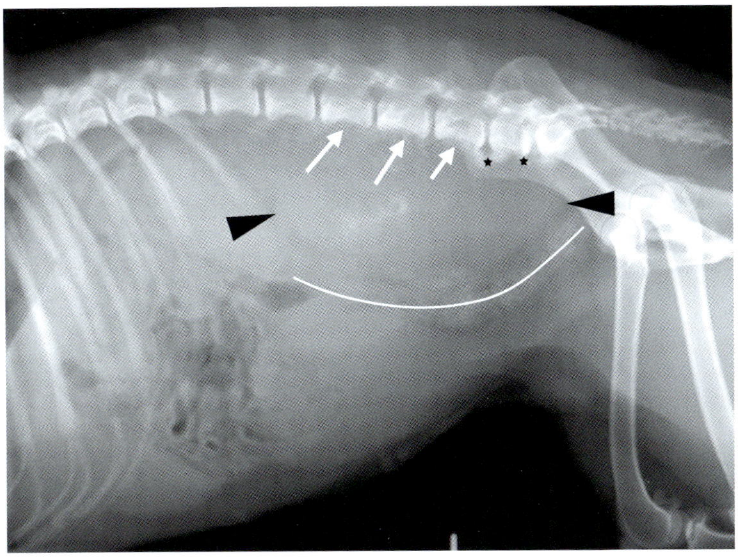

Fig. 12.21 Left lateral view of the abdomen in a dog with severe enlargement of the iliosacral lymph centre ventral to the fourth through seventh lumbar vertebrae (arrowheads) with amorphous mineralization within the lymph nodes, spiculated periosteal reaction ventral to the adjacent vertebral bodies (arrows) and secondary ventral displacement of the descending colon (white line). Spondylosis deformans associated with the sixth and seventh lumbar vertebrae and the first sacral vertebra is incidental (stars). Diagnosis was metastasis of anal sac gland adenocarcinoma (L = left).

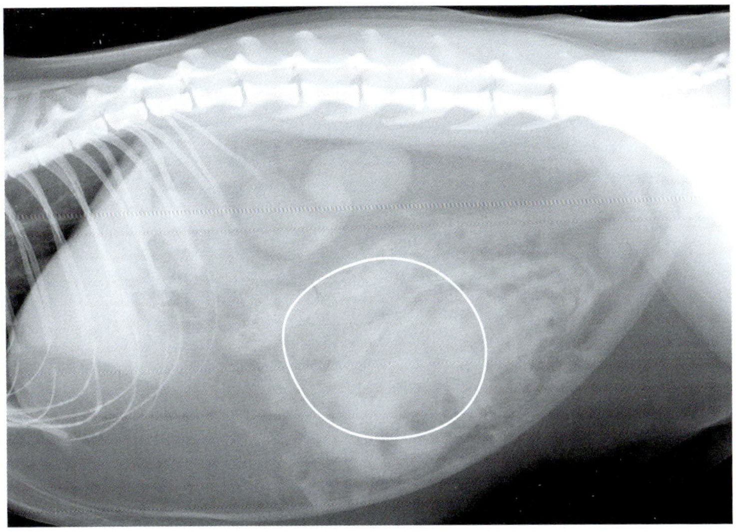

Fig. 12.22 Left lateral view of the abdomen in a cat with mild to moderate enlargement of the mesenteric lymph nodes. A poorly circumscribed soft-tissue opaque region without associated displacement of adjacent intestinal segments is recognized in the mid abdomen (circle). There is streaky loss of serosal margin detail in the adjacent part of the abdomen due to concurrent mild peritoneal effusion. Cytological diagnosis was lymphoma.

feline mast cell tumour, and enteritis/enterocolitis of different aetiologies). Inflammatory disorders generally result in less severe enlargement than neoplastic lesions, and lymph node enlargement is often not recognized on survey radiographs.

In rare cases, enlarged lymph nodes may have **altered radiographic opacity**. This may be seen for example with dystrophic mineralization secondary to lymph node necrosis, or with metastatic mineralization of lymph node metastases (e.g. metastasis from perianal tumours, which may also be associated with periosteal reaction of the adjacent vertebrae and pelvic bones; see Fig. 12.21).

Abdominal ultrasound is more sensitive than radiographs in the identification of lymph nodes that are only slightly enlarged (Fig. 12.23). In addition to assessment of size, structure, shape and echogenicity of the lymph nodes, this technique also allows evaluation of the other abdominal organs and acquisition of ultrasound-guided fine-needle aspirates or biopsies for definitive diagnosis.

12.6 Diseases of the pancreas

The normal pancreas is not usually visible radiographically, and radiographic abnormalities seen with pancreatic disease are not pathognomonic (Frank and Mahaffey 2007; Graham et al. 2007; Owens and Biery 1999).

The appearance of **pancreatic masses** (such as pseudocysts, abscesses, nodular hyperplasia and neoplasia; Fig. 12.24 and 12.25; see also section 11.4) varies with their size and location (right or left lobe of the pancreas, pancreatic body). **Pancreatitis** may also result in mass-like pancreatic enlargement.

Pancreatic tumours include adenomas, adenocarcinomas, insulinomas and, rarely, metastases. Adenocarcinomas are often aggressive and at time of diagnosis have often metastasized to regional lymph nodes, stomach, duodenum or liver. Depending on the size and location of the pancreatic mass, it may interfere with gastric outflow or result in obstruction of the common bile duct and icterus.

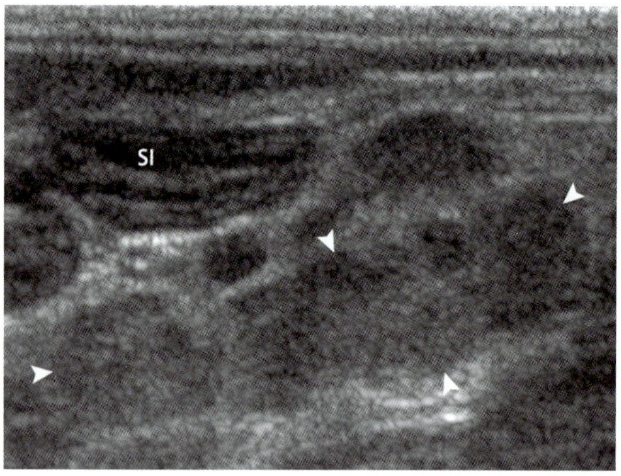

Fig. 12.23 B-Mode ultrasound image of a group of slightly enlarged jejunal lymph nodes (arrowheads). Cytological diagnosis was reactive lymphadenitis. (SI = small intestine)

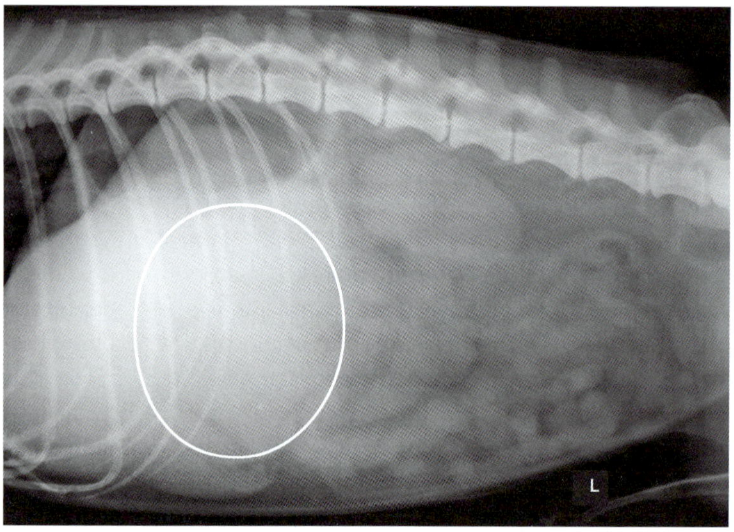

Fig. 12.24 Left lateral radiograph of the abdomen in a dog with pancreatic carcinoma. A region of increased soft-tissue opacity is recognized in the cranial abdomen (circle), the gastric axis and duodenum are not clearly visualized (L = left).

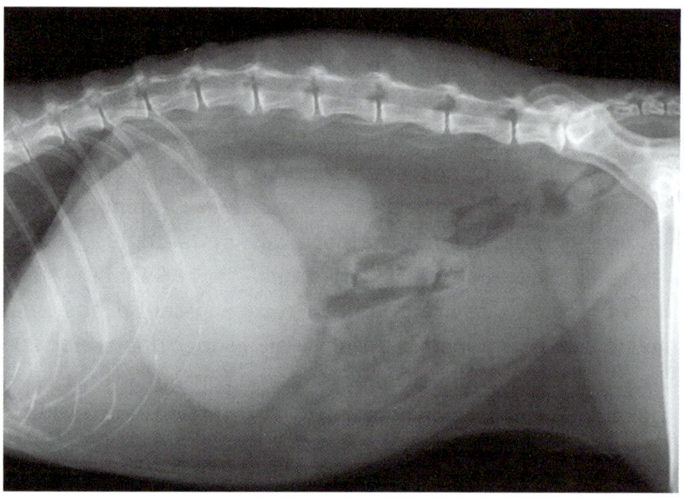

a

Fig. 12.25 Right lateral a and ventrodorsal b radiographs of the abdomen in a cat with pancreatic carcinoma. A large soft-tissue opaque mass is noted in the mid-cranial abdomen which results in cranial displacement of the stomach and caudal displacement of the small intestine. (Courtesy of Dr William H. Adams, University of Tennessee)

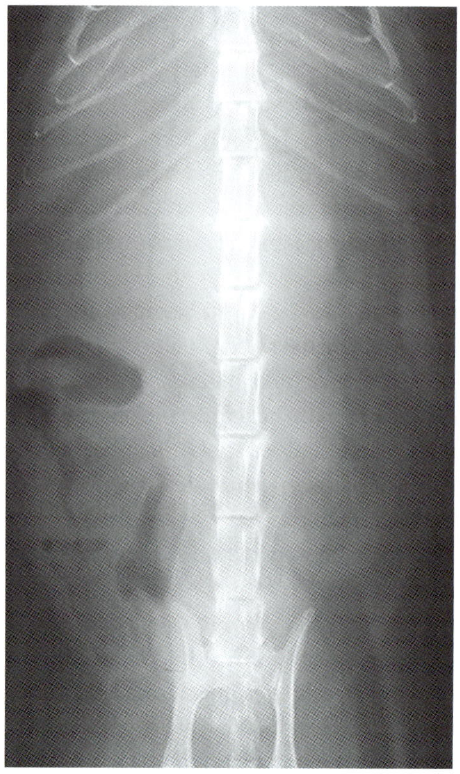

b

RADIOGRAPHIC FINDINGS Masses originating from the right lobe of the pancreas or pancreatic body are most conspicuous on abdominal radiographs. These may result in displacement of the descending duodenum towards the right and of the pyloric antrum towards the left. The associated widening of the gastroduodenal angle and caudal displacement of the transverse colon are best seen on a ventrodorsal view. On a lateral view, dorsal displacement of the duodenum is the most prominent finding. Concurrent abdominal effusion, peritonitis or carcinomatosis lead to loss of serosal margin detail especially in the cranial and mid abdomen.

Clinically, a distinction is made between **acute and chronic pancreatitis**. Radiographically, **chronic pancreatitis** may yield only minor radiographic abnormalities or none at all. With **acute pancreatitis** (with or without associated pancreatic necrosis), focal loss of serosal margin detail in the cranial mid abdomen may be noted due to concurrent abdominal effusion (Fig. 12.26). Additionally, a mass effect similar to that described above for tumours and a rigid, gas-distended duodenum may be noted (Fig. 12.26 and 12.27; Ruaux 2003).

In **cats**, radiographic signs of pancreatitis are even more subtle than in dogs. In some cases, concurrent cholangiohepatitis may result in mild hepatomegaly, or pleural effusion may be noted if the inflammation extends into the thoracic cavity.

As the radiographic findings described here are nonspecific and often very subtle, abdominal ultrasound is indicated in any case where pancreatic disease is of concern.

Ultrasound has a higher sensitivity than abdominal radiographs in the diagnosis of pancreatic abnormalities, especially in dogs and also to a lesser degree in cats. However, even ultrasound findings are often nonspecific, and fine-needle aspirates or biopsies are sometimes needed for a definitive diagnosis (Fig. 12.28 and 12.29; Ruaux 2003).

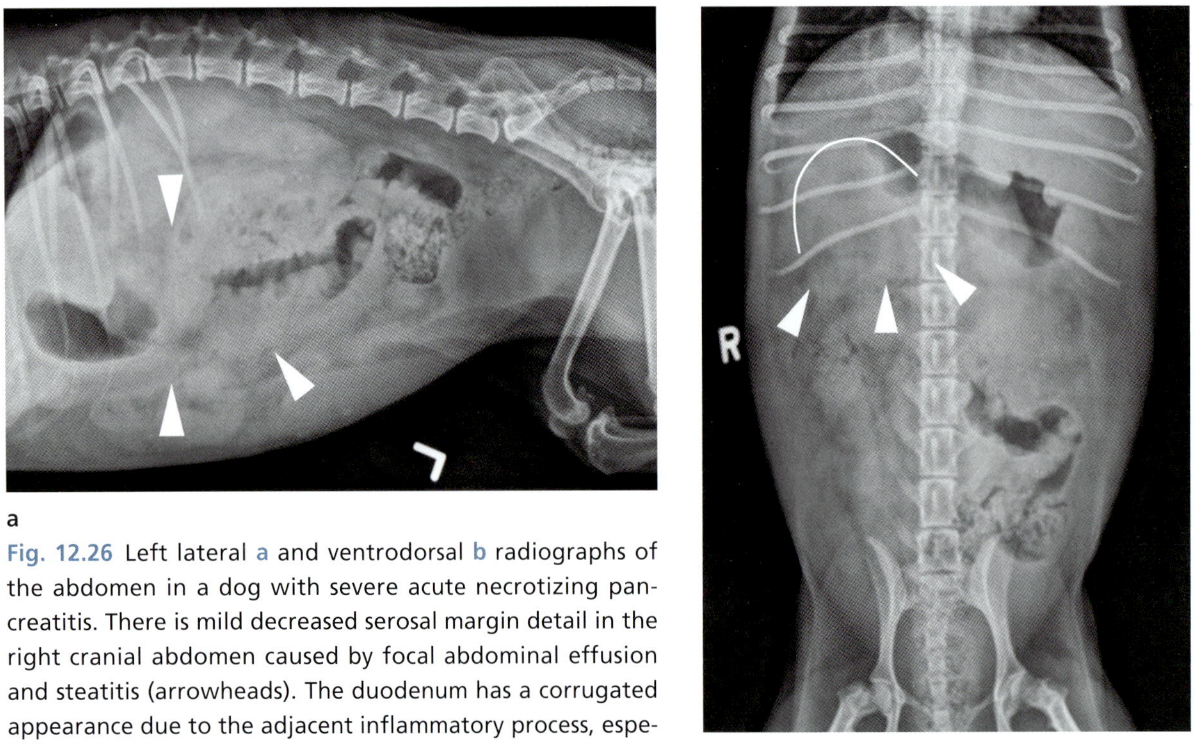

a

b

Fig. 12.26 Left lateral a and ventrodorsal b radiographs of the abdomen in a dog with severe acute necrotizing pancreatitis. There is mild decreased serosal margin detail in the right cranial abdomen caused by focal abdominal effusion and steatitis (arrowheads). The duodenum has a corrugated appearance due to the adjacent inflammatory process, especially seen on the lateral view. The gastroduodenal angle (curved line) is widened and rounded. Despite the severity of the disease process, radiographic changes are rather subtle. Incidental findings in this patient include mineralized foci associated with the kidneys and degenerative joint disease of coxofemoral and stifle joints (L = left; R = right).

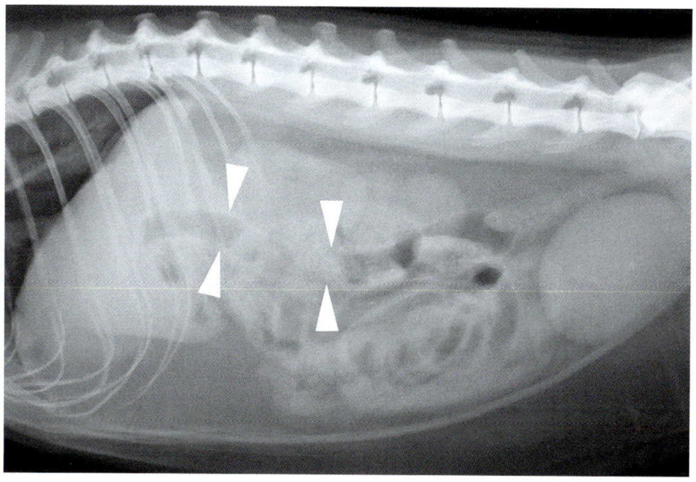

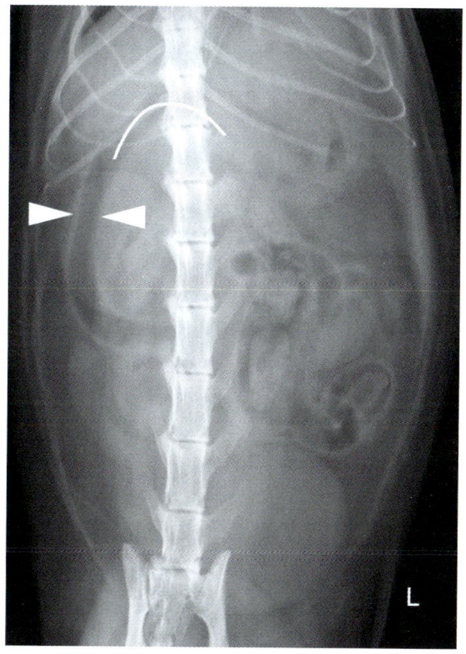

a

b

Fig. 12.27 Left lateral a and ventrodorsal b views of the cranial abdomen in a cat with pancreatitis. The descending duodenum is rigid and gas-filled (arrowheads). The gastroduodenal angle (curved line) is widened.

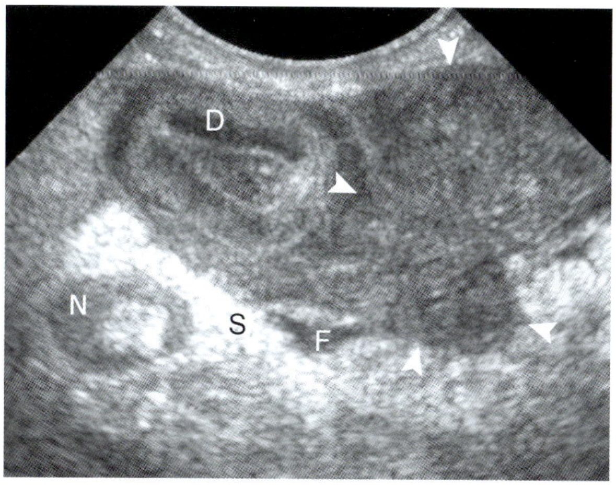

Fig. 12.28 B-mode ultrasound image in a dog with a severely enlarged pancreas characterized by an irregular contour and hypoechoic parenchyma (arrowheads). Additional regional abnormalities include diffusely hyperechoic fat consistent with steatitis (S), mild accumulation of free abdominal fluid (F), a necrotic focus of abdominal fat (N) and dilatation and thickening of the duodenum (D) consistent with duodenitis. Histological diagnosis was pancreatitis.

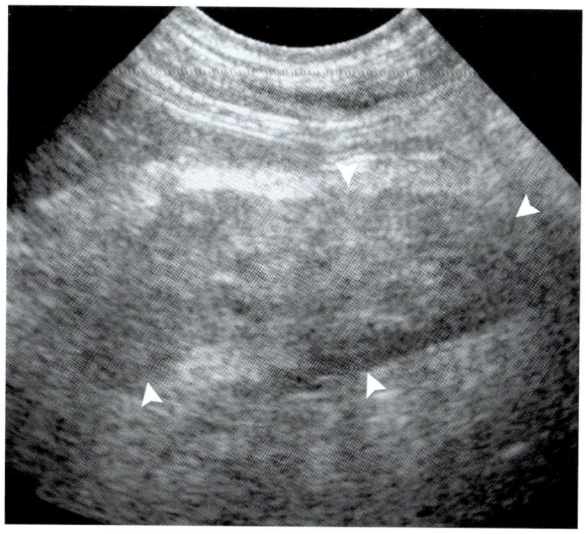

Fig. 12.29 B-mode ultrasound image of the cat shown in Fig. 12.27 with a hypoechoic, mildly patchy and enlarged pancreas, which also has an irregular contour (arrowheads). Histological diagnosis was pancreatitis.

References and further reading

Baldo CF, Garcia-Pereira FL, Nelson NC, Hauptman JG, Shih AC. Effects of anesthetic drugs on canine splenic volume determined via computed tomography. Am J Vet Res 2012; 73(12): 1715–19.

Bezuidenhout AJ. The lymphatic system. In: Evans HE, de Lahunta A (eds). Miller's Anatomy of the Dog. St. Louis: Saunders Elsevier 2013; 535–62.

Frank PM, Mahaffey MB. The peritoneal space. In: Thrall DE (ed.). Textbook of Veterinary Diagnostic Radiology. Philadelphia: WB Saunders 2007; 647–66.

Graham JP, Berry CR, Thrall DE. Interpretation paradigms for the abdomen – canine and feline. In: Thrall DE (ed). Textbook of Veterinary Diagnostic Radiology. Philadelphia: WB Saunders 2007; 626–44.

Moon Larson M. The liver and spleen. In: Thrall DE (ed.). Textbook of Veterinary Diagnostic Radiology. Philadelphia: WB Saunders 2007; 667–92.

Owens JM, Biery DN. Radiographic Interpretation for the Small Animal Clinician. Baltimore: Williams & Wilkins 1999.

Ruaux CG. Diagnostic approaches to acute pancreatitis. Clin Tech Small Anim Pract 2003; 18(4): 245–9.

Santilli RA, Gerboni G. Diagnostic imaging of congenital portosystemic shunts in dogs and cats: a review. Vet J 2003; 166(1): 7–18.

Sonnenfield JM, Armbrust LJ, Radlinsky MA, Chun R, Hoskinson JJ, Kennedy GA. Radiographic and ultrasonographic findings of liver lobe torsion in a dog. Vet Radiol Ultrasound 2001; 42(4): 344–6.

Vollmerhaus B, Roos H. Speiseröhre, Magen, Darm, Darmanhangsdrüsen. In: Frewein J, Gasse H, Leiser R, Roos H, Thomé H, Vollmerhaus B, Waibl H (eds). Lehrbuch der Anatomie der Haustiere. Vol 2. Eingeweide. Stuttgart: Parey Verlag 2004a; 103–213

Vollmerhaus B. Milz. In: Frewein J, Gasse H, Leiser R, Roos H, Thomé H, Vollmerhaus B, Waibl H (eds). Lehrbuch der Anatomie der Haustiere. Vol 2. Eingeweide. Stuttgart: Parey Verlag 2004b; 215–22.

Vollmerhaus B. Lymphatisches System. In: Habermehl KH, Vollmerhaus B, Wilkens H, Waibl H (eds). Lehrbuch der Anatomie der Haustiere. Vol 3. Kreislaufsystem, Haut und Hautorgane, 4th edn. Stuttgart: Parey Verlag 2005; 276–374.

Weber NA. Chronic primary splenic torsion with peritoneal adhesions in a dog: Case report and literature review. J Am Vet Med Assoc 2000; 36, 390–4.

13

Digestive tract (including contrast procedures)

Silke Hecht and William H. Adams

13.1 Anatomy and indications

13.1.1 Anatomy

The radiographic evaluation of the digestive tract includes the cervical and thoracic oesophagus as well as stomach, small and large intestine. An example of normal radiographic abdominal gastrointestinal anatomy can be found in Figure 13.1. As survey radiographs are of limited value for evaluation of many gastrointestinal tract lesions, advanced imaging procedures (ultrasound, contrast studies and increasingly computed tomography; CT) are often needed for further evaluation. This chapter will cover the normal anatomy of the digestive tract and contrast procedures.

Oesophagus

The cervical oesophagus extends from the larynx to the thoracic inlet. Within the thorax, the oesophagus is located within the mediastinum dorsal and to the left of the trachea. It enters the abdominal cavity at the oesophageal hiatus and connects to the stomach. The oesophagus is usually not visible on survey thoracic radiographs. However, a small amount of intraluminal gas or fluid is a common physiological finding (Fig. 13.2).

Stomach

The stomach is located in the cranial abdomen and is in close contact with the liver, pancreas, spleen and small intestine. The fundus (left dorsal), body and pylorus (including antrum; right ventral) can be distinguished radi-

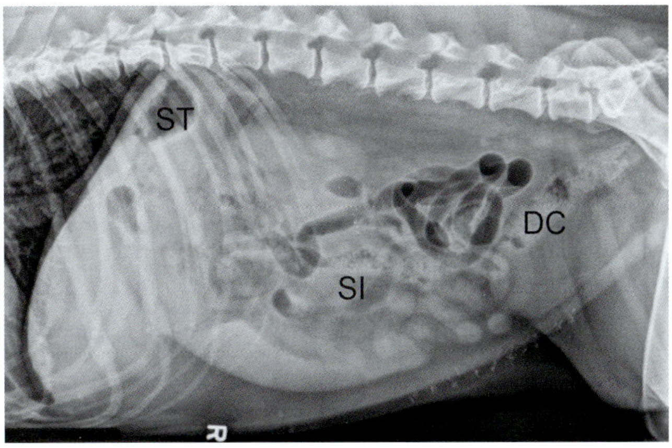

a

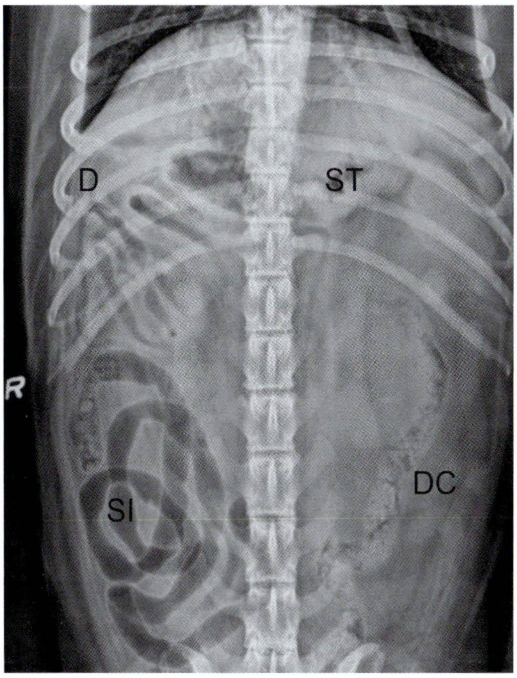

b

Fig. 13.1 Lateral **a** and ventrodorsal **b** abdominal radiographs in a normal dog. The location of various gastrointestinal tract segments is indicated (ST = stomach, D = descending duodenum, SI = small intestine, DC = descending colon). The caecum is not clearly visible. The stomach only contains a small amount of gas (R = right).

ographically. The appearance of the stomach is extremely variable and dependent on multiple factors (species, breed, degree of distention, contents, patient positioning and abnormalities of adjacent structures) as follows.

- The stomach in dogs extends into both the left and right abdomen while it is located mostly to the left of the midline in cats (Fig. 13.3).
- While the stomach in deep-chested dogs is often completely contained within the costal arch, it often extends beyond that level in shallow-chested breeds.
- Gastric position is significantly influenced by gastric contents (Fig. 13.4).
- Due to redistribution of luminal contents with gravity, the pylorus contains fluid on a right lateral view and gas on a left lateral view (Fig. 13.5).
- Abnormalities of adjacent organs (e.g. hepatomegaly or masses originating from the pancreas) commonly affect the position and appearance of the stomach due to displacement or, less often, invasion.

A fluid-filled pylorus appears as a round soft-tissue opacity structure in the cranioventral abdomen on a right lateral view. This should not be confused with a foreign body or abdominal mass.

Evaluation of gastric wall thickness is often not possible on survey radiographs due to silhouetting with intraluminal contents (ingesta or fluid) or extraluminal soft-tissue opaque structures.

Small intestine

The small intestine is formed by the duodenum, jejunum and ileum. The descending **duodenum** originates from the pylorus and extends along the right abdominal wall (dog) or paramedian (cat) caudally to the duodenal flexure. The ascending duodenum connects to the jejunum. The descending duodenum is the only small intestinal segment that can usually be identified confidently on survey radiographs due to its connection

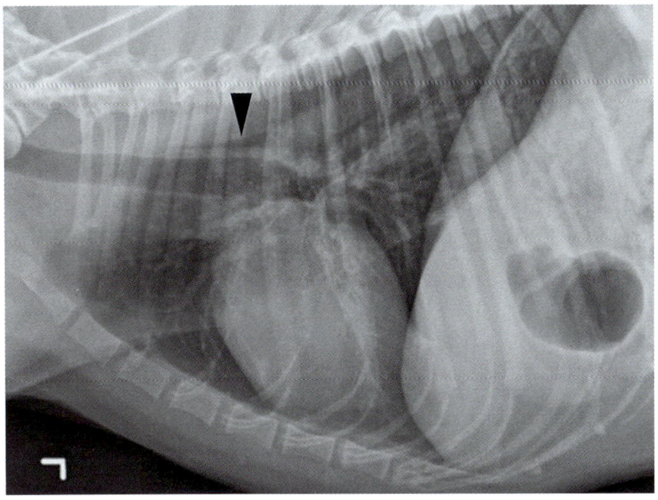

Fig. 13.2 Normal oesophagus in a dog. A small amount of intraluminal gas seen dorsal to the trachea allows identification of the oesophagus (arrowhead), which is otherwise not visible (L = left).

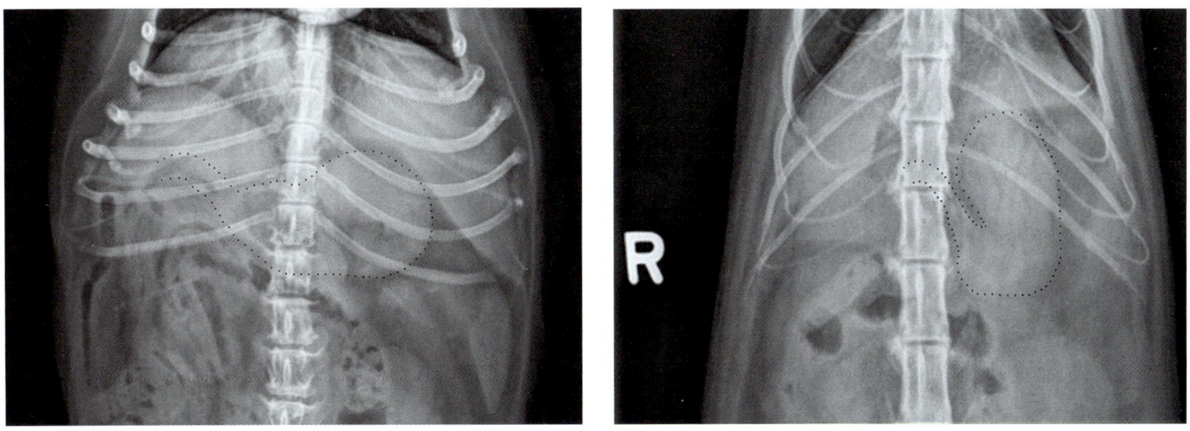

a b

Fig. 13.3 Illustration of species-specific differences in gastric position on ventrodorsal abdominal radiographs. The outer gastric margin is outlined by small dots. The stomach extends into the left and right abdomen in dogs a and is located almost entirely to the left of the midline in cats b.

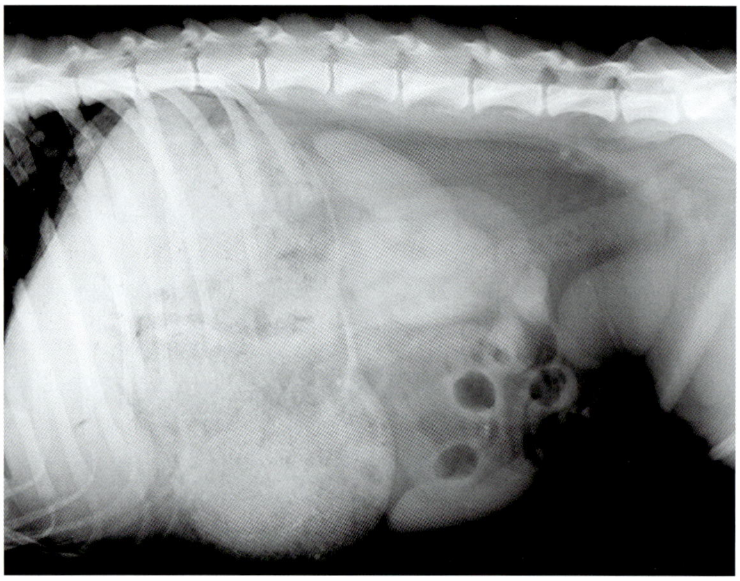

Fig. 13.4 Effect of luminal contents on gastric position. In contrast to the dog shown in Fig. 13.1, the stomach in this dog is distended with granular ingesta and extends beyond the costal arch.

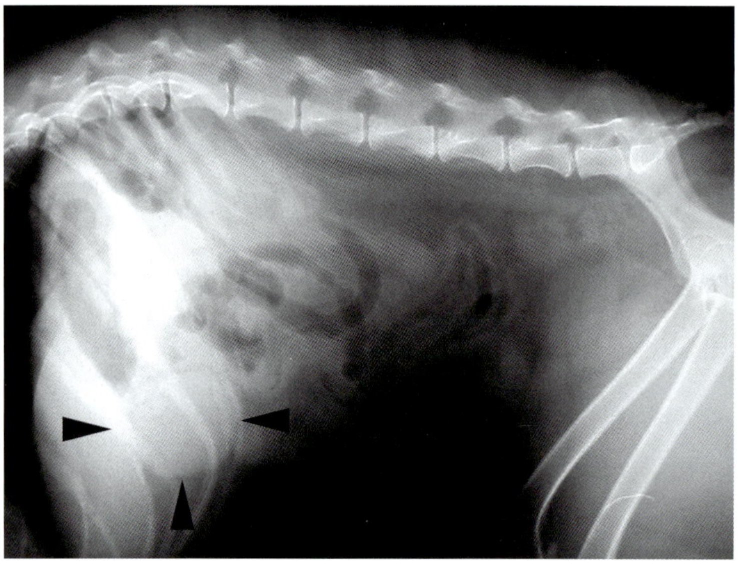

a

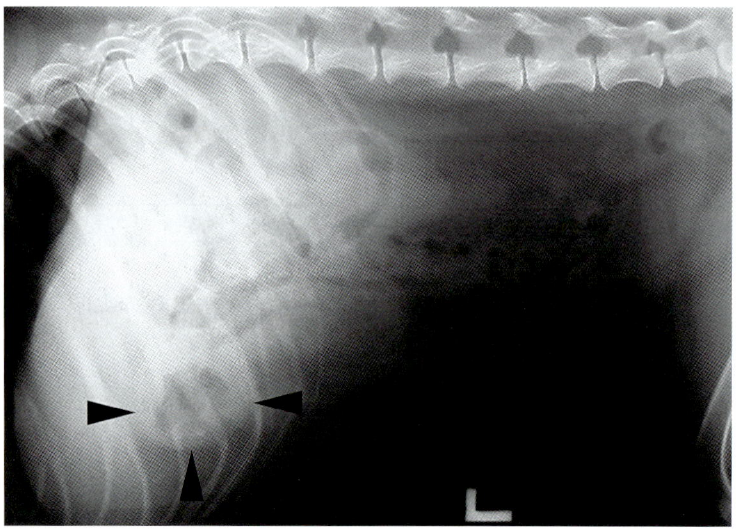

b

Fig. 13.5 Physiological change in radiographic appearance of the stomach based on positioning.

a On the right lateral view, the pylorus contains fluid and appears as a homogeneous circular structure with soft-tissue opacity in the cranioventral abdomen (arrowheads). This should not be confused with a foreign body or tumour.

b On the left lateral view, the pylorus contains gas (arrowheads). (L = left)

to the stomach and consistent position on a ventrodorsal view. It may contain gas and be visible on a left lateral view. However, redistribution of luminal contents with intraluminal fluid accumulation within the descending duodenum on a right lateral view hampers identification.

The **jejunum** is highly variable in position and often occupies most of the peritoneal cavity. In obese cats there is a tendency for small intestine to accumulate in the right mid abdomen, which should not be confused with intestinal plication ('bunching') caused by a linear foreign body.

The **ileum** connects the jejunum and large intestine and is not visualized as a separate structure on plain radiographs.

Small intestinal diameter is somewhat variable. Several publications report a normal small intestinal diameter in dogs and cats, either as an absolute value or in relation to other structures.

- The small intestinal diameter in **dogs** should not exceed twice the diameter of a rib, 1.6 times the height of the fifth lumbar vertebral body on a lateral view, or the width of a lumbar vertebral body on a ventrodorsal view.
- The small intestinal diameter should not exceed 12 mm in **cats**.

It is important to note that radiographic diagnosis of pathological **intestinal dilatation** is challenging and to some degree subjective, and that a diagnosis especially of partial intestinal obstruction may require additional imaging.

The appearance of the small intestine is not only influenced by position and diameter but also by intestinal contents. The intestinal lumen may be empty or contain gas and/or fluid. While a larger proportion of small intestinal segments in dogs tends to contain gas, the intestine in cats is usually mostly empty or contains fluid.

The small intestine should not typically contain **radiopaque ingesta**, as the pylorus functions as a filter and limits transition of solid particles from the stomach into the intestine. However, small opaque 'foreign bodies' such as sand, bone fragments and small rocks within the small intestine are common, especially in dogs, and are usually an incidental finding.

Small intestinal wall thickness cannot be reliably evaluated on survey radiographs due to the physiological presence of gas and fluid within the lumen and the distribution of intraluminal contents with gravity. Gas rises to the nondependent part of a small intestinal loop and forms a 'bubble', while fluid accumulates in the dependent portion. Intraluminal fluid silhouettes with the intestinal wall on radiographs, mimicking intestinal wall thickening (Fig. 13.6).

Silhouetting of intraluminal fluid with the intestinal wall can mimic wall thickening. Assessment of intestinal wall thickness on plain abdominal radiographs is usually not possible.

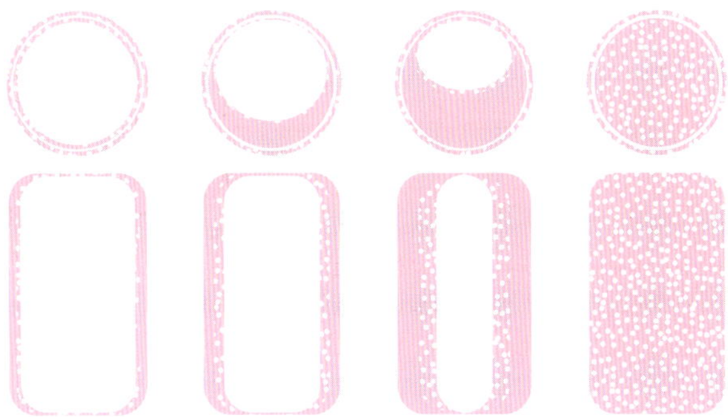

1 2 3 4

a

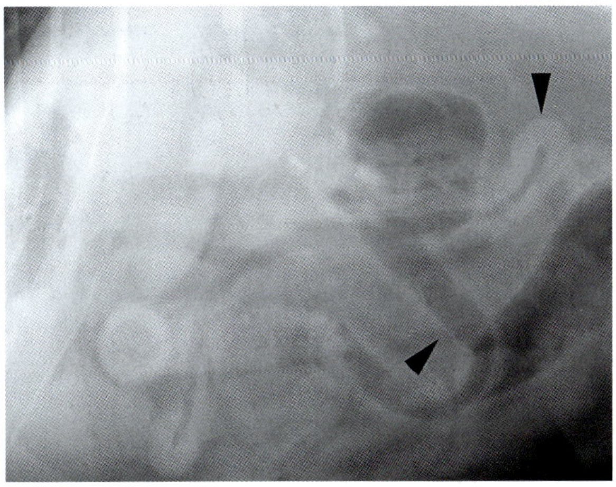

b

Fig. 13.6 Effect of intraluminal gas and fluid on appearance of the intestinal wall.

a The schematic drawing illustrates how the presence of intraluminal fluid may mimic thickening of the intestinal wall. The top row shows cross-sectional images of gas and/or fluid-filled intestinal segments. The bottom row illustrates the appearance of these intestinal segments on radiographs. (1) The wall of an intestinal segment containing only gas appears thin. (4) A completely fluid-filled intestinal segment is of homogeneous soft-tissue opacity with no visible walls. (2, 3) The presence of both fluid and gas within the lumen may give the impression of variable wall thickening.

b Detail of a lateral abdominal radiograph in a normal dog. Jejunal segments contain variable proportions of gas and fluid, resulting in the impression of differences in wall thickness (arrowheads).

Large intestine

The large intestine consists of the caecum, colon and rectum. The **caecum** marks the border between the small and large intestine. It is often seen as a corkscrew-shaped gas-filled structure in the right craniodorsal abdomen in dogs (Fig. 13.7). It is not usually visible in cats owing to the small size of the comma-shaped organ in this species.

The **colon** has three components: the ascending colon is located in the right cranial abdomen; the transverse colon is located caudal and parallel to the stomach; and the descending colon extends caudally along the left abdominal wall. The course of the colon resembles a question mark on the ventrodorsal view (Fig. 13.7b).

The border between the colon and **rectum** is not radiographically visible and is located approximately at the pelvic inlet or within the pelvic canal.

The radiographic appearance of the colon varies with its contents. In normal animals, it may be empty or contain gas or formed faecal material. The large intestine is distensible, and a radiographic diagnosis of pathological dilatation may be difficult. As a rule of thumb, **colonic diameter** should not be wider than 1.5 times the length of the seventh lumbar vertebral body. The large intestinal wall is thin and cannot usually be distinguished from intraluminal faecal matter. With fluid in the large intestinal lumen (in patients with diarrhoea), the radiographic evaluation of wall thickness is limited, in a similar manner to that described above for the small intestine.

13.1.2 Indications

Indications for a radiographic examination of the gastrointestinal tract overlap with general indications for radiographic evaluation of the abdomen. Clinical signs that may be seen with gastrointestinal disorders include:

- vomiting
- regurgitation
- diarrhoea
- inappetence
- abdominal pain
- distended abdomen
- haematemesis
- melena
- weight loss.

13.2 Radiographic technique and positioning

Information on radiographic technique and positioning for general abdominal radiography can be found in Chapter 11. This chapter will provide an overview of commonly used contrast procedures for the digestive tract, and some that are used less often.

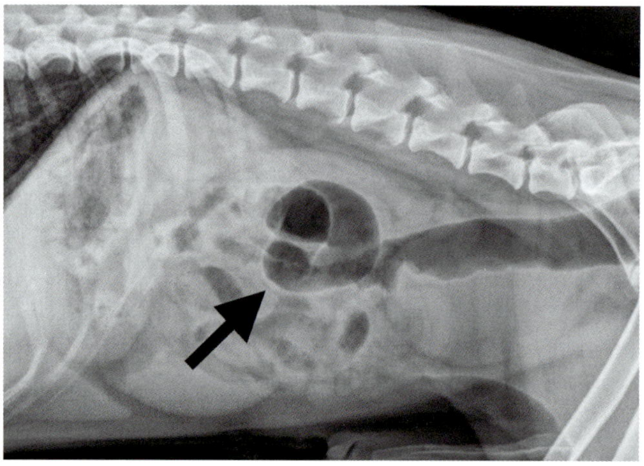

a

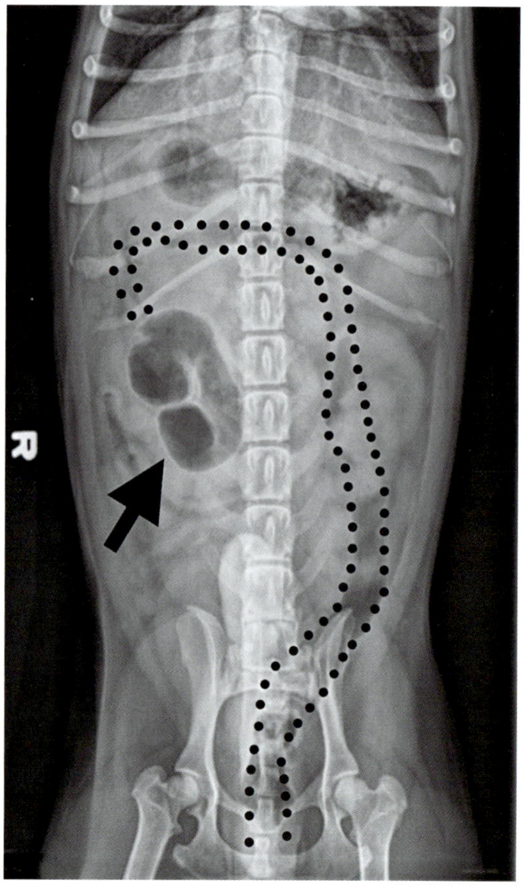

Fig. 13.7 Lateral a and ventrodorsal b abdominal radiographs in a normal dog. The caecum appears as a gas-filled corkscrew-shaped structure in the right cranial to mid abdomen (arrow). The course of the colon and rectum (dotted lines) resembles a question mark on the ventrodorsal view. b

As described in section 13.1.1, survey radiographs are of limited value in the evaluation of the gastrointestinal tract. They do not usually allow assessment of wall thickness, mucosal lesions, infiltrative diseases and intestinal motility. Even intraluminal foreign bodies or mural mass lesions such as tumours may not be recognized on plain radiographs unless they are very large, radiopaque and/or result in complete intestinal obstruction. Oesophagography remains an excellent procedure for evaluation of the oesophagus. Other contrast studies of the gastrointestinal tract have lost popularity due to increasing availability of and expertise in ultrasonography and endoscopy of the gastrointestinal tract. However, they remain valuable in the evaluation of motility disorders or when ultrasound and/or endoscopy are unavailable.

13.2.1 Introduction

There are three basic types of contrast procedures:

- positive contrast studies
- negative contrast studies
- double contrast studies.

Positive contrast studies are most commonly used in the evaluation of the small animal digestive tract. Positive contrast media contain elements with a high atomic number (barium or iodine). These materials have increased X-ray absorption compared to surrounding structures and appear metal opaque on radiographs. A summary of the most commonly used contrast media is found in Table 13.1.

Contrast media for **negative contrast studies** include room air or CO_2. These gaseous materials result in decreased absorption of X-rays compared to surrounding structures and thus are of gas opacity on the resultant radiographs. One disadvantage of negative contrast studies of the gastrointestinal tract is inability to distinguish gas administered as a contrast medium from gas naturally present in the gastrointestinal tract. Additionally, loss of negative contrast medium through 'vomiting' or 'defecation' cannot be detected. For those reasons, negative contrast studies of the digestive tract are limited to the identification of the position of the stomach or colon.

Double contrast studies allow evaluation of the mucosal surface and the diagnosis of mural or intraluminal lesions of the stomach and colon/rectum (foreign bodies, strictures, tumours, ulcers etc.). The administration of positive contrast medium (optimally, barium sulphate suspension due to its excellent mucosal coating properties) is followed by instillation of gas.

A summary of contrast procedures available for evaluation of different sections of the digestive tract can be found in Table 13.2.

13.2.2 Oesophagography

This contrast procedure may aid in the evaluation of swallowing disorders, regurgitation, and mediastinal masses seen on survey radiographs. The procedure should optimally be performed under fluoroscopy as a diagnosis of functional abnormalities (e.g. cricopharyngeal dyssynchrony, oesophageal motility disorders) and intermittent lesions (e.g. sliding hiatal hernia) is only possible in real time. Fluoroscopic oesophagography using a horizontal beam is the best technique to mimic and evaluate physiological swallowing (Fig. 13.8) but is not feasible in most veterinary practices due to the need for specialized equipment. Additionally, like any horizontal beam technique, horizontal beam oesophagography results in an increased radiation dose to the examiner and should be limited to cases where a diagnosis cannot be established by other means. In many oesophageal disorders (e.g. foreign body or vascular ring anomaly), a diagnosis can be made by means of two-view thoracic radiographs obtained after contrast medium administration. In these cases, radiographic oesophagography becomes a feasible and useful diagnostic tool for small animal practitioners.

Material

The following material is needed.

- Syringes (number and size depend on the size of the animal and the indication).
- Positive contrast medium (typically barium sulphate suspension ± paste, less commonly iodinated contrast media).
- Canned food ± kibble mixed with positive contrast medium.

The choice of contrast medium depends on the indication for the study. In many instances, the examination has to be performed several times using different contrast materials in the same patient.

- The mucosal surface is best evaluated using barium sulphate suspension or paste.
- Some oesophageal diseases may affect the passage of liquid differently than the passage of solid food. For example, liquid barium suspension may easily pass an oesophageal stricture, while partial oesophageal obstruction will become evident when kibble coated with barium is administered.

With suspicion of oesophageal perforation, iodinated contrast medium is given preference over barium suspension. However, iodinated contrast media should otherwise be avoided due to their poor mucosal coating abilities and often bitter taste. Additionally, some iodinated contrast agents are hyperosmolar, which may result in pulmonary oedema if aspiration occurs during the procedure.

Table 13.1 Overview of contrast media used for evaluation of the digestive tract. (Modified from Hecht 2004a)

Contrast medium	Advantages	Disadvantages	Applications
Barium sulphate suspension	Established reference values for normal gastrointestinal (GI) transit times Good contrast Excellent delineation of the mucosal margin Remains in suspension Physiologically inert and not osmotically active No dilution within the gastrointestinal tract Affordable	Aspiration may result in pneumonia or pulmonary granulomas. Should be administered with a tube if possible (aspiration of a small amount usually clinically insignificant) May cause granulomas or adhesions in mediastinum or peritoneal cavity (should not be used with suspected perforation) Should not be used immediately prior to endoscopy	Contrast medium of choice for most examinations of the digestive tract: Oesophagram (administration as liquid, paste and mixed with food) Gastrogram (positive or double contrast study) Upper GI contrast study Colonogram (positive or double contrast study)
Barium sulphate powder	Cheap	Has to be mixed with fluid prior to use Flocculation Limited evaluation of mucosa	Not recommended
BIPS (barium impregnated polyethylene spheres)	Barium impregnated markers of a defined size and administered in a defined number Administration with food possible Established reference values for normal GI transit times	Do not allow evaluation of mucosal surface	Suspected ileus Assessment of GI transit times Generally inferior to barium sulphate suspension
Ionic iodinated contrast media	Rapid GI transit times Do not result in severe complications following leakage into the mediastinum or peritoneal cavity	Unpredictable GI transit times Inadequate mucosal coating Hypertonic water is drawn into intestinal lumen; may cause patient dehydration Causes pulmonary oedema with aspiration and should not be given orally! May be absorbed into the blood stream and excreted through the kidneys	Upper GI contrast study performed immediately prior to endoscopy Upper GI contrast study or oesophagram in cases of suspected perforation
Nonionic iodinated contrast media	Rapid GI transit times Do not result in severe complications following aspiration, leakage into the mediastinum or peritoneal cavity Low osmolarity no dilution in GI tract No negative side effects for patient Very safe	Expensive Inadequate coating of the mucosal surface	Upper GI contrast study performed immediately prior to endoscopy Upper GI contrast study or oesophagram in cases of suspected perforation High-risk patients

Table 13.2 Overview of contrast studies of the digestive tract and indications.

Contrast study	Indications	Figures
Oesophagram ('barium swallow')	Regurgitation Swallowing disorders; inability or reluctance to swallow liquid and/or solid food Abnormal findings on thoracic radiographs such as mediastinal mass lesions or abnormal amount or distribution of oesophageal intraluminal gas	13.8, 13.18, 13.20
Gastrogram	Localization of the stomach, e.g. with suspected diaphragmatic rupture or with cranial abdominal mass lesions of undetermined origin and aetiology Suspected gastric foreign body Evaluation of the gastric mucosa, e.g. with suspected neoplasia or ulcer	13.12, 13.28, 13.30
Upper GI contrast study	Evaluate position of the gastrointestinal tract Vomiting Diarrhoea Weight loss Melena Abdominal masses of undetermined origin	13.11, 13.13, 13.14, 13.27, 13.38
Colonogram	Determine position of colon and rectum Diarrhoea Tenesmus Suspected/possible intussusception Melena	13.15, 13.40

Modified from Hecht (2004a, 2004b).

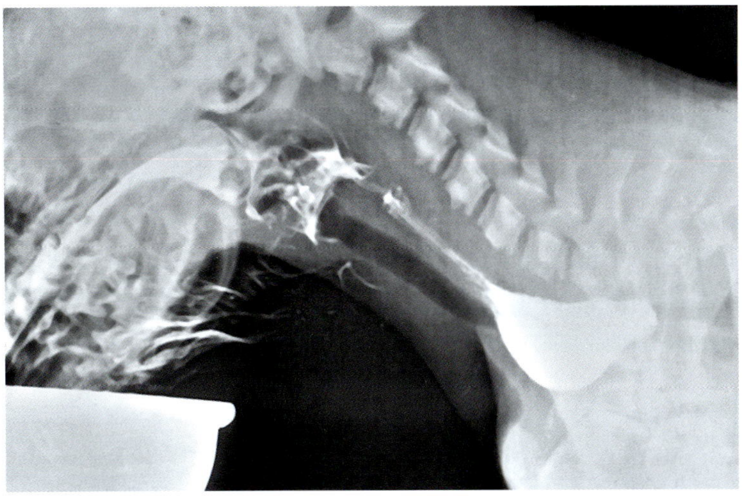

Fig. 13.8 Horizontal beam oesophagram (barium swallow) in a young dog. Positive contrast medium (barium sulphate suspension) outlines the oral cavity, pharynx and oesophagus. (From Hecht 2004a)

The contrast medium dose is highly variable and depends on patient size, indication and the presence, type and location of the lesion. A rough starting point may be a dose of 5–20 ml; however, this may have to be increased.

Procedure

Unless it is an emergency, the patient should be fasted for 12–24 hours. Water can be offered during this time.

If possible, the procedure should be performed without sedation, as sedative drugs affect oesophageal motility and may cause relaxation of the gastro-oesophageal sphincter, which increases the risk for gastro-oesophageal reflux and aspiration pneumonia. If sedation is unavoidable, a small dose of acepromazine may be administered (e.g. 0.05 mg/kg).

Following survey radiographs of the neck and thorax (opposite lateral and ventrodorsal views), contrast medium is administered as follows:

- liquid contrast medium (approximately 5–20 ml)
- barium paste
- canned food mixed with positive contrast medium ('barium burger')
- kibble mixed with positive contrast medium.

Each swallowing episode is either monitored by means of fluoroscopy, or a lateral radiograph is acquired. Ventrodorsal views are usually acquired in a mildly oblique fashion to avoid superimposition of the oesophagus with the spine. In some cases (e.g. oesophageal foreign body), a diagnosis is possible after the first phase, and the procedure can be aborted. In other instances, individual phases of the procedure may have to be repeated to fully evaluate mild or questionable abnormalities. The procedure should be aborted if marked resistance of the patient to the examination or dyspnoea are noted, in order to minimize a risk of contrast medium aspiration.

Regardless of the results of the contrast study, thoracic radiographs should be obtained following the procedure to rule out aspiration of contrast medium.

Interpretation

Following successful initiation of swallowing, contrast medium rapidly reaches the stomach. While the oesophagus in normal dogs exhibits longitudinal striations due to mucosal folds (Fig. 13.9a), the caudal third of the feline oesophagus is characterized by a 'herring bone' pattern (Fig. 13.9b). Abnormal findings during the study may include focal or generalized oesophageal dilatation, filling defects (e.g. due to tumours or intraluminal foreign bodies), stenosis, mucosal defects or leakage of contrast medium due to perforation. These abnormalities are covered under oesophageal diseases (see section 13.3).

Possible complications

Aspiration of contrast medium usually results from hasty contrast medium administration or from the patient's inability to swallow the material. Aspiration of a very small amount of barium sulphate suspension usually has no significant consequences; however, aspiration of a large amount of barium sulphate suspension or of a hypertonic iodinated contrast medium may be lethal (Fig. 13.10).

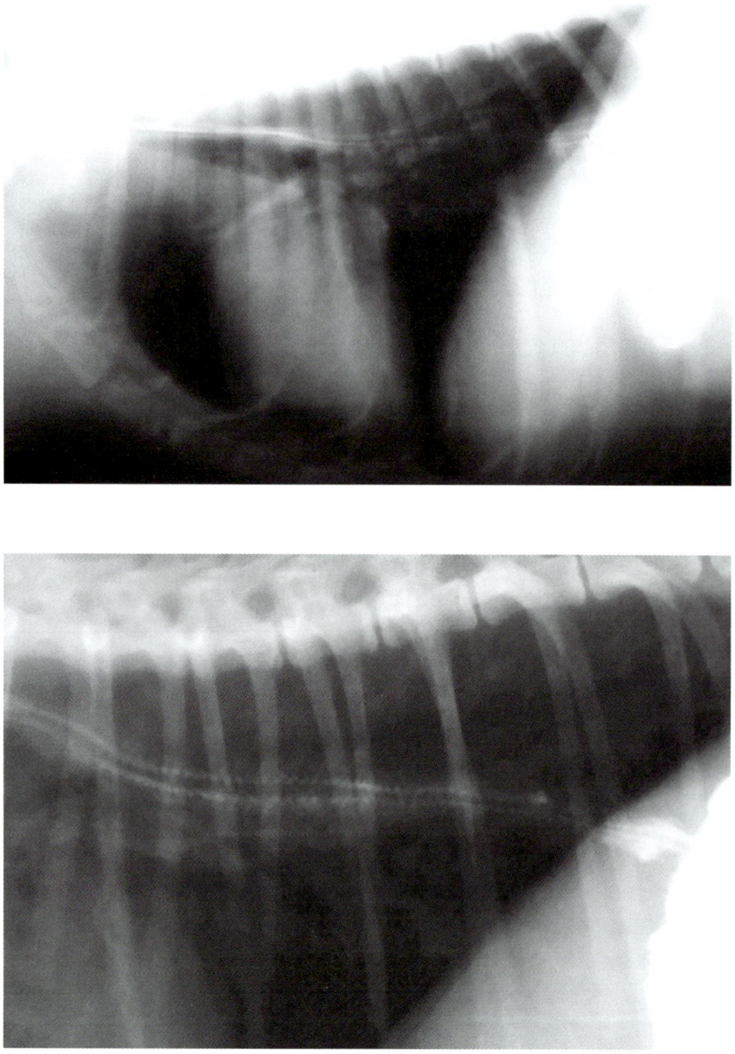

a

b

Fig. 13.9 Species differences on a normal oesophagram.
a Normal oesophagram in a dog. Longitudinal mucosal folds are a normal finding in this species. (Courtesy of Tufts Cummings School of Veterinary Medicine)
b Normal oesophagram in a cat. The caudal third of the oesophageal mucosa has a characteristic herring bone appearance, which should not be confused with oesophagitis. (Courtesy of Tufts Cummings School of Veterinary Medicine)

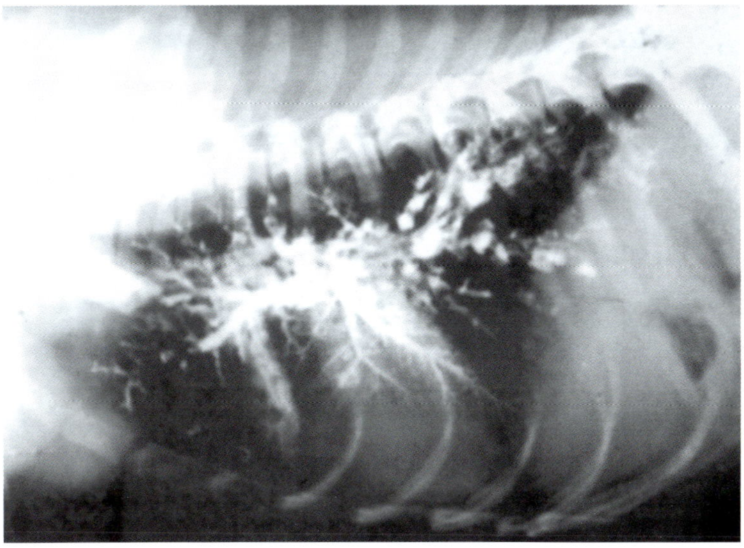

Fig. 13.10 Aspiration of a large amount of barium sulphate suspension. Positive contrast medium outlines the bronchial tree, smaller airways and part of the pulmonary parenchyma in this dog. (From Hecht 2004a)

Even though mediastinal infection due to leakage of food and other contaminants is probably more harmful to a patient with **oesophageal perforation** than the leakage of contrast medium, the contrast procedure should be avoided or performed with iodinated contrast media if an oesophageal tear is suspected.

13.2.3 Contrast examination of the stomach and small intestine

A dedicated contrast examination of the stomach is referred to as '**gastrogram**', while the examination of stomach and small intestine is typically referred to as '**upper gastrointestinal (GI) contrast study**'.

Indications include:

- determination of the position of gastrointestinal tract segments (e.g. with poor serosal detail due to ascites)
- vomiting
- diarrhoea
- abdominal mass lesions
- melena
- haematemesis
- weight loss
- abdominal pain
- assessment of gastrointestinal motility.

There are few **contraindications** for a contrast examination of the gastrointestinal tract. These include definitive radiographic evidence of gastrointestinal obstruction or perforation, and incessant vomiting.

Motility of the gastrointestinal tract, gastric emptying time and gastrointestinal transit time are variable and depend on multiple factors. As gastrointestinal passage of liquid contrast medium is different from solid ingesta, studies have been performed to investigate if solid markers impregnated with contrast medium ('**barium impregnated polyethylene spheres**'; **BIPS**) allow more accurate assessment of gastrointestinal motility. However, as this method proved to be inferior to the traditional gold standard of scintigraphy for the diagnosis of subtle motility disorders, it will not be discussed further in this chapter.

Double contrast gastrography is a special technique used for evaluation of gastric mucosa. Following initial administration of a small amount of barium sulphate suspension (approximately 2 ml/kg), the stomach is filled with air. This procedure is rarely used in practice and is inferior to endoscopy.

The **contrast medium** of choice for routine upper GI contrast studies is barium sulphate suspension. Ionic or non-ionic iodinated contrast agents should only be used in case of suspected gastrointestinal perforation or immediately before endoscopy. Following contrast medium administration, radiographs are obtained on a regular basis to evaluate the passage of contrast medium through the gastrointestinal tract. If fluoroscopy is available, intermittent fluoroscopic assessment of gastrointestinal motility may be performed, depending on clinical suspicion and initial findings.

Material

The following material is needed.

- Syringe(s).
- Orogastric tube (and mouth gag) or nasogastric tube (and liquid local anaesthetic) and lube. Contrast medium should always be administered via a tube to minimize risk of aspiration and assure administration of a sufficient amount of contrast medium. This is especially important in patients notoriously resistant to oral administration of liquids (cats!). The length of the tube is estimated before the procedure by measuring the distance from the nares to the costal arch.

Correct placement within the stomach can be verified by means of palpation, auscultation (blowing into the tube should result in a bubbly sound) or a radiograph.

- Positive contrast medium.
  - Barium sulphate suspension: 5 ml/kg (large dogs) to 15 ml/kg (small dogs and cats).
  - Ionic iodinated contrast media: 2–3 ml/kg (undiluted).
  - Nonionic iodinated contrast media: 10 ml/kg (1:2 or 1:3 dilution).
- Possibly a radiolucent compression device. This is a wooden or plastic (Plexiglas) stirring spoon or paddle which may aid in separation of small intestinal segments filled with contrast medium from a lesion. Gentle pressure over the area of interest displaces intestinal segments peripherally and allows visualization of a foreign body, tumour or other (obstructive) lesion (Fig. 13.11).

Procedure

1. Patient preparation (except in emergency cases).
   - Fasting for 24 hours with free access to water.
   - If necessary, enema 2–4 hours prior to contrast medium administration.
   - If necessary, emptying of urinary bladder.
2. Sedation or anaesthesia should be avoided if possible as they affect gastrointestinal tract motility. If necessary, use of the following protocols has been advocated.
   - Dog:
     - acepromazine 0.02–0.1 mg/kg s.c., i.m. or i.v. (3 mg maximum) ± butorphanol 0.05 mg/kg s.c., i.m. or i.v. (4.5 mg maximum).
   - Cat:
     - ketamine 2.7 mg/kg + acepromazine 0.05 mg/kg i.m.
     - or ketamine 5.5 mg/kg
     - or ketamine 2.7 mg/kg + diazepam 0.1 mg/kg.

   Note that assessment of gastric emptying time or gastrointestinal transit time may not be possible at all or may be limited in a sedated patient.
3. Opposite lateral and ventrodorsal survey radiographs.
4. Contrast medium administration via orogastric or nasogastric tube (contrast medium dose listed above).
5. The radiographic protocol following contrast medium administration can be found in Table 13.3.

Evaluation

EVALUATION OF MOTILITY AND TRANSIT TIMES As mentioned above, assessment of gastrointestinal motility by means of an upper GI contrast study has limitations. On fluoroscopic examination, there should be **three to five symmetric gastric contractions per minute**. **Regular peristaltic waves** should be noted throughout the small intestine. **Gastrointestinal motility** is not only affected by pathological processes but also medications and other factors such as stress. As a rule of thumb, gastric emptying time should be approximately 1–4 hours, and contrast medium should have vacated the small intestine after 5 hours (dog) and 3 hours (cat), respectively. **Delayed transit times** may indicate a functional problem (functional ileus) or an intestinal obstruction (mechanical ileus). **Intestinal atony** occurring after long-standing intestinal obstruction may be indistinguishable from a paralytic ileus. **Decreased transit times** may, for example, be noted with hyperperistalsis due to acute gastroenteritis.

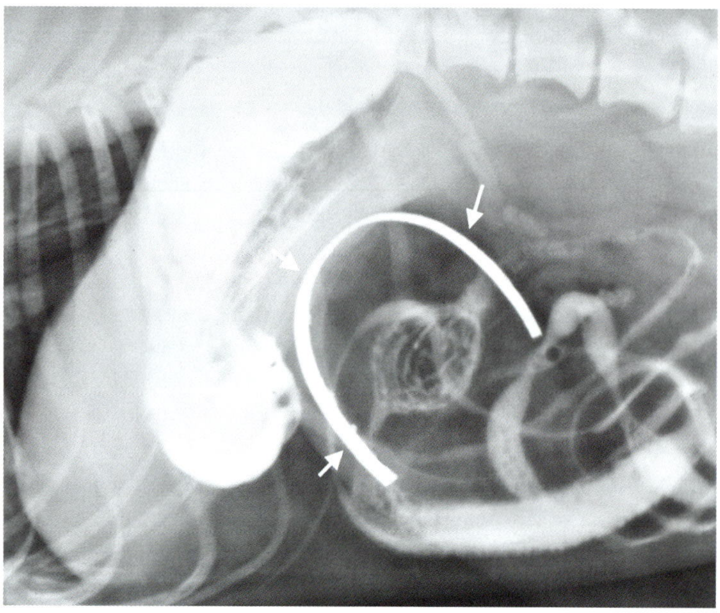

Fig. 13.11 Application of abdominal pressure for improved visualization of an intestinal foreign body. Positive contrast medium adheres to the rough surface of an intraluminal structure (peach pit). Contrast medium passes the foreign body with only minor intestinal dilatation proximal to the lesion, consistent with incomplete/partial obstruction. On initial radiographs (not shown), intestinal segments filled with contrast medium were superimposed with the foreign body, hampering identification. A wooden spoon with a metallic rim (arrows) was used to apply pressure and separate the area of interest from adjacent intestinal segments. (From Hecht 2004b)

Table 13.3 Gastrointestinal transit times of various contrast media in dogs and cats.

	Barium	Iodinated contrast media	Radiographs*	Contrast medium visible in**:
Dog	Immediately	Immediately	VD/DV/LL/RL	Stomach
	15 minutes		VD/RL	Stomach, small intestine
	30 minutes	15 minutes	VD/RL	Stomach, small intestine
	1 hour		VD/RL	Stomach, small intestine
	2 hours	30 minutes	VD/RL	Stomach, small intestine
	4 hours	1 hour	VD/RL	Small and large intestine
Cat	Immediately	Immediately	VD/DV/LL/RL	Stomach
	5 minutes	5 minutes	VD/RL	Stomach, duodenum
	30 minutes	30 minutes	VD/RL	Small intestine
	60 minutes	60 minutes	VD/RL	Small and large intestine

From Hecht (2004b).

Notes: * VD = ventrodorsal; DV = dorsoventral; LL = left lateral; RL = right lateral (additional views may be helpful in some cases); ** variable.

Additional views may have to be acquired later than indicated above. The study is considered complete when the stomach is completely empty, and all of the contrast medium has reached the colon.

EVALUATION OF THE STOMACH The gastric wall is smooth, with the exception of physiological linear to serpentine rugal folds. Depending on patient positioning, contrast medium and air show gravity dependent distribution within the gastric lumen (Fig. 13.12). Normal rugal folds, contraction waves and accumulation of intraluminal secretions may mimic pathological changes of the gastric wall. Definitive diagnosis of a lesion requires repeat radiographs with persistence of abnormalities throughout the study.

EVALUATION OF THE SMALL INTESTINE The small intestinal mucosal surface is generally smooth or has fine fimbriations (Fig. 13.13). One physiological exception are **duodenal 'pseudo-ulcers'** seen especially in young **dogs**. These represent focal lymphatic aggregates in the antimesenteric mucosal surface which appear as regular square filling defects during the contrast study. The small intestinal wall is uniformly thin, without evidence of focal or generalized thickening. Small intestinal diameter is relatively uniform and should not exceed the reference ranges listed in section 13.1.1. Peristaltic waves appear as intermittent symmetric regions of luminal narrowing which change in position on subsequent radiographs. It is important to note that the duodenum and proximal jejunum in cats may assume the appearance of a 'string of pearls' due to strong and regular intestinal contractions (Fig. 13.14). This should not be confused with intestinal plication due to a linear foreign body. As described for the stomach, incidental variations and artefacts may mimic intestinal disease. Diagnosis of a true lesion requires persistence of an abnormality on repeat radiographs.

Possible complications

The most important complication of an upper GI contrast study is **aspiration** of contrast medium occurring secondary to inappropriate tube placement, during oral contrast medium administration, or following vomiting.

A second important complication is **granulomatous peritonitis** secondary to leakage of barium sulphate suspension into the peritoneal cavity in patients with intestinal perforation. This problem is not observed with iodinated contrast agents.

13.2.4 Contrast examination of the large intestine (colonogram)

The most common indication for a colonogram in small animal practice today is determination of the exact position of an **intestinal foreign body** (within small or large intestine). This can easily be accomplished by performing a negative contrast study. A positive contrast study will also yield the desired result. Colonoscopy is the best procedure for evaluation of **colonic mucosa**. A double contrast colonogram may be substituted for this technique in select cases.

Material

The following material is needed.

- Catheter (optimally with cuff to seal the rectum to the outside) and lube.
- Infusion bag or other device to allow instillation of contrast medium into the colon with gravity.
- Positive contrast medium: approximately 10–20 ml/kg (variable!) barium sulphate suspension, diluted 1:1 with warm water.

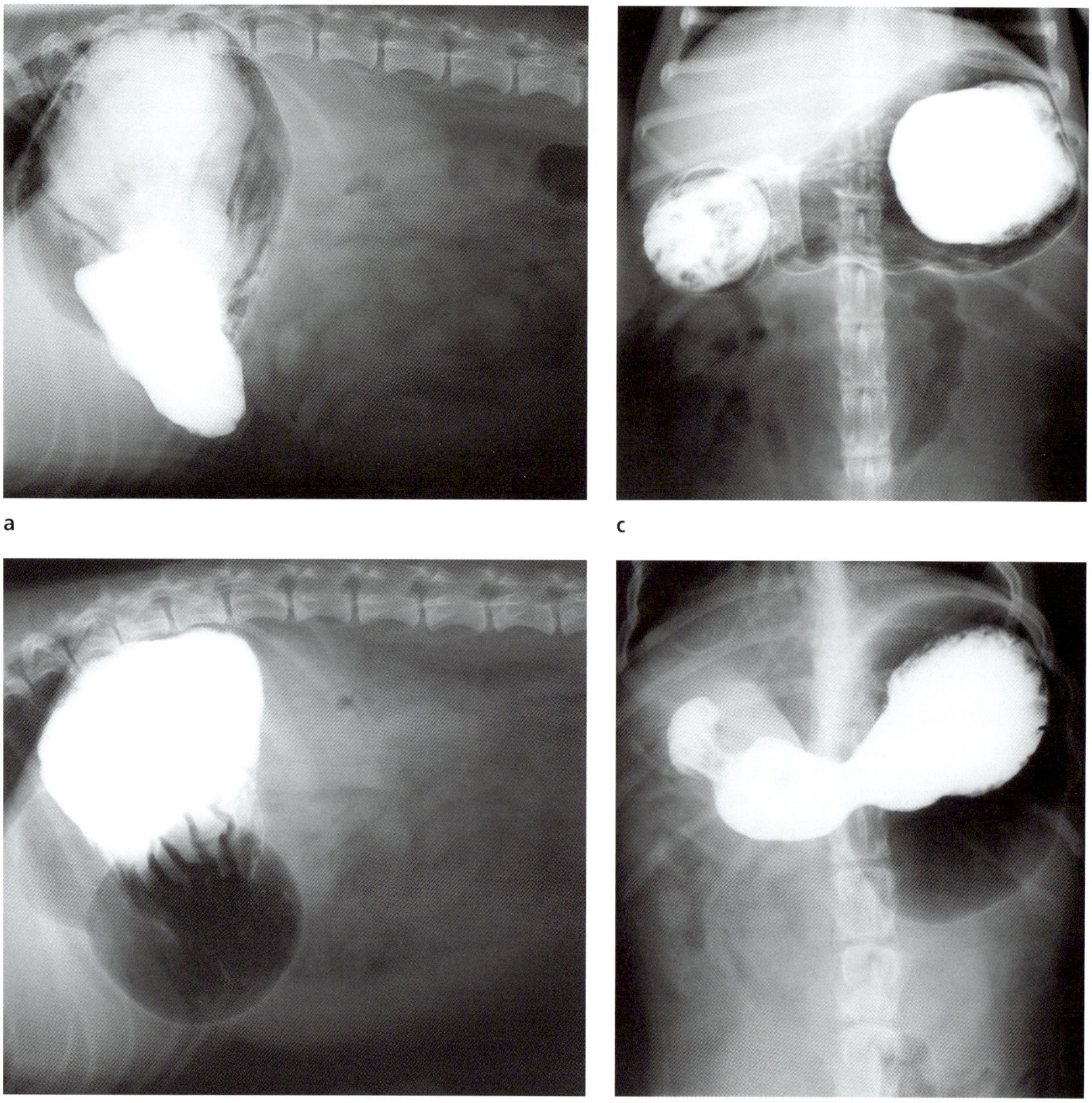

a c

b d

Fig. 13.12 Distribution of intraluminal contrast medium and air in the stomach of a normal dog is dependent on positioning.

a On the right lateral view, contrast medium accumulates in the dependent portion (pylorus) while air rises to the fundus.

b On the left lateral view, the fundus is filled with contrast medium and the pylorus with air.

c On the ventrodorsal view, contrast medium accumulates in the dorsal parts of the stomach (fundus and pylorus). The gastric body is ventrally located and contains air.

d On the dorsoventral view, most of the contrast medium accumulates within the gastric body. The fundus is gas-filled.

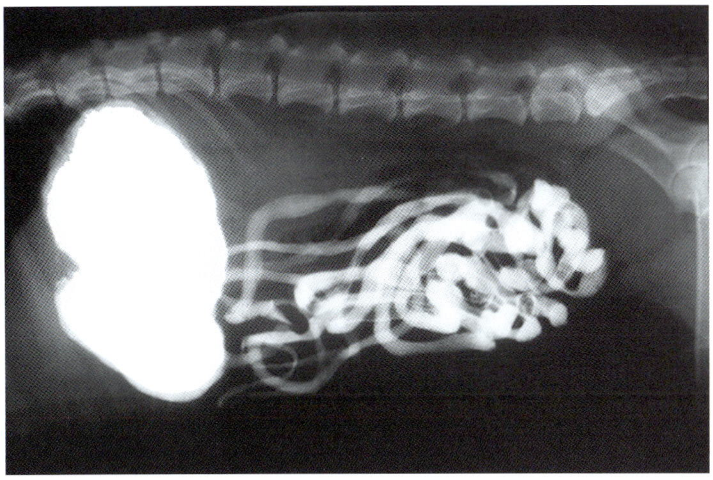

a

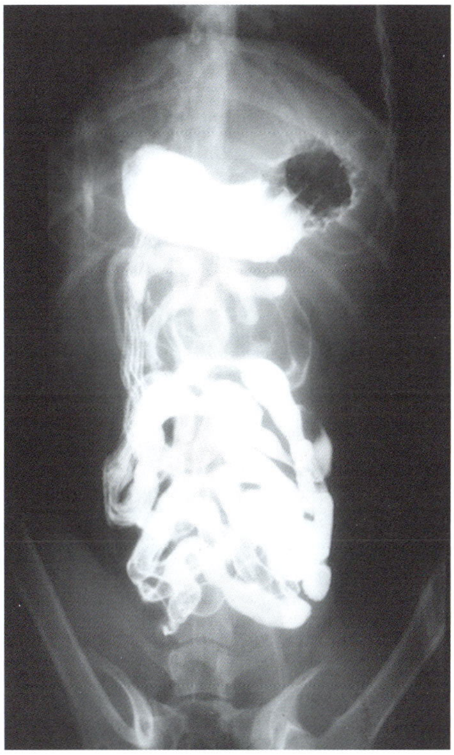

b

Fig. 13.13 Lateral a and ventrodorsal b abdominal radiographs during an upper GI contrast study in a normal dog. Contrast medium was administered 1 hour prior to obtaining these radiographs. Most of the small intestine is filled with contrast medium. The small intestinal wall is of even thickness, the mucosal surface is smooth, and there is no evidence of intestinal dilatation or abnormal filling defects.

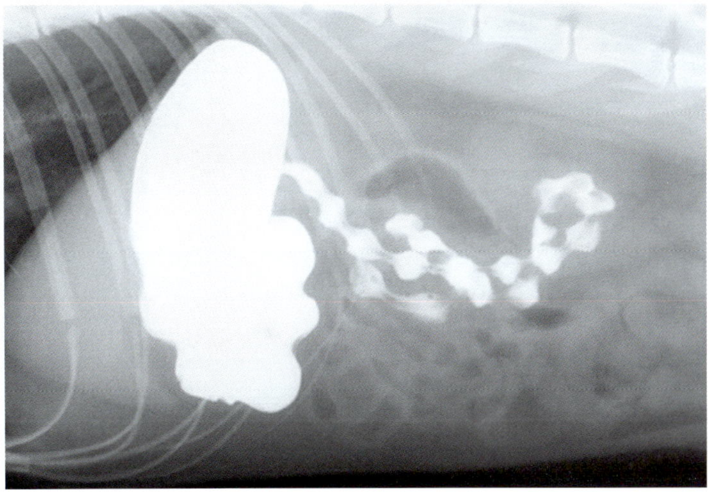

a

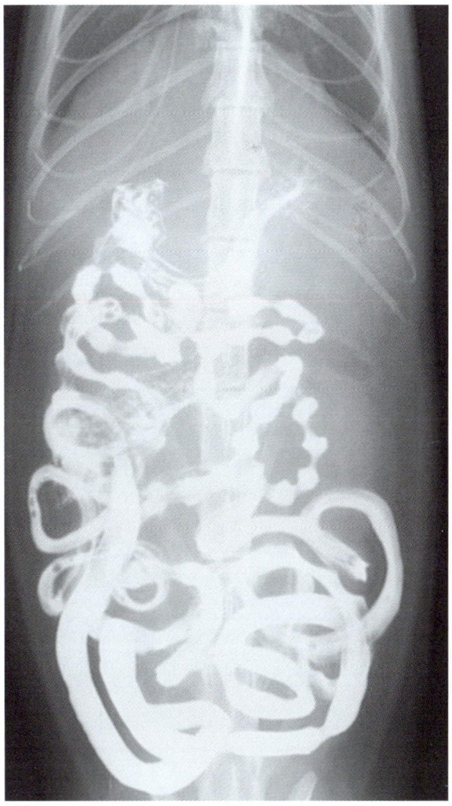

b

Fig. 13.14 Normal upper GI contrast study in a cat. Radiographs were obtained immediately a and 20 minutes b after contrast medium administration. Note strong peristaltic contractions of the duodenum and proximal jejunum which result in a 'string of pearls' sign. This should not be confused with a linear foreign body!

Contrast medium should be instilled into the colon with gravity rather than being injected under pressure, to avoid backflow into the small intestine and to minimize the risk of intestinal damage. For a double contrast colonogram, the entire amount of positive contrast medium is administered initially and is subsequently evacuated before filling the colon with air. This ensures even mucosal coating throughout the entire length of the large intestine.

Procedure

1. Patient preparation (except in emergency cases).
   - Fasting for at least 24 hours with free access to water.
   - Regular enemas until colon and rectum are completely empty.
2. General anaesthesia (usually not needed for a negative contrast colonogram performed to determine location of the colon and position of a foreign body).
3. Opposite lateral and ventrodorsal survey radiographs.
4. Insertion of the catheter and blocking of the cuff.
5. Instillation of positive contrast medium. Adequate filling of the colon can be monitored by means of fluoroscopy. Alternatively, a ventrodorsal abdominal radiograph can be acquired after an initial contrast medium dose of 10 ml/kg has been administered. The colon should be mildly distended throughout its entire length.
6. Radiographs: lateral, ventrodorsal, ± opposite lateral and oblique ventrodorsal.
7. ± evacuation of the colon and filling with air for a double contrast study.

Evaluation

The normal colon is in an adequate position, homogeneously fills with contrast medium, and has a smooth thin wall (Fig. 13.15). Possible abnormalities include abnormal position and length, intraluminal filling defects, strictures and mural lesions.

Possible complications

The most serious complication of the procedure is **colonic rupture** due to overdistention of the colon, overinflation of the cuff or trauma during contrast medium administration. Underlying diseases of the colonic mucosa (e.g. neoplastic infiltration) or pre-existent iatrogenic lesions (e.g. due to prior biopsy or repeat enemas) may predispose for colonic rupture. Overdistention of the intestinal wall during the procedure must be avoided by all means to minimize the risk of perforation.

Procedural complications which are not harmful to the patient but will limit the diagnostic quality of the contrast study include the following.

- Large intestinal spasms, which are especially severe following prior enemas or if using cold contrast medium. These may mimic mucosal lesions.
- Backflow of contrast medium into the ileum and jejunum.
- Leakage of contrast material to the outside and patient contamination resulting in radiographic artefacts.

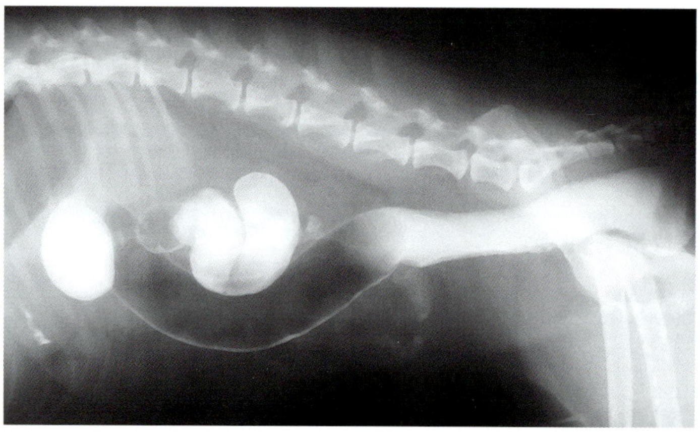

a

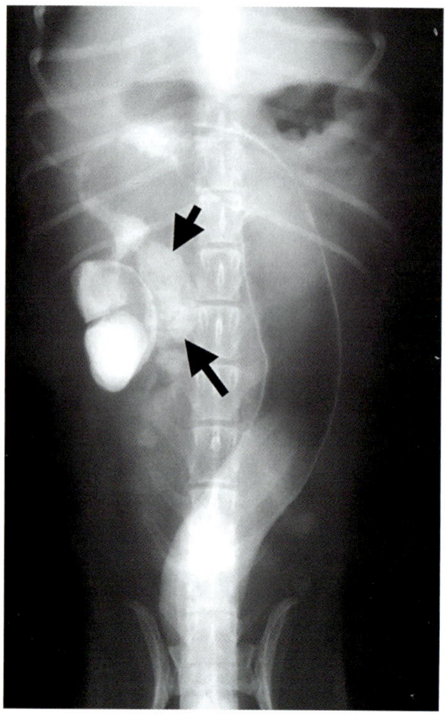

b

Fig. 13.15 Lateral a and ventrodorsal b abdominal radiographs during a double contrast colonogram in a normal dog. The mucosal surface is coated with a thin layer of positive contrast medium and appears thin and smooth, without evidence of mural or intraluminal filling defects. On the ventrodorsal view, intraluminal foreign material is associated with a small intestinal segment between the caecum and spine (arrows).

13.3 Disorders of the oesophagus

13.3.1 Megaoesophagus

Pathological dilatation of the oesophagus may be generalized or focal. Unlike most other oesophageal diseases, a radiographic diagnosis is usually possible on survey radiographs without requiring contrast medium administration.

Generalized megaoesophagus

Generalized megaoesophagus may be congenital or acquired, secondary to an underlying disease process (endocrine, toxic or autoimmune causes), or idiopathic. Dogs of all ages may be affected. This condition is uncommon in cats. The underlying cause of megaoesophagus is usually not evident on thoracic radiographs, necessitating further patient workup.

RADIOGRAPHIC FINDINGS A tubular structure containing gas, fluid and / or ingesta is present in the dorsal mediastinum. The enlarged oesophagus often results in ventral displacement of the trachea on a lateral view and widening of the mediastinum on a ventrodorsal view (Fig. 13.16). Summation of the ventral oesophageal wall and the dorsal wall of the trachea may give the erroneous impression of a thickened tracheal wall ('tracheal stripe sign'). Aspiration pneumonia is a common concurrent finding in patients with megaoesophagus.

Focal dilatation of the oesophagus

Focal dilatation of the oesophagus may be caused by increased intraluminal pressure (e.g. secondary to chronic partial obstruction) or by traction from the outside (pulsation or traction diverticulum). A relatively common cause of focal megaoesophagus is a vascular ring anomaly at the heart base (e.g. persistent right aortic arch), resulting in compression of the oesophagus and chronic partial obstruction. Affected animals usually present at a young age and often when transitioning from liquid to solid food.

RADIOGRAPHIC FINDINGS Thoracic radiographs in affected animals demonstrate marked oesophageal dilatation cranial to the heart with focal luminal narrowing at the level of the vascular anomaly at the heart base (Fig. 13.17). Mild oesophageal dilatation caudal to the obstructive lesion and concurrent aspiration pneumonia are common.

13.3.2 Oesophageal stricture

Strictures usually occur secondary to injury to the oesophageal mucosa with subsequent scarring, fibrosis and luminal narrowing. Underlying causes may include prior oesophageal foreign body, surgical intervention, gastro-oesophageal reflux, and inflammatory or neoplastic infiltration of the oesophageal wall.

Fig. 13.16 Generalized megaoesophagus in a dog.
a On the right lateral view, the oesophagus appears as a gas-dilated structure extending throughout the entire length of the dorsal mediastinum (arrowheads). The trachea is displaced ventrally. The ventral wall of the oesophagus silhouettes with the dorsal margin of the trachea, resulting in erroneous impression of tracheal wall thickening ('tracheal stripe sign'). An alveolar pattern associated with the ventral aspect of both subsegments of the left cranial lung lobe (arrows) is consistent with aspiration pneumonia.
b On the ventrodorsal view, there is generalized widening of the mediastinum (arrowheads).

a

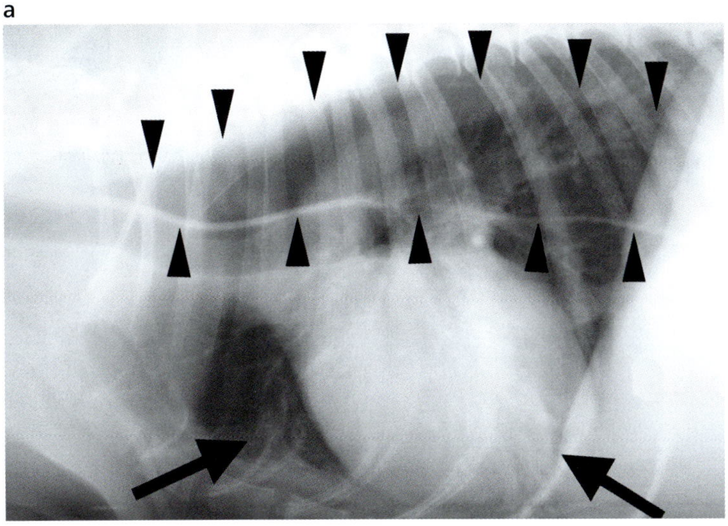

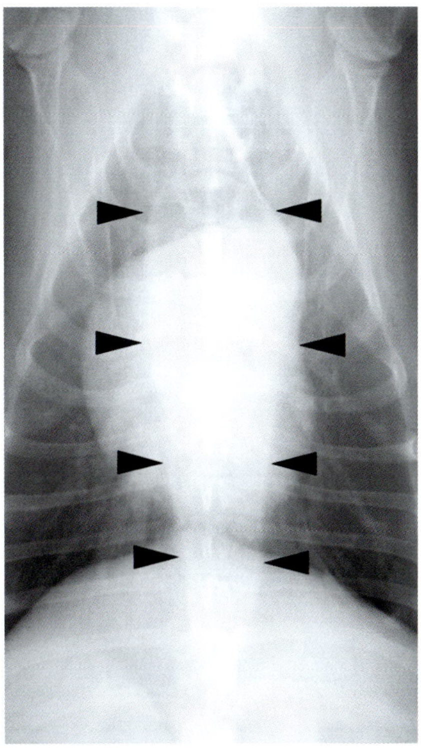

b

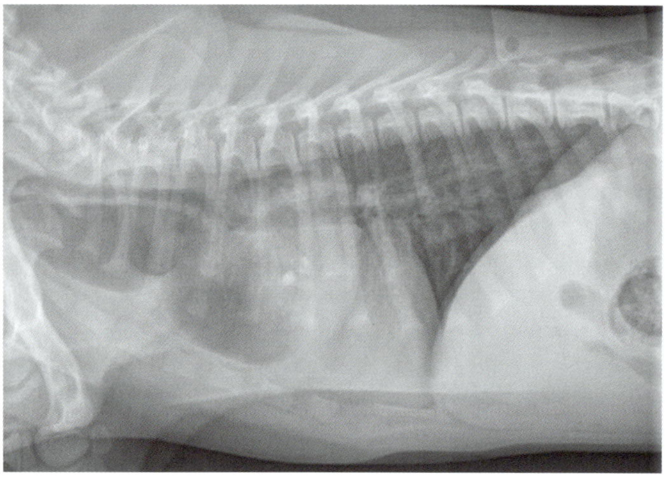

a

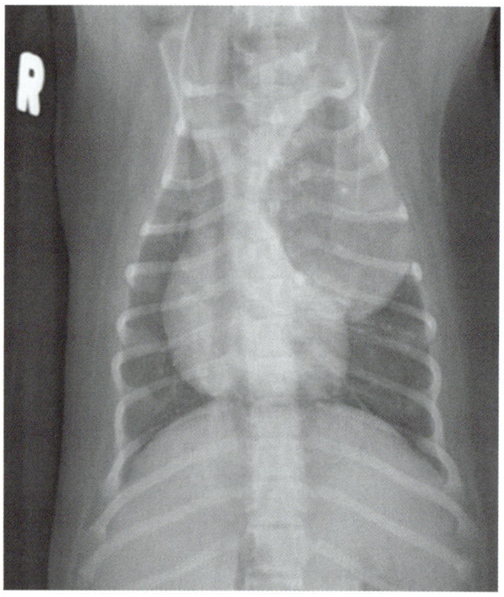

b

Fig. 13.17 Lateral a and ventrodorsal b thoracic radiographs in a 2-month-old Miniature Dachshund. There is severe focal oesophageal dilatation due to a vascular ring anomaly and resultant oesophageal obstruction at the level of the heart base. The oesophagus cranial to the heart is severely distended with gas, fluid and ingesta, which results in displacement of the trachea. (R = right)

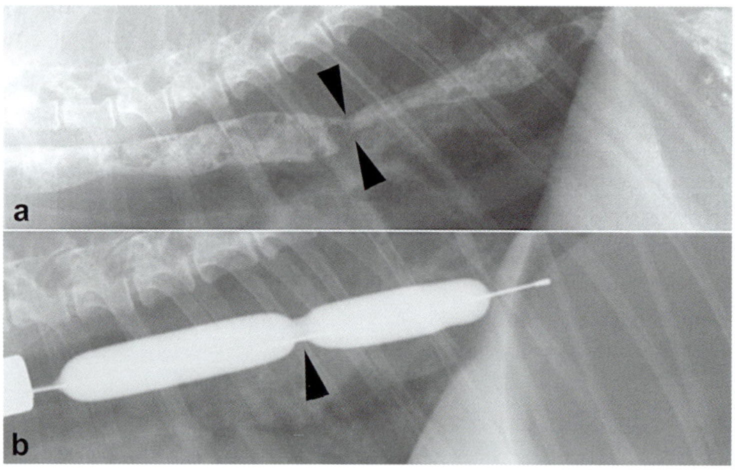

Fig. 13.18 Oesophageal stricture in a dog 2 months after extraction of an oesophageal foreign body.
a The oesophagram (administration of positive contrast medium mixed with canned food) demonstrates moderate focal circumferential narrowing of the oesophageal lumen (arrowheads). An evaluation of the mucosal contour is not possible and would require use of barium sulphate suspension or paste.
b Lateral thoracic radiograph obtained during balloon dilation of the stricture. A balloon filled with contrast medium has been placed within the caudal oesophagus. The stricture results in focal narrowing of the oesophageal lumen (arrowhead).

Radiographic findings Survey radiographs are often normal or may show variable degrees of oesophageal dilatation cranial to the stricture. An oesophagram demonstrates luminal narrowing with or without an irregular mucosal contour (Fig. 13.18).

13.3.3 Foreign bodies

Diagnosis of a **radiopaque** oesophageal foreign body is usually possible on plain radiographs (Fig. 13.19). Radiographic findings include a mineral or bone opaque structure within the oesophageal lumen. Oesophageal dilatation cranial to the lesion is common.

Non-opaque foreign bodies are a diagnostic challenge and may require a contrast study for visualization. An oesophagram shows an intraluminal filling defect and variable degrees of oesophageal dilatation.

A possible severe complication of an oesophageal foreign body is oesophageal perforation, which may result in mediastinitis, pneumomediastinum and/or formation of a broncho-oesophageal fistula.

13.3.4 Oesophageal neoplasia

Tumours of the oesophagus are rare in small animal patients. The most common tumour types are carcinomas and smooth muscle tumours (leiomyoma, leiomyosarcoma).

Oesophageal osteosarcomas may develop in dogs secondary to *Spirocerca lupi* infection, and should be con-

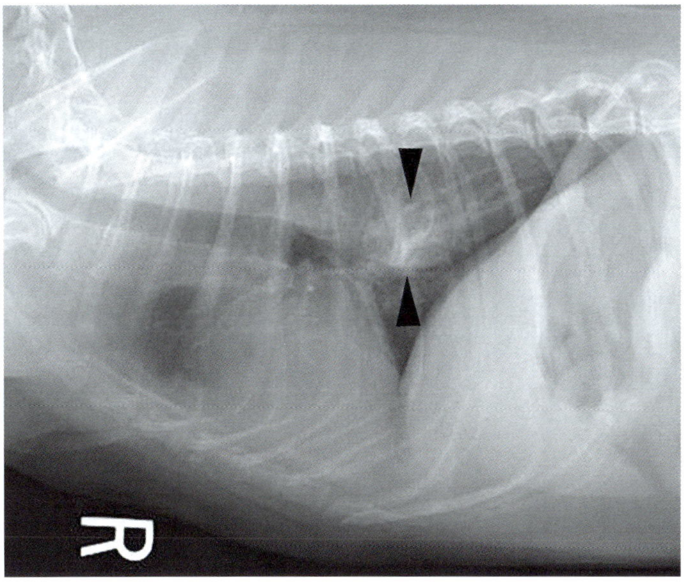

a

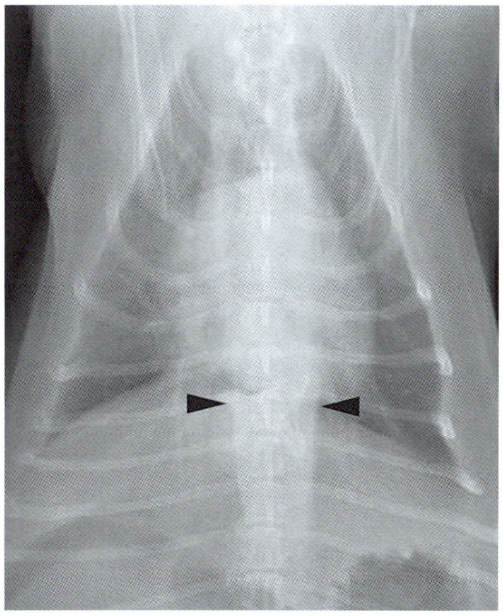

b

Fig. 13.19 Lateral a and ventrodorsal b thoracic radiographs in a dog with a caudal oesophageal foreign body (bone). The caudodorsal mediastinum is increased in opacity and widened (arrowheads). Concurrent oesophageal dilatation cranial to the intraluminal lesion commonly seen with this condition is not present in this patient. (R = right)

sidered as a possible differential diagnosis in animals from endemic areas.

RADIOGRAPHIC FINDINGS Depending on its size, opacity and position, an oesophageal tumour may resemble a mediastinal mass of a different aetiology, an oesophageal foreign body (see section 13.3.3) or a hiatal hernia (see section 13.3.5) on survey radiographs. An oesophagram is helpful in identifying tumour association with the oesophageal wall and intraluminal or extraluminal tumour extension (Fig. 13.20).

Following radiographic identification of an oesophageal mass, tissue sampling is required for a definitive diagnosis and therapy planning. Fine-needle aspiration or biopsy can be performed by means of endoscopy, ultrasound or CT guidance, or surgery depending on lesion location.

13.3.5 Hiatal hernia and gastro-oesophageal intussusception

Hiatal hernia

Incompetence of the oesophageal hiatus allows herniation of part of the stomach into the thoracic cavity. A **paraoesophageal hernia** is characterized by maintained physiological position of the gastro-oesophageal sphincter caudal to the diaphragm and herniation of part of the stomach through the oesophageal hiatus adjacent to the sphincter. With a **true hiatal hernia**, the gastro-oesophageal sphincter and part of the stomach are both displaced cranially through the hiatus. The hernia may be permanent and clinically significant, or intermittent and often incidental (**'sliding hiatal hernia'**).

RADIOGRAPHIC FINDINGS A hiatal hernia appears as a soft-tissue opacity mass lesion in the caudodorsal mediastinum immediately cranial to the diaphragm. It may on occasion be difficult to distinguish from a caudal mediastinal mass of a different aetiology. Concurrent dorsal and lateral displacement of the stomach, extension of intraluminal gastric gas into the hernia, or intermittent nature of a lesion which is seen on some but not all radiographic projections usually aids in diagnosis (Fig. 3.21). Permanent and paraoesophageal hernias may require an oesophagram to confirm the presence of part of the stomach in the caudal mediastinum and to demonstrate the location of the gastro-oesophageal sphincter.

A sliding hiatal hernia may be an incidental finding and should not be confused with a caudal mediastinal mass or oesophageal foreign body. However, some hiatal hernias may result in clinical signs (regurgitation), necessitating further workup.

Gastro-oesophageal intussusception

With this condition there is complete or partial herniation of the stomach into the oesophageal lumen. This is usually a life-threatening emergency and associated with a poor prognosis even with immediate surgical intervention. This disease is rare and predominantly affects young dogs, with a predilection for German Shepherd Dogs.

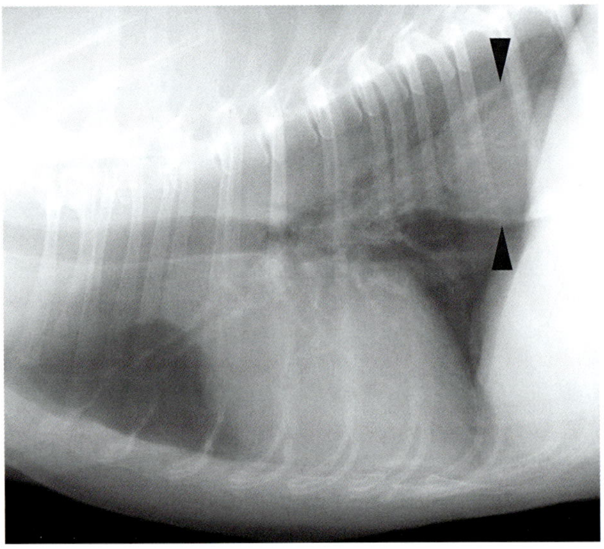

a

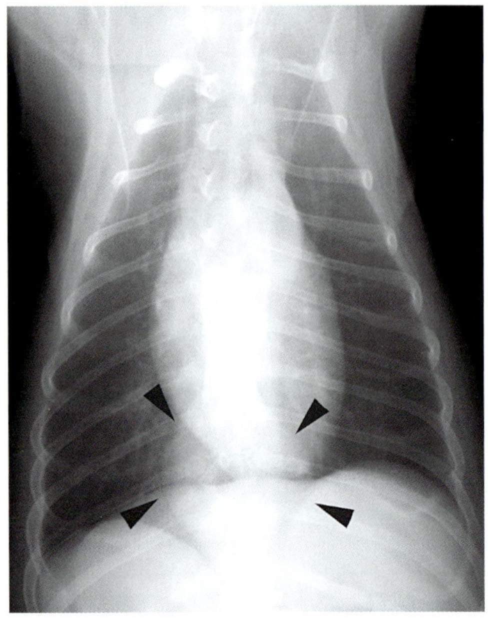

b

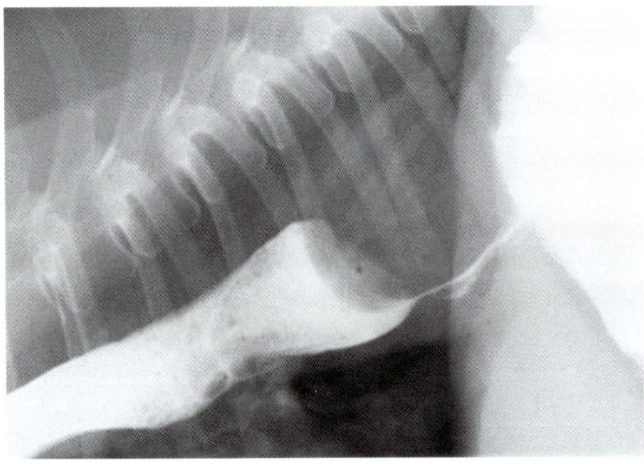

c

Fig. 13.20 Tumour of the caudal oesophagus in a dog.

a, b On lateral und ventrodorsal views, there is a focal soft-tissue opacity mass associated with the caudal mediastinum (arrowheads).

c The oesophagram proves mural origin of the lesion with extra- and intraluminal extension and resultant partial oesophageal obstruction. Histological diagnosis was leiomyoma.

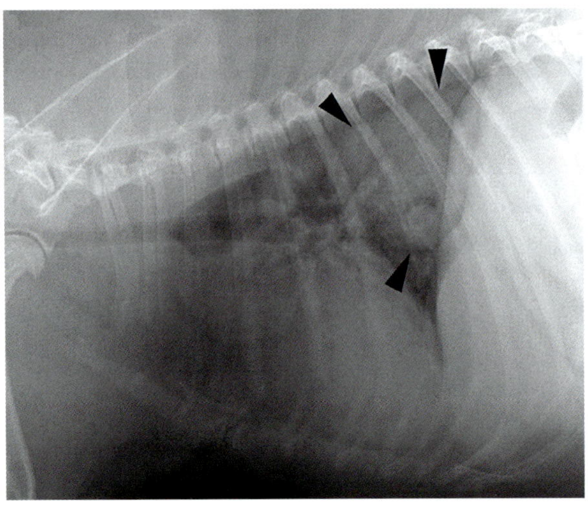

a

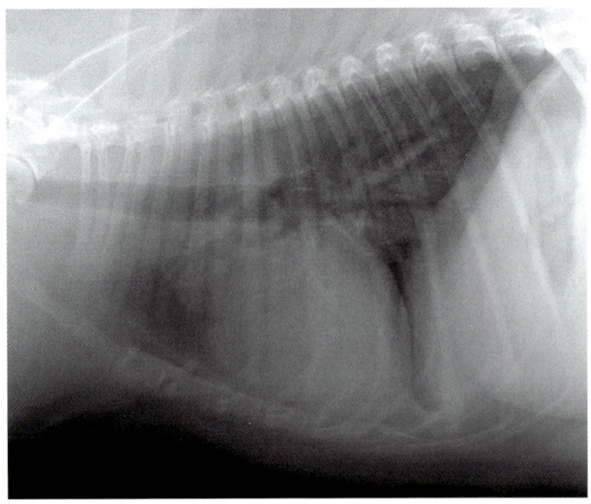

b

Fig. 13.21 Sliding hiatal hernia in a dog.

a On the initial right lateral thoracic radiograph, a large soft-tissue opacity mass lesion is associated with the caudodorsal mediastinum (arrowheads). The oesophagus cranial to the lesion contains gas.

b The mediastinal mass lesion is no longer present on the recheck radiograph obtained a few hours later.

RADIOGRAPHIC FINDINGS Thoracic radiographs reveal severe dilatation of the oesophagus with gas cranially and soft-tissue opaque material caudally (Fig. 13.22). The stomach is absent from the abdomen or abnormally small. The diagnosis is usually straightforward. In questionable cases (e.g. to distinguish a herniated stomach from a large oesophageal foreign body) an oesophagram may be helpful.

13.4 Disorders of the stomach

13.4.1 Changes in gastric position

Enlargement or mass lesions of organs near the stomach such as liver or pancreas result in displacement of the stomach from its normal position and/or in alteration of the normal gastric contour. Examples can be found in Chapters 11 and 12.

13.4.2 Gastric dilatation (GD) and gastric dilatation with volvulus (GDV)

Gastric dilatation with or without volvulus is a common problem especially in large-breed dogs. Differentiation between mere dilatation and volvulus is important, as **GDV** represents an indication for emergency surgery while **GD** may be treated conservatively.

With gastric dilatation and volvulus, the pylorus is displaced along the ventral abdominal wall towards the left and dorsally, while it remains in a physiological position in the right abdomen in cases of gastric dilatation.

RADIOGRAPHIC FINDINGS Identification of the position of the pylorus is key for a diagnosis of GD versus GDV. Diagnosis is usually possible on three-view abdominal radiographs (opposite lateral and ventrodorsal views). Oral contrast medium administration may be beneficial in select cases.

With **gastric dilatation,** the stomach is moderately to severely distended with gas, fluid or food ('food bloat'). The stomach is in a normal position (Fig. 13.23a).

With **gastric dilatation and volvulus**, the stomach is typically severely distended with gas. Pyloric displacement towards the left and craniodorsally is best demonstrated on a right lateral view and results in projection of a soft-tissue opaque fold over the gastric lumen ('compartmentalization'; Fig. 13.23b). Common concurrent findings include splenomegaly due to congestion, and gas distention of the oesophagus and small intestine. Gas inclusions within the gastric wall previously attributed to gastric wall necrosis do not appear to be a negative prognostic indicator according to recent studies.

13.4.3 Foreign bodies

A radiographic diagnosis of a **radiopaque** gastric foreign body is usually easily made on plain radiographs (Fig. 13.24). To further evaluate the exact position and extent of visible foreign material (e.g. when deciding between endoscopy and surgery as treatment options), positional radiographs with or without oral administration of a small amount of positive contrast medium may be helpful.

A diagnosis of **non-opaque** gastric foreign material, especially in the fundus, is difficult. It may appear similar to normal ingesta or may be masked by the concurrent presence of food. Repeat radiographs after fasting for 12–24 hours may be helpful in these cases. Normal ingesta should have been evacuated from the stomach at this point. Persistence of soft-tissue opaque material within the stomach increases the suspicion of foreign material. Persistence of soft-tissue opaque material in the stomach in a vomiting or anorexic patient also raises concern about the presence of foreign material (Fig. 13.25). Equivocal cases may require advanced imaging (ultrasound) or (double contrast) gastrography for further evaluation.

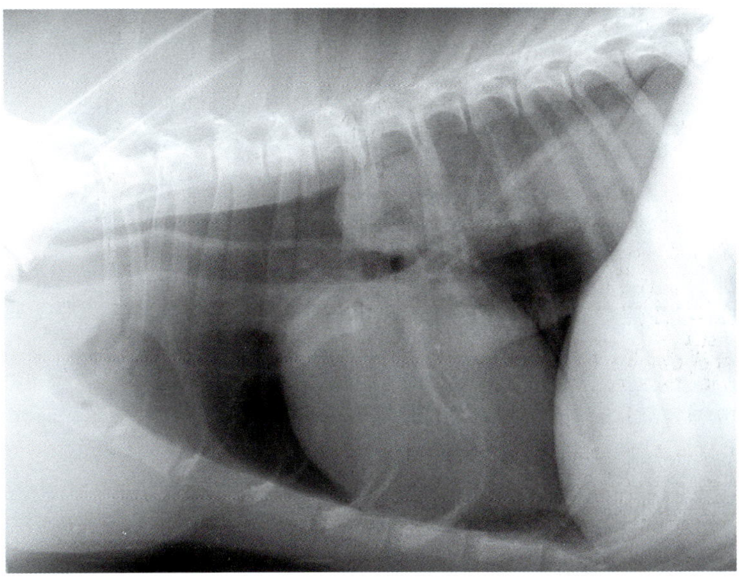

Fig. 13.22 Gastro-oesophageal intussusception in a dog. A large soft-tissue opaque intraluminal structure is associated with the caudal oesophagus. The oesophagus cranial to the lesion is gas dilated.

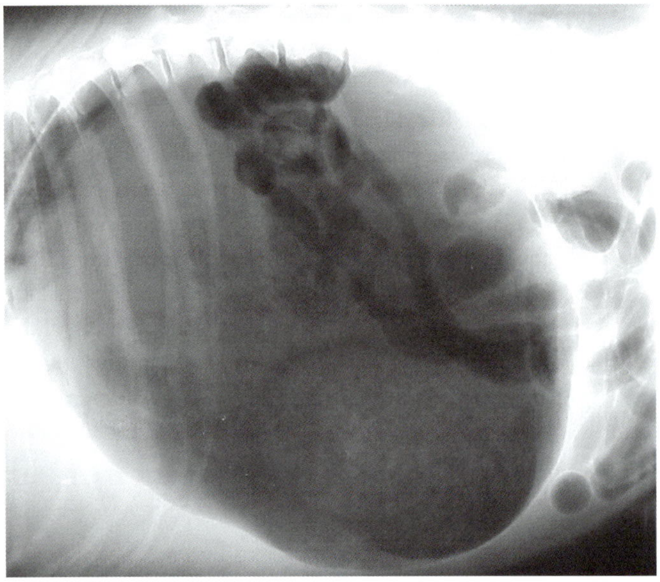

a

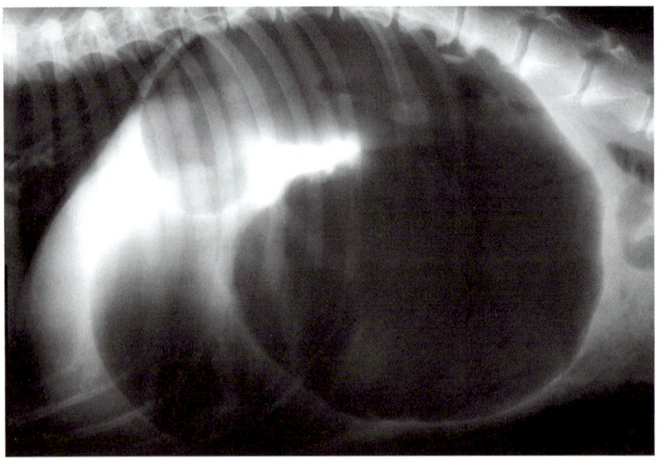

b

Fig. 13.23 Gastric dilatation (GD) versus gastric dilatation and volvulus (GDV). a The right lateral abdominal radiograph in this dog with GD shows severe distention of the stomach, mostly with gas and a moderate amount of ingesta. The pylorus is in a normal position (i.e. in the dependent portion of the abdomen and thus not visible). There is no evidence of gastric compartmentalization. b The right lateral abdominal radiograph in this dog with GDV also shows severe gas distention of the stomach. The pylorus is displaced into the left dorsal abdomen and filled with gas. A linear soft-tissue opacity fold separates the pylorus from the caudoventrally located fundus ('compartmentalization').

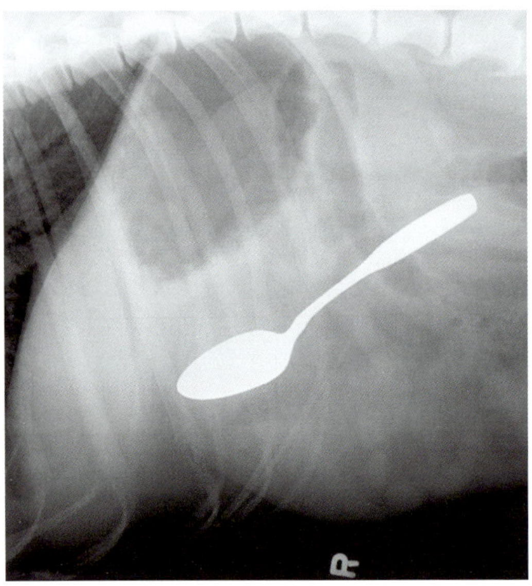

a

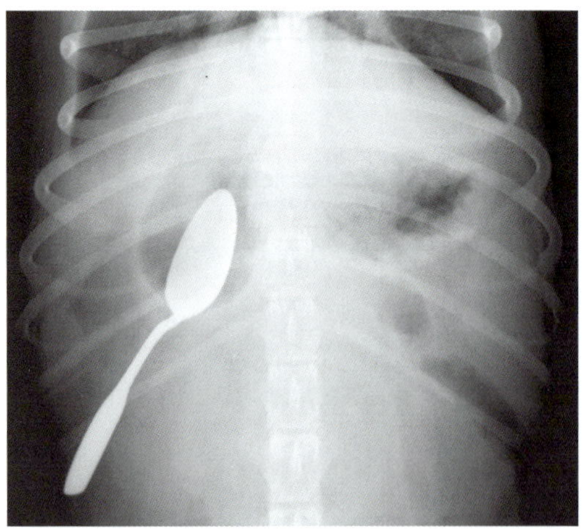

b

Fig. 13.24 Lateral a and ventrodorsal b abdominal radiographs in a dog with a metal opaque gastric foreign body. A spoon is located within the stomach and extends into the proximal duodenum. It is unknown which food was originally associated with the spoon and lead to its ingestion.

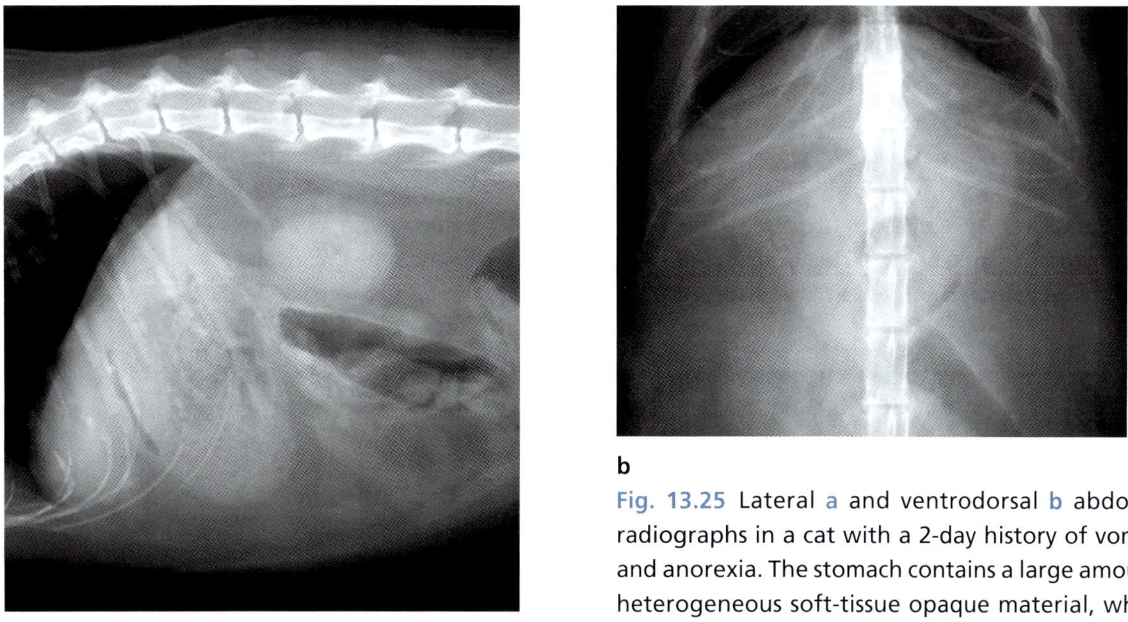

a

b

Fig. 13.25 Lateral a and ventrodorsal b abdominal radiographs in a cat with a 2-day history of vomiting and anorexia. The stomach contains a large amount of heterogeneous soft-tissue opaque material, which is inconsistent with normal ingesta based on the history. The ultimate diagnosis was a large hairball.

Foreign material within the pylorus may cause partial or complete **gastric outflow obstruction** and result in marked dilatation of the stomach with fluid and gas (see section 13.4.4). Diagnosis of pyloric foreign material is often possible on a left lateral view where intraluminal gas rises to the nondependent portion of the stomach and surrounds the foreign body.

13.4.4 Pyloric obstruction (gastric outflow obstruction)

Gastric outflow obstruction may be acute (e.g. secondary to foreign body ingestion; see section 13.4.3) or have a chronic (progressive) course.

Chronic pyloric obstruction is usually caused by an anatomic abnormality (such as pyloric hypertrophy, neoplasia, inflammation or fibrosis) or less likely may be functional (pylorospasm). Most chronic gastric outflow obstructions are partial and progress over time.

Radiographic findings The stomach is moderately to severely distended with fluid and some gas (Fig. 13.26). The cause of gastric outflow obstruction is usually not visible on survey radiographs unless an obvious pyloric mass is noted.

> While the stomach is distended with gas in cases of GD/GDV, it contains mostly fluid in cases of gastric outflow obstruction.

A **contrast study** of the gastrointestinal tract demonstrates delayed gastric emptying and may aid in identification of an obstructive lesion. Possible findings include gastric wall thickening, ulceration and mural mass lesions (Fig. 13.27).

Radiographs are no substitute for a histological diagnosis. Depending on the nature of the obstructive lesion, tissue samples may be obtained by means of ultrasound, endoscopy or laparotomy.

13.4.5 Gastric ulcers

Gastric ulcers are not visible on survey abdominal radiographs. As mentioned above, contrast gastrography has largely been replaced by ultrasonography and endoscopy. However, if these technologies are unavailable, a positive contrast or preferably a double contrast gastrogram may aid in diagnosis. Gastric ulcers form craters in the gastric wall which retain contrast medium even after gastric emptying has occurred (Fig. 13.28). Additional findings include focal gastric wall thickening and flattening of adjacent rugal folds.

> Gastric ulcers may be secondary to infiltrative gastric disease (e.g. neoplasia) or may be a primary condition. Benign and malignant gastric ulcers cannot be distinguished radiographically!

13.4.6 Infiltrative disorders and mass lesions of the stomach

Diffuse thickening of the gastric wall may be seen with neoplasia, inflammation or gastric wall oedema.

Radiographic findings Survey radiographs are usually unrewarding except in severe cases. A contrast study may show generalized smooth or nodular thickening of the gastric wall with altered appearance of the rugal folds. Due to normal variations of the radiographic appearance of the stomach related to contractility and the presence and distribution of luminal ingesta and secretions, a suspected lesion has to be verified on several successive radiographs.

Focal mass lesions of the stomach are rather rare and usually neoplastic in aetiology (adenocarcinoma, lymphoma, leiomyoma / leiomyosarcoma / gastrointestinal stromal tumour, etc.). Inflammatory masses such as granulomas and abscesses are uncommon.

Radiographic findings A tumour of a certain size may be visible on survey radiographs if the remainder of the stomach is gas-filled (Fig. 13.29). Large and / or circumferential pyloric tumours may result in gastric outflow obstruction and subsequent fluid distention of the stomach (see section 13.4.4).

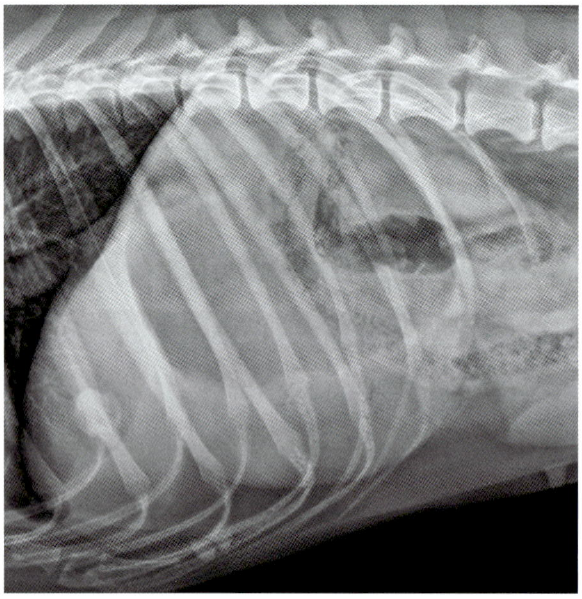

a

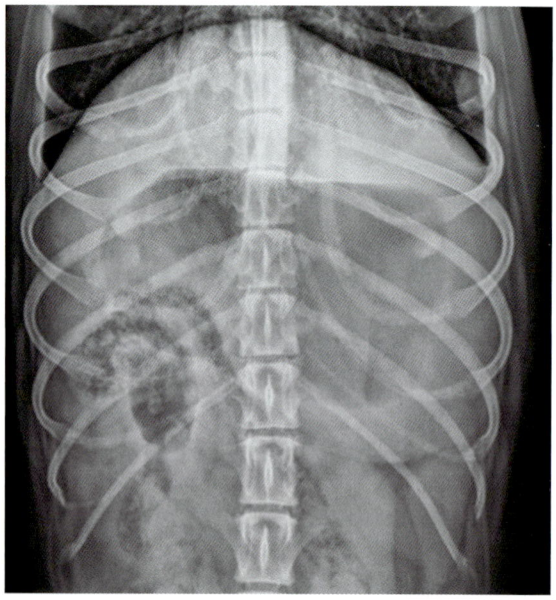

b

Fig. 13.26 Partial gastric outflow obstruction in a dog: lateral a and ventrodorsal view b. The stomach is moderately dilated, contains both fluid and gas, and is in a normal position. A severe gastritis with pyloric ulcer was diagnosed by means of endoscopy.

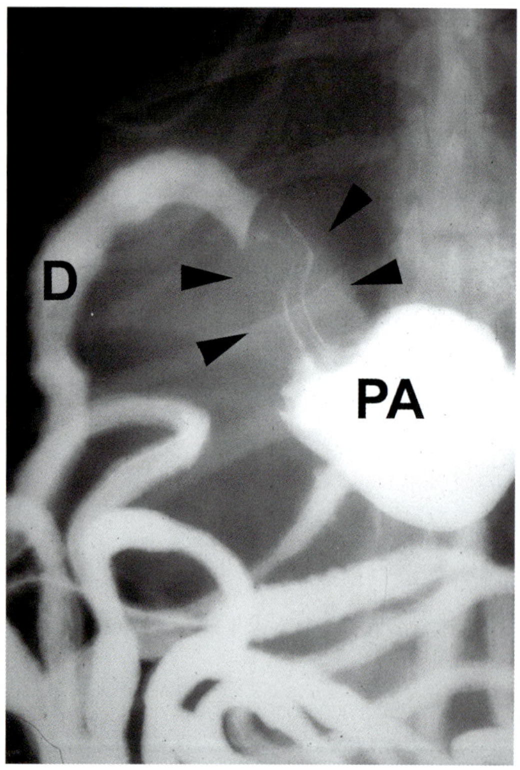

Fig. 13.27 Detail of a ventrodorsal abdominal radiograph obtained during an upper GI contrast study in a dog with chronic progressive partial pyloric outflow obstruction. There is circumferential thickening of the gastric wall at the pylorus (arrowheads), resulting in marked luminal narrowing (recognized by thin lines of contrast medium) compared to the proximal pyloric antrum (PA) and distal descending duodenum (D). Contrast medium can pass the lesion, consistent with partial obstruction. Histological diagnosis was lymphoma.

Fluid accumulation within the pylorus on a right lateral view or intraluminal soft-tissue opaque foreign material may give the wrong impression of a gastric mass. Positional radiographs, abdominal ultrasound or a gastrointestinal contrast study may be necessary for a definitive diagnosis of a mural gastric mass lesion.

When performing a gastrogram, a gastric tumour appears as a peripheral wall associated filling defect with a smooth or ulcerated surface (Fig. 13.30). Radiographic differentiation of different tumour types is not possible; however, some tumour types exhibit certain features that allow prioritization of differential diagnoses.

- **Adenocarcinomas** predominantly affect the lesser curvature and pyloric antrum and are commonly ulcerated.
- **Lymphomas** are more common in cats than in dogs. They are typically more extensive and larger than adenocarcinomas or may be diffusely infiltrative.
- **Leiomyomas** are smoothly marginated, commonly located in the region of the cardia, and grow exophytically. They rarely result in obstruction and may be incidental.
- Cytology or histopathology are always needed for a definitive diagnosis!

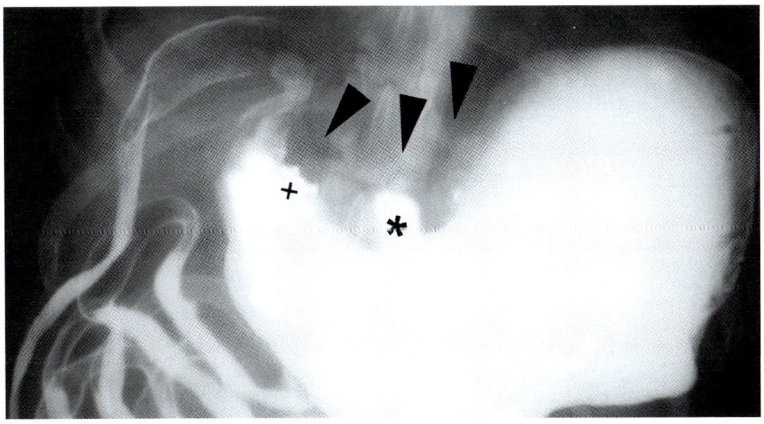

Fig. 13.28 Gastric ulcer in a dog. Detail of a ventrodorsal abdominal radiograph obtained following administration of positive contrast medium shows thickening of the gastric wall at the level of the lesser curvature (arrowheads), a deep crater at the level of the gastric body (*), and an irregular mucosal contour in the region of the pylorus (cross). A radiographic distinction between benign and malignant ulcers is not possible!

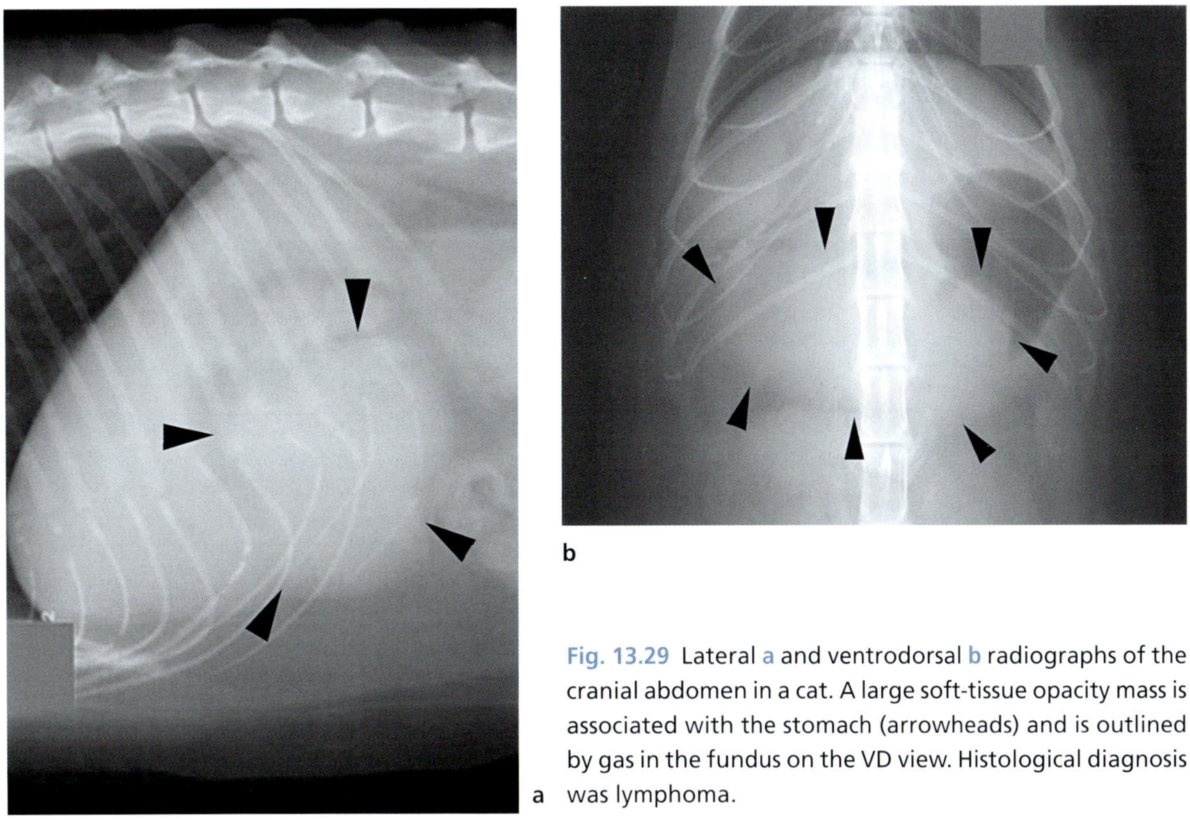

Fig. 13.29 Lateral a and ventrodorsal b radiographs of the cranial abdomen in a cat. A large soft-tissue opacity mass is associated with the stomach (arrowheads) and is outlined by gas in the fundus on the VD view. Histological diagnosis was lymphoma.

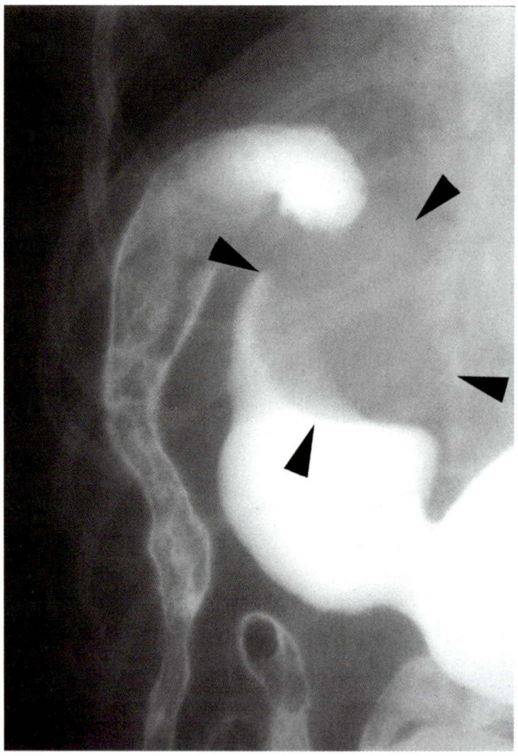

Fig. 13.30 Gastric tumour in a dog. The detail of a ventrodorsal abdominal radiograph obtained following positive contrast medium administration shows a wall associated, rounded, smoothly marginated and exophytic mural filling defect in the region of the pylorus (arrowheads). Histological diagnosis was leiomyoma.

13.4.7 Gastric perforation

Gastric perforation may occur secondary to a variety of gastric diseases (e.g. gastric ulcer, ulcerated tumour of the gastric wall, gastric foreign body, GDV), abdominal trauma or interventional procedures (e.g. placement of a gastric tube, endoscopy with biopsies). A radiographic diagnosis of subsequent pneumoperitoneum, abdominal effusion and peritonitis is usually straightforward (see Chapter 11).

13.5 Disorders of the small intestine

13.5.1 Ileus

Various definitions of ileus are found in the literature. In general, it refers to an inability of the intestine to properly transport ingesta. It may be caused by an obstructive lesion (**mechanical ileus**) or may be secondary to a motility disorder (**paralytic ileus**). A differentiation of these conditions is important from a therapeutic and prognostic standpoint.

Mechanical (obstructive) ileus

Physical blockage of the intestine may be caused by intraluminal structures (e.g. foreign bodies, large parasite load), mural abnormalities (e.g. neoplasia, stricture, severe inflammation) or extraluminal lesions (strangulation). Intestinal obstruction may be **complete** or **partial**. Animals with a complete obstruction typically present with acute and severe clinical signs including vomiting, anorexia and abdominal pain. The clinical course with partial obstruction is often chronic.

Radiographic findings Small intestinal segments proximal to the obstructive lesion are moderately to severely distended with gas and/or fluid while intestines distal to the obstruction are of normal diameter ('two populations of bowel'). Dilated small intestinal segments often appear stacked and may be arranged in hairpin turns (Fig. 13.31 and 13.32). The intestine is initially hyperperistaltic but will become flaccid with persistent obstruction.

With chronic partial obstruction, larger particles (e.g. sand and stones a few millimetres in diameter) which are usually able to pass through the GI tract may accumulate proximal to the lesion. This is referred to as a 'gravel sign' (Fig. 13.33). The most common cause is a slow growing intestinal tumour.

Mechanical ileus is a surgical indication. A diagnosis is often possible on survey radiographs, especially in acute cases. Equivocal cases may require additional imaging (ultrasound or an upper GI contrast study). These procedures not only allow a definitive diagnosis of an obstructive lesion, they also aid in assessment of the type of obstruction (intraluminal, mural or extraluminal), degree of intestinal obstruction, gastrointestinal transit time, intestinal peristalsis and indicators of intestinal perforation.

Paralytic (functional) ileus

With paralytic ileus there is decreased intestinal motility to a degree that prevents normal gastrointestinal passage of ingesta. Possible causes include a primary neuromuscular intestinal dysfunction, abdominal trauma, inflammation or infection, or recent abdominal surgery.

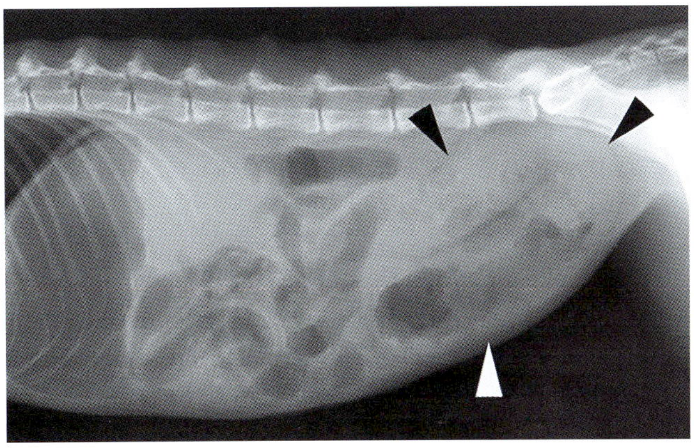

a

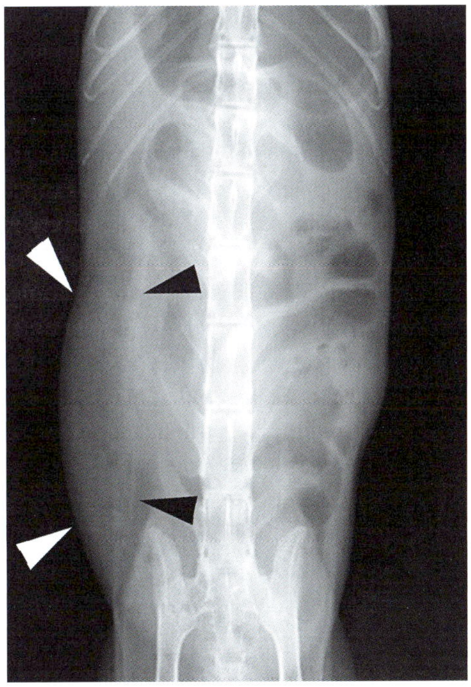

b

Fig. 13.31 Obstructive ileus in a cat. The stomach and part of the small intestine are moderately to markedly dilated with gas. Several intestinal segments are stacked, and some are arranged in hairpin turns. A small intestinal segment distended with foreign material is seen in the caudal abdomen, cranial to the pelvic inlet on the lateral view a and in the right caudal abdomen on the ventrodorsal view b (arrowheads). This segment has a U-shaped course and is separate from the descending colon.

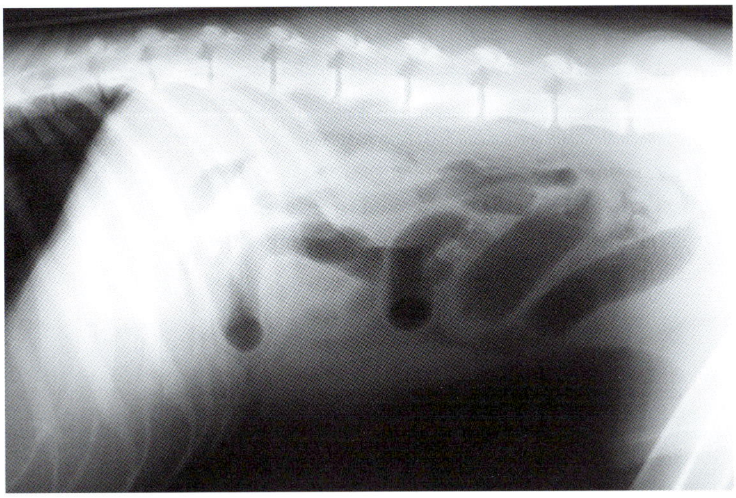

Fig. 13.32 Obstructive ileus in a dog. Several small intestinal segments within the caudal and ventral abdomen are severely dilated and stacked on top of each other, while other small intestinal segments in the cranial and dorsal abdomen are of normal diameter ('two populations of bowel').

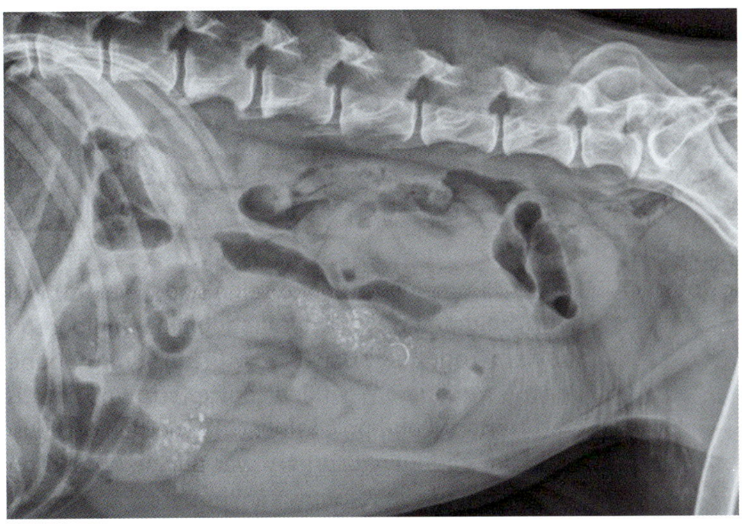

Fig. 13.33 Lateral abdominal radiograph in a dog showing numerous small mineral opaque fragments within a gas and fluid dilated small intestinal segment. This is a sign of a chronic partial obstruction, in which larger particles accumulate proximal to a lesion, while fluid and normal ingesta are able to pass ('gravel sign'). The most common cause is a slow growing intestinal tumour. In this patient, exploratory laparotomy yielded the diagnosis of a chronic partial foreign body obstruction with earlier perforation and scar tissue formation.

RADIOGRAPHIC FINDINGS Radiographs may be fairly normal or show generalized mild to moderate dilatation of the small intestine (possibly including stomach or large intestine). Intestinal segments are flaccid (adynamic) and arranged in smooth rounded turns ('lazy loops') (Fig. 13.34). An upper GI contrast study is usually not indicated, as a diagnosis is possible on survey radiographs. However, it may be performed in ambiguous cases to rule out mechanical ileus as a surgical indication. Findings include marked prolongation in transit time and diffuse intestinal dilatation.

Abdominal trauma or inflammatory disease processes such as peritonitis may result in a focal intestinal motility disorder. The resultant segmental small intestinal dilatation is difficult to distinguish from a true mechanical ileus. A thorough history, additional radiographic abnormalities such as ascites, and further imaging (abdominal ultrasound or upper GI contrast study) may aid in diagnosis.

13.5.2 Foreign bodies

As discussed in section 13.4.3, **radiopaque** foreign bodies are usually easily recognized on survey radiographs (Fig. 13.35).

A diagnosis of **non-opaque** foreign bodies is more difficult. With complete intestinal obstruction, radiographic findings of mechanical ileus predominate, usually without definitive identification of the underlying cause. Identification of partially obstructive or nonobstructive foreign bodies usually requires further imaging. With injury to the intestinal wall (e.g. secondary to a sharp-edged foreign body or intestinal necrosis), abdominal radiographs may show signs of peritonitis and/or pneumoperitoneum.

The radiographic diagnosis of an intestinal foreign body does not necessarily represent a surgical indication, as many foreign bodies are able to pass. The finding has to be considered in light of clinical signs and other radiographic findings (i.e. evidence of obstruction or peritonitis).

An upper GI contrast study can be helpful in equivocal cases, especially if there is no evidence of obstructive ileus on survey radiographs. With complete intestinal obstruction, contrast medium does not pass beyond the level of the foreign body. With a partially obstructive foreign body, contrast medium is able to pass the lesion and allows identification of its intraluminal location (see Fig. 13.11).

A special type of small intestinal foreign body is a **linear foreign body** (e.g. string, cloth, linear clothing such as underwear, etc.). Part of the foreign body becomes lodged in the proximal gastrointestinal tract (typically oral cavity/sublingual in cats and within the stomach in dogs), while the free end trails down the intestinal tract. As soon as aborad transport of the foreign body is halted, the intestine starts 'crawling' up the foreign body. This results in 'ribbon candy' or accordion-like intestinal plication. A diagnosis is usually possible on survey radiographs. Intestinal segments appear 'bunched' (Fig. 13.36) and contain mostly fluid as well as multiple discontinuous gas opacities, which are often comma-shaped.

13.5.3 Intussusception

With intussusception there is invagination of a segment of intestine (**intussusceptum**) into an adjacent portion

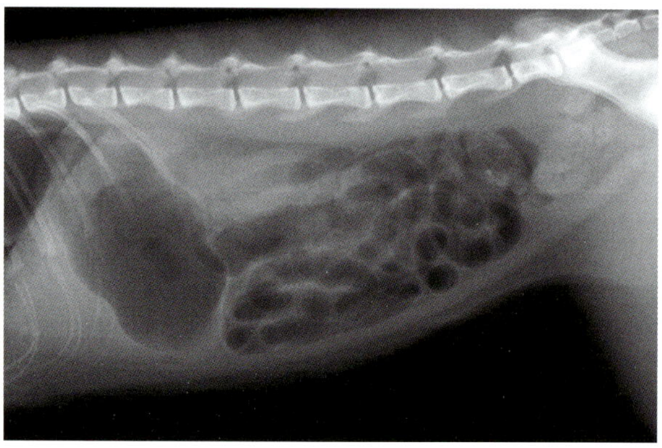

Fig. 13.34 Paralytic ileus in a cat with dysautonomia. The stomach and small intestine are gas-filled throughout. Small intestinal segments are of even diameter and arranged in rounded curves.

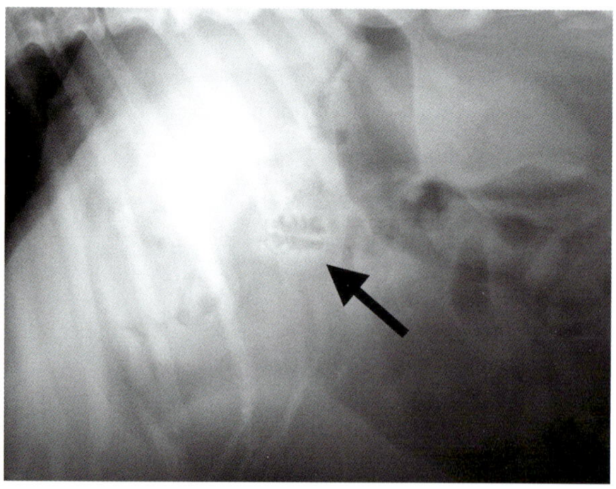

Fig. 13.35 Small intestinal foreign body (walnut) in a dog. The detail of the lateral abdominal radiograph shows a rounded structure with an almost bone opaque rim and a gas-filled centre (arrow). There is no current radiographic evidence of mechanical ileus. However, abdominal surgery was pursued based on the severity of clinical signs.

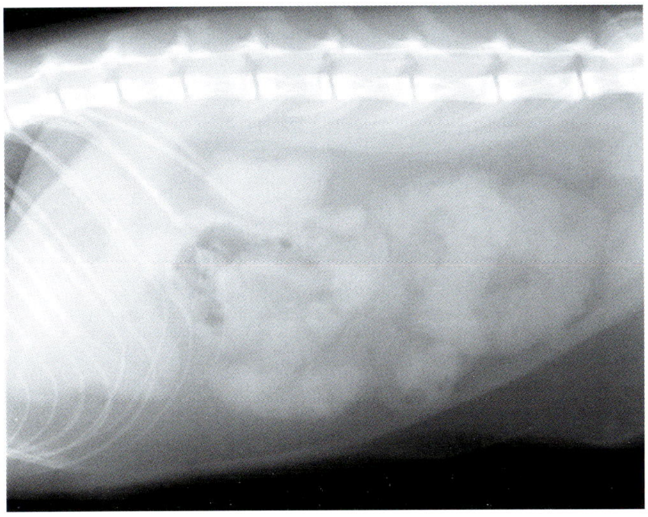

a

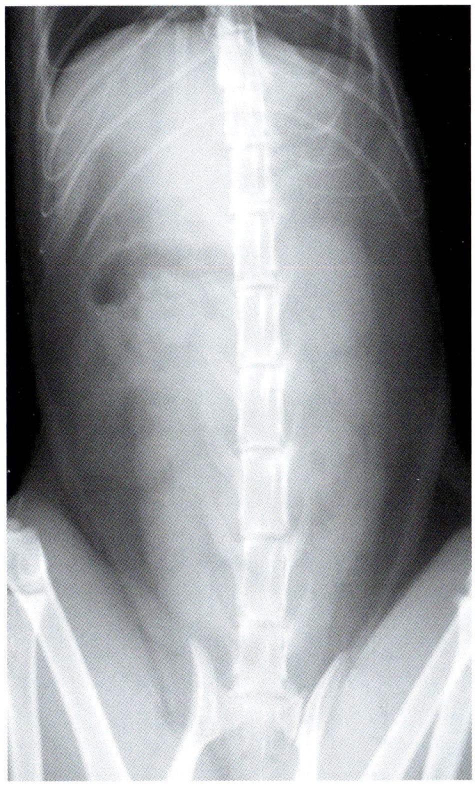

b

Fig. 13.36 Lateral a and ventrodorsal b abdominal radiographs in a cat with a linear foreign body. The entire small intestine is plicated and located in the right ventral abdomen. The intestine mostly contains fluid; occasional discontinuous intraluminal gas foci are also present.

(**intussuscipiens**), resulting in complete or partial mechanical ileus. This problem may occur secondary to abnormal intestinal motility or infiltrative intestinal diseases, or it may be idiopathic. Even though an intussusception can occur in any gastrointestinal tract segment, the small intestine and the transition zone between small and large intestine are most commonly affected.

Radiographic findings Radiographic findings vary depending on the location and underlying cause of the intussusception as well as the presence and degree of intestinal obstruction: with small intestinal intussusception, the small intestine is typically filled with fluid. Concurrent signs of obstructive ileus are common. Differentiation from other obstructive disease processes is often impossible. Air filling of small intestine sometimes facilitates visualization of a sausage-like, blind-ended intraluminal structure consistent with the intussusceptum. An upper GI contrast study may demonstrate the intussusceptum lying within the intussuscipiens; however, intestinal oedema and swelling seen especially with long-standing intussusception may limit entry of contrast medium between the intestinal segments. Radiographic abnormalities consistent with obstructive ileus predominate in these cases. Radiographic findings seen with intussusception of small into large intestine are discussed in section 13.6.3.

13.5.4 Small intestinal volvulus

Rotation of the small intestine around the cranial mesenteric root leads to complete small intestinal obstruction both cranially and caudally and to compromise of the vascular supply. Radiographic abnormalities include severe generalized gas dilatation of the small intestine with a stacked appearance of intestinal segments.

13.5.5 Infiltrative disorders of the small intestine

As discussed for the stomach (see section 13.4.6), the small intestinal wall may be affected by neoplastic or inflammatory (infectious or noninfectious) disease processes. As a rule of thumb, most intestinal tumours (lymphoma, adenocarcinoma, leiomyoma, leiomyosarcoma, gastrointestinal stromal tumour, etc.) tend to cause a focal intestinal mass lesion, while inflammatory disease processes tend to involve longer sections or affect the entire length of the intestine. However, some neoplastic processes may be extensive or generalized (e.g. lymphoma in cats), and some inflammatory or benign processes may result in focal abnormalities (e.g. feline eosinophilic sclerosing fibroplasia). Due to the overlap in radiographic abnormalities found with benign and malignant infiltrative intestinal diseases, a cytological or histopathological examination is needed for a definitive diagnosis.

RADIOGRAPHIC FINDINGS Survey radiographs are often inconclusive, as silhouetting of intraluminal fluid and ingesta with the intestinal wall prohibits accurate evaluation of intestinal wall thickness. Mild generalized intestinal wall thickening common with inflammatory intestinal diseases cannot therefore be reliably diagnosed on survey radiographs. Even focal intestinal masses have to reach a certain size for radiographic visualization and determination of their association with intestine (Fig. 13.37).

Due to the difficulty in intestinal mass lesion identification on survey radiographs, other radiographic abnormalities such as mechanical ileus, concurrent organ abnormalities (e.g. enlarged lymph nodes or hepatosplenomegaly with lymphoma) or signs of peritonitis/pneumoperitoneum with intestinal perforation may predominate at the time of patient presentation.

An **upper GI contrast study** is valuable in the diagnosis of infiltrative intestinal diseases and allows evaluation of gastrointestinal transit time and peristalsis, intestinal wall thickness, lesion extent, mucosal surface and the presence and degree of intestinal obstruction.

As mentioned above, there is an overlap between radiographic abnormalities seen with inflammatory and neoplastic infiltrative diseases of the intestinal wall. With **inflammatory conditions**, abnormalities typically affect longer intestinal segments or the entire length of the intestinal tract. Gastrointestinal transit time is often decreased, and the intestine may appear hyperperistaltic. The intestinal wall may be of normal thickness or mildly thickened. An irregular mucosal surface and spastic contractions of the intestinal wall are common (Fig. 13.38a). Deep mucosal defects (ulceration) and partial or complete intestinal obstruction are rare.

Most **intestinal neoplasms** result in focal areas of wall thickening/mural masses. A radiographic differentiation of different tumour types is not possible. Intestinal adenocarcinomas tend to cause circumferential luminal narrowing with irregular mucosal surface due to ulceration ('apple core appearance') (Fig. 13.38b). Concurrent intestinal obstruction is common. Intestinal lymphoma is often more extensive and may or may not be associated with obstruction. Leiomyomas do not typically result in intestinal obstruction due to their exophytic growth and may be incidental findings.

13.6 Disorders of the large intestine

The same principles and limitations of radiographic examination of the small intestine also apply to the large intestine. Survey radiographs are often unrewarding, necessitating use of advanced imaging (ultrasound, contrast colonogram) or colonoscopy. The radiographic appearance and position of the colon are affected by normal variations (e.g. retroperitoneal fat deposits) and disease processes of adjacent structures (e.g. sublumbar lymph nodes), which must be distinguished from primary large intestinal diseases.

13.6.1 Megacolon

Normal colonic diameter is variable and to some degree dependent on individual factors such as feeding and frequency of defecation. The diagnosis of megacolon should not be made just on the basis of a patient presenting with a large amount of faecal matter within the colon, as this may also be caused by dehydration, for example. However, persistent or recurrent constipation with dilatation of the colon with faecal matter is compatible with megacolon. This may occur secondary to spinal anomalies, metabolic disorders, mechanical luminal narrowing of the pelvic canal (e.g. secondary to a pelvic fracture) and other causes. The predominant radiographic finding is severe dilatation of the colon with faeces.

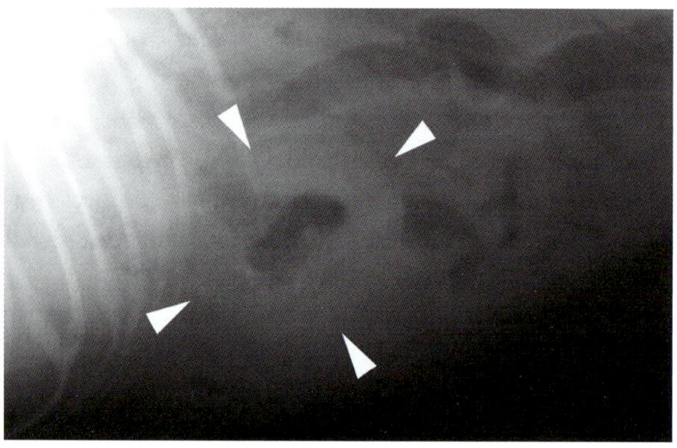

a

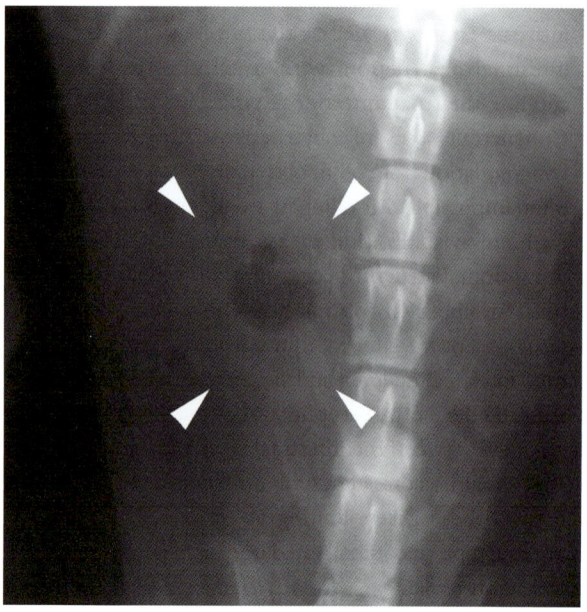

b

Fig. 13.37 Detail of lateral a and ventrodorsal b abdominal radiographs in a dog with an intestinal tumour (lymphoma). Note a soft-tissue opacity mass with central gas accumulation in the right ventral abdomen (arrowheads).

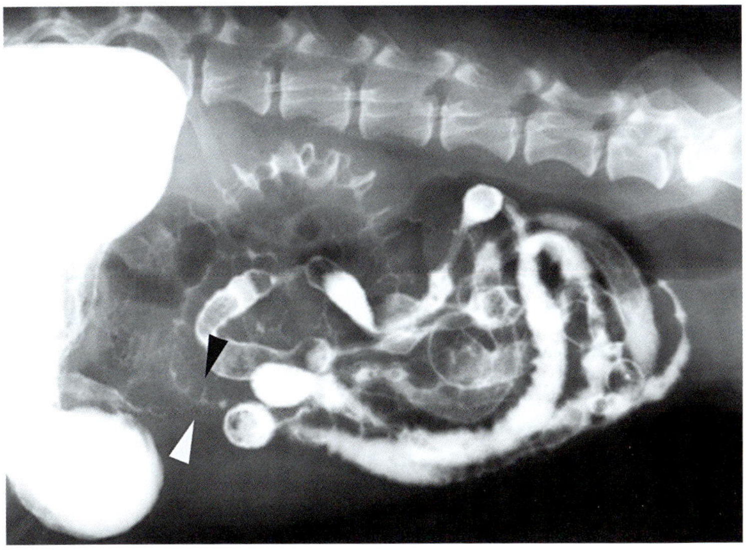

a

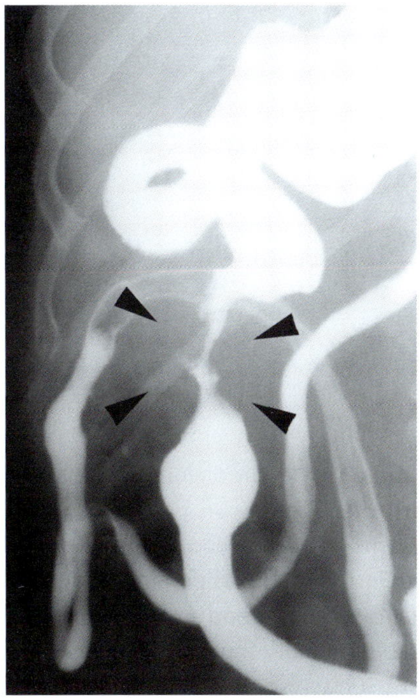

b

Fig. 13.38 Diagnosis of infiltrative small intestinal diseases by means of an upper GI contrast study.
a Inflammatory bowel disease in a dog. The radiograph was obtained 30 minutes after administration of contrast medium. Gastrointestinal transit time is decreased, the intestine is hyperperistaltic and some small intestinal segments appear spastic. Multifocal small intestinal wall thickening is identified (arrowheads). There is no evidence of intestinal obstruction or ulceration. Histological diagnosis was idiopathic chronic inflammatory bowel disease with muscular hypertrophy.
b Duodenal neoplasia in a dog. The radiograph was obtained a few minutes after contrast medium administration. There is a focal circumferential mural mass associated with the descending duodenum (arrowheads). The intestinal lumen is narrowed, the mucosal surface is irregular, and the appearance of the lesion resembles an 'apple core'. Despite luminal narrowing there is no current evidence of complete intestinal obstruction. Histological diagnosis was an ulcerated adenocarcinoma.

A maximum colonic diameter to length of L5 ratio >1.48 has been proposed as a good indicator of megacolon in cats. Depending on the underlying cause, concurrent findings may include spinal or pelvic abnormalities.

13.6.2 Congenital anomalies

Congenital large intestinal anomalies are rare in small animals and include atresia of the anus or colon and rectovaginal fistulas. Survey radiographs are typically unrewarding. A diagnosis is made based on a combination of clinical examination findings and contrast procedures (colonogram, fistulogram).

13.6.3 Intussusception

Intussusception of small or large intestinal segments into the colon is relatively common and may be idiopathic or occur secondary to neuromuscular conditions or infiltrative intestinal diseases. Especially in older cats, it is often associated with neoplasia at the ileocaecocolic junction.

Radiographic findings Survey radiographs are often unremarkable. However, if the colon is air-filled, the intussusceptum may be visible within the proximal colon where it appears as a fairly homogeneous sausage-like intraluminal structure with a rounded edge that is bordered by a concave gaseous margin (Fig. 13.39). If intussusception results in complete intestinal obstruction, radiographic signs of mechanical ileus predominate. A positive or negative contrast colonogram may be helpful in equivocal cases and will show the intussusceptum as an intraluminal filling defect with a rounded, blind edge.

13.6.4 Infiltrative disorders of the large intestine

As described for the small intestine, neoplastic and non-neoplastic infiltrative diseases may affect the large intestine.

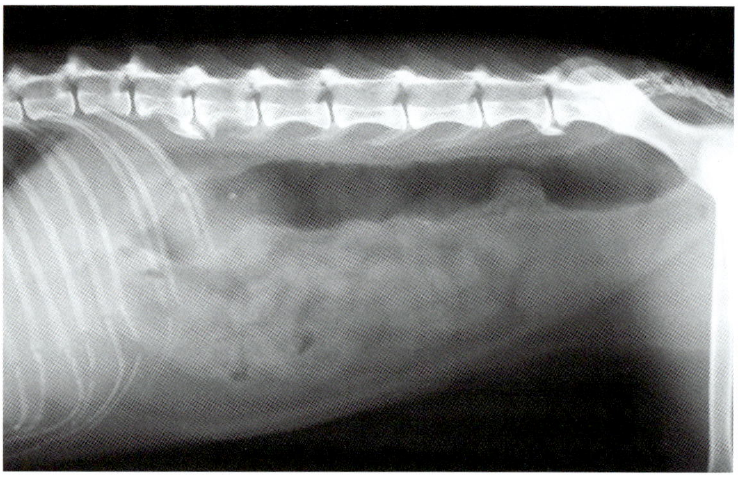

a

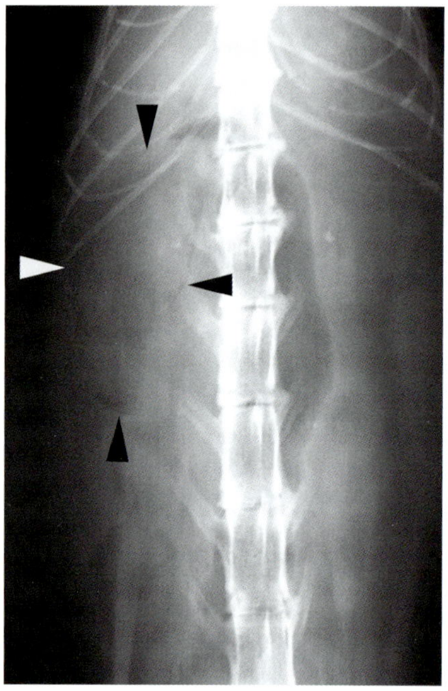

b

Fig. 13.39 Ileocaecocolic intussusception in a 14-year-old cat.
a On the lateral abdominal radiograph, the descending colon contains mostly air and a small amount of peripheral faecal matter. The ascending and transverse colon are not visible. Renal mineralization and lumbar spondylosis deformans are incidental.
b On the ventrodorsal view, an elongated, blind-ended, 'sausage-like' intraluminal structure with soft-tissue opacity is present within the descending and proximal transverse colon, consistent with the intussusceptum (arrowheads). The gas column within the descending and transverse colon abruptly terminates at the border of the lesion. Surgical resection and anastomosis was performed. The histological examination of removed intestine yielded a diagnosis of lymphocytic plasmacytic enteritis but no evidence of neoplasia.

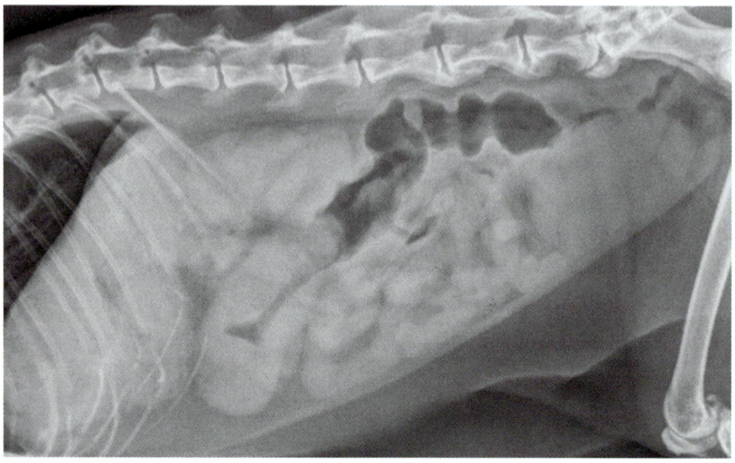

a

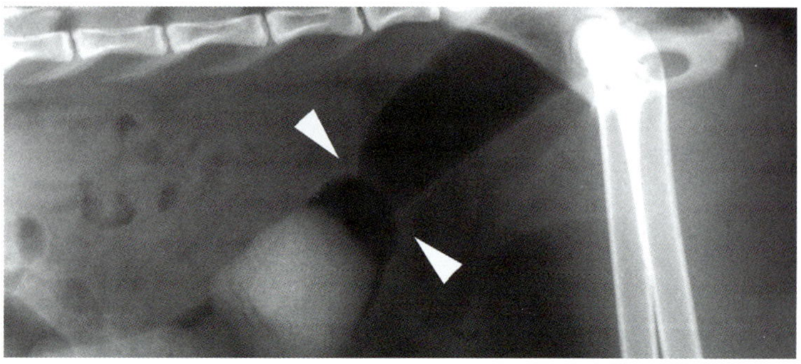

b

Fig. 13.40 Diagnosis of infiltrative large intestinal diseases.
a Lateral abdominal radiograph in a cat. The caudal part of the descending colon is empty/air-filled. The cranial descending colon and the transverse colon are moderately to severely thickened. Histological diagnosis was lymphoma. Degenerative lumbar spinal changes and degenerative disease of the stifle joint are incidental.
b Negative contrast colonogram in a cat. There is marked focal circumferential narrowing of the descending colon (arrowheads), consistent with a stricture. The descending colon proximal to the lesion is distended with formed faecal matter and gas.

RADIOGRAPHIC FINDINGS Survey radiographs may demonstrate obstipation secondary to luminal narrowing, or fluid accumulation within the colonic lumen. Diagnosis of underlying infiltrative colonic disease is usually not possible. However, in severe cases and/or if the colon is air-filled, colonic wall thickening or mass lesions may be visible (Fig. 13.40a).

Further diagnostics include imaging or endoscopy. A (double contrast) colonogram allows identification and characterization of a mural large intestinal lesion (Fig. 13.40b).

As discussed above, abnormalities such as intestinal wall thickening, stricture, ulceration or mass may be caused by benign or malignant processes, necessitating histopathology or cytology for definitive diagnosis in many cases.

References and further reading

Brawner WR, Bartels JE. Contrast radiography of the digestive tract. Indications, techniques and complications. Vet Clin North Am Small Anim Pract 1983; 13: 599–26.

Evans S. Double versus single contrast gastrography in the dog and cat. Vet Radiol 1983; 24: 6–10.

Hall JA, Watrous BJ. Effect of pharmaceuticals on radiographic appearance of selected examinations of the abdomen and thorax. Vet Clin North Am Small Anim Pract 2000; 30: 349–77.

Hecht S. Die Kontrastmitteluntersuchung des Verdauungstraktes. Part 1: Grundlagen, Kontrastmittel, Ösophagographie. Tierärztl Prax (K) 2004a; 32: 322–8.

Hecht S. Die Kontrastmitteluntersuchung des Verdauungstraktes. Part 2: Gastrographie, Passage, Irrigoskopie. Tierärztl Prax (K) 2004b; 32: 389–94.

Kleine LJ, Lamb CR. Comparative organ imaging: The gastrointestinal tract. Vet Radiol 1989; 30: 133–41.

McNeel SV. The small bowel. In: Thrall DE (ed.). Textbook of Veterinary Diagnostic Radiology. Philadelphia: Saunders 1994; 524–43.

O'Brien T. Radiographic Diagnosis of Abdominal Disorders in the Dog and Cat. Philadelphia: Saunders 1978.

Owens JM, Biery DN. Radiographic Interpretation for the Small Animal Clinician. Baltimore: Williams & Wilkins 1999.

Selting KA. Intestinal tumors. In: Withrow SJ, Vail DM (eds). Withrow and MacEwen's Small Animal Clinical Oncology, 4th edn. St. Louis: Saunders Elsevier 2007; 491–503.

Stickle RL, Love NE. Radiographic diagnosis of esophageal diseases in dogs and cats. Semin Vet Med Surg 1989; 4: 179–87.

Thrall DE. Textbook of Veterinary Diagnostic Radiology. Philadelphia: WB Saunders 2002.

Trevail T, Gunn-Moore D, Carrera I, Courcier E, Sullivan M. Radiographic diameter of the colon in normal and constipated cats and in cats with megacolon. Vet Radiol Ultrasound 2011; 52: 516–20.

Ticer JW. Radiographic Technique in Veterinary Practice. Philadelphia: Saunders 1984.

Wallack ST. The Handbook of Veterinary Contrast Radiography. Solana Beach, CA: San Diego Veterinary Imaging, Inc 2003.

Watrous BJ. Clinical presentation and diagnosis of dysphagia. Vet Clin North Am Small Anim Pract 1983; 13: 437–59.

Weissman A, Penninck D, Webster C, Hecht S, Keating J, Craig LE. Ultrasonographic and clinicopathological features of feline gastrointestinal eosinophilic sclerosing fibroplasia in four cats. J Fel Med Surg 2013; 15: 148–54.

Wyse CA, McLellan J, Dickie AM, Sutton DG, Preston T, Yam PS. A review of methods for assessment of the rate of gastric emptying in the dog and cat: 1898–2002. J Vet Intern Med 2003; 17: 609–21.

Zwingenberger AL, Marks SL, Baker TW, Moore PF. Ultrasonographic evaluation of the muscularis propria in cats with diffuse small intestinal lymphoma or inflammatory bowel disease. J Vet Intern Med 2010; 24: 289–92.

14 Urogenital tract (including contrast procedures)

Silke Hecht and George A. Henry

14.1 Anatomy and indications

14.1.1 Anatomy

The radiographic evaluation of the urinary tract includes the kidneys, ureters, urinary bladder and urethra. Female reproductive organs evaluated radiographically include the ovaries, uterus and, with limitations, the vagina. The prostatic gland is typically the only male reproductive organ evaluated radiographically. However, abnormal position or enlargement of the testicles may be noted, and possible underlying conditions will be covered in this chapter. The penis and prepuce are also visible on radiographs. Survey radiographs have limitations in the diagnosis of urogenital tract diseases, and further imaging procedures such as contrast medium studies or ultrasound are often needed for detailed evaluation. This section will cover the radiographic anatomy of the urogenital tract on survey radiographs and contrast procedures.

Kidneys

The kidneys are located in the retroperitoneal space between the 13th thoracic and the 4th lumbar vertebra. They are of soft-tissue opacity, smoothly marginated, ovoid, and in well-nourished animals clearly delineated by retroperitoneal fat (Fig. 14.1a). The right kidney is located to the right of the spine and is in contact with the renal fossa of the caudate process of the liver. The left kidney is located to the left of the spine and further

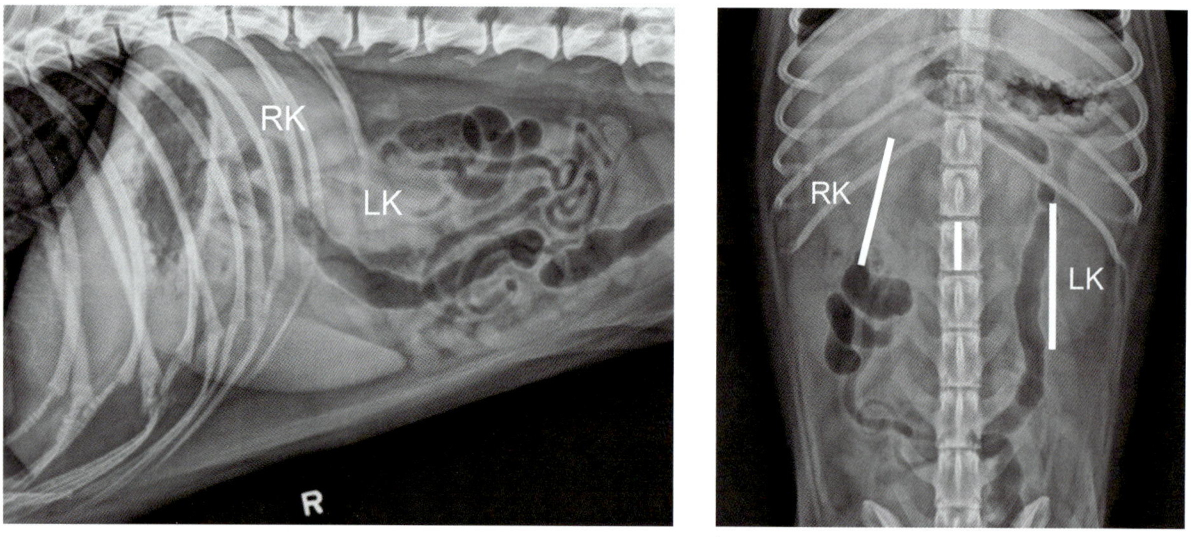

a b

Fig. 14.1 Lateral a and ventrodorsal b radiographs of the abdomen in a normal dog. The right kidney (RK) is located cranial and slightly dorsal to the left kidney (LK) and is in contact with the caudate process of the liver. The kidneys are clearly visible as they contrast with adjacent retroperitoneal fat. Relative renal size is judged on a ventrodorsal view by comparing its length to the length of the left vertebral body (L2): LK = 3 × L2; RK = 2.8 × L2.

caudal than the right kidney. It is fairly mobile and may be found in a more ventral location than expected in some animals.

Renal size is evaluated by comparing the length of a kidney to the length of the second lumbar vertebral body (L2) on a ventrodorsal view. Normal renal size in **dogs** is 2.5–3.5 × L2 (Fig. 14.1b). Normal renal length in **cats** has traditionally been reported as 2.4–3.0 × L2. However, more recent studies have shown a significant association of renal size with reproductive status, and reference values have been adjusted accordingly: normal renal length is 1.9–2.6 × L2 in neutered and spayed cats, and 2.1–3.2 × L2 in intact cats.

Normal kidneys are usually of homogeneous soft-tissue opacity. However, in fat cats a central region of decreased opacity may be noted, which is attributed to peripelvic fat deposition (Fig. 14.2).

> Peripelvic fat deposition in the kidneys of fat cats should not be confused with pathological gas inclusions.

Ureters

These are not visible on survey radiographs in normal animals but can be evaluated by means of excretory urography (see section 14.2.1).

Urinary bladder

The urinary bladder is located in the caudoventral abdomen and may extend caudally into the pelvic canal. It is of homogeneous soft-tissue opacity, smoothly marginated and delineated by surrounding peritoneal fat. It consists of a rounded cranial **apex**, a **body,** and a caudal **neck** that tapers towards the pelvic inlet (Fig. 14.3). The size and shape of the urinary bladder are highly variable and depend on the degree of filling. There are no published reference values for minimum or maximum urinary bladder size in dogs and cats.

Urethra

The urethra originates at the bladder neck. It is not visible on survey radiographs in normal animals, but may be visualized and evaluated by means of urethrography (see section 14.2.2).

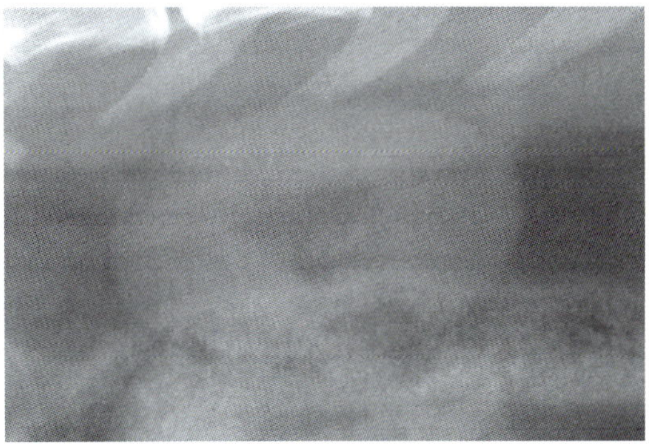

a

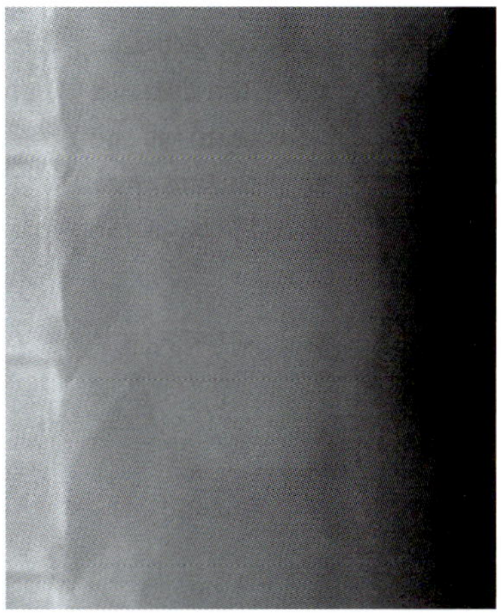

b

Fig. 14.2 Close-up of a lateral a and a ventrodorsal b abdominal radiograph in a normal cat. The central region is less opaque than the periphery due to the presence of peripelvic fat.

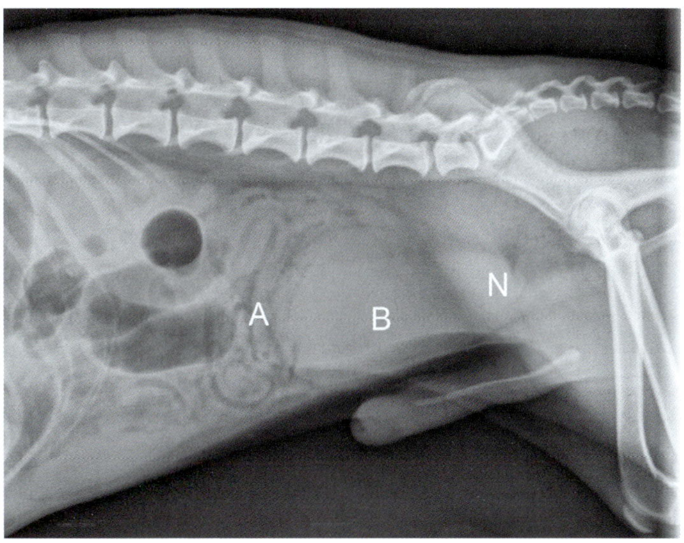

Fig. 14.3 Lateral view of the caudal abdomen in a dog. The urinary bladder is located cranial to the pelvis (A = apex, B = body, N = neck).

Ovaries, uterus and vagina

The normal ovaries are located in immediate proximity to the caudal poles of the kidneys. They are not usually visible on survey radiographs owing to their small size. Similarly, a normal nongravid uterus and the vagina are not usually visible. Particularly in fat animals, a normal uterus may on occasion be seen as a thin structure of soft-tissue opacity located between the urinary bladder and the descending colon (see Fig. 11.4). The radiographic appearance of the uterus during pregnancy is covered in section 14.5.1.

Prostatic gland

The appearance of the normal prostate in dogs varies with age, status (intact or neutered) and, to some degree, breed.

The prostate in **neutered dogs** is small and inconspicuous, and is often not visible on radiographs due to its small size and intrapelvic position. If visible, it appears as a thin oval structure of soft-tissue opacity immediately caudal to the urinary bladder.

The prostate in **intact dogs** is usually clearly visible. It appears as a round, soft-tissue opaque, smoothly marginated structure caudal to the urinary bladder, located either in the caudoventral abdomen or (partially) within the pelvic canal. The prostate increases in size with age. On a lateral view, it should not exceed 70% of the distance between the pubis and the cranioventral margin of the sacrum (Fig. 14.4a). It may be difficult to delineate on a ventrodorsal view, where it should not exceed 50% of the transverse pelvic canal diameter (Fig. 14.4b).

The prostate is not visible in **cats**.

Testicles, penis and prepuce

As mentioned in section 14.1.1, these structures are not usually evaluated radiographically. The scrotum may be noted as soft-tissue opaque structure in the inguinal region in intact dogs. Visible testicles, the penis and prepuce should not be mistaken for pathological structures.

14.1.2 Indications

In general, indications for a radiographic examination of the urogenital tract overlap with those for general abdominal radiography. Specific indications for evaluation of the urinary tract include azotaemia, haematuria, dysuria, pollakiuria and stranguria. Indications for contrast studies of the urinary tract are covered in section 14.2. Specific indications for a radiographic evaluation of the female reproductive tract include vaginal discharge, pregnancy, and abdominal mass lesions in female intact dogs. Specific indications for a radiographic evaluation of the male reproductive tract include prostatic enlargement and/or pain, difficulty urinating and caudal abdominal mass lesions.

14.2 Radiographic technique and positioning

Radiographic technique and positioning for general abdominal radiography are described in Chapter 11. This section will cover the basic principles for contrast studies of the urinary tract.

Different types of contrast procedures (**positive, negative and double contrast studies**) have already been discussed in Chapters 11 and 13. Contrast studies of the urinary tract that are easily performed in practice include **excretory urography**,

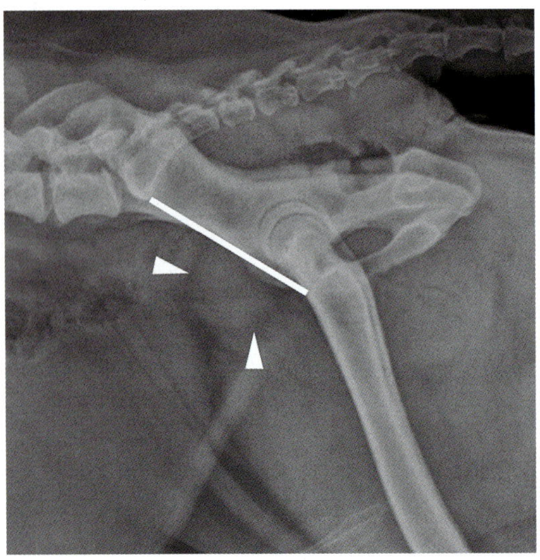

a

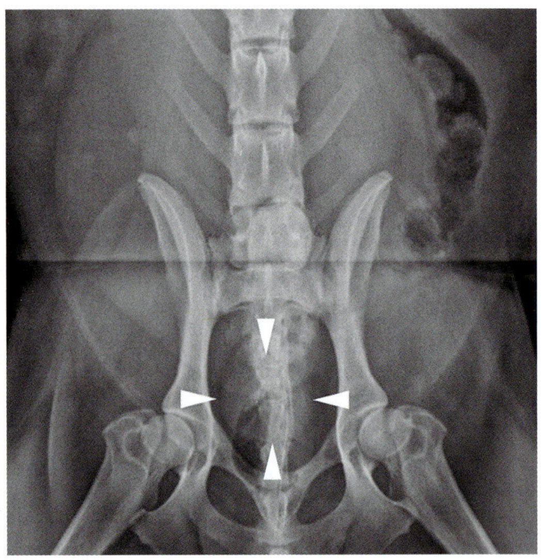

b

Fig. 14.4 Lateral a and ventrodorsal b radiographs of the abdomen in a 2-year-old male intact dog. The prostate (arrowheads) is surrounded by fat and easily recognized. On the lateral view, it measures approximately 60% of the height of the pelvic inlet (white line). On the ventrodorsal view, it occupies approximately 50% of the transverse pelvic diameter.

retrograde cystography and urethrography. Even though abdominal ultrasound is often preferred for evaluation of the urinary tract in small animals, these contrast studies may be superior to ultrasonography for certain indications (localization of the urinary bladder when cystic or mass lesions are present in the caudal abdomen, suspected rupture of a kidney, ureter, urinary bladder or urethra, and diagnosis of ectopic ureters and urethral diseases).

Additional contrast procedures for the urinary tract include **antegrade pyelography**, **antegrade urethrography** and **computed tomography (CT) excretory urography**. However, these procedures are rarely performed in practice as they are technically demanding, may require specialized equipment, and/or raise concerns with regards to radiation safety or adverse effects.

14.2.1 Excretory urography (EU)/intravenous pyelography (IVP)

Iodinated contrast medium is administered intravenously and is excreted with urine following glomerular filtration by the kidneys. This procedure allows evaluation of the kidneys, ureters and (with limitations) the urinary bladder.

Indications

The main indication for excretory urography is evaluation of the ureters (suspected ureteral obstruction, ectopia or rupture). The technique can also be used to visualize the kidneys and urinary bladder if those are not visible on survey radiographs (e.g. due to poor abdominal detail in animals with ascites, or due to abdominal mass lesions). Lastly, the degree and pattern of renal contrast medium accumulation and excretion allow an approximate assessment of renal function.

Contrast medium

Any iodinated contrast medium labelled for intravenous use and excreted through the kidneys can be used for this procedure. Ionic contrast agents are considered safe for use in most animals. However, if the procedure is to be performed in high-risk patients (e.g. old cats with heart and/or renal damage), nonionic (more expensive) contrast agents are preferred. Adverse effects following intravenous administration of contrast medium are less common in veterinary patients than in humans; however, certain precautions should be taken.

Contraindications

The most important contraindication for excretory urography is **dehydration** or **oliguria,** as the injection of iodinated contrast medium may cause acute renal failure in these patients. The study should be delayed until the animal is adequately hydrated. Decreased renal function is not considered a true contraindication. However, the increase in contrast medium dose required to achieve adequate contrast uptake by the kidneys increases the risk of adverse effects. In the rare case of known allergy to iodine, iodinated contrast agents should not be administered.

Adverse effects

The most important and severe adverse effects of the intravenous administration of contrast medium are **hypotension** and **acute renal failure**. Affected animals show initially good contrast medium uptake in the renal parenchyma, but the renal pelvis and ureter fail to fill with contrast medium. The kidneys accumulate more and more contrast medium over time, resulting in a progressive increase rather than a decrease in renal opacity. Contrast-induced renal failure is reversible with aggressive intravenous fluid therapy, which should be instituted immediately. Based on our experience, this complication is rare in adequately hydrated animals. Other possible adverse effects include **nausea/vomiting** (not observed in patients under general anaesthesia) and **allergic reactions**.

Procedure

1. Bloodwork (including serum urea and creatinine) and urinalysis (including culture and sensitivity).
   - Diagnosis and correction of dehydration.
   - Adjustment of contrast medium dose in patients with azotaemia.
   - Iodinated contrast media affect growth of some bacteria in culture. Urine culture and sensitivity is of limited value after an excretory urogram has been performed.
2. Adequate patient preparation (unless emergency).
   - Fasting for 24 hours with free access to water.
   - ± enema to evacuate rectum and colon. This is especially important if the examination is performed to determine the presence of ectopic ureters.
   - Placement of an intravenous catheter and intravenous fluid administration in case of dehydration.
3. Sedation or general anaesthesia.
   - General anaesthesia is recommended especially in patients with suspected ectopic ureters as multiple radiographs with variable positioning require extensive manipulation of the animal. It is also recommended if abdominal compression may be necessary for improved evaluation of the renal pelves.
   - Minimization of nausea and vomiting.
   - Preferable from a radiation safety perspective (examiner can leave the room during radiographs).
4. Intravenous fluid administration throughout the duration of the procedure.
5. Lateral and ventrodorsal survey radiographs.
6. Placement of a urinary catheter and filling of the urinary bladder with negative contrast medium (gas) prior to excretory urography increases the contrast between bladder lumen and positive contrast medium within the ureters. This may aid in the diagnosis of ectopic ureters.

7. Intravenous contrast medium bolus.
   - Dose (independent of contrast medium): 880 mg iodine/kg.
   - In azotaemic patients (urea >100 mg/dl, creatinine >4 mg/dl): double contrast medium dose.
8. Radiographs:
   - Ventrodorsal and lateral radiographs immediately following contrast medium injection and after 5, 10, 20 (± 40, 60) minutes.
   - ± oblique views of the urinary bladder after 10 minutes to evaluate termination of the ureters.
   - The timing of the radiographs varies depending on the indication and if/when the clinical question has been satisfactorily answered. For example, a ureteral avulsion may be noted very early in the study, while partial ureteral obstruction in a patient with chronic renal insufficiency may not be evident until later due to delayed contrast medium excretion.

Interpretation

The quality of the contrast study depends on the ability of the kidneys to clear contrast medium from the blood (glomerular filtration) and to concentrate it in the renal parenchyma (reabsorption of water and electrolytes in the proximal renal tubules). A schematic illustration of a physiological radiographic sequence during excretory urography is shown in Fig. 14.5. Sequential radiographs obtained during excretory urography in a normal dog are shown in Fig. 14.6.

NEPHROGRAM (FILTRATION PHASE)

- The nephrogram can be subdivided into two phases:
  - **vascular phase** (passage of contrast medium through the renal vessels):
    - very early (5–10 seconds following injection of contrast medium) and thus often not documented radiographically
    - cortex more opaque than medulla.
  - **tubular phase** (contrast medium accumulates in the renal tubules following glomerular filtration).
- The maximum contrast accumulation within the kidneys is reached after 10–30 seconds. If the contrast study is performed for **evaluation of renal parenchyma** (e.g. to assess for filling defects indicating cysts or renal tumours), radiographs obtained immediately after contrast administration, after 1 minute and after 5 minutes provide the best results.
- The **degree of contrast medium uptake** and thus the radiopacity of the kidneys on radiographs depends on several factors:
  - hydration status of the patient
  - plasma osmolality
  - renal function
  - renal blood supply (this explains decreased contrast medium uptake, e.g. in case of heart failure).
- Renal opacity decreases over 1–3 hours. After 2 hours, a persistent nephrogram is only visible in approximately 25% of healthy dogs. The **duration of the nephrogram** is proportional to the contrast medium dose administered. Additional factors include glomerular filtration rate, unobstructed ureteral clearance of urine, and adequate renal blood supply (including systemic blood pressure).
- The only **physiological filling defects** within the kidney are the renal pelvis and peripelvic fat deposits.

PYELOGRAM (EXCRETORY PHASE)

- Excretion of contrast medium and reabsorption of water results in increased concentration of contrast medium in the collecting system. The collecting system is increased in opacity compared to the renal parenchyma.
- The **renal pelves** and **ureters** are visible shortly after contrast medium administration (typically 1–3 minutes following the nephrogram). Due to successive excretion of contrast medium, the collecting system may remain visible for several hours. However, evaluation of the pyelogram is best performed within the first hour of the study.
- The renal pelves and ureters can usually be evaluated without further patient manipulation. However, to improve visualization of the **pelvic diverticula** (e.g. for diagnosis of pyelonephritis or small renal calculi), abdominal compression may be necessary. This can be accomplished by tightly wrapping the animal's abdomen in a bandage or blanket. The applied abdominal pressure results in backflow of contrast medium into the renal pelves and pelvic diverticula, which improves visualization of these structures.
- The **diameter** of the renal pelves and diverticula should not exceed 1–2 mm, and ureteral diameter should not exceed 2–3 mm.
- Fluoroscopic evaluation during the pyelogram phase allows evaluation of **ureteral peristalsis**. This is not possible on static radiographs.

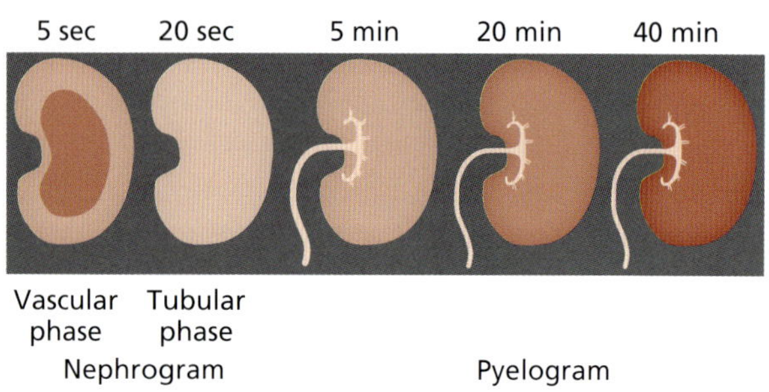

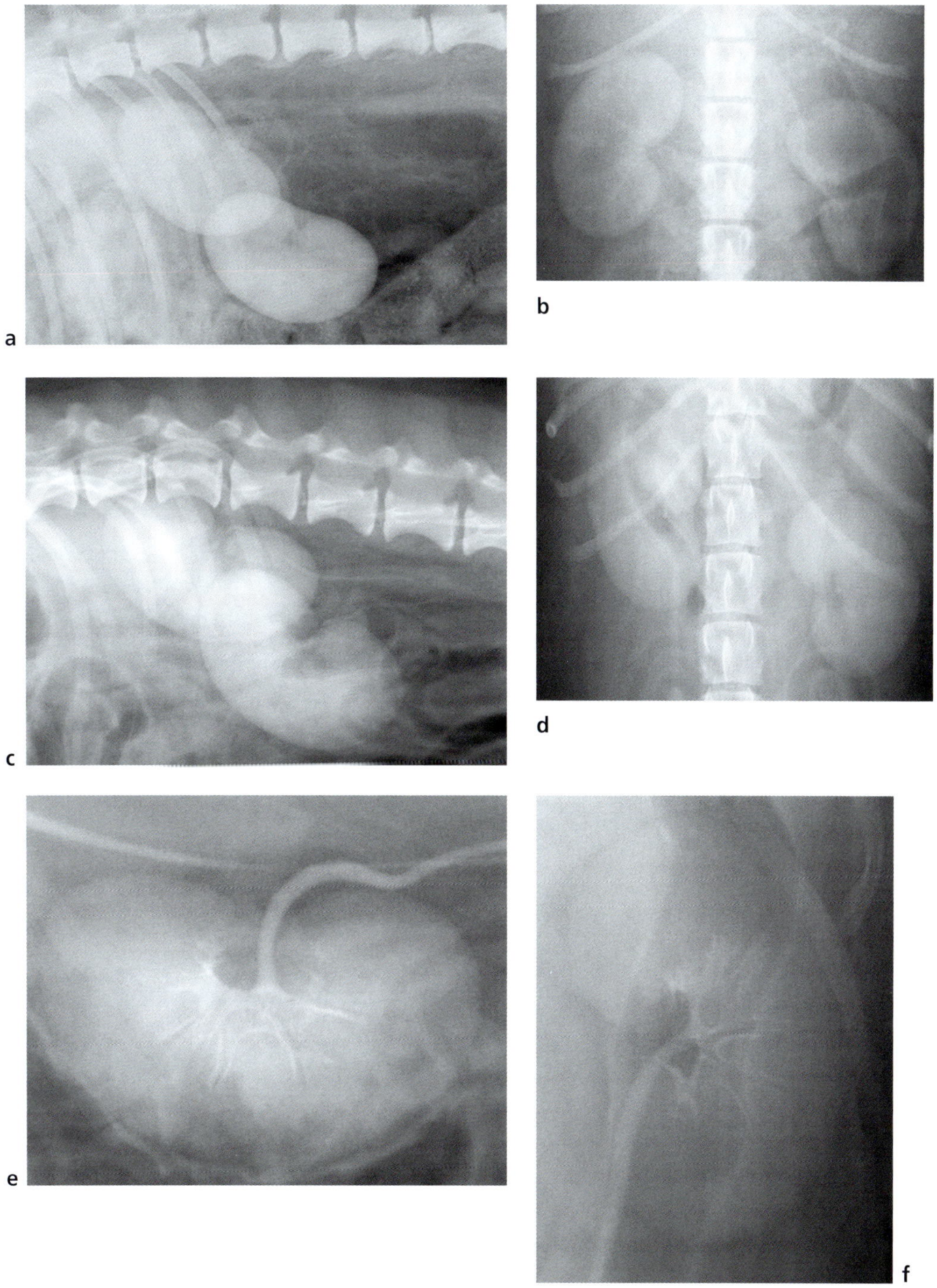

Fig. 14.6 Phases of normal excretory urography.

a, b Vascular phase of the nephrogram: Contrast medium is visible within the abdominal vasculature. The renal cortex is more opaque than the medulla.

c, d Tubular phase of the nephrogram: The kidneys are of homogeneously increased opacity. The renal pelves and ureters are indistinctly visible but at this point only contain a very small amount of contrast medium.

e, f Pyelogram phase: The renal pelves and ureters are filled with contrast medium and are more opaque than the renal parenchyma. The diverticula of the renal pelves are evenly filled with contrast medium and uniformly thin.

Fig. 14.5 Schematic illustration of normal excretory urography phases. The initial nephrogram phase (consisting of a very short vascular and subsequent tubular phase) is characterized by strong renal contrast medium uptake. Renal opacity decreases during the pyelogram phase. Contrast medium is excreted and outlines the renal pelvis, ureter and urinary bladder.

A schematic illustration of common pathological findings during excretory urography is provided in Fig. 14.7. Possible findings during the nephrogram and pyelogram phases are summarized in Tables 14.1 and 14.2, respectively.

14.2.2 Cystography and urethrography (retrograde)

These procedures involve retrograde instillation of contrast medium into the urinary bladder (**cystography**) and/or urethra (**urethrography**). A cystogram can be performed as a negative contrast study, positive contrast study or double contrast study (Fig. 14.8). A **urethrogram** is performed using positive contrast medium (Fig. 14.9).

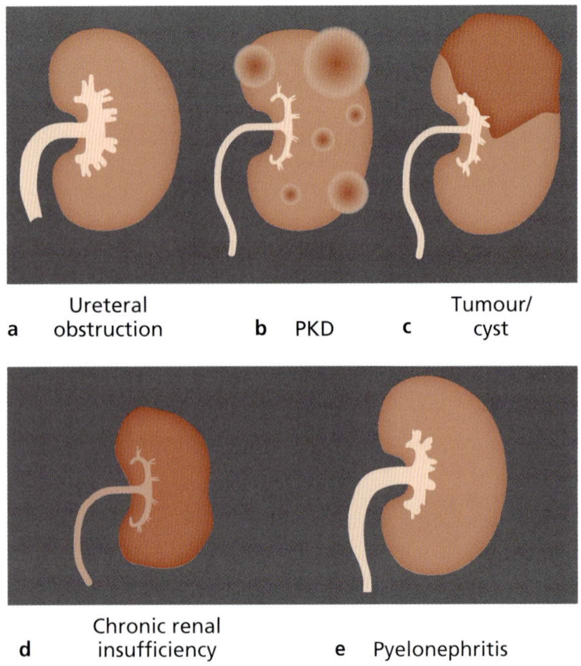

Fig. 14.7 Schematic overview of typical pathological findings during excretory urography.
a Uniform dilatation of the renal pelvis and proximal ureter is indicative of an obstructive lesion.
b Numerous round, smooth filling defects within renal parenchyma are commonly seen with cysts (e.g. polycystic kidney disease). However, solid lesions (e.g. metastasis) cannot be entirely excluded.
c A solitary irregularly marginated filling defect is most consistent with renal neoplasia (e.g. carcinoma).
d A small, irregularly marginated kidney with decreased contrast medium uptake is a typical finding in chronic/end-stage renal disease.
e Irregular margination of a dilated renal pelvis is indicative of pyelonephritis.

Indications for cystography/urethrography include persistent haematuria, stranguria, pyuria, crystalluria, proteinuria, dysuria and persistent or recurrent urinary tract infections. A contrast study may also be considered if the urinary bladder cannot be identified on an abdominal radiograph, or cannot be distinguished from caudal abdominal mass lesions. Even though abdominal ultrasound is now commonly used instead of contrast examinations for many of the above indications, cystography/urethrography remains the method of choice in the diagnosis of suspected bladder or urethral rupture.

Negative contrast cystography

There are only a few indications for a negative contrast study of the urinary bladder (Fig. 14.8a). This method allows quick and easy localization of the urinary bladder. It is also useful in the diagnosis of certain intraluminal filling defects (bladder calculi); however, it is inferior to double contrast cystography for this indication. A negative contrast cystography is often used as a complementary technique when performing an excretory urogram (see section 14.2.1). Especially in patients with haematuria, the use of CO_2 rather than room air is recommended due to its improved solubility in blood and thus decreased risk of gas embolism.

Positive contrast cystography

This technique can be used to localize the urinary bladder and assess bladder wall integrity. Any iodinated contrast medium approved for intravenous application may be used. Contrast medium is diluted 1:10 with sterile physiological saline solution (Fig. 14.8b).

Double contrast cystography

This is the preferred technique for most indications, as it provides the best visualization of the mucosa and any intraluminal structures.

Table 14.1 Possible findings during the nephrogram phase of an excretory urogram.

Finding	Description
Renal morphology	
Decreased size	Many chronic renal diseases result in atrophy of the renal parenchyma over time. In addition to small kidney size, decreased contrast medium uptake is noted during excretory urography. The changes may be unilateral or bilateral.
Enlargement	An increase in size of one kidney can result from obstruction (hydronephrosis), inflammatory or neoplastic infiltration, as well as compensatory hypertrophy due to contralateral renal insufficiency. Enlargement of both kidneys may result from inflammatory conditions (e.g. interstitial nephritis or pyelonephritis), neoplasia (e.g. lymphoma), or less commonly from bilateral obstruction.
Abnormal shape and contour	These can result from many different conditions including mass lesions or chronic infarcts.
Abnormal location and number	Abnormal position of a kidney (renal ectopia), missing or supernumerary kidneys are rare and often incidental.
Homogeneity of contrast medium uptake and filling defects	Regions of decreased contrast medium uptake compared to adjacent normal strongly enhancing parenchyma may be seen with cysts, focal masses (e.g. neoplasia), nephroliths and infarcts. With hydronephrosis, the remaining parenchyma may form a variably thin contrast enhancing rim around the dilated renal pelvis.
Contrast medium uptake (onset, degree and decrease)	
Adequate initial contrast medium uptake followed by successive decrease in radiopacity	Normal
Moderate to adequate initial contrast medium uptake followed by successive increase in radiopacity	Contrast-induced renal failure, systemic hypotension (contrast-induced), acute renal obstruction (including contrast-induced precipitation of protein in renal tubules)
Moderate to adequate initial contrast medium uptake that remains unchanged over time	Acute renal tubular necrosis, contrast-induced renal failure, systemic hypotension (contrast-induced), ethylene glycol toxicity
Poor initial contrast medium uptake followed by successive decrease in radiopacity	Polyuric renal failure, inadequate dose of contrast medium administered
Poor initial contrast medium uptake followed by successive increase in radiopacity	Acute extrarenal obstruction, systemic hypotension (pre-existing prior to contrast medium administration), renal ischaemia
Poor initial contrast medium uptake that remains unchanged over time	Primary chronic glomerular dysfunction, severe generalized renal disease
No nephrogram	Unilateral: Renal aplasia, prior nephrectomy, renal artery occlusion Bilateral: Inadequate dose of contrast medium, paravenous injection of contrast medium

Table 14.2 Possible findings during the pyelogram phase of an excretory urogram.

Finding	Description
Renal pelvis and/or ureteral morphology	
Enlargement	While mild dilatation of the renal pelvis may be seen with inflammatory conditions (pyelonephritis), moderate to marked renal pelvis and ureteral dilatation is usually indicative of an obstructive process. Possible underlying aetiologies include urinary calculi, haematuria, an increased amount of cells and protein in urine (e.g. with pyelonephritis), iatrogenic causes and bladder tumours in the region of the trigone. Ectopic ureters are often partially obstructed and increase in diameter over time.
Abnormal shape and contour	Inflammation of the renal pelvis (pyelonephritis) usually results in an irregular contour of the renal pelvis with plump or uneven sized pelvic diverticula. Space-occupying lesions bordering the renal pelvis, such as cysts or neoplastic lesions, may also affect its appearance.
Abnormal location	One of the most common indications for excretory urography is urinary incontinence due to suspected ectopic ureters. Instead of terminating in the urinary bladder at the bladder neck, the abnormal ureter connects to the urethra or vagina, and contrast medium accumulates within these structures. A diagnosis is unfortunately often difficult due to concurrent abnormal position of the urinary bladder within the pelvic canal, oblique course of the ureters through the bladder wall, or the presence of several ureteral openings with an intramural course. Bilateral ureteral ectopia poses an additional diagnostic challenge. Filling of the urinary bladder with negative contrast medium prior to excretory urography is recommended as it increases the contrast between ureter and bladder lumen. Oblique views are usually required in addition to standard lateral and ventrodorsal radiographs.
Filling defects	Material within the renal pelvis or ureter (urinary calculi, neoplastic tissue, blood clots or pus) appears as filling defects of variable size and shape within surrounding contrast medium. Ureteral peristalsis has to be distinguished from true filling defects. In contrast to ureteral pathology, peristaltic waves are absent or are present in a different location on successive radiographs and are not associated with pre-stenotic ureteral dilatation.
Contrast medium leakage	Ureteral avulsion/rupture most commonly occurs secondary to abdominal trauma and is characterized by contrast medium leakage into the surrounding soft tissues.
Contrast medium uptake (onset, degree and decrease) (Usually concurrent with abnormal nephrogram)	
Decreased contrast medium uptake	Inability of the kidney to concentrate urine
Persistent contrast medium uptake	Ureteral obstruction

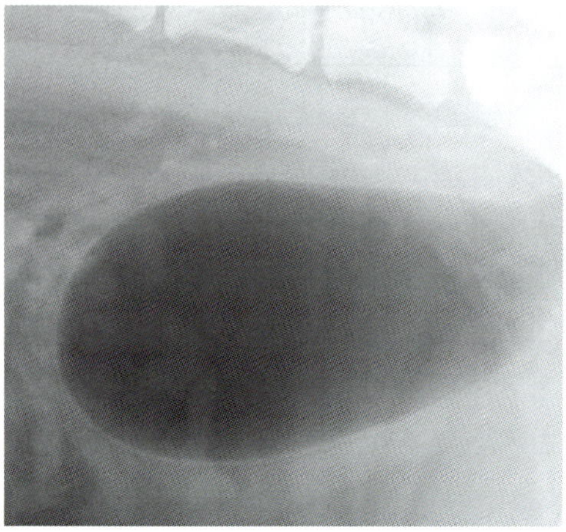

a

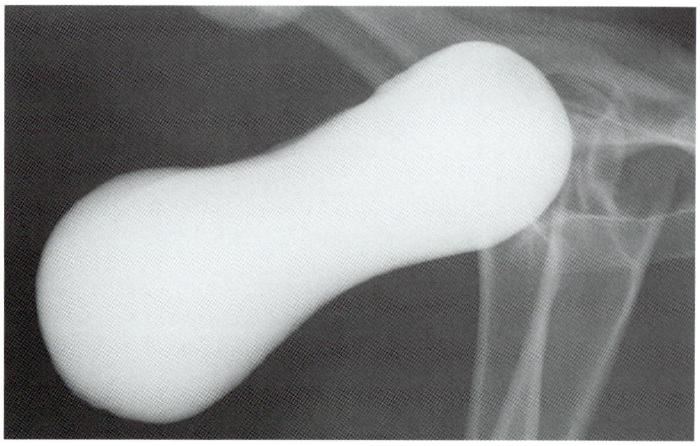

b

PROCEDURE

Urinalysis and bacteriological evaluation of urine should be performed before the contrast study due to the risk of introducing bacteria during the procedure, and as growth of certain bacteria in culture may be affected by contrast medium.

1. Patient preparation, except in emergency cases.
   - Fasting for 24 hours with free access to water.
   - If necessary, evacuation of the rectum and colon (enema) 2–4 hours prior to the procedure.
2. Preparation of necessary materials.
   - Catheter (balloon catheter preferred, size dependent on patient), three-way stopcock, sterile gel, potentially lidocaine, potentially speculum for female dogs.
   - Sterile gloves.
   - Contrast medium.
   - Positive contrast study: Iodinated contrast medium (diluted 1:10); dogs 4–10 ml/kg, cats 10–50 ml total.
   - Negative contrast study: Gaseous contrast medium (room air or CO_2); same volume as listed for positive contrast study.
   - Double contrast study: Iodinated contrast medium (dogs 3–10 ml total, cats 0.5–1 ml total) and gaseous contrast medium (room air or CO_2; dogs 4–10 ml/kg, cats 10–50 ml total).
3. Sedation or anaesthesia.
   - Improved diagnostic quality of radiographs, decreased stress for both examiner and patient.
   - Especially recommended for elective procedures requiring multiple sets of radiographs and special (oblique) projections.
   - Advantageous from a radiation safety perspective as the examiner can leave the room during acquisition of radiographs.
4. Lateral and ventrodorsal survey radiographs of the abdomen. Left lateral recumbency is recommended to trap any gas emboli in the right atrium.
5. Placement of the urinary catheter.
   - Aseptic catheterization of the urinary bladder.
   - Inflation of the balloon and withdrawal of the catheter tip to the region of the trigone.
   - Connection of the catheter to a three-way stopcock.
   - Evacuation of the urinary bladder. Repeat flushing of the urinary bladder with sterile saline may be helpful, especially if detailed evaluation of the mucosal surface is desired.
6. Contrast medium administration (double contrast study).
   - Injection of negative contrast medium until bladder feels firm on palpation (variable dose, see above).
   - Injection of positive contrast medium.
   - Rotation of the patient to ascertain even coating of the mucosal surface with contrast medium.
7. Radiographs: Ventrodorsal, lateral ± oblique (45°).

INTERPRETATION

PHYSIOLOGICAL AND INCIDENTAL FINDINGS Unless stated otherwise, findings are for double contrast cystography.

- Incomplete filling of the urinary bladder results in the impression of an irregularly marginated and thickened wall. With moderate filling of the urinary bladder (4 ml contrast medium/kg) the mucosal surface smoothens, and reliable measurements of

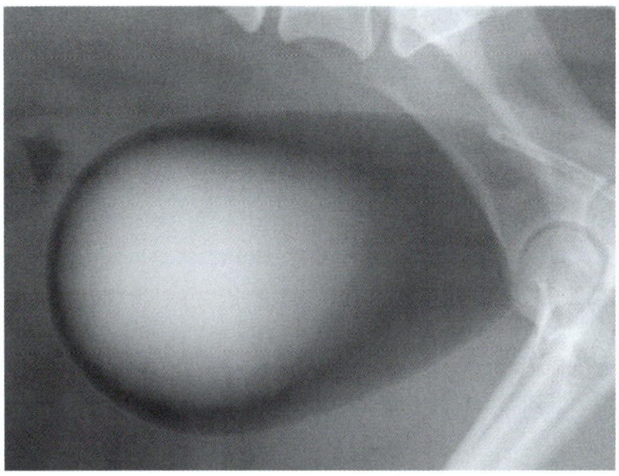

c

Fig. 14.8 Normal cystogram.
a Negative contrast cystogram. The urinary bladder is filled with gas and radiolucent. This technique is most commonly used to localize a urinary bladder not visible on survey radiographs, or as an adjunct when performing excretory urography. It may also aid in the diagnosis of non-opaque cystic calculi.
b Positive contrast cystogram. The urinary bladder is filled with positive contrast medium. This technique may be used to localize the urinary bladder and to evaluate bladder wall integrity.
c Double contrast cystogram. The urinary bladder contains mostly gas and a small amount of positive contrast medium. This technique allows evaluation of wall abnormalities and intraluminal filling defects and is thus the preferred method for most indications.

bladder wall thickness become possible (Fig. 14.8c). The bladder wall should measure approximately 1 mm in thickness in cats and up to 2 mm in thickness in dogs.
- Positive contrast medium accumulates in a 'pool' in the dependent portion of the urinary bladder. Any filling defects will appear less opaque compared to the surrounding contrast medium.
- **Reflux of contrast medium into the ureters** may be an incidental finding in young dogs with any type of cystography, and has to be distinguished from pathological reflux such as seen with ureteritis/ pyelonephritis.

Gas bubbles injected during the procedure appear as rounded radiolucent filling defects within the pool of contrast medium, which can lead to confusion with pathological filling defects (bladder calculi). If there is any doubt, radiographs should be repeated following repositioning of the patient. Gas bubbles change in size and shape and often become confluent to form larger bubbles. Bladder stones change in position but not in shape, size or number!

PATHOLOGICAL FINDINGS Unless stated otherwise, findings are for double contrast cystography.
- Intraluminal filling defects (less opaque than the surrounding pool of positive contrast medium): Free filling defects (e.g. calculi or intraluminal blood clots) change in position with repositioning of the patient. Wall associated (mural) filling defects (e.g. wall adherent blood clots, neoplasia, or polyps of the bladder wall) remain in place following repositioning of the patient.
- Thickening and irregular margination of the bladder wall: Inflammation, haemorrhage, neoplasia, fibrosis and other infiltrative diseases of the urinary bladder wall.
- Abnormal position of the urinary bladder (seen on positive, negative and double contrast studies): Congenital anomalies (pelvic bladder), caudal abdominal mass lesions, abdominal or perineal hernia with displacement of the urinary bladder.
- Leakage of contrast medium into the peritoneal cavity (best seen with positive contrast cystography): Bladder rupture (secondary to trauma or spontaneously secondary to chronic infiltrative wall disease).
- Rounded or triangular focal outpouching at the bladder apex: urachal diverticulum.

Note that a cystogram is often normal in cases of acute cystitis and in feline lower urinary tract disease!

Urethrography

This technique is often performed in conjunction with cystography. Indications, patient preparation and material are identical to the information provided for cystography. Unlike cystography, urethrography is only performed using positive contrast medium (diluted or undiluted). The dose of contrast medium is variable and depends on the indication, patient size, and the type of lesion/time of diagnosis. In cats and female dogs, 5–30 ml is usually sufficient, while the dose needed in large male dogs may be as high as 100 ml or more.

PROCEDURE

Patient preparation, pre-procedural laboratory analysis, anaesthesia, survey radiographs and catheterization of the urinary bladder are identical to cystography.

- **Pre-procedural distention of the urinary bladder:** If urethrography is performed and the urinary bladder is empty, contrast medium tends to follow the path of least resistance and stream into the urinary bladder. Adequate assessment of the urethral mucosa is only possible with adequate distension of the urethra. Pre-procedural distension of the urinary bladder (preferably with positive contrast medium in a 1:10 solution) increases resistance during the injection and results in adequate urethral dilatation.
- **Positioning of the catheter within the urethra:** Ideally, a balloon type catheter should be used to minimize the risk of contrast medium reflux during the injection. However, inflation of the balloon must be performed with caution and only for limited time periods to avoid damage to the urethral mucosa. Owing to the length of their urethra, the procedure usually has to be performed in several steps in male dogs, which involves repeat contrast medium injections during successive catheter withdrawals. For example, the first injection may be performed from the level of the ischiatic arch, the second from the caudal aspect of the os penis, and the third from the tip of the penis. If catheterization of the urinary bladder is not possible (e.g. due to complete urethral obstruction), the catheter is advanced as far as possible before contrast medium is injected, and is then withdrawn for further injections.
- **Examination technique:** In contrast to cystography, the examiner has to remain in the room during this procedure, and strict adherence to radiation safety principles is mandatory. One to three radiographs are obtained with the patient in lateral recumbency during continued or repeat contrast medium injection, without changing the position of the catheter. Alternatively, the injection can be performed with fluoroscopic monitoring. Repetition of radiographs without change in catheter position minimizes the

risk of artefacts (e.g. gas bubbles or urethral spasms that may mimic true filling defects). The injection may be repeated and an oblique ventrodorsal projection obtained if necessary. As mentioned above, in large male dogs the catheter is withdrawn to the next level after an adequate examination of the first region has been completed.

- Urethral catheterization may be difficult in female dogs. If satisfactory positioning of the urinary catheter in the urethra is not possible, a **vaginourethrography** may be performed as an alternative to a true urethrogram. With this procedure, the catheter is positioned in the caudal vagina and contrast medium is injected. Following complete filling of the vagina, contrast medium reflux into the urethra is usually observed. The injection has to be performed under relatively high pressure to overcome the resistance of the external urethral sphincter. To avoid contrast medium leakage to the outside, the vagina has to be occluded, which can be accomplished using an atraumatic (bowel) clamp, for example.

INTERPRETATION

Physiological and incidental findings

- The mucosal surface should generally be smooth (Fig. 14.9). Physiological persistent wall associated filling defects include the **colliculus seminalis** in male animals and the **urethral crest in cats** (Fig. 14.9a).
- Occasional intraluminal physiological filling defects (gas bubbles) should be transient and change or disappear with repeat injections.
- The urethra in female animals is shorter and generally wider than in male animals (Fig. 14.9b, c).
- The prostatic portion of the urethra is often wider than the remainder of the urethra in male dogs.
- Linear reflux of contrast medium into the prostate is a common finding in male intact dogs. This has to be distinguished from contrast medium accumulation in pathological prostatic cavities such as abscesses or cysts.
- When performing vaginourethrography in female animals, parts of the female reproductive tract become visible along with the urethra (Fig. 14.9d).

Anatomists and radiologists use a different terminology when subdividing the urethra in male dogs. In radiographic terminology, the urethra is subdivided into the **prostatic** urethra (from the urinary bladder to the caudal margin of the prostatic gland), the **membranous** urethra (from the prostate to the ischium) and the **penile** urethra. The anatomic subdivision distinguishes the **pelvic** urethra (again subdivided into a pre-prostatic and prostatic portion) and the **cavernous** urethra. Unless stated otherwise, this chapter will use radiographic terminology.

Pathological findings

- Filling defects: Calculi, blood clots, gas bubbles, neoplasia, inflammation, strictures.
- Thickening and irregularity of the mucosal surface: Inflammation, neoplasia, haemorrhage, fibrosis.
- Leakage of contrast medium: Urethral rupture (usually traumatic, possibly secondary to urethral pathology).

14.2.3 Other contrast studies

Antegrade pyelography

This technique has been described as a method to distinguish obstructive from nonobstructive dilatation of the renal pelvis. Particularly with acute ureteral obstruction, renal function is often reduced to such a degree that adequate contrast medium accumulation and concentration within the renal collecting system and ureter cannot be achieved with conventional excretory urography. In addition, contrast medium is often diluted within the renal pelvis and/or dilated ureter, so that a confident diagnosis of a partial or intermittent obstruction is not possible even with maintained renal function.

In antegrade pyelography, positive contrast medium is directly injected into the dilated renal pelvis using ultrasound guidance. This technique can be combined with diagnostic pyelocentesis (aspiration of urine directly from the abnormal renal pelvis). Adequate filling of the ureter is monitored by means of fluoroscopy or frequent repeat radiographs. **Advantages** include a high concentration of contrast medium in the renal pelvis and ureter, with a concurrent decrease in overall contrast medium dose compared to excretory urography. This minimizes the risk of systemic adverse effects. However, the technique is not without **risks**. The examination is performed under general anaesthesia, which may be problematic in patients with renal disease. Potential risks of renal puncture and direct injection of contrast medium include haemorrhage, leakage of potentially infected urine into the retroperitoneal space, and ureteral obstruction due to displacement of blood clots or inflammatory products from the renal pelvis into the ureter. This technique should thus be limited to specialty practices prepared to adequately address any adverse effects.

Antegrade urethrography

This technique may be considered as an alternative to retrograde urethrography in cases where urethral catheterization is not possible, or if the urethra is too short to allow adequate positioning of the catheter tip and balloon. The urinary bladder has to be filled with an adequate amount of positive contrast medium prior to the procedure. This can be accomplished either in retrograde fashion via a

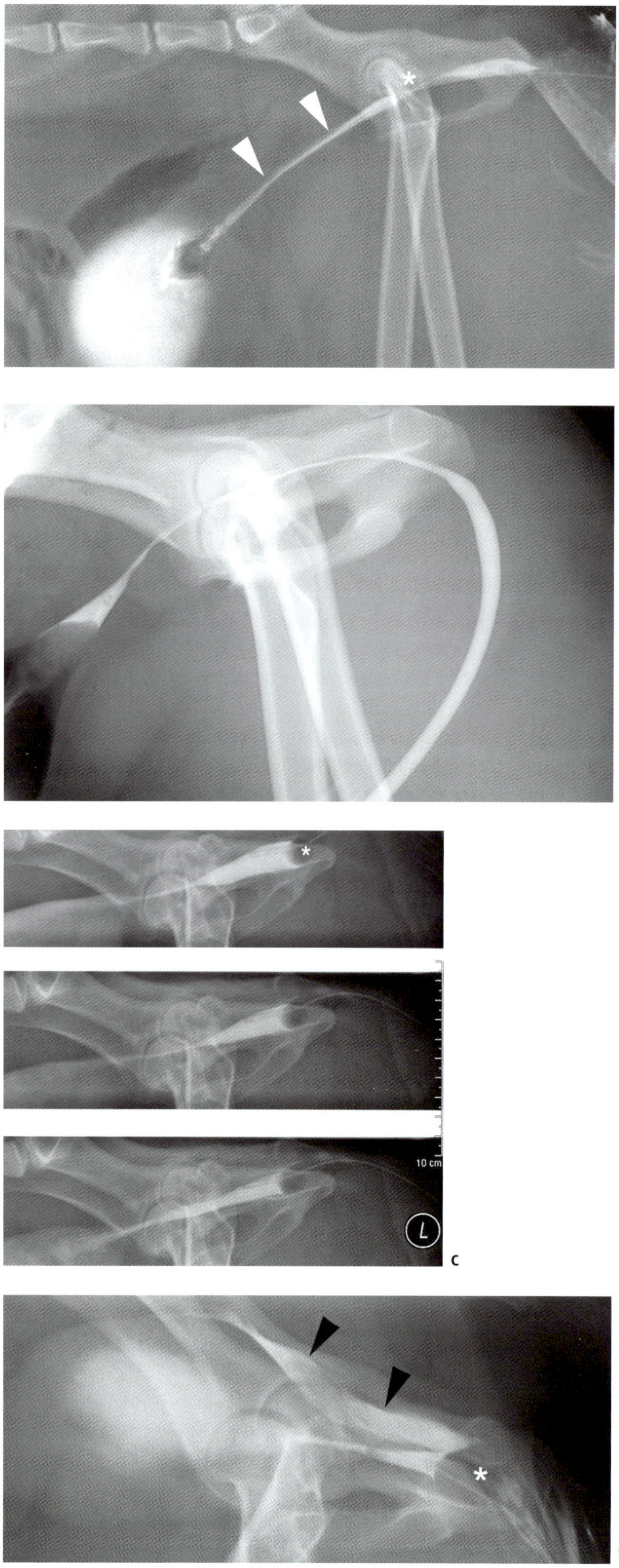

a b c d

Fig. 14.9 Normal urethrogram.

a Urethrogram in a male cat. The urethra is of uniform diameter and smoothly marginated. The urethral crest is recognized as a linear filling defect along the dorsal urethral margin (arrowheads). A focal indentation in the dorsal urethra represents the colliculus seminalis (*), which is indistinct in this animal. These filling defects are physiological and should not be confused with abnormal wall thickening or a mural mass.

b Urethrogram in a male dog. During this procedure, the urinary catheter was successively withdrawn and contrast medium injected repeatedly to allow evaluation of all portions of the urethra. Mild narrowing of the prostatic and membranous urethra compared to the penile urethra noted on this image is an artefact which was not present when the catheter was positioned at the level of the ischiatic arch.

c Urethrogram in a female dog. The catheter has been placed in the most caudal part of the urethra (balloon marked by * on top image). These three radiographs were obtained in rapid succession and show physiological intermittent variations in urethral diameter (L = left).

d Vaginourethrogram in a female dog with pelvic bladder. The catheter was unable to be positioned in the short urethra and is placed in the vestibule of the vagina (balloon marked with *). This results in concurrent contrast medium filling of the urethra and the vagina (arrowheads).

catheter or indirectly by performing an excretory urogram. Subsequently, (manual) pressure is applied to the urinary bladder until urine is successfully expressed. The urethra is evaluated either fluoroscopically or radiographically during bladder evacuation. This technique is often frustrating: adequate expression of the urinary bladder and thus urine flow is often difficult to accomplish with the patient in lateral recumbency. Coordination with radiographs or fluoroscopy may be challenging. Additionally, at least one of the examiner's hands is often very close to or even within the primary beam, which is unacceptable from a radiation safety perspective.

CT excretory urography

The diagnostic accuracy of excretory urography in the evaluation of ectopic ureters can be improved by combining the technique with abdominal computed tomography. This technique is limited to hospitals with access to CT equipment.

14.3 Renal and ureteral diseases

The technique and basic interpretation principles of excretory urography are covered in section 14.2.1. This chapter will cover survey radiographic and select excretory urographic abnormalities seen in renal and ureteral diseases.

14.3.1 Abnormalities in renal number and position

The inability to identify both kidneys in their expected positions on survey radiographs is typically related to patient or technical factors rather than a pathological condition. Common causes include lack of intra-abdominal fat, deep-chested patient conformation, silhouetting of the right kidney with hepatic parenchyma, a large volume of ingesta within the gastrointestinal tract, and inadequate exposure factors.

True (congenital) anomalies such as **renal aplasia**, **fusion of the kidneys** ('horseshoe kidney') or **renal ectopia** are rare and may be incidental. Prior **nephrectomy** is a potential differential diagnosis for an absent kidney, but this information is usually provided in the history. **Abdominal mass lesions** originating from the liver, ovaries or adrenal glands may result in renal displacement and are far more common reasons for renal displacement than true renal ectopia.

14.3.2 Abnormalities in renal size and shape

Many different renal diseases affect the size and shape of the kidneys, and a definitive diagnosis of the underlying disease process is rarely possible. Abdominal ultrasound or excretory urography may be helpful in narrowing the list of differential diagnoses; however, ultrasonographic or excretory urographic abnormalities are also rarely pathognomonic. In particular, diffuse infiltrative renal diseases (inflammatory, metabolic or neoplastic) have similar imaging features, and the results of other tests as well as renal fine-needle aspiration cytology or biopsy may be needed for a definitive diagnosis. Another important consideration is that acute renal diseases, in particular, may not be associated with any radiographic abnormalities, requiring further diagnostic tests for diagnosis. An overview of differential diagnoses for changes in renal size and shape is provided in Table 14.3.

> Normal radiographs do not rule out renal disease!

14.3.3 Abnormalities in renal opacity

A (multi)focal increase in renal opacity is common. Differential diagnoses include **renal calculi/mineralization** along the collecting system and **dystrophic mineralization** of renal parenchymal lesions such as cysts or neoplasms. A generalized increase in renal radiographic opacity is an uncommon finding and may be associated with diffuse mineralization of the renal parenchyma (**nephrocalcinosis**). Recent intravenous administration of iodinated contrast medium will also result in a diffuse increase in renal opacity.

A decrease in renal opacity is rare. Differential diagnoses include **abscess/infection with gas-producing bacteria** and **vesicoureteral reflux** of gas in patients with emphysematous cystitis or following negative contrast cystography.

14.3.4 Pyelonephritis

Abdominal radiographs in patients with acute pyelonephritis may be normal or reveal unilateral or bilateral renomegaly, with or without concurrent retroperitoneal effusion (Fig. 14.10). Chronic pyelonephritis typically results in small and irregularly marginated kidneys. Abdominal ultrasound or excretory urography may aid in diagnosis and show renal pelvis dilatation with uneven width and irregular margination of the pelvic recesses (Fig. 14.11).

14.3.5 Chronic renal disease

Patients with chronic renal disease commonly have small and irregularly marginated kidneys (Fig. 14.12). Concurrent renal mineralization or nephrolithiasis are common. Excretory urography is typically not needed for diagnosis. Expected findings include decreased contrast medium accumulation within the renal parenchyma, and poor opacification of the renal pelvis and ureter due to decreased renal function (Fig. 14.11).

14.3.6 Hydronephrosis and hydroureter

Hydronephrosis and hydroureter refer to dilatation of the renal pelvis and ureter, respectively. In human medicine, a distinction is made between obstructive and nonobstructive hydronephrosis. However, in veterinary medicine this

Table 14.3 Differential diagnoses for abnormal renal size and shape.

Renal size and shape	Disease process	Possible concurrent radiographic findings	Excretory urography helpful
Enlarged with normal contour	Acute inflammatory renal diseases (pyelonephritis, glomerulonephritis, interstitial nephritis)	Retroperitoneal effusion	±
	Diffuse infiltrative neoplasia (e.g. lymphoma in cats)	Other organ anomalies (hepatomegaly etc.)	±
	Hydronephrosis	Underlying cause (e.g. ureteral calculus) may be visible	±
	Compensatory hypertrophy	Contralateral kidney small or absent	+
	Portosystemic shunt	Small size of the liver, urolithiasis	–
	Perinephric pseudocysts	–	+
	Other renal diseases (metabolic, e.g. amyloidosis, parenchymal mass lesions not resulting in changes to renal contour, etc.)	Variable	±
Enlarged with abnormal contour	Focal or multifocal parenchymal mass lesions such as cysts, abscesses, neoplasia or haematomas	Variable	+
	Infiltrative diseases (e.g. lymphoma, FIP)	Variable	±
	Others (perinephric pseudocysts, renal infarcts)	Variable	±
Small with normal contour	Congenital renal diseases such as hypoplasia or dysplasia	If unilateral, compensatory hypertrophy of contralateral kidney is common	±
	Chronic renal disease	Variable	±
Small with abnormal contour	Chronic (end-stage) renal disease	Variable, renal mineralization or nephrolithiasis is common	±

Note: FIP = feline infectious peritonitis.

terminology is typically reserved for conditions resulting in partial or complete obstruction of the urinary outflow tract. The obstructive lesion may be located anywhere between the renal pelvis and the urinary bladder and may be intraluminal (e.g. renal or ureteral calculus, blood clot or inflammatory debris secondary to pyelonephritis), mural (e.g. neoplastic or inflammatory wall lesion) or extraluminal (e.g. adjacent retroperitoneal mass or iatrogenic ureteral ligation).

Radiographic findings Depending on severity of renal pelvis dilatation, hydronephrosis may result in unilateral or bilateral renomegaly visible on survey radiographs (Fig. 14.13). Identification of the underlying cause may on occasion be possible (e.g. ureteral calculus; Fig. 14.14). Excretory urography findings with mild to moderate hydronephrosis and maintained renal function include contrast enhancement of renal parenchyma and contrast medium accumulation within the dilated renal pelvis (Fig. 14.15). With severe hydronephrosis, a peripheral rim of contrast enhancement may be observed in the remaining renal parenchyma; however, a pyelogram is typically not achieved due to both a decrease in renal function and dilution of contrast medium within the distended renal pelvis. Normal ureters are not visible on survey radiographs. However, severely dilated ureters may appear as soft-tissue opaque, tubular and tortuous structures in the retroperitoneal space. Assuming adequate renal function, distended ureters are easily identified with excretory urography (Fig. 14.15).

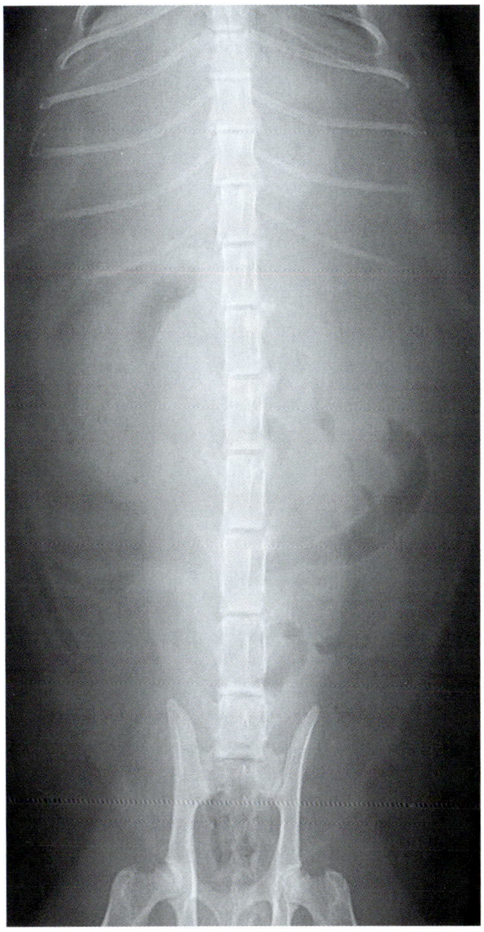

a

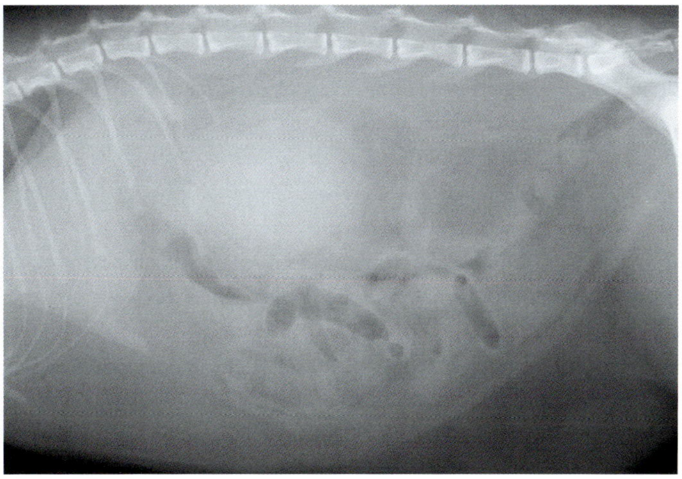

b

Fig. 14.10 Acute pyelonephritis in a cat. The ventrodorsal a and lateral b radiographs of the abdomen show moderate bilateral renomegaly and rounding of the kidneys. Streaky loss of detail in the retroperitoneal space resulting in poor visualization of the kidneys is consistent with retroperitoneal effusion.

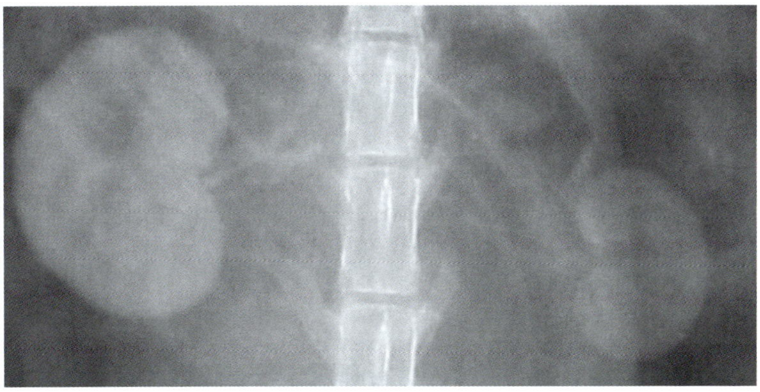

a

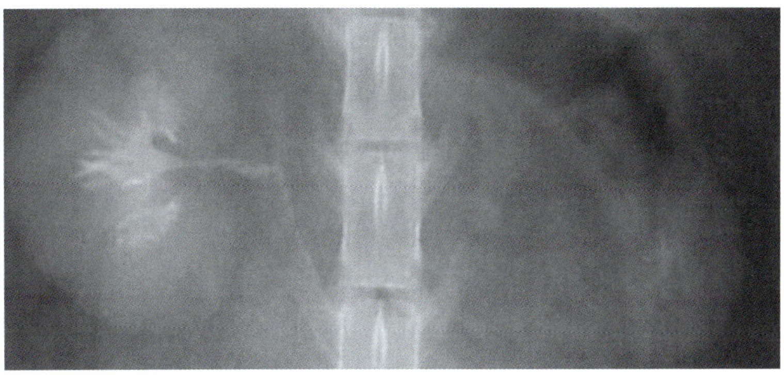

b

Fig. 14.11 Ventrodorsal radiographs of the cranial abdomen in a cat immediately a (nephrogram) and 30 minutes after intravenous injection of iodinated contrast medium b (pyelogram). The left kidney is smaller than the right and has decreased contrast medium uptake and excretion. The right renal pelvis is of irregular shape, with uneven size of the pelvic diverticula. The diagnosis was left-sided chronic renal insufficiency/end-stage kidney disease and right-sided pyelonephritis. (Courtesy of Tufts University School of Veterinary Medicine)

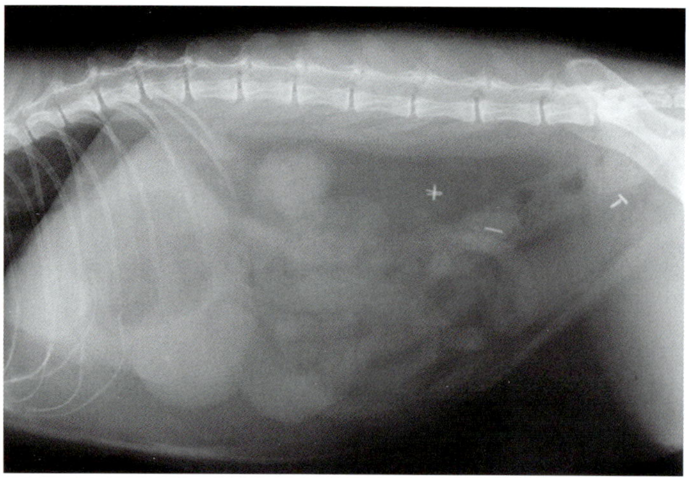

a

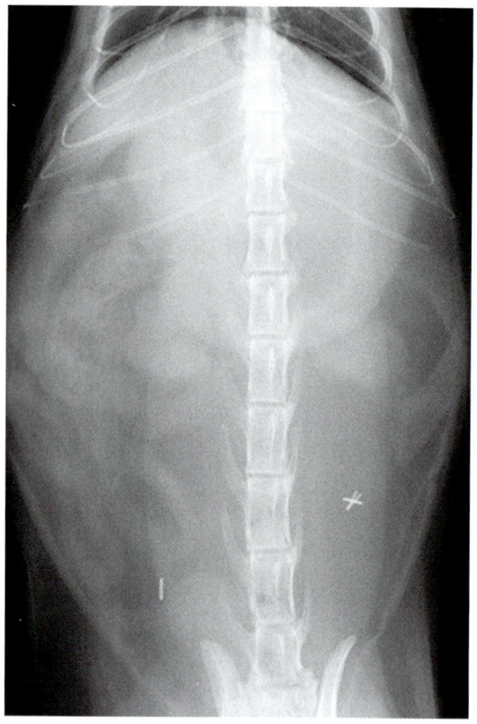

b

Fig. 14.12 Lateral a and ventrodorsal b abdominal radiographs in a cat with end-stage kidney disease. Both kidneys are very small and markedly irregularly marginated. Note gas and fluid dilatation of the stomach due to concurrent duodenal obstruction by a hairball.

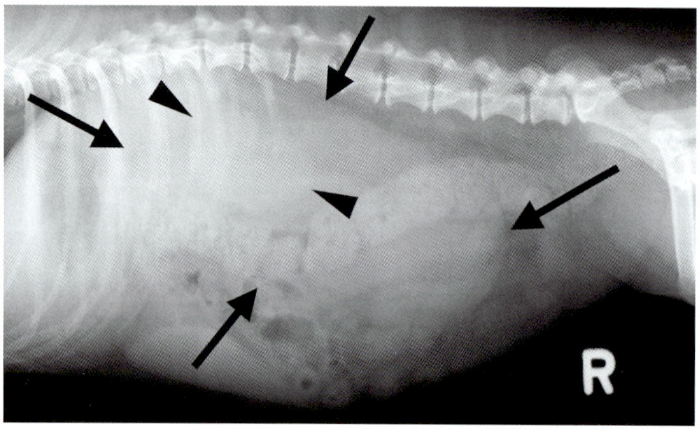

a

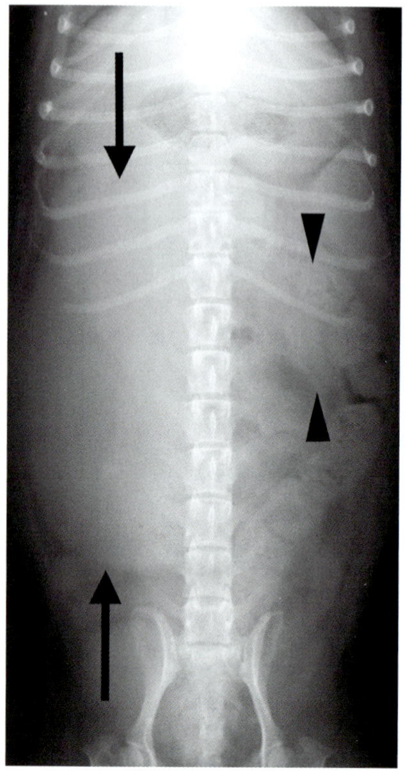

b

Fig. 14.13 Lateral a and ventrodorsal b abdominal radiographs in a dog with severe right hydronephrosis secondary to inadvertent ureteral ligation during ovariohysterectomy. The right kidney (arrows) is severely enlarged compared to the left kidney (arrowheads) and smoothly marginated (R = right).

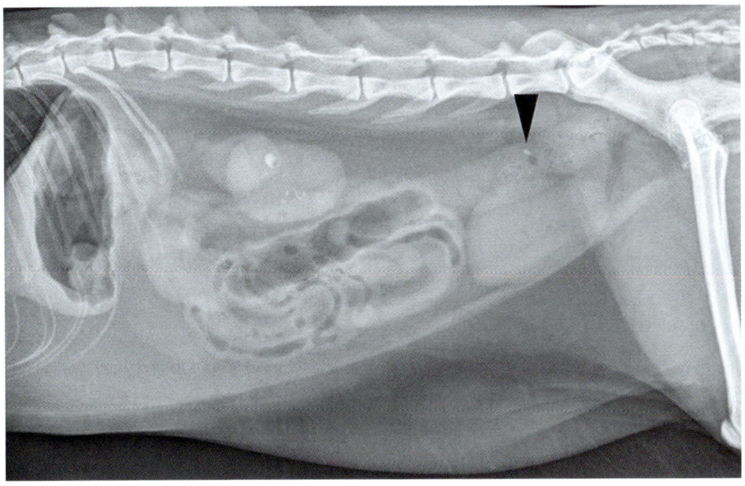

a

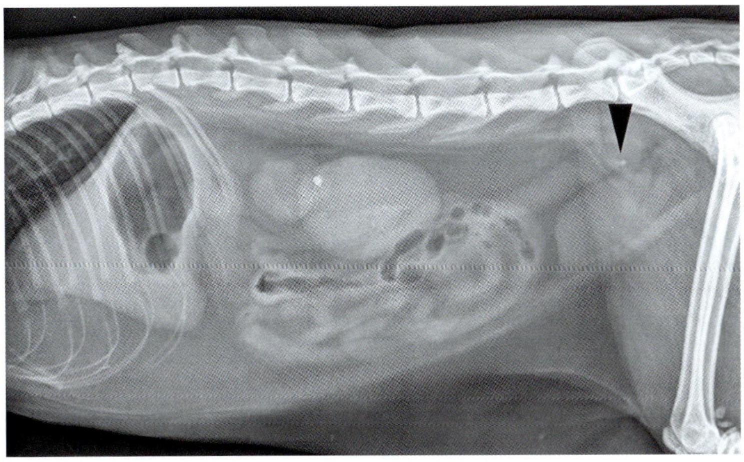

b

Fig. 14.14 Lateral abdominal radiographs in a cat with hydronephrosis secondary to ureteral obstruction.

a Radiographic abnormalities on the initial radiograph at presentation include a very small and irregularly marginated right kidney, bilateral renal mineralization/nephrolithiasis, and a punctate mineral opacity in the plane of the caudal ureters dorsal to the urinary bladder and superimposed with the colon (arrowhead).

b On recheck radiographs one day later, there is notable enlargement of the left kidney compared to the previous radiograph (5.2 versus 4.4 cm length). Previously noted nephrolithiasis, small size and irregular shape of the right kidney, and mineral opaque focus dorsal to the urinary bladder (arrowhead) are unchanged. Suspected severe chronic renal disease, bilateral nephrolithiasis, and left-sided hydronephrosis and hydroureter due to obstruction by a small ureteral calculus were confirmed by means of ultrasonography.

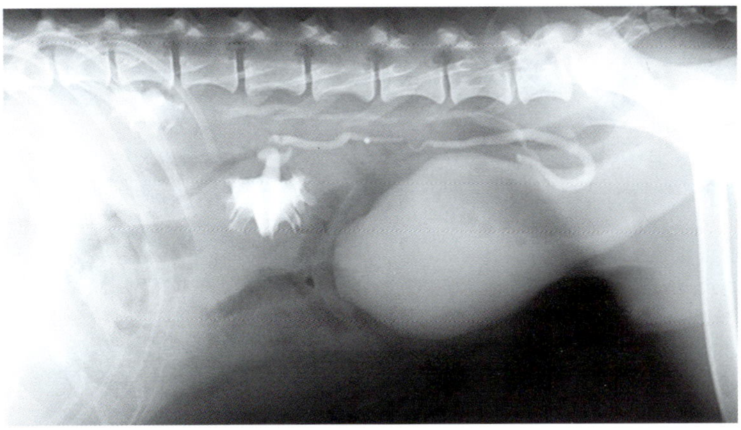

a

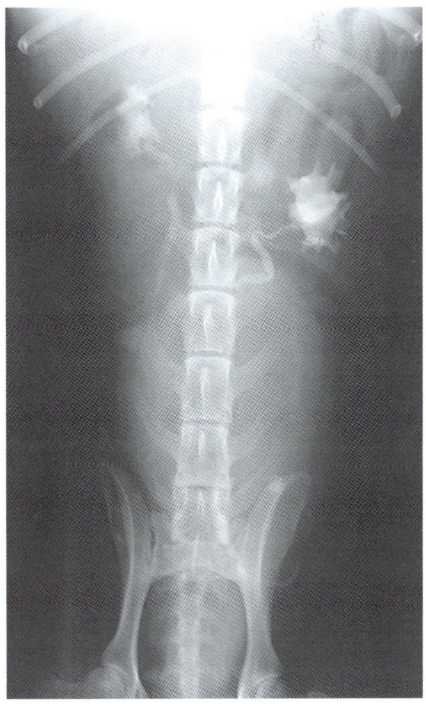

b

Fig. 14.15 Moderate bilateral hydronephrosis and hydroureter in a dog. The lateral a and ventrodorsal b radiographs obtained during the pyelogram phase of an excretory urogram show dilatation of the renal pelves and ureters bilaterally. The underlying cause is not evident on these radiographs.

14.3.7 Polycystic kidney disease (PKD)

This is a congenital condition most commonly seen in Persian cats. The number and size of renal cysts increase with age. Single or multiple renal cysts may also develop in patients with degenerative renal disease.

RADIOGRAPHIC FINDINGS Advanced polycystic kidney disease results in bilateral enlargement and irregular contour of the kidneys (Fig. 14.16). Excretory urography demonstrates numerous round, well-circumscribed parenchymal filling defects.

14.3.8 Perirenal pseudocysts

With perirenal pseudocysts, there is unilateral or bilateral subcapsular or pericapsular fluid accumulation. Even though this condition is rare in comparison to other renal diseases, it is an important differential diagnosis for renomegaly. Perirenal pseudocysts are most commonly seen in older neutered cats. They may be associated with chronic renal disease, result in abdominal enlargement or be asymptomatic.

RADIOGRAPHIC FINDINGS Survey radiographs show unilateral or bilateral enlargement of the renal silhouette (often severe), with a smooth or less commonly an irregular contour (Fig. 14.17). Abdominal ultrasound or excretory urography will show a normal or small kidney with normal architecture in the centre of the large surrounding non-contrast-enhancing cystic structure.

14.3.9 Renal neoplasia

Renal neoplasms may be diffusely infiltrative (e.g. lymphoma in cats) or cause focal or multifocal renal nodules or masses (e.g. carcinoma, haemangiosarcoma, metastases).

RADIOGRAPHIC FINDINGS Imaging findings with renal tumours are highly variable, ranging from normal to unilateral or bilateral renomegaly with maintained normal or altered renal contour (Fig. 14.18). The organ of origin may be difficult to identify with very large renal tumours (Fig. 14.19). Excretory urography, abdominal ultrasound or cross-sectional imaging may be helpful in these instances. With excretory urography, focal or multifocal renal tumours are typically characterized by heterogeneous, decreased or absent contrast enhancement compared to normal renal parenchyma (Fig. 14.20). The pyelogram phase may also be abnormal, when renal parenchymal lesions bordering the collecting system deform the contour of the renal pelvis. Excretory urography findings with diffuse infiltrative neoplasia are variable and, among other factors, dependent on remaining renal function.

14.3.10 Renal and ureteral calculi

Urolithiasis is common in dogs and cats.

RADIOGRAPHIC FINDINGS A diagnosis on survey radiographs is easy if uroliths are radiopaque and have reached a certain size (typically 1–2 mm). Renal and ureteral cal-

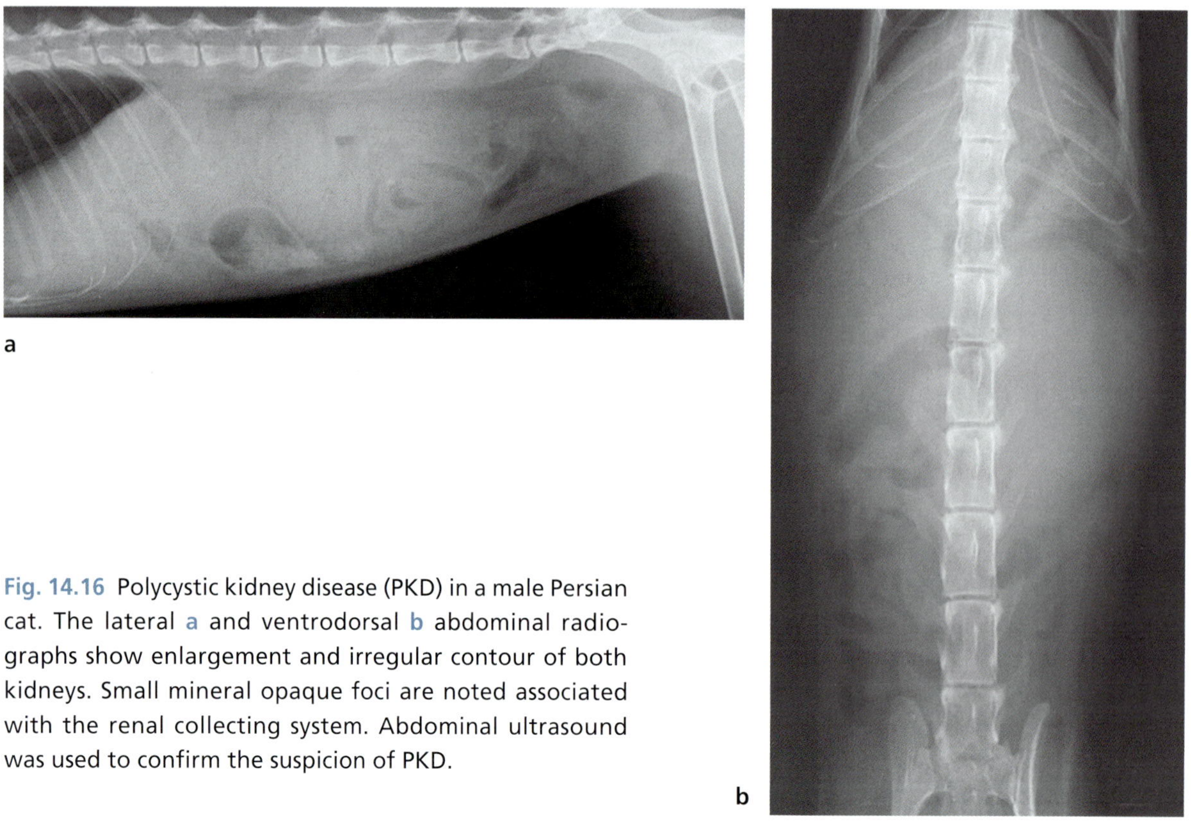

a

b

Fig. 14.16 Polycystic kidney disease (PKD) in a male Persian cat. The lateral a and ventrodorsal b abdominal radiographs show enlargement and irregular contour of both kidneys. Small mineral opaque foci are noted associated with the renal collecting system. Abdominal ultrasound was used to confirm the suspicion of PKD.

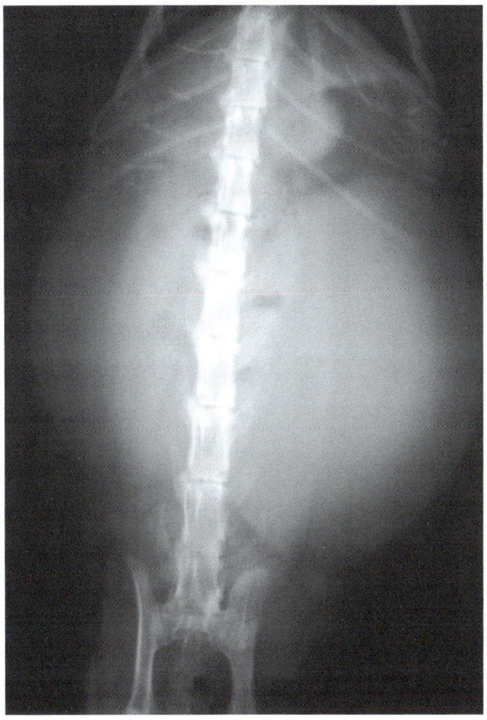

a

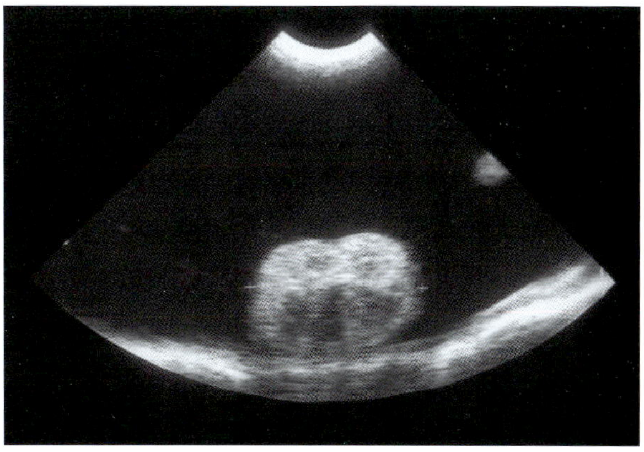

b

Fig. 14.17 Perirenal pseudocysts in a cat.
a On the ventrodorsal radiographs, there is severe enlargement of both renal silhouettes. The 'kidneys' have a normal shape and are smoothly marginated.
b On abdominal ultrasound, the kidneys were found to be rather small and surrounded by fluid contained within well-defined cavities ('pseudocysts').

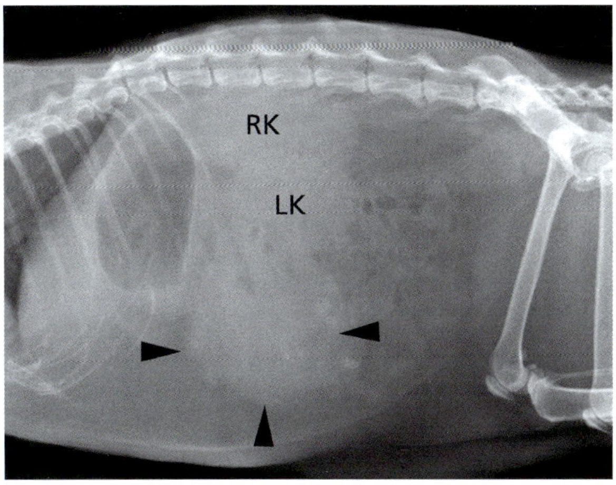

a

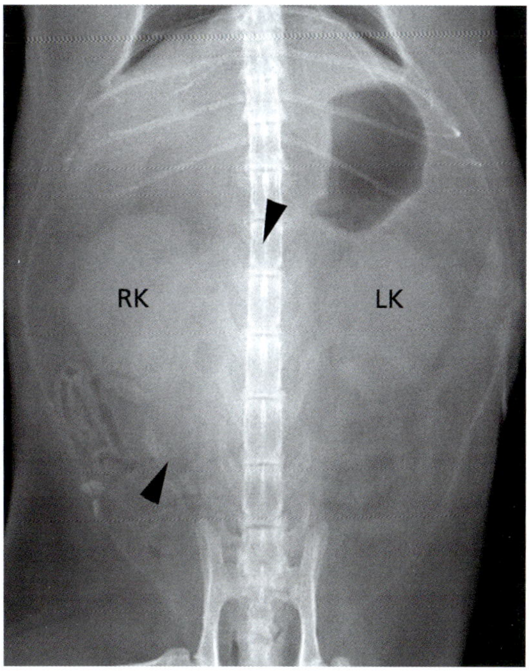

b

Fig. 14.18 Renal lymphoma in a cat. Rounding and irregular contour of both kidneys is noted on lateral a and ventrodorsal b abdominal radiographs. The left kidney (LK) is at the upper limits of normal for size, the right kidney (RK) is enlarged. In addition, an intestinal mass is noted in the ventral abdomen (arrowheads). The diagnosis was made based on ultrasound-guided fine-needle aspirates.

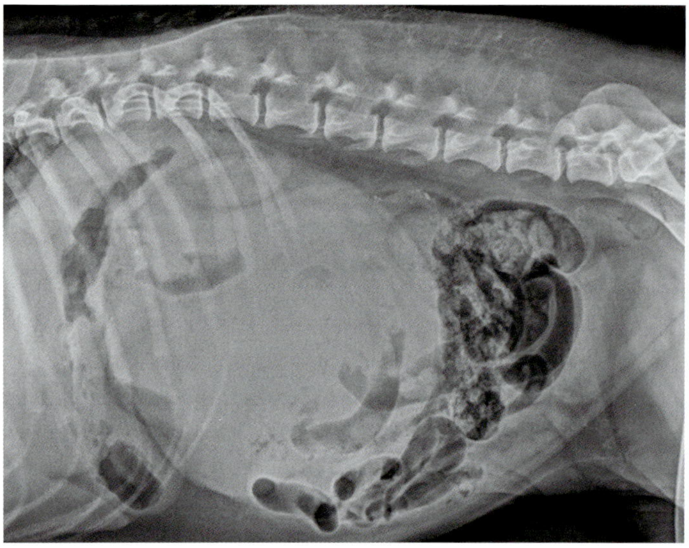

a

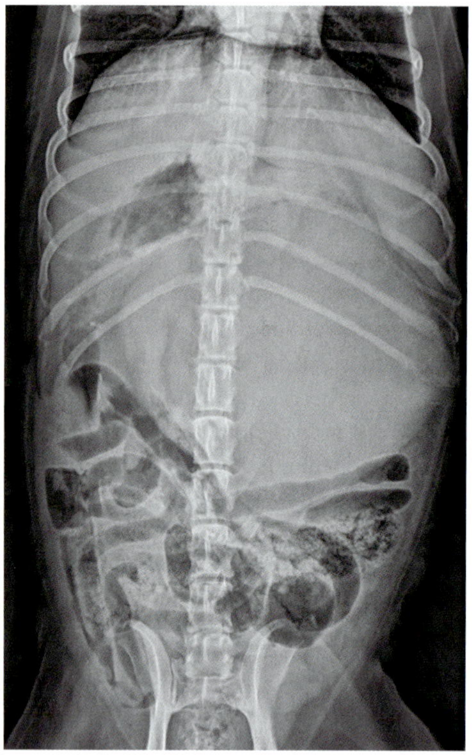

b

Fig. 14.19 Very large tumour of the left kidney (cystadenocarcinoma).

a On the lateral view, the severely enlarged left kidney occupies a majority of the cranial abdomen and results in cranial displacement of the gastric axis and caudal displacement of the small intestine. The right kidney is in normal position.

b On the ventrodorsal view, the mass occupies the entire cranial and mid abdomen and extends across the midline towards the right. A normal left kidney is not visible. The organ of origin may on occasion be difficult to determine with a mass of this size, and abdominal ultrasound or excretory urography may aid in identifying renal origin.

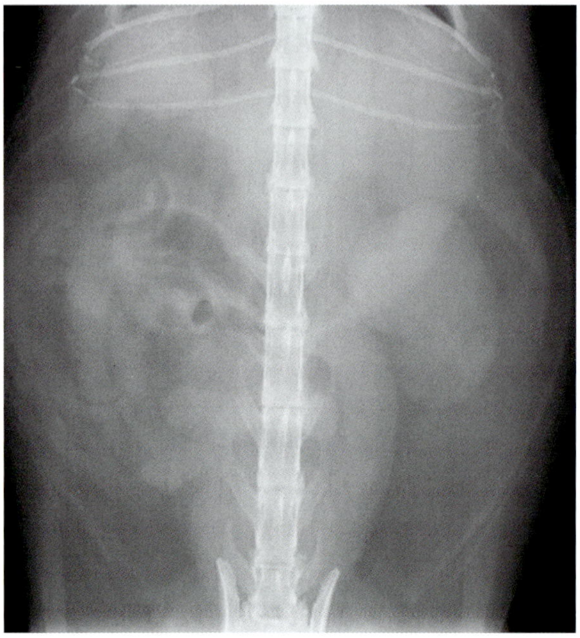

a

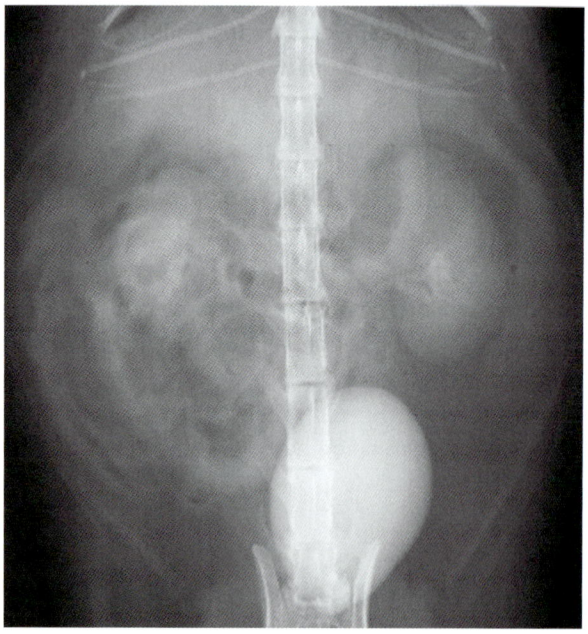

b

Fig. 14.20 Left renal tumour (adenocarcinoma) in a cat.

a The cranial pole of the left kidney has an unusual contour on the ventrodorsal view with a notable bulge.

b This abnormal region has decreased contrast medium uptake on excretory urography compared to more normal-appearing renal parenchyma caudally.

culi appear as solitary or multiple well-circumscribed, mineral opaque structures in the plane of the kidneys and/or retroperitoneal space (see Fig. 14.14). Possible concurrent findings include signs of chronic pyelonephritis or hydronephrosis/hydroureter.

> The size of a renal or ureteral calculus is not an accurate predictor of the presence or absence of urinary tract obstruction. This determination can only be made based on concurrent radiographic abnormalities (hydronephrosis and/or hydroureter) or following advanced imaging tests (Fig. 14.21; see also Fig. 14.14).

Advanced imaging including ultrasound or excretory urography allows further evaluation for possible urinary tract obstruction and for concurrent or additional diseases such as pyelonephritis (Fig. 14.21). It is also helpful in the diagnosis of non-opaque urinary calculi not visible on survey radiographs.

14.3.11 Renal or ureteral rupture

These conditions are most commonly seen following trauma and result in urine leakage into the retroperitoneal space.

RADIOGRAPHIC FINDINGS Survey radiographs show streaky loss of detail in the retroperitoneal space. Other concurrent findings indicative of abdominal trauma (e.g. peritoneal effusion or musculoskeletal trauma such as vertebral fractures) are possible. Excretory urography is indicated if ureteral avulsion or renal rupture are suspected, and allows accurate lesion localization. The contrast procedure shows leakage of contrast medium into the retroperitoneal space at the site of injury (Fig. 14.22).

14.3.12 Ectopic ureter

This congenital condition is most commonly diagnosed in female large-breed dogs. One or both ureters terminate in the urethra or vagina rather than in their physiological position at the trigone of the urinary bladder. This may be an isolated lesion or associated with other conditions such as pelvic bladder and short urethra.

RADIOGRAPHIC FINDINGS The evaluation of a patient with ectopic ureters is a diagnostic challenge. Cystoscopy or CT excretory urography are more accurate than radiographic excretory urography. Survey radiographs are typically unrewarding. With (partial) ureteral obstruc-

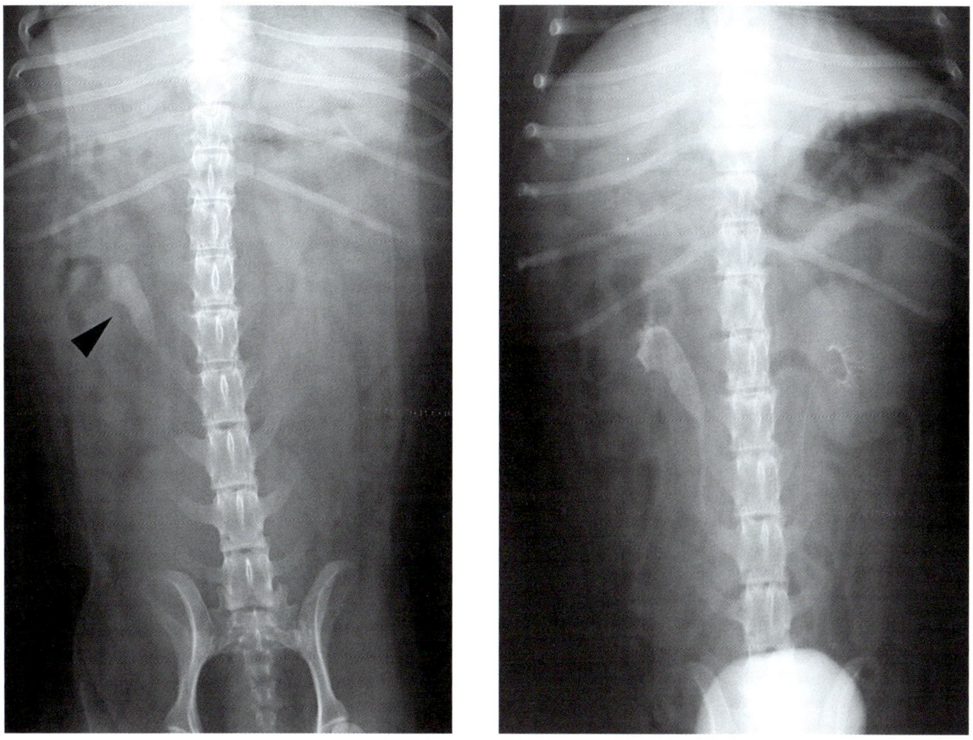

a b

Fig. 14.21 Large renal calculus in a dog.
a On the ventrodorsal abdominal radiograph, a mineral opaque calculus is clearly visible and extends from the right renal pelvis into the proximal ureter (arrowhead).
b On excretory urography, there is mild irregular widening of the renal pelvis, indicative of pyelonephritis. However, the ureter distal to the calculus is filled with contrast medium and of normal width, ruling out ureteral obstruction.

tion, hydronephrosis and/or hydroureter may be evident. A small and/or pelvic urinary bladder may not be visible or may be seen within the pelvic canal. In addition to these abnormalities, excretory urography may demonstrate abnormal termination of the ureters and/or abnormal contrast medium accumulation within the vagina or urethra (Fig. 14.23 and 14.24).

14.4 Diseases of the urinary bladder and urethra

Disorders of the lower urinary tract are common in dogs and cats and may be isolated conditions or associated with concurrent diseases of the kidneys and/or ureters. With few exceptions, survey radiographs are unrewarding. Excretory urography may on occasion allow a diagnosis of urinary bladder disease; however, abdominal ultrasound, cystography and/or urethrography are usually necessary for full evaluation. The technique and basic principles of interpretation of these contrast studies are described in section 14.2.2. This chapter will discuss select diseases of the urinary bladder and urethra.

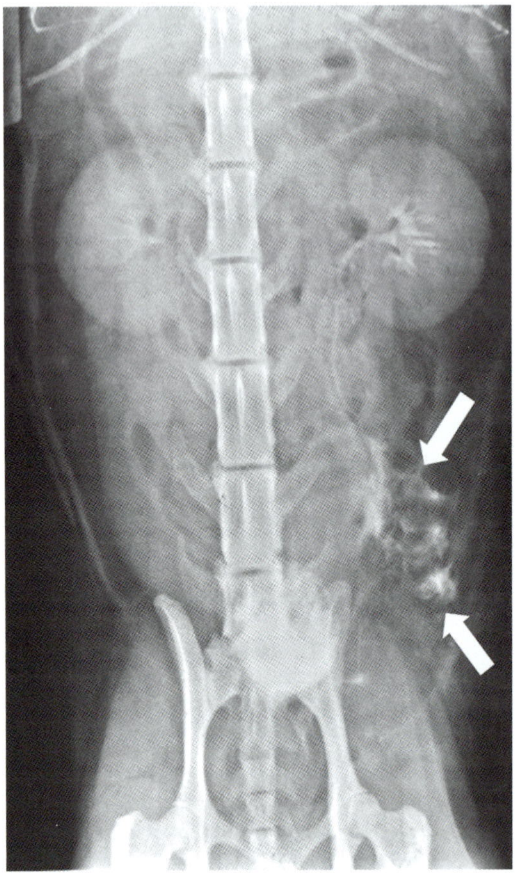

Fig. 14.22 Excretory urography in a cat with left ureteral rupture following abdominal trauma. Accumulation of positive contrast medium is noted in the left caudal abdomen/retroperitoneal space (arrows).

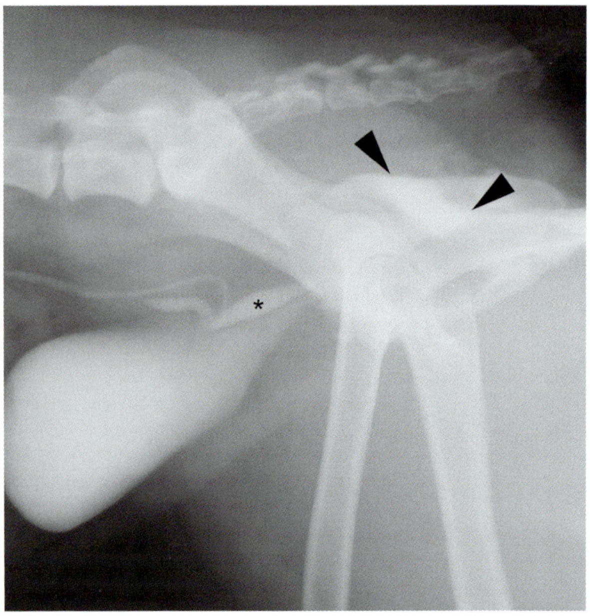

Fig. 14.23 Unilateral ectopic ureter in a dog. The abnormal ureter (*) is dilated and enters the pelvic canal dorsal to the bladder neck rather than entering the bladder neck at the level of the trigone. Contrast medium accumulation is noted within the vagina (arrowheads), which is abnormal and compatible with ectopic ureter.

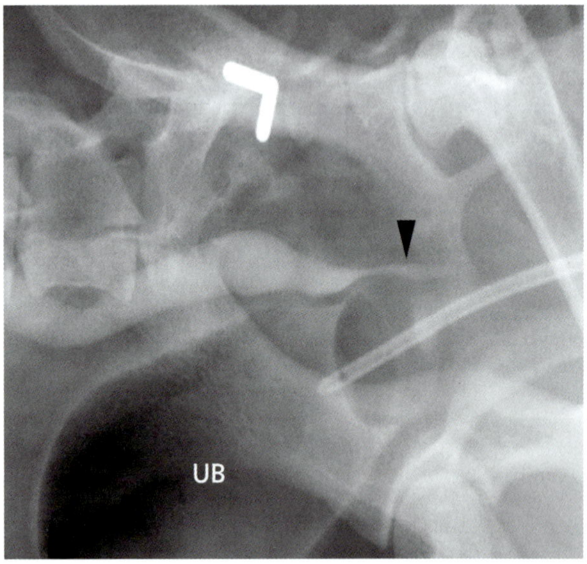

Fig. 14.24 Bilateral ectopic ureters in a dog. On this oblique view of the caudal abdomen, the dilated left ureter (arrowhead) bypasses the bladder neck and enters the pelvic canal. The urinary bladder (UB) has been filled with air for improved visualization of positive contrast medium within the ureters. The urinary catheter with inflated balloon has been left in place. The right ureter in this patient was also found to be ectopic (L = left).

14.4.1 Cystitis and urethritis

Survey radiographs are usually not helpful in the diagnostic workup of inflammatory diseases of the urinary bladder and urethra aside from allowing identification of opaque bladder or urethral calculi. One exception is **emphysematous cystitis**. This condition is predominantly but not exclusively seen in patients with diabetes mellitus and is characterized by gas accumulation within the urinary bladder lumen and wall due to infection with gas-producing bacteria (Fig. 14.25).

Cystography and urethrography yield variable results in patients with lower urinary tract infections. In acute cases, imaging studies may be normal or show intraluminal filling defects such as blood clots and/or bladder calculi. With severe and chronic cases, thickening of the urinary bladder wall may be noted, especially at the level of the apex, and the mucosal surface may appear irregular (Fig. 14.26).

Polypoid cystitis is a special type of inflammatory bladder disease that results in the formation of wall associated polypoid mass lesions (Fig. 14.27). Unlike malignant bladder tumours, these polyps are most commonly located in the cranioventral aspect of the urinary bladder. However, bladder tumours have to be considered as a differential diagnosis.

Granulomatous urethritis is a rare inflammatory condition. Urethrography shows numerous irregular mural filling defects and thickening of the urethra, mimicking urethral neoplasia.

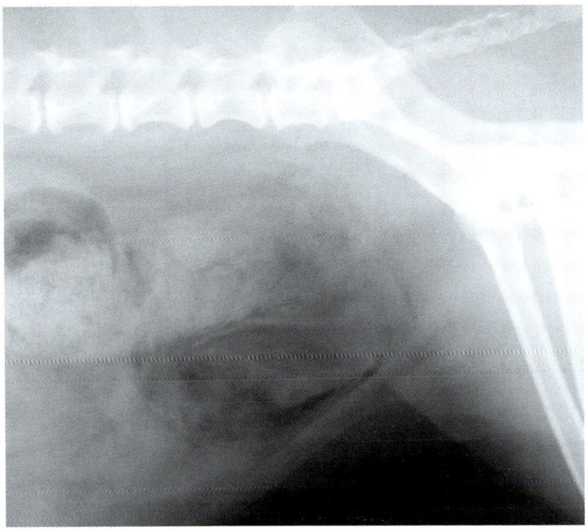

Fig. 14.25 Emphysematous cystitis in a dog. Gas accumulation is noted within the lumen as well as the wall of the urinary bladder. This condition is diagnosed most commonly but not exclusively in diabetic patients.

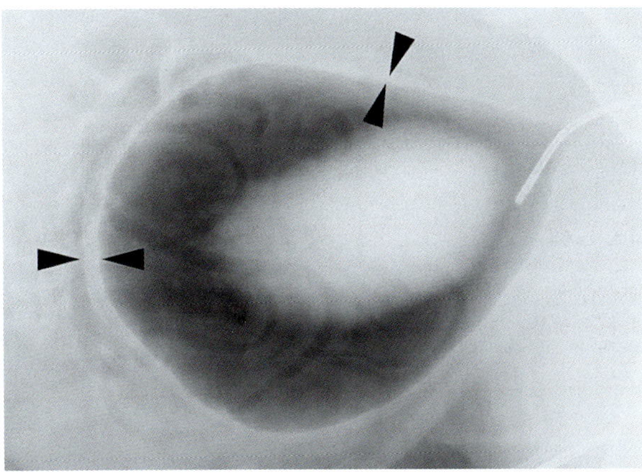

Fig. 14.26 Chronic cystitis in a dog (double contrast cystogram). The bladder wall at the level of the apex is thickened compared to the body (arrowheads), and the mucosal margin is mildly irregularly marginated.

14.4.2 Bladder and urethral calculi

The diagnosis of **opaque** urinary calculi is usually straightforward (Fig. 14.28). Urethral calculi located within the pelvic canal may be difficult to identify due to superimposition with osseous structures (Fig. 14.29). Additional (oblique) views may aid in visualization. **Non-opaque** calculi may not be visible on survey radiographs and require further imaging (ultrasound, cystography and/or urethrography) for diagnosis (Fig. 14.30). The contrast study will show urinary calculi as filling defects within the surrounding pool of contrast medium. Possible concurrent radiographic abnormalities include renal or ureteral calculi and indicators of cystitis and/or pyelonephritis.

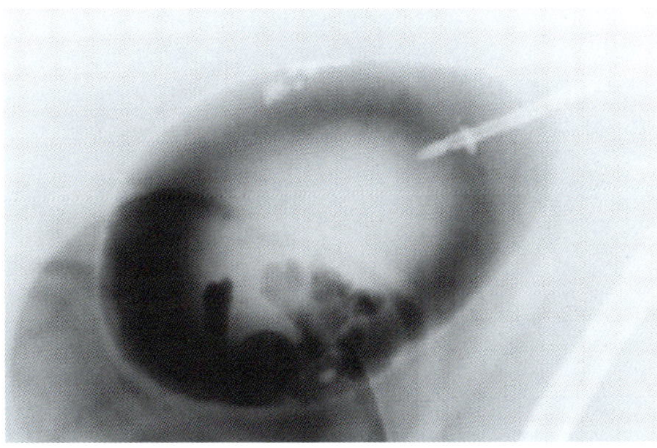

Fig. 14.27 Polypoid cystitis in a dog. On double contrast cystography, there are numerous polypoid and cauliflower-like mass lesions in the region of the cranioventral urinary bladder wall which appear as filling defects within the surrounding pool of contrast medium. Even though the appearance of these lesions is atypical for bladder neoplasia such as transitional cell carcinoma, malignant conditions cannot be excluded based on imaging.

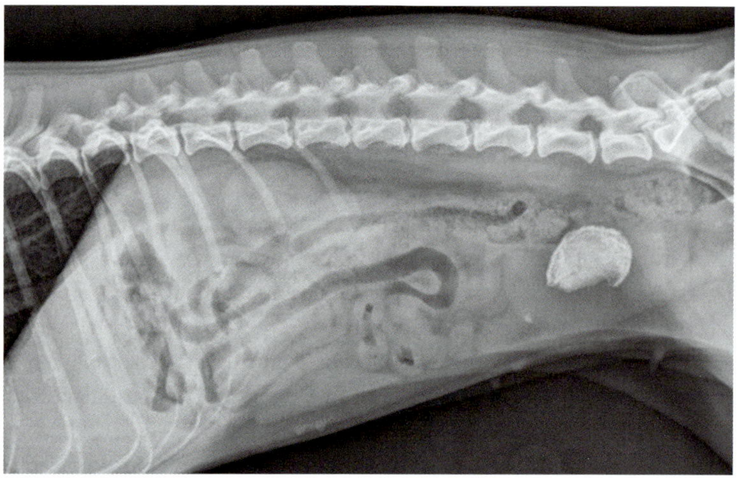

Fig. 14.28 Very large bladder calculus in a dog. This diagnosis is easily possible on a survey radiograph as the calculus is of mineral opacity.

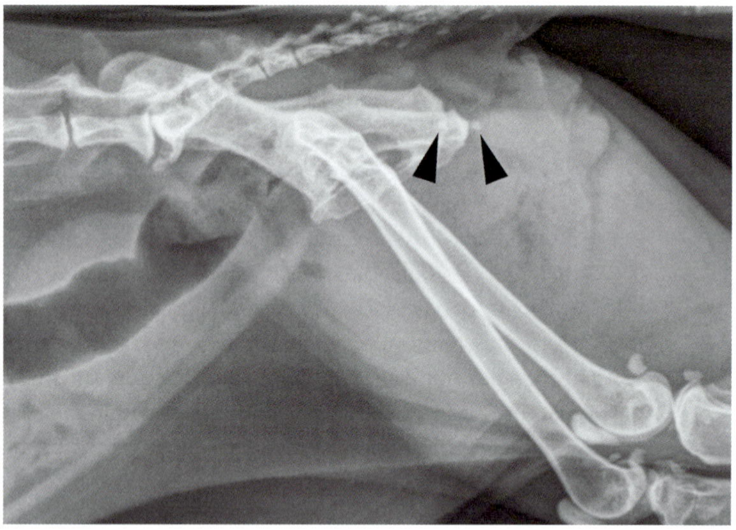

Fig. 14.29 Multiple small mineral opaque urethral calculi in a male cat (arrowheads). On this lateral view they are partially superimposed with the osseous pelvis and difficult to identify. Oblique views may aid in identification in questionable cases.

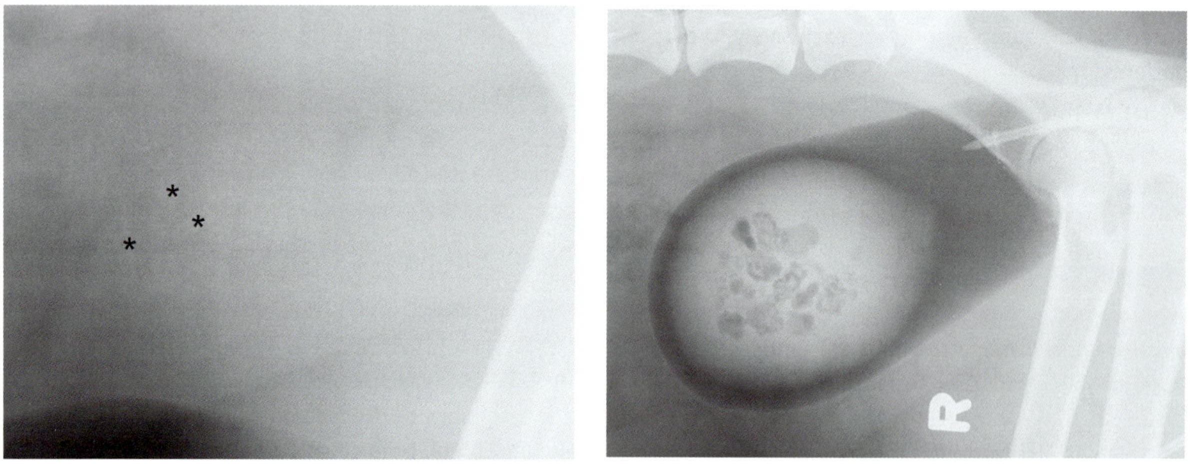

a b

Fig. 14.30 Radiolucent bladder calculi in a dog.

a On the survey radiograph, very faint foci of increased opacity are visible in the plane of the urinary bladder (*); however, distinct bladder calculi are not visible.

b On the double contrast cystogram, bladder calculi appear as numerous irregularly marginated filling defects within the pool of positive contrast medium (R = right).

On conventional radiographs, struvite, calcium oxalate and silicate stones are radiopaque, while cystine and urate stones are not radiopaque. On digital radiographs, particularly large cystine and urate stones may be visible. Mixed calculi have a variable radiographic appearance.

14.4.3 Bladder and urethral neoplasia

The most common tumour type of the lower urinary tract in dogs and cats is **transitional cell carcinoma**. Other less common tumours include other carcinomas, sarcomas and benign tumours such as leiomyomas.

RADIOGRAPHIC FINDINGS Survey radiographs are typically unrewarding. Dystrophic mineralization of the tumour may on occasion be noted and may lead to confusion with urinary calculi. Metastases to sublumbar lymph nodes are common, and bone metastases to the lumbar spine and pelvis may on occasion be noted. Tumours in the region of the bladder neck may result in ureteral obstruction and cause hydroureter and hydronephrosis (see section 14.3.6). Cystography and urethrography show focal or multifocal thickening of the urinary bladder or urethral wall and more or less extensive wall associated filling defects (Fig. 14.31).

Even though transitional cell carcinoma has a predisposition for the region of the urinary bladder trigone, it may affect any portion of the urinary bladder or urethra. Conversely, not every mass lesion at the level of the bladder neck is a transitional carcinoma. A definitive diagnosis requires cytology or histopathology.

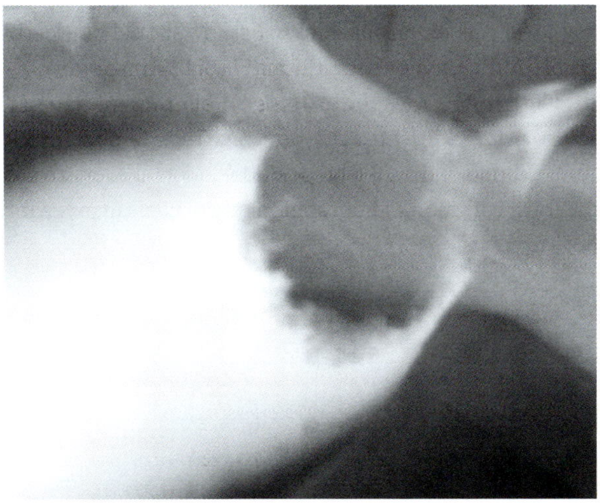

Fig. 14.31 Tumour at the level of the bladder neck in a dog. On a double contrast cystogram, there is an irregularly marginated large filling defect in the region of the bladder neck and extending caudally into the urethra. The histological diagnosis was transitional cell carcinoma.

14.4.4 Urachal diverticulum

The urachus connects the apex of the urinary bladder to the umbilicus during fetal development. It regresses after birth. A small focal diverticulum may remain visible at the urinary bladder apex in some animals and may be incidental or associated with recurrent episodes of cystitis.

RADIOGRAPHIC FINDINGS Survey radiographs are usually normal, or the urinary bladder may have an unusual contour. Cystography shows an irregular cranial bladder contour or a round to triangular diverticulum of variable size associated with the bladder apex (Fig. 14.32).

14.4.5 Bladder or urethral rupture

A bladder or urethral rupture is usually traumatic in aetiology (e.g. blunt abdominal trauma or iatrogenic following catheterization or biopsy). Underlying diseases of the bladder wall (inflammatory or neoplastic) can also result in perforation.

RADIOGRAPHIC FINDINGS The predominant finding in a patient with bladder rupture on survey radiographs is loss of serosal margin detail due to leakage of contrast medium into the peritoneal cavity. Depending on the location of a urethral tear, abdominal radiographs may show loss of serosal detail or may be normal. Positive contrast cystography/urethrography is the diagnostic method of choice to confirm or rule out a perforation of the lower urinary tract. Leakage of contrast medium from the urinary bladder or urethra, respectively, is noted (Fig. 14.33).

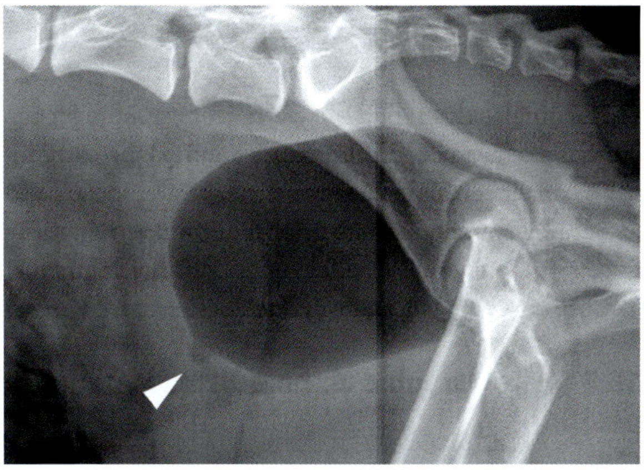

Fig. 14.32 Urachal diverticulum in a dog. A small focal outpouching of the bladder at the level of the apex is visible on a negative contrast cystogram (arrowhead).

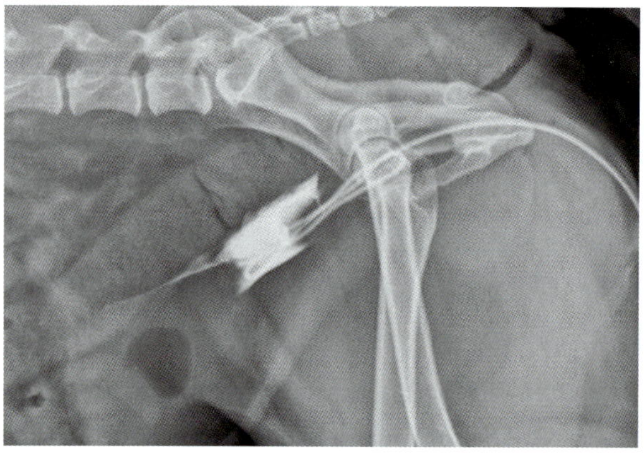

Fig. 14.33 Rupture of the urethra immediately caudal to the bladder neck in a female dog. Endoscopic biopsies of the urethra had been performed previously in this patient to confirm a clinical suspicion of a urethral tumour. On urethrography there is evidence of contrast medium leakage into the abdominal cavity, allowing identification and localization of urethral perforation. Note folding of the catheter within the urethral lumen, which could have been avoided by estimation of appropriate catheter length prior to its insertion. The gas opacity focus within the urinary bladder is consistent with prior endoscopy.

14.5 Pregnancy and diseases of the female reproductive tract

14.5.1 Pregnancy

Normal pregnancy

Even though abdominal ultrasound has largely replaced survey radiographs in pregnancy diagnosis, radiographs still play a role in the evaluation of pregnant dogs and cats. Radiographs are usually preferred over ultrasound for the following indications.

- Determination of the number of fetuses.
- Postpartum evaluation of the uterus to rule out residual fetuses.
- Evaluation of fetal position with dystocia.
- Assessment of fetal size in relation to pelvic canal diameter.
- Identification of fetal oversize.

Abdominal ultrasound is preferred for early pregnancy diagnosis, assessment of fetal viability and in utero diagnosis of congenital anomalies.

Some variability exists in the literature regarding radiographic findings in different **stages of pregnancy**. A summary of expected radiographic findings can be found in Table 14.4. In dogs, the gravid uterus becomes radiographically visible approximately 30 days after the luteinizing hormone (LH) peak and at this point is indistinguishable from a fluid-filled uterus (such as seen with pyometra) (Fig. 14.34a). In cats, the gravid uterus becomes visible between the 25th and 30th day of pregnancy. A definitive radiographic diagnosis of pregnancy is possible once **fetal mineralization** is apparent. In dogs, early skeletal mineralization becomes apparent on approximately the 45th and in cats on the 38th day of pregnancy. In comparison, ultrasonographic identification of gestation chambers is possible as early as day 20 in dogs and day 10 in cats, and the embryo as well as cardiac activity are recognized on approximately day 25 in dogs and day 18 in cats. Fetal ossification begins with the vertebrae and progresses to the appendicular skeleton. The teeth are the last structures to become radiographically visible and appear shortly before the end of pregnancy (approximately day 61 in dogs and day 58 in cats). Osseous fetal structures should be clearly visible at the time of parturition (Fig. 14.34b).

Abnormal pregnancy

Fetal death, abnormal fetal position and fetal oversize are the most common radiographic abnormalities in pregnant dogs and cats.

Table 14.4 Radiographic findings in different stages of pregnancy in dogs and cats.

Radiographic findings	Dog	Cat
Uterus visible	Day 30 (28–34)	Day 25–30
Fetal mineralization noted (beginning with axial followed by appendicular skeleton)	Day 45 (43–46)	Day 38 (36–40)
Teeth visible	Day 61 (58–63)	Day 58

Note: Data are based on luteinizing hormone (LH) peak in dogs, and last date of breeding in cats.

An ultrasonographic diagnosis of **fetal death** is possible immediately following cessation of cardiac activity. A radiographic diagnosis is based on loss of normal fetal position, collapse of bony structures or gas accumulations within the fetus or uterus (Fig. 14.35). These abnormalities may be evident as early as 6 hours but are often not recognized until 1 or 2 days after fetal death.

Mummified fetuses may be found months to years after fetal death and appear as shrunken and malaligned structures with partial skeletal maceration.

Abnormal fetal position and fetal oversize are two of many possible causes of **dystocia**, and can be diagnosed based on radiographs. Even though mathematical formulas have been developed to determine adequate fetal dimensions in relation to the mother's pelvic canal diameter, the diagnosis of fetal oversize is often based on subjective assessment.

14.5.2 Ovarian diseases

As mentioned in section 14.1.1, normal ovaries are not visible radiographically. All ovarian disorders important from a radiographic perspective (cysts, tumours, granulomas, abscesses) result in varying degrees of ovarian enlargement. Enlarged ovaries are visible caudal (and lateral) to the kidneys and typically appear as soft-tissue opacity nodules or masses (Fig. 14.36; see also Fig. 11.24).

Larger ovarian masses tend to descend ventrally within the abdominal cavity, which makes identification of the organ of origin difficult or impossible. Many ovarian diseases result in hormonal imbalances, and concurrent findings such as thickening or fluid filling of the uterus, or development of mammary tissue, are common.

Radiographic findings Different types of ovarian mass lesions cannot generally be distinguished radiographically. Epithelial tumours (e.g. adenocarcinoma), mesenchymal tumours, and sex cord stromal tumours (e.g. granulosa cell tumour) are typically of homogeneous soft-tissue opacity. Germ cell tumours (e.g. teratoma) are often characterized by enormous size and multifocal mineralized or ossified regions. Ovarian cysts and granulomas tend to be smaller than abscesses or tumours. However, as with many other conditions, cytology or histopathology are necessary for a definitive diagnosis.

14.5.3 Diseases of the uterus

Uterine disorders can be subdivided into two categories: intraluminal fluid accumulation (pyometra, mucometra, hydrometra and haemometra) and mural lesions (generalized wall thickening and uterine masses).

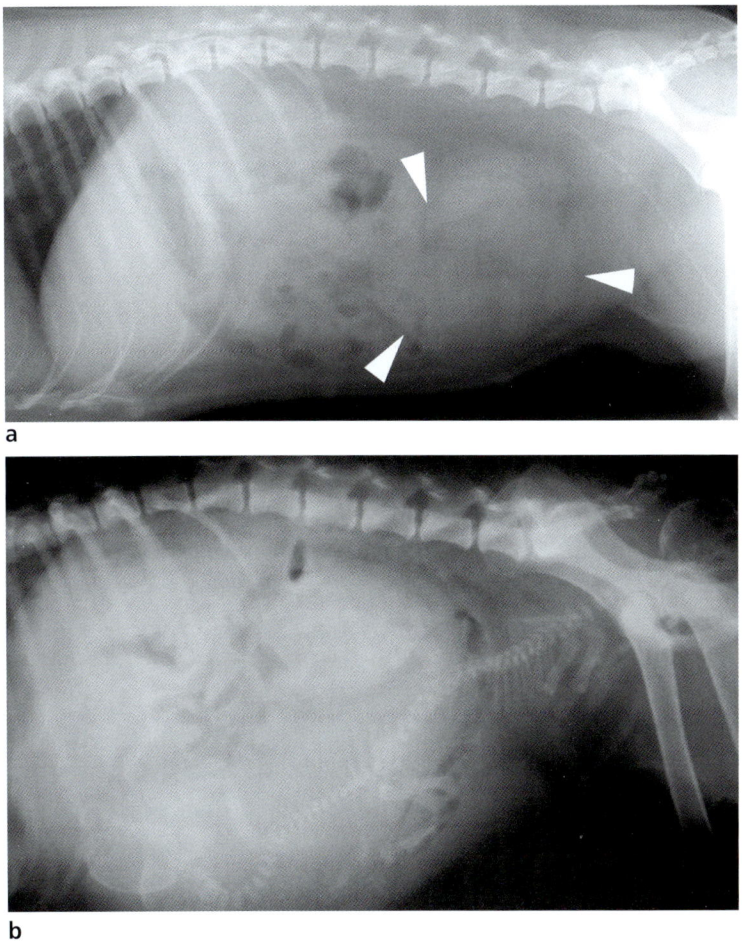

a

b

Fig. 14.34 Normal pregnancy in a dog.
a On this radiograph obtained during the middle trimester, the uterus is enlarged and appears as a tubular structure with homogeneous soft-tissue opacity in the mid and caudal abdomen (arrowheads). Differentiation between mid-term pregnancy and fluid filling of the uterus (e.g. pyometra) is not possible based on radiographs.
b The radiograph obtained at the time of parturition demonstrates three intact ossified fetuses, one of which has already entered the pelvic canal.

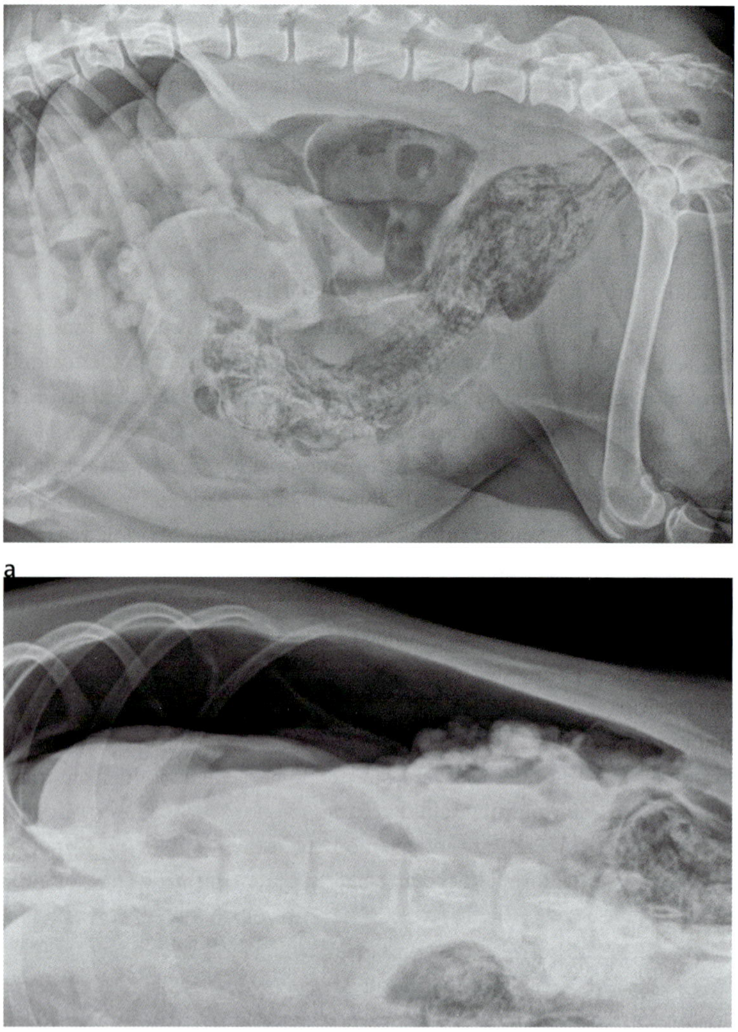

a

b

Fig. 14.35 Fetal death, emphysematous uterus and pneumoperitoneum in a dog.
a On the lateral view, a collapsed and macerated fetus surrounded by intraluminal gas is identified within the uterus. Additionally, numerous gas opacity foci located outside the gastrointestinal tract are present in the craniodorsal abdomen. Note developed mammary tissue ventral to the abdominal wall, consistent with advanced pregnancy.
b Even though this horizontal beam view was not necessary for diagnosis in this dog, as pneumoperitoneum was diagnosed on standard radiographs, it provides an impressive demonstration of the large amount of free abdominal gas accumulating in the nondependent portion of the abdomen. Exploratory laparotomy confirmed the radiographic findings of fetal death, emphysematous metritis and uterine perforation with subsequent pneumoperitoneum.

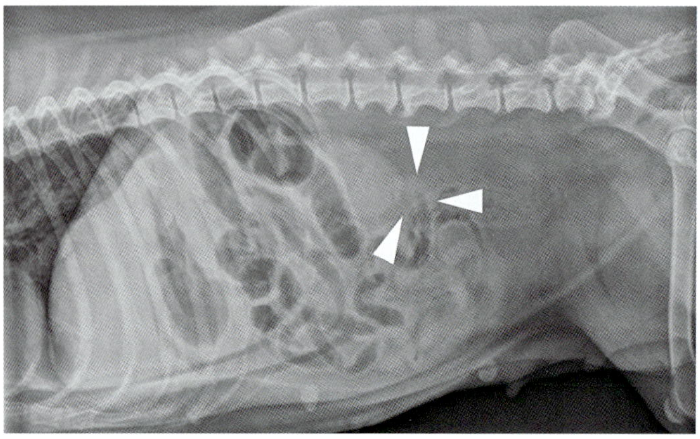

a

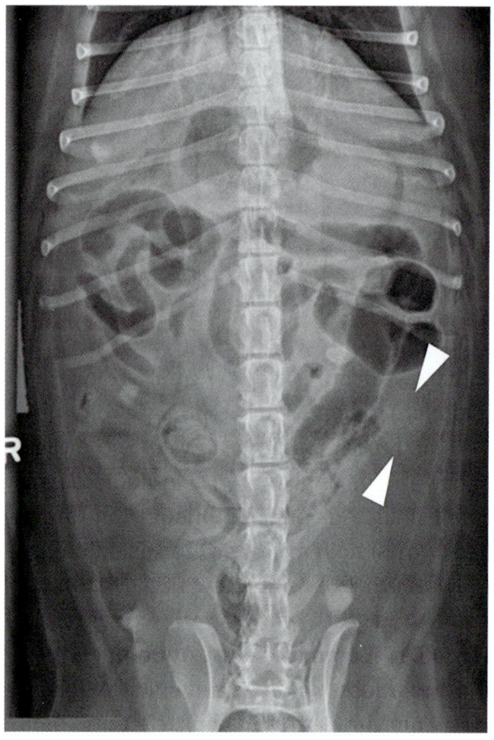

b

Fig. 14.36 Cystic ovaries in a dog. Lateral a and ventrodorsal b abdominal radiographs show an irregularly shaped, rounded, soft-tissue opacity structure caudal and lateral to the left kidney (arrowheads). The right kidney and region of the right ovary are obscured by superimposed intestinal segments. Note large mamillae associated with the ventral abdominal wall indicative either of prior pregnancy or hormonal imbalances. Abdominal ultrasonography yielded a diagnosis of bilateral ovarian cysts (R = right).

Pyometra, mucometra, hydrometra and haemometra

These conditions result in abnormal fluid accumulation within the uterus. Even though a definitive radiographic diagnosis is not usually possible, the history and clinical examination findings may aid in appropriate prioritization of differential diagnoses. Dogs with pyometra commonly present with putrid vaginal discharge and a fever, while hydrometra and mucometra are commonly incidental findings in asymptomatic dogs and cats. Haemorrhage into the lumen of the uterus (haemometra) may occur, for example secondary to trauma, coagulopathy or neoplastic infiltration of the uterine wall.

RADIOGRAPHIC FINDINGS Radiographic distinction of these conditions is not possible. The enlarged uterus appears as a tubular structure with homogeneous soft-tissue opacity between the urinary bladder and descending colon. It extends from the pelvic canal cranially and ventrally into the abdominal cavity (Fig. 14.37).

> Different types of intraluminal uterine fluid accumulation and normal mid-term pregnancy cannot be distinguished radiographically.

Severe distention of the uterus may result in **uterine rupture** and radiographic loss of serosal margin detail.

With **emphysematous pyometra**, there is gas accumulation within the lumen and/or wall of the uterus. This is most commonly seen secondary to fetal death (see Fig. 14.35), but may also occur as an isolated condition due to infection with gas-producing bacteria.

Infection of the uterine stump in spayed animals (**'stump pyometra'**) results in a blind ending soft-tissue opacity pouch or mass lesion between the urinary bladder and the descending colon. Affected animals present with similar clinical signs to animals with true pyometra.

Mural thickening and mass lesions of the uterus

Diffuse wall thickening of the uterus, such as seen with endometritis or cystic endometrial hyperplasia, is difficult to identify on abdominal radiographs. Radiographs are normal in mild cases. In more severe cases, or if concurrent intraluminal fluid accumulation is present, generalized thickening of the uterus is evident, which cannot be distinguished from other causes of intraluminal fluid accumulation such as pyometra.

Mass lesions originating from the uterus are rare. Differential diagnoses include uterine neoplasms (leiomyoma/leiomyosarcoma, adenocarcinoma, etc.), granulomas, abscesses and cystic lesions. These masses vary in their appearance based on size and location. Masses originating from the uterine body or the caudal horns are located dorsal to the urinary bladder and ventral to the descending colon (Fig. 14.38). Even though a normal vagina is not visible radiographically, larger masses of vaginal origin may extend from the pelvic canal cranially into the abdomen, and are indistinguishable from caudal uterine masses. Masses originating from more cranial parts of the uterus are typically located in the mid and ventral abdomen. Depending on their size and location, the organ of origin may be difficult to determine. Uterine masses are commonly associated with concurrent intraluminal fluid accumulation, which may result in an erroneous diagnosis of, for example, pyometra.

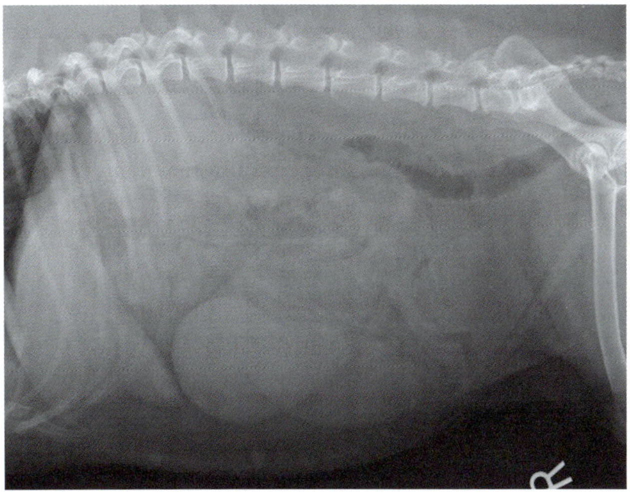

a

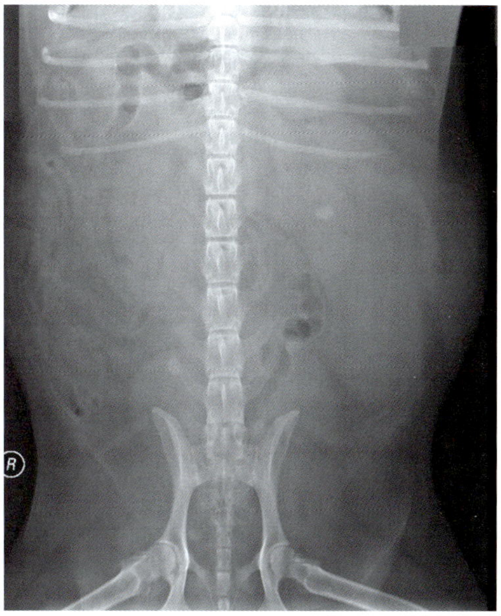

b

Fig. 14.37 Pyometra in a dog. The enlarged uterus is visible as a homogeneous soft-tissue opaque tubular structure on both lateral a and ventrodorsal b abdominal radiographs. The dilated uterine horns extend from the pelvic inlet into the mid to cranioventral abdomen (R = right).

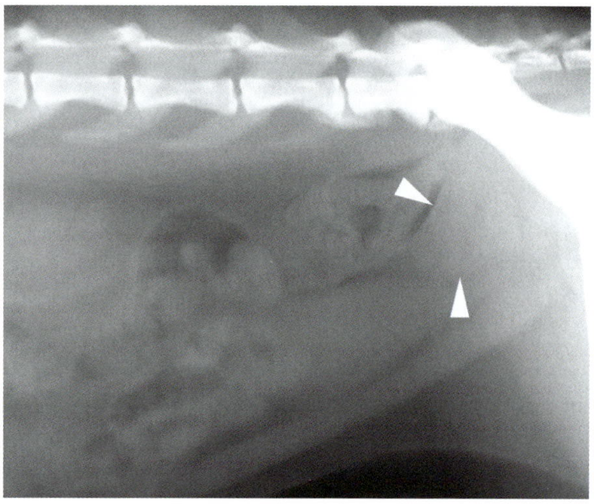

Fig. 14.38 Uterine stump granuloma in a spayed female cat. A homogeneous soft-tissue opaque blind ending mass lesion is visible between the urinary bladder and descending colon (arrowheads). Additional differential diagnoses for this finding would include a uterine stump tumour or a stump pyometra. The diagnosis was made based on ultrasound-guided fine-needle aspiration. Lumbar spondylosis deformans is incidental.

14.6 Diseases of the male reproductive tract

Diseases of the male reproductive tract in small animals are almost exclusively seen in male dogs. Only a few isolated case reports describe reproductive tract abnormalities in male cats. Information provided in this chapter refers to dogs unless stated otherwise.

14.6.1 Diseases of the prostatic gland

Prostatic diseases typically result in enlargement of the prostate and/or paraprostatic abnormalities. As mentioned above, normal prostate size varies with age and reproductive status.

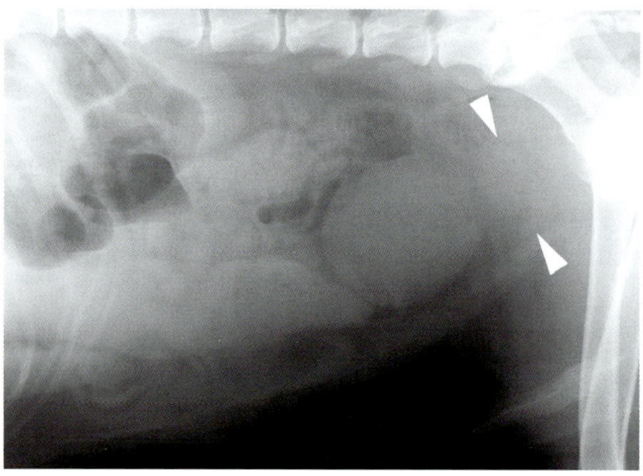

Fig. 14.39 Benign prostatic hyperplasia in an intact male dog. The prostate (arrowheads) is enlarged, homogeneous and smoothly marginated.

The prostate in intact dogs is considered enlarged when its height exceeds 70% of the pelvic inlet on a lateral view, and when its width exceeds 50% of the transverse pelvic canal diameter on a ventrodorsal view. The diagnosis of prostatic enlargement is more subjective in neutered dogs. As a normal prostate is not visible in most neutered dogs, increased conspicuity of the gland is considered an indicator of prostatomegaly.

In general, **prostatomegaly** is a nonspecific finding and is not pathognomonic for any specific type of prostatic disease. However, patient signalment and history as well as additional findings such as regional (sublumbar) lymphadenopathy may aid in prioritization of differential diagnoses. Distinction between an enlarged prostate and adjacent mass lesions such as paraprostatic cysts may be difficult in some patients. Abdominal ultrasound or cystography may aid in identification of the urinary bladder in these cases.

> Different underlying aetiologies of prostatomegaly cannot be distinguished on survey radiographs. Certain concomitant findings may aid in prioritization of differential diagnoses. Signalment and history, clinical examination findings and abdominal ultrasound may also yield additional information. However, a definitive diagnosis requires fine-needle aspiration or biopsy.

Benign prostatic hyperplasia (BPH) and prostatic cysts

Virtually any older intact male dog is affected by some degree of prostatic hyperplasia with cysts, and this condition may or may not cause clinical signs. Abnormalities in urination and defecation (dysuria, stranguria and constipation) may develop with increasing prostate size and formation of larger cystic lesions.

RADIOGRAPHIC FINDINGS The prostate is moderately to markedly enlarged, but typically maintains smooth margins and a rounded shape (Fig. 14.39). There is no evidence of regional metastasis or associated focal peritonitis.

Prostatitis and prostatic abscesses

Inflammation of the prostate also results in prostatic enlargement. Aetiological agents include bacteria and, in endemic areas, fungal organisms. Intact dogs are more commonly affected than neutered animals.

RADIOGRAPHIC FINDINGS Regional peritonitis may result in focal loss of serosal detail adjacent to the enlarged prostate (Fig. 14.40). Infection with gas-producing bacteria is rare, but may result in gas accumulation within the prostatic parenchyma.

With increasing availability of ultrasound in veterinary practice, retrograde cystography is nowadays rarely performed in the diagnostic workup of patients with suspected prostatitis. Possible findings with this procedure are abnormal reflux of contrast medium into the prostatic gland, and contrast medium accumulation in cavitary lesions (abscess cavities).

Paraprostatic cysts

Paraprostatic cysts (aka 'cystic uterus masculinus') result from fluid accumulation within remnants of the Mullerian duct system. This is predominantly seen in intact older large-breed dogs; however, a true breed predisposition does not exist.

RADIOGRAPHIC FINDINGS Paraprostatic cysts appear as tubular, blind ending, soft-tissue opacity structures in the caudoventral abdomen. They can reach considerable size, and may on occasion be difficult to distinguish from the adjacent urinary bladder and prostate (Fig. 14.41a). Abdominal ultrasound or cystography may aid in identification of the urinary bladder in these cases (Fig. 14.41b). Dystrophic mineralization of the cyst wall may be seen in chronic cases, and may mimic mineralization of the urinary bladder wall or urinary bladder calculi.

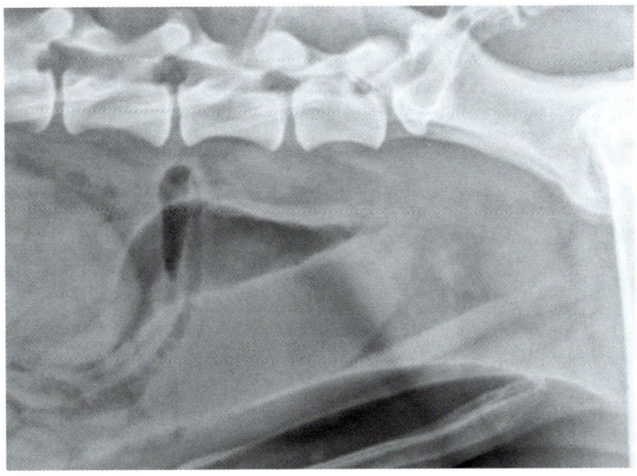

Fig. 14.40 Prostatitis and prostatic abscesses in a male intact dog. Radiographic abnormalities include prostate enlargement and poor serosal margin detail in the caudal abdomen with soft-tissue streaking of the caudal abdominal fat, consistent with regional peritonitis/steatitis.

Prostatic neoplasia

Even though prostatic neoplasia may affect intact animals, it is more common in neutered dogs. The primary differential diagnosis for a neutered dog presenting with prostatomegaly is thus prostatic neoplasia. The most common tumour types are adenocarcinoma and transitional cell carcinoma (originating from the prostatic urethra). Other tumour types are uncommon.

RADIOGRAPHIC FINDINGS The prostatic gland is enlarged and, in contrast to other conditions, is typically irregularly marginated. Focal or multifocal dystrophic mineralization of prostatic parenchyma is common. The finding of an enlarged, mineralized prostate in a neutered dog, with or without evidence of metastases to sublumbar lymph nodes, lumbosacral vertebrae and pelvis, is virtu-

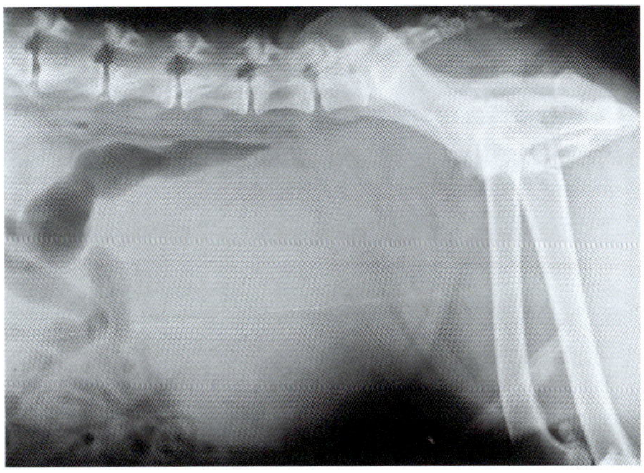

a

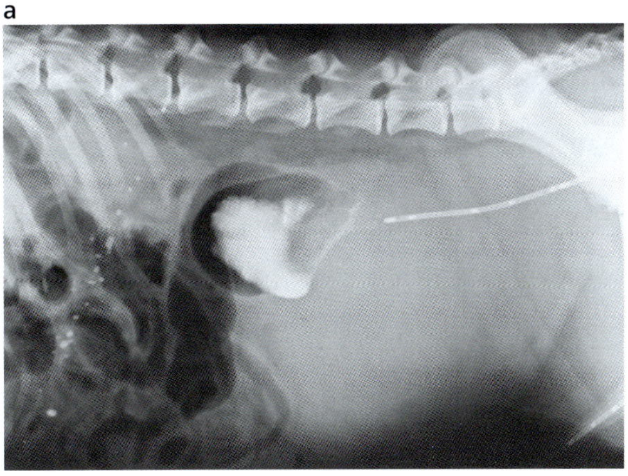

b

Fig. 14.41 Paraprostatic cyst in a dog.
a On the lateral survey radiographs, there is a large mass lesion of homogeneous soft-tissue opacity within the caudal abdomen. This structure is indistinguishable from the urinary bladder and prostatic gland.
b Following the injection of air and positive contrast medium, the urinary bladder is identified and is displaced cranially and dorsally by the large mass lesion. Exploratory laparotomy confirmed the presumptive diagnosis of paraprostatic cysts.

ally pathognomonic for prostatic neoplasia (Fig. 14.42; see also Chapter 7, Fig. 7.47). However, cytology or histopathology are needed for a definitive diagnosis.

14.6.2 Other diseases of the male reproductive tract

Testicular diseases are typically not amenable to radiographic diagnosis. A possible exception is cryptorchidism.

RADIOGRAPHIC FINDINGS Non-neoplastic inguinal or abdominal testicles are typically not visible on survey radiographs due to their small size. Neoplastic retained testicles (Sertoli cell tumours or seminomas) appear as inguinal or abdominal soft-tissue opacity mass lesions. Abdominal neoplastic testicles are commonly located in the mid-ventral to caudal abdomen (Fig. 14.43). Concurrent indicators of hyperoestrogenism or other hormonal imbalance (enlarged nipples and prostate) are common, especially with Sertoli cell tumours. Torsion of an intra-abdominal neoplastic testicle typically results in mild abdominal effusion adjacent to the abdominal mass.

Suggested reading

Adin CA, Herrgesell EJ, Nyland TG, Hughes JM, Gregory CR, Kyles AE, Cowgill LD, Ling GV. Antegrade pyelography for suspected ureteral obstruction in cats: 11 cases (1995–2001). J Am Vet Med Assoc 2003; 222: 1576–81.

Boyd JS. The radiographic identification of the various stages of pregnancy in the domestic cat. J Small Anim Pract 1971; 12: 501–6.

Feeney D, Anderson KL. Radiographic imaging in urinary tract disease. In: Bartges J, Polzin DJ (eds). Nephrology and Urology of Small Animals. Ames: Wiley Blackwell 2011; 97–127.

Feeney D, Thrall D, Barber D. Normal canine excretory urogram: effects of dose, time and individual dog variation. Am J Vet Res 1979; 40: 1596–1604.

Feeney DA, Barber DL, Osborne CA. The functional aspects of the nephrogram in excretory urography: a review. Vet Radiol 1982; 23: 42–5.

Hecht S. Nephropyelocentesis and antegrade pyelography. In: Bartges J, Polzin DJ (eds). Nephrology and Urology of Small Animals. Ames: Wiley Blackwell 2011; 43–5.

Hecht S, McCarthy RJ, Tidwell AS. What is your diagnosis? Ectopic kidney in a cat. J Am Vet Med Assoc 2005; 227: 223–4.

Johnston GR, Feeney DA. Comparative organ imaging:- – Lower urinary tract. Vet Radiol 1984; 25: 146–53.

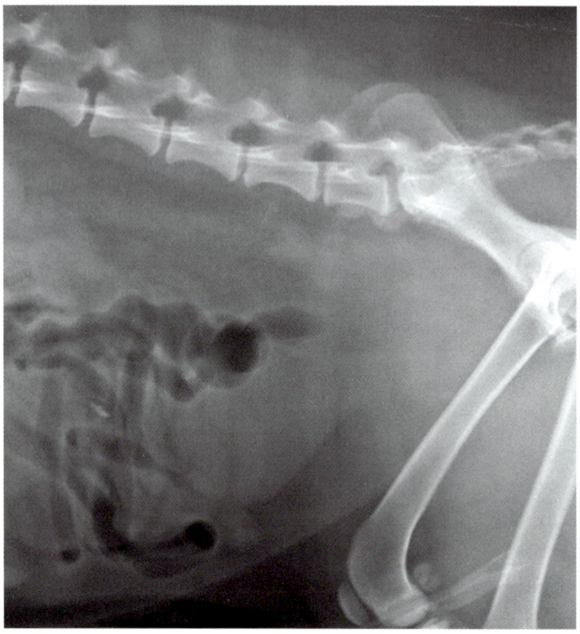

Fig. 14.42 Prostatic neoplasia (adenocarcinoma) in a male neutered dog. The prostate is enlarged and irregularly marginated. There is an irregular soft-tissue opacity mass lesion ventral to the caudal lumbar spine (L6 through the sacrum). Note also irregular periosteal new bone formation along the ventral margin of the seventh lumbar vertebra and the sacrum. These findings are virtually pathognomonic for prostatic neoplasia with metastases to sublumbar lymph nodes and spine.

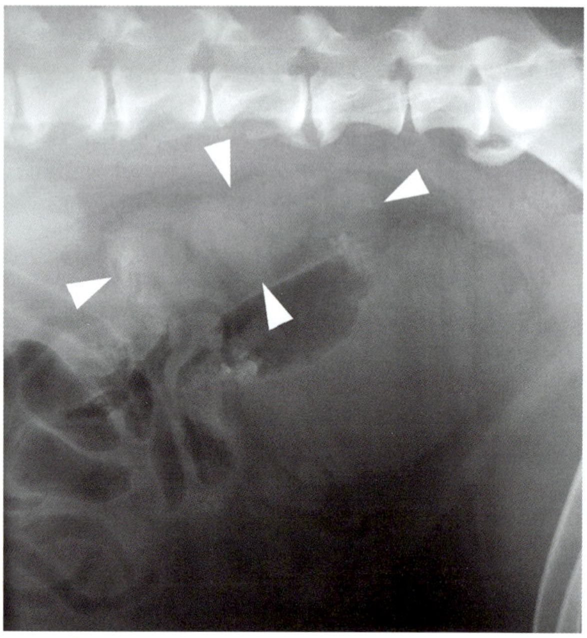

Fig. 14.43 Abdominal cryptorchidism in a dog. The retained testicles (arrowheads) are visible in the plane of the caudal retroperitoneal space. They are enlarged and irregularly marginated, indicative of neoplastic transformation. Histopathological examination was consistent with bilateral Sertoli cell tumour. Caudal lumbar spondylosis deformans is incidental.

O´Brien T. Radiographic Diagnosis of Abdominal Disorders in the Dog and cat. Philadelphia: Saunders 1978.

Owens JM, Biery DN. Radiographic Interpretation for the Small Animal Clinician, 2nd edn. Baltimore: Williams & Wilkins 1999.

Pobisch R. Röntgendiagnostik in der Chirurgie. In: Schebitz H, Brass W (eds). Allgemeine Chirurgie. Berlin: Parey 1975; 86–9.

Pugh CR, Rhodes WH, Biery DN. Contrast studies of the urogenital system. Vet Clin North Am Small Anim Pract 1993; 23: 281–306.

Rendano VR. Radiographic evaluation of fetal development in the bitch and fetal death in the bitch and queen. In: Kirk RW (ed.). Current Veterinary Therapy, Vol VIII. Philadelphia: WB Saunders 1983: 947–52.

Rivers BJ, Walter PA, Polzin DJ. Ultrasonographic-guided, percutaneous antegrade pyelography: Technique and clinical application in the dog and cat. J Am Anim Hosp Assoc 1997; 33: 61–8.

Rozear L, Tidwell AS. Evaluation of the ureterovesicular junction using helical computed tomographic excretory urography in healthy dogs. Vet Radiol Ultrasound 2003; 44: 155–64.

Schebitz H, Wilkens H. Atlas der Röntgenanatomie von Hund und Katze, 4th edn. Berlin: Parey 1986.

Shiroma JT, Gabriel JK, Carter RL, Scruggs SL, Stubbs PW. Effect of reproductive status on feline renal size. Vet Rad Ultrasound 1999; 40: 242–5.

Thrall DE. Textbook of Veterinary Diagnostic Radiology, 4th edn. Philadelphia: W.B. Saunders 2002.

Tiedemann K, Henschel E. Early radiographic diagnosis of pregnancy in the cat. J Small Anim Pract 1973; 14: 567–72.

Ticer JW. Radiographic Technique in Veterinary Practice. Philadelphia: Saunders 1984.

Waibl H, Mayrhofer E, Matis U, Brunnberg L, Köstlin R (eds). Atlas der Röntgenanatomie der Katze (founded by Schebitz H, Wilkens H). Stuttgart: Parey 2004.

Waibl H, Mayrhofer E, Matis U, Brunnberg L, Köstlin R (eds). Atlas der Röntgenanatomie des Hundes (founded by Schebitz H, Wilkens H), 2nd edn. Stuttgart: Parey 2005.

Wallack ST. The Handbook of Veterinary Contrast Radiography. Solana Beach, CA: San Diego Veterinary Imaging Inc 2003.

General principles of orthopaedic radiology

15

Silke Hecht, Federica Morandi and Gregory B. Daniel

15.1 Anatomy and indications

15.1.1 Anatomy

A solid knowledge base of the normal radiographic anatomy of the musculoskeletal system is extremely important to be able to differentiate physiological structures (and normal variants) from pathological changes. This book does not replace a radiographic atlas or a textbook of anatomy and physiology, but will provide a brief overview of important concepts of orthopaedic radiology.

Overview

Bone consists of cellular structures and an extracellular matrix.

Cellular structures of bone are responsible for production, maintenance and remodelling of bone tissue. These cells include **osteoblasts** (bone producing cells), **osteocytes** (osteoblasts following integration into the bone matrix) and **osteoclasts** (bone resorbing cells). Bone matrix consists of inorganic components (65%; predominantly calcium phosphate in the form of **hydroxyapatite crystals**) and organic **osteoid** (35%; predominantly type I collagen fibres).

MACROSCOPIC ANATOMY Two types of bone structure can be distinguished, the exterior cortex (*substantia compacta* and *substantia corticalis*) and the central spongy or cancellous bone (*substantia spongiosa*). The compacta surrounds the central medullary cavity, the corticalis the epiphyses which contain spongiosa. As corticalis and compacta are radiographically indistinguishable, they will be combined under the term 'cortex' in this chapter.

The articular surfaces of bone are covered by cartilage. The nonarticular surfaces are covered by periosteum, and the inner surface by endosteum.

Generally, bones can be subdivided according to:

- location (axial versus appendicular skeleton)
- development (endochondral versus intramembranous ossification)
- shape (long bones, short bones, flat bones or irregular bones).

BONE SHAPES Long bones constitute the majority of bones in the appendicular skeleton. They develop from separate centres of ossification (**diaphysis** and proximal and distal **epiphyses** separated by growth plates/ **physes**). The transition zone between epiphysis and diaphysis is termed **metaphysis** (Fig. 15.1). Short bones are, for example, found in the carpus and tarsus. Flat bones are formed by two compact bone plates which surround a thin layer of spongiosa (**diploe**). Examples include the bones of the skull and the scapula.

SESAMOID BONES These are regions of bone formation that develop in areas where tendons (or ligaments) glide over an underlying osseous structure. Some sesamoid bones are present in all mammals (e.g. patella and sesamoid bones of the gastrocnemius and popliteal muscles in the stifle joint, sesamoid bones of the metacarpophalangeal joints and metatarsophalangeal joints), while others are only found in some animals (e.g. sesamoid bone of the supinator muscle lateral to the elbow joint, sesamoid bone of the extensor carpi obliquus muscle/abductor pollicis longus muscle medial to the carpus).

OSSIFICATION CENTRES AND GROWTH PLATES The linear region between the metaphysis and epiphysis (**physis**) is responsible for the longitudinal growth of a long bone. Many bones have additional separate centres of ossification at the insertion sites of tendinous structures (**apophyses**). These contribute to the characteristic contour of a long bone, but not to its longitudinal growth. Examples include the olecranon tuber of the ulna, the medial humeral epicondyle, the greater trochanter of the femur and the tibial tuberosity.

Radiographic findings Generally, bones have a very radiopaque peripheral cortex and a less opaque central region (medullary cavity and spongiosa) (Fig. 15.2). The cortex is fairly homogeneous except for thin oblique radiolucent lines representing vascular channels. These are located at characteristic locations for each specific bone and should not be confused with fracture lines (Fig. 15.3). Bones are modelled into characteristic shapes with protrusions, indentations, curves and articular surfaces depending on the origin and insertion of tendons and ligaments, the type and degree of load bearing, and articulation with adjacent osseous structures. The specific radiographic anatomy of the front and hind limbs is covered later in this chapter.

The **periosteum, endosteum, articular cartilage, joint capsule** and most associated **soft-tissue structures** (e.g. ligaments) are not radiographically visible or cannot be distinguished from adjacent tissues. Evaluation of these structures therefore often requires the use of other imaging modalities such as ultrasound, computed tomography (CT) or magnetic resonance imaging (MRI). However, the radiographic appearance of some soft-tissue anomalies and the possible effects of soft-tissue lesions on osseous structures are covered in this chapter.

Radiographic evaluation of the musculoskeletal system in immature animals This is especially challenging, as open physes may mimic fractures (Fig. 15.4).

The time of physeal closure differs from physis to physis, as well as between dogs and cats. As determination of normal versus abnormal physes is essential in the radiographic assessment of young animals (e.g. differentiation of a normal physis from a traumatic lesion, identification of premature physeal closure secondary to trauma, or identification of delayed physeal closure in the case of metabolic disorders such as congenital hypothyroidism), it is advisable to keep a table with normal physeal closure times handy (Tables 15.1 and 15.2). Following physeal closure, prior growth plates remain visible as thin lines of increased opacity (**'physeal scars'**).

In the following sections the reader will find semi-schematic images illustrating the normal radiographic

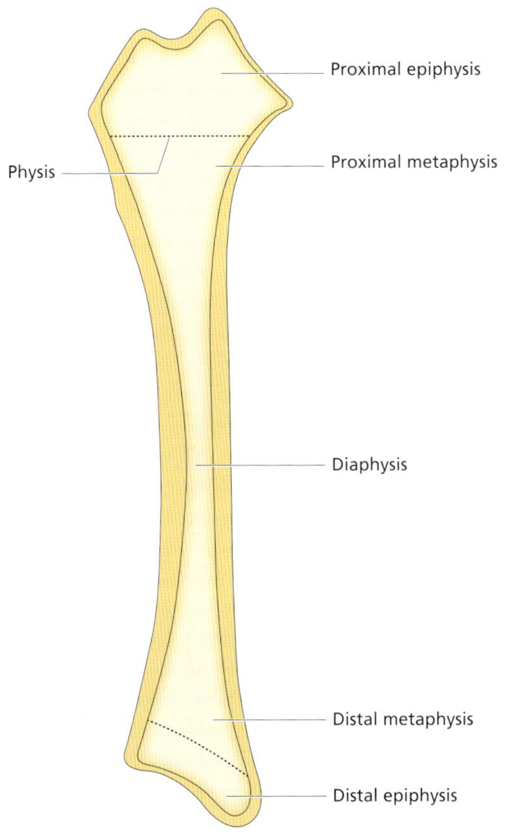

Fig. 15.1 Schematic illustration showing long bone anatomy.

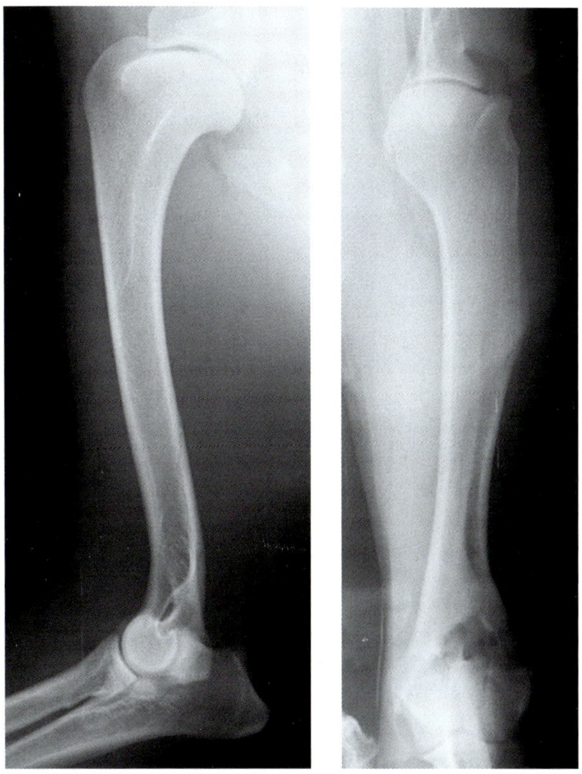

a b

Fig. 15.2 Lateral a and craniocaudal b radiographs of a normal long bone (humerus) in a dog. The peripheral cortex surrounds the central less opaque medullary cavity and spongiosa. Periosteum, endosteum, joint cartilage and capsule as well as adjacent soft-tissue structures, such as ligaments, are not visible.

anatomy of front and hind limbs. These are mostly based on radiographs of dogs. Important species-specific differences between dogs and cats are covered at the end of each section. The anatomy of the head, spine and thoracic wall is covered in Chapters 6, 7 and 9, respectively.

Forelimbs including shoulder girdle

The shoulder girdle and forelimbs consist of the following **osseous structures**:

- scapula
- humerus
- radius and ulna
- carpal bones (intermedioradial carpal bone, ulnar carpal bone, accessory carpal bone and carpal bones I–IV)
- metacarpal bones I–V
- phalanges I–III
- clavicle (only in cats).

Joints of the forelimb include:

- shoulder joint (scapulohumeral joint)
- elbow joint (cubital joint)
- carpus
- metacarpophalangeal joints
- proximal and distal interphalangeal joints.

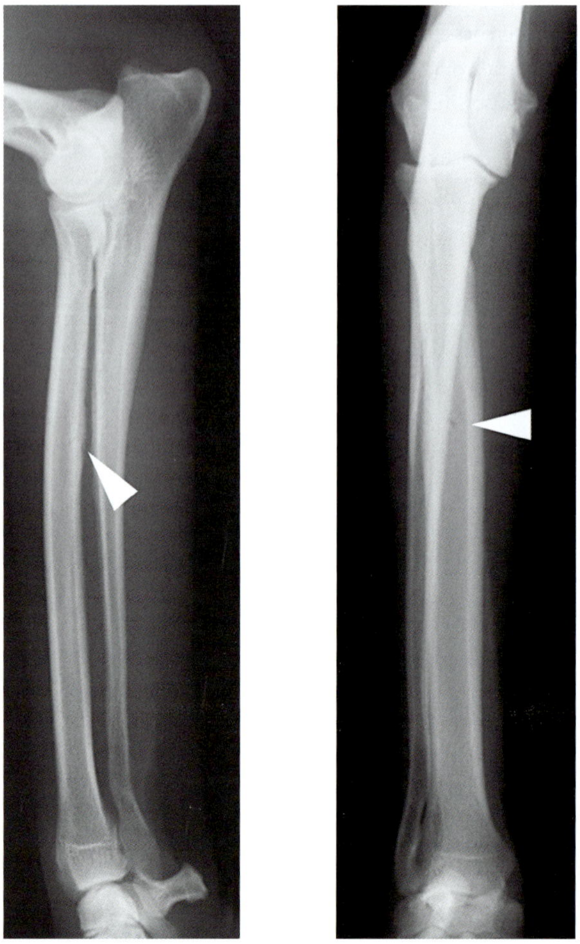

a b

Fig. 15.3 Lateral a and craniocaudal b radiographs of the antebrachium in a dog. A thin oblique radiolucent line is associated with the caudal cortex of the radius at the margin between the proximal and middle thirds (arrowheads). This is a normal vascular channel and should not be confused with a pathological abnormality such as a fracture.

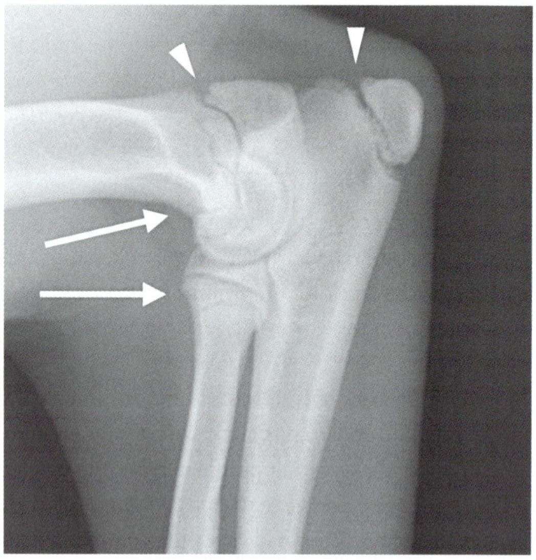

Fig. 15.4 Lateral radiograph of the elbow joint in a 5-month-old dog. The open physes of the distal humerus and proximal radius (arrows) as well as the apophyseal physes of the medial humeral epicondyle and the olecranon tuber (arrowheads) appear as distinct radiolucent lines.

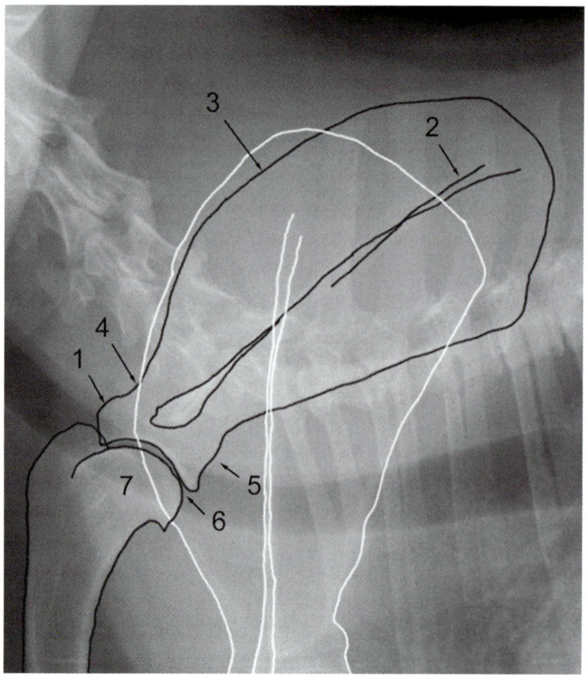

a

Table 15.1 Important physeal closure times of the forelimb in dogs and cats.

Osseous structure		Approximate age at physeal closure and fusion of separate centres of ossification (months)	
		Dog	Cat
Scapula	Supraglenoid tubercle	3–7	3.5–6
Humerus	Proximal epiphysis	10–15	18–24
	Distal epiphysis	5–8	4
	Fusion of lateral and medial aspect of the humeral condyle	5	3.5–7
	Medial epicondyle	5–6	4–6
Radius	Proximal epiphysis	5–11	5–7
	Distal epiphysis	6–12	14–25
Ulna	Olecranon tuber	5–10	9–14
	Anconeal process	3–5	
	Distal epiphysis	6–12	14–25
Carpus	Intermedioradial carpal bone	3–4	
	Accessory carpal bone	3–6	4–7
Metacarpus	Proximal epiphysis of metacarpal I	6–7	9–11
	Distal epiphysis of metacarpals II–V	5–7	7–12
Proximal and middle phalanges	Proximal epiphysis	5–7	6–9

Note: Data from Chapman 1965; de Lahunta and Habel 1986; Hare 1972; I. Horvath 1983; Pomriaskynski-Kobozieff and Kobozieff 1954; Smith and Allcock 1960; Sumner-Smith 1966; Thrall and Robertson 2011; Ticer 1975; Van Sickle 1966.

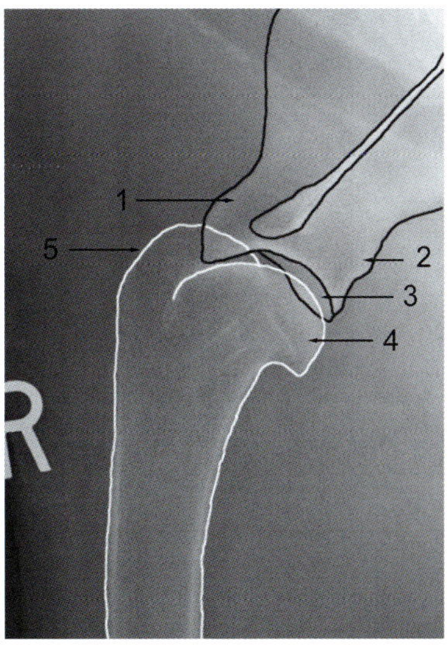

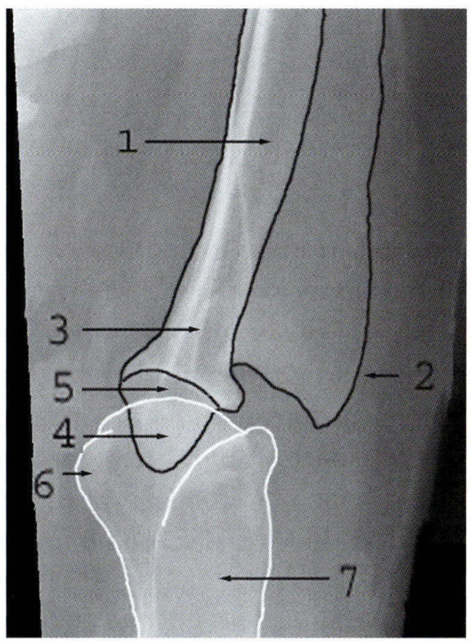

Fig. 15.5 Normal radiographic anatomy of the shoulder joint. a Lateral view of the scapula. 1 Supraglenoid tubercle, 2 Scapular spine, 3 Cranial margin of the scapula, 4 Scapular notch/neck of the scapula, 5 Infraglenoid tubercle, 6 Joint space, 7 Humeral head. b Lateral view of the shoulder joint. 1 Supraglenoid tubercle, 2 Infraglenoid tubercle, 3 Joint space, 4 Head of the humerus, 5 Greater tubercle of humerus (R = right). c Caudocranial view of the shoulder joint. 1 Scapula, 2 Acromion, 3 Neck of the scapula, 4 Cranial part of the glenoid cavity, 5 Joint space, 6 Lesser tubercle of the humerus, 7 Body of the humerus. (Courtesy of Dr Ryan King, Dr Andrea Matthews and Dr James Sutherland-Smith, Tufts University Cummings School of Veterinary Medicine)

Table 15.2 Important physeal closure times of the hind limb in dogs and cats.

Osseous structure		Approximate age at physeal closure and fusion of separate centres of ossification (months)	
		Dog	Cat
Pelvis	Physes between ilium, ischium, pubis and acetabular bone	4–6	8–9
	Iliac crest	15–66	>26
	Ischiatic tuber	8–14	>26
	Pelvic symphysis	30–72	
Femur	Head	6–9	7–12
	Greater trochanter	6–9	7–14
	Lesser trochanter	8–13	8–15
	Distal epiphysis	6–12	17–20
Tibia	Tibial tuberosity	8–10	17–22
	Proximal epiphysis	6–15	12–21
	Distal epiphysis	5–11	10–14
	Medial malleolus	4–5	
Fibula	Proximal epiphysis	6–12	13–21
	Distal epiphysis	5–13	10–14
Tarsus	Calcanean tuber	3–8	7–15
Metatarsus	Distal epiphysis metatarsals II–V	5–7	8–12
Proximal and middle phalanges	Proximal epiphysis	5–7	6–9

Note: Data from Chapman 1965; de Lahunta and Habel 1986; Hare 1972; A. Horvath 1983; Smith 1969; Smith and Allcock 1960; Sumner-Smith 1966; Thrall and Robertson 2011; Ticer 1975.

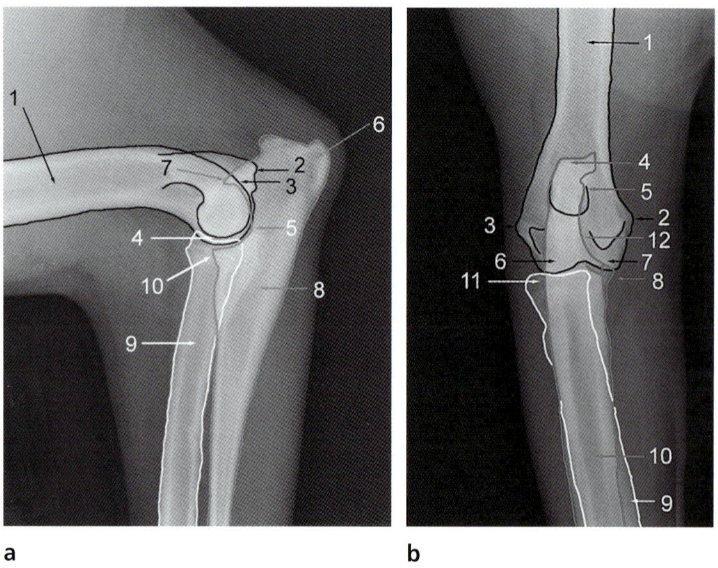

Fig. 15.6 Normal radiographic anatomy of the elbow joint.
a Lateral view of the elbow joint. 1 Humerus, 2 Medial humeral epicondyle, 3 Lateral humeral epicondyle, 4 Joint space, 5 Ulnar trochlear notch, 6 Olecranon, 7 Anconeal process, 8 Ulna, 9 Radius, 10 Medial coronoid process of the ulna.
b Craniocaudal view of the elbow joint. 1 Humerus, 2 Medial humeral epicondyle, 3 Lateral humeral epicondyle, 4 Olecranon, 5 Anconeal process, 6 Lateral aspect of the humeral condyle (capitulum), 7 Medial aspect of the humeral condyle (trochlea), 8 Medial coronoid process of the ulna, 9 Radius, 10 Ulna, 11 Head of the radius, 12 Ulnar trochlear notch. (Courtesy of Dr Ryan King, Dr Andrea Matthews and Dr James Sutherland-Smith, Tufts University Cummings School of Veterinary Medicine)

Sesamoid bones are found associated with the elbow joint, carpus, metacarpophalangeal joints and distal interphalangeal joints.

Semi-schematic images of the normal radiographic anatomy of the forelimb are shown in Figures 15.5 to 15.7.

DIFFERENCES IN RADIOGRAPHIC ANATOMY OF THE FORELIMB BETWEEN DOGS AND CATS While cats have a distinct thin ossified clavicle (Fig. 15.8), dogs typically only have a cartilaginous remnant which rarely shows evidence of mineralization.

A pronounced coracoid process of the scapula is seen in cats (Fig. 15.8b).

On radiographs of the feline elbow joint, the supratrochlear foramen connecting the olecranon fossa with the radial fossa seen in dogs (Fig. 15.9a) is absent, and cats have a supracondylar foramen associated with the distomedial aspect of the humerus instead (Fig. 15.9b). This is important as the median nerve and brachial artery pass through this opening, and may be involved in cases of distal humeral fractures.

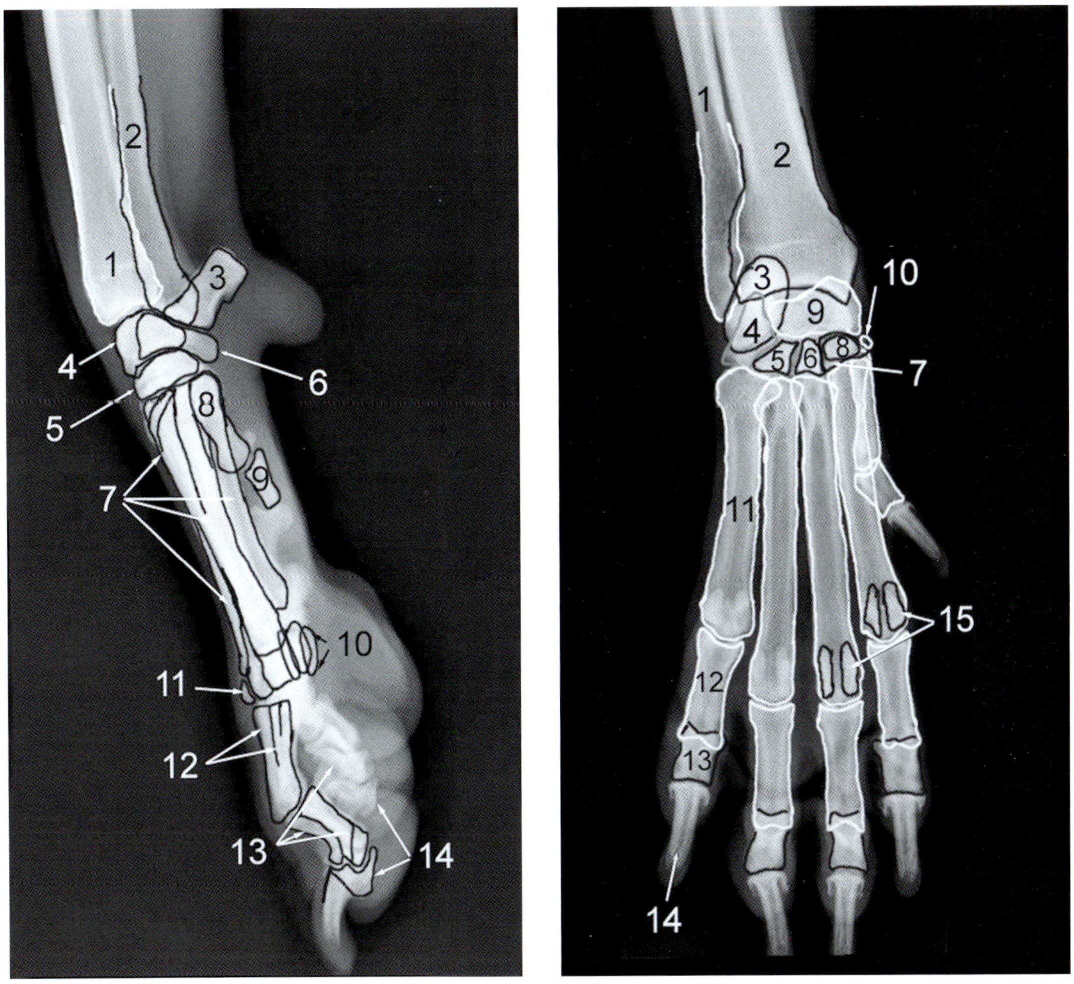

a b

Fig. 15.7 Normal radiographic anatomy of the carpus and manus.

a Lateral view of the carpus and manus. 1 Radius, 2 Ulna, 3 Accessory carpal bone, 4 Intermedioradial carpal bone, 5 Carpal bones I–IV (superimposed), 6 Ulnar carpal bone, 7 Metacarpal bones II–V (superimposed), 8 Metacarpal I, 9 Phalanx I of the first digit, 10 Proximal sesamoid bones of the metacarpophalangeal joints, 11 Dorsal sesamoid bone of the metacarpophalangeal joint, 12 Proximal phalanges (superimposed), 13 Middle phalanges (superimposed), 14 Distal phalanges (superimposed).

b Dorsopalmar view of carpus and manus. 1 Ulna, 2 Radius, 3 Accessory carpal bone, 4 Ulnar carpal bone, 5 Carpal bone IV, 6 Carpal bone III, 7 Carpal bone II, 8 Carpal bone I, 9 Intermedioradial carpal bone, 10 Sesamoid bone of the abductor pollicis longus/extensor carpi obliquus muscle, 11 Metacarpal V, 12 Proximal phalanx of the fifth digit, 13 Middle phalanx of the fifth digit, 14 Distal phalanx of the fifth digit, 15 Proximal sesamoid bones of the metacarpophalangeal joints.

(Courtesy of Dr Ryan King, Dr Andrea Matthews and Dr James Sutherland-Smith, Tufts University Cummings School of Veterinary Medicine)

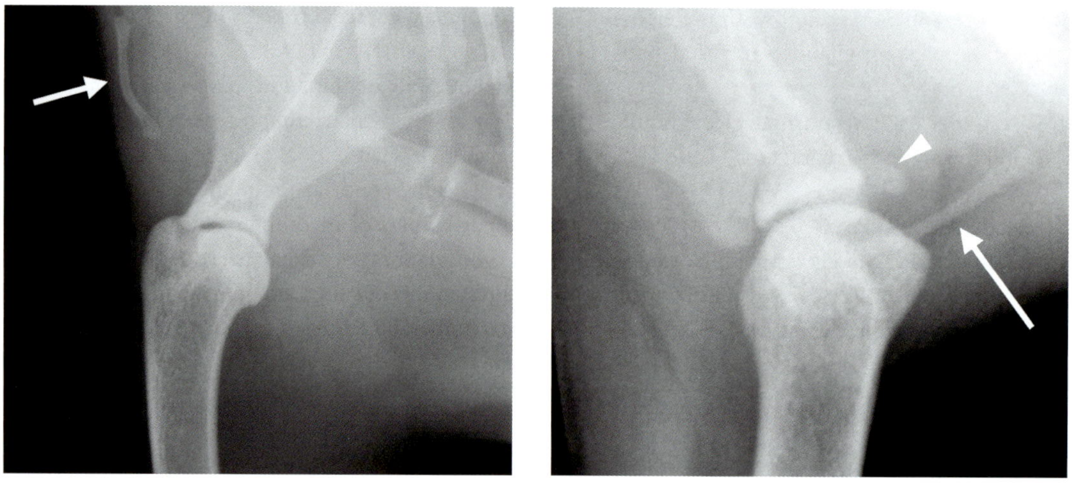

a b

Fig. 15.8 Lateral a and caudocranial b radiographs of the shoulder joint in a cat. The clavicle (arrow) is clearly visible cranial and medial to the joint. This structure is typically cartilaginous in dogs and not visible on radiographs. Additionally, a prominent coracoid process is noted associated with the distal scapula (arrowhead).

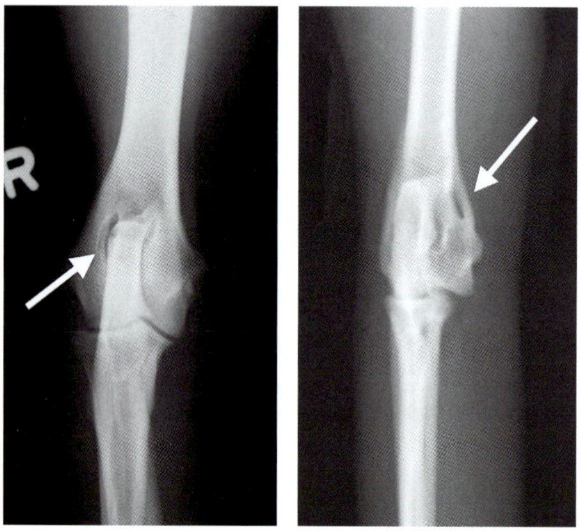

a b

Fig. 15.9 Species-specific anatomic differences in the distal humerus.

a Craniocaudal radiograph of the elbow joint in a dog. A round radiolucent region within the olecranon fossa (arrow, partially obscured by the superimposed olecranon) corresponds to the supratrochlear foramen (R = right).

b Craniocaudal radiograph of the elbow joint in a cat. The oval radiolucent region associated with the distal medial humerus (arrow) corresponds to the supracondylar foramen. The median nerve and brachial artery pass through this opening.

Hind limbs including pelvic girdle

The pelvic girdle and hind limb consists of the following osseous structures:

- pelvis
- femur
- tibia and fibula
- tarsal bones (talus, calcaneus, central tarsal bone and tarsal bones I–IV)
- metatarsal bones I–V
- phalanges I–III.

Joints of the hind limb include:

- sacroiliac joint
- hip joint (coxofemoral joint)
- stifle joint
- tarsus
- metatarsophalangeal joints
- proximal and distal interphalangeal joints.

Sesamoid bones are found associated with the stifle joint, the metatarsophalangeal joints and the distal interphalangeal joints.

Semi-schematic images of the normal radiographic anatomy of the hind limb are shown in Figures 15.10 to 15.12.

In contrast to the forelimb, there are no significant differences between the radiographic anatomy of the hind limb in cats and dogs.

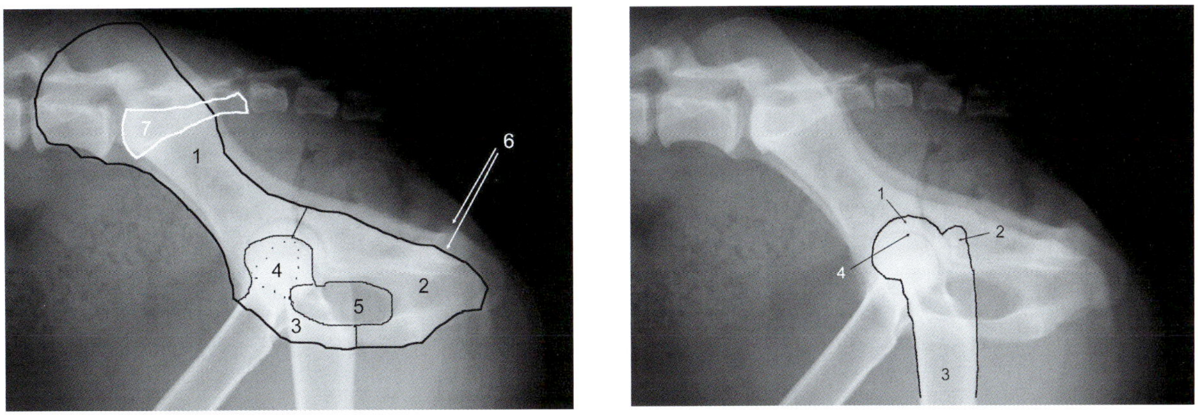

a b

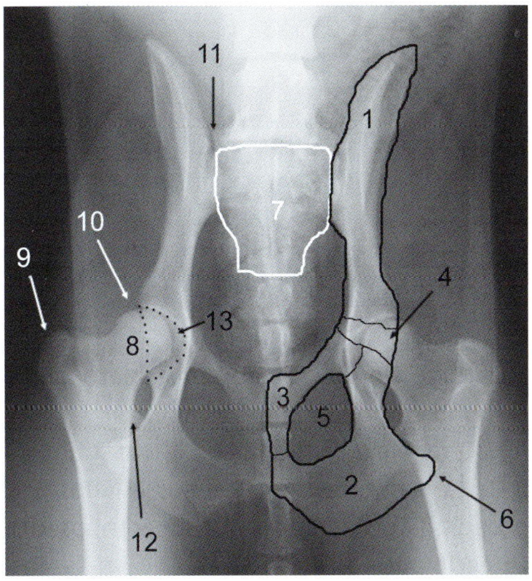

c

Fig. 15.10 Normal radiographic anatomy of the pelvis and coxofemoral joints.

a Lateral view of the pelvis. 1 Ilium, 2 Ischium, 3 Pubis, 4 Area of acetabular bone (superimposed with head of the femur), 5 Obturator foramen, 6 Right and left ischiatic tuber, 7 Body of the sacrum.

b Lateral view of the pelvis. 1 Head of the femur that is distant from the plate, 2 Greater trochanter, 3 Body of the femur, 4 Joint space of the coxofemoral joint closer to the plate.

c Ventrodorsal view of the pelvis. 1 Ilium, 2 Ischium, 3 Pubis, 4 Area of acetabular bone (superimposed with head of the femur), 5 Obturator foramen, 6 Ischiatic tuber, 7 Sacrum, 8 Head of the femur, 9 Greater trochanter, 10 Joint space of the coxofemoral joint, 11 Sacroiliac joint, 12 Lesser trochanter, 13 Acetabulum.

Fig. 15.11 Normal radiographic anatomy of the stifle joint.

a Lateral view of the stifle joint. 1 Margin of the femoral trochlea, 2 Patella, 3 Sesamoid bones of the gastrocnemius muscle (fabellae), 4 Lateral and medial femoral condyles (superimposed), 5 Popliteal sesamoid bone, 6 Intercondylar eminence, 7 Head of the fibula, 8 Body of the fibula, 9 Tibial crest, 10 Tibial tuberosity, 11 Patellar ligament, 12 Infrapatellar fat pad.

b Craniocaudal view of the stifle joint. 1 Patella, 2 Body of the femur, 3 Medial sesamoid bone of the gastrocnemius muscle (medial fabella), 4 Medial femoral epicondyle, 5 Medial tibial condyle, 6 Intercondylar eminence, 7 Tibial crest, 8 Body of the fibula, 9 Head of the fibula, 10 Lateral tibial condyle, 11 Medial femoral epicondyle, 12 Lateral sesamoid bone of the gastrocnemius muscle (lateral fabella). (Courtesy of Dr Ryan King, Dr Andrea Matthews and Dr James Sutherland-Smith, Tufts University Cummings School of Veterinary Medicine)

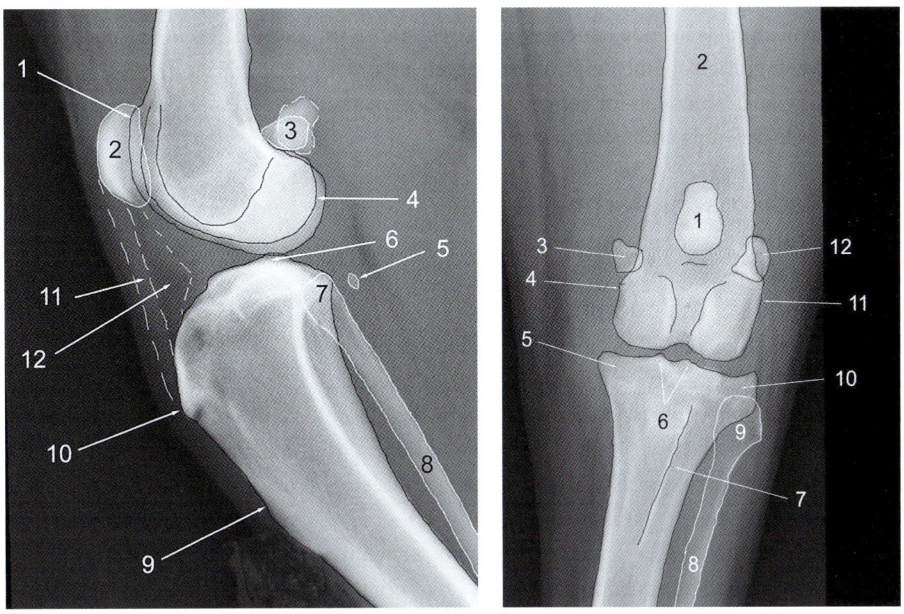

a b

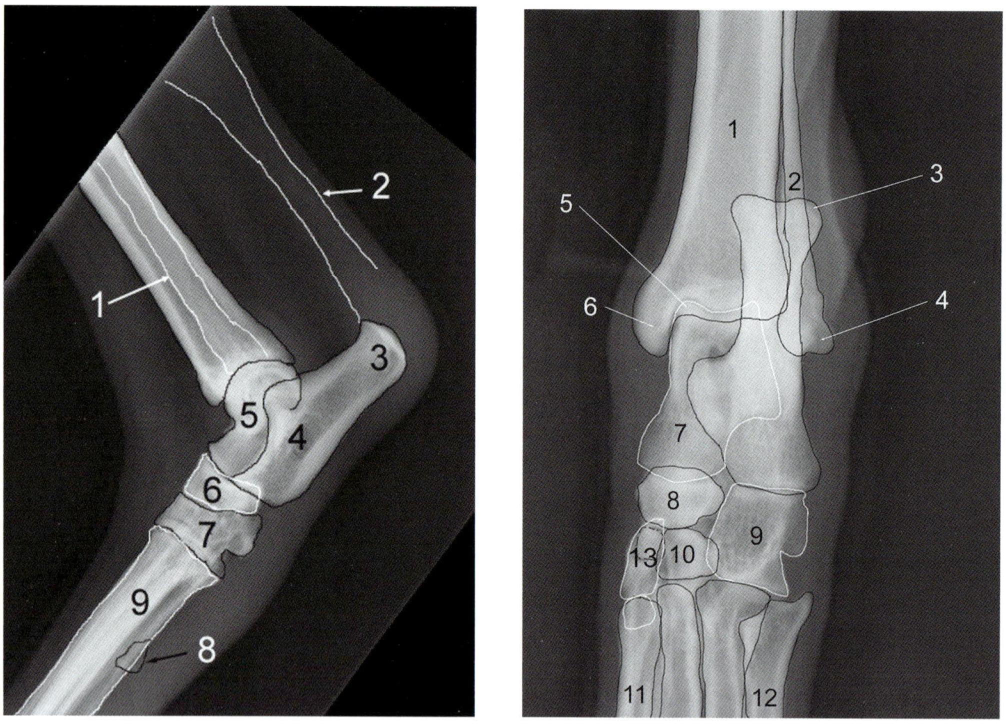

a b

Fig. 15.12 Normal radiographic anatomy of the tarsus (anatomy of metatarsus and digit corresponds to forelimb anatomy).
a Lateral view of the tarsus. 1 Distal fibula (superimposed with tibia), 2 Calcanean tendon, 3 Calcanean tuber, 4 Calcaneus, 5 Talus, 6 Central tarsal bone and tarsal bone IV (superimposed), 7 Tarsal bones I–IV (superimposed), 8 Metatarsal I (rudimentary), 9 Metatarsals II–V (superimposed).
b Dorsoplantar view of the tarsus. 1 Tibia, 2 Fibula, 3 Calcanean tuber, 4 Lateral malleolus, 5 Tarsocrural joint, 6 Medial malleolus, 7 Talus, 8 Central tarsal bone, 9 Tarsal bone IV, 10 Tarsal bone III, 11 Metatarsal II, 12 Metatarsal V, 13 Tarsal bones I–III (superimposed).
(Courtesy of Dr Ryan King, Dr Andrea Matthews and Dr James Sutherland-Smith, Tufts University Cummings School of Veterinary Medicine)

15.1.2 Indications

Indications for radiographic examination of the extremities in small animals include lameness, pain, reluctance to move, swelling, angular limb deformities, uneven length of extremities, and evaluation for congenital / developmental anomalies in breeding and working dogs.

15.2 Radiographic technique and positioning

15.2.1 Standard radiographs

A bone technique should be used for evaluation of the extremities (high in contrast, i.e. low in kVp) (see section 2.2). For radiographs of structures proximal to the elbow and stifle joint, a **grid** is typically used, while radiographs of the distal limb are typically acquired using a tabletop technique.

With conventional film–screen radiography, **exposure factors** may have to be varied to allow optimal evaluation of osseous structures (often resulting in overexposure of soft tissues) and soft tissues (often resulting in underexposure of bone), respectively.

> With conventional radiography, a mildly overexposed radiograph may still be diagnostic for evaluation of soft tissues and small structures (e.g. periosteal surface) if a strong light source (i.e. hot lamp) is available. However, an underexposed radiograph cannot be used for evaluation of osseous structures. Even though digital radiographs are more forgiving, care should still be taken to optimize radiographic technique.

A single radiograph may occasionally suffice to establish a diagnosis in a given patient (e.g. single lateral view of the proximal humerus in a dog with osteosarcoma). However, radiographs in **at least two projections** are necessary for most indications. These are routinely acquired with orthogonal beam direction (Fig. 15.13 to 15.16). Lateral

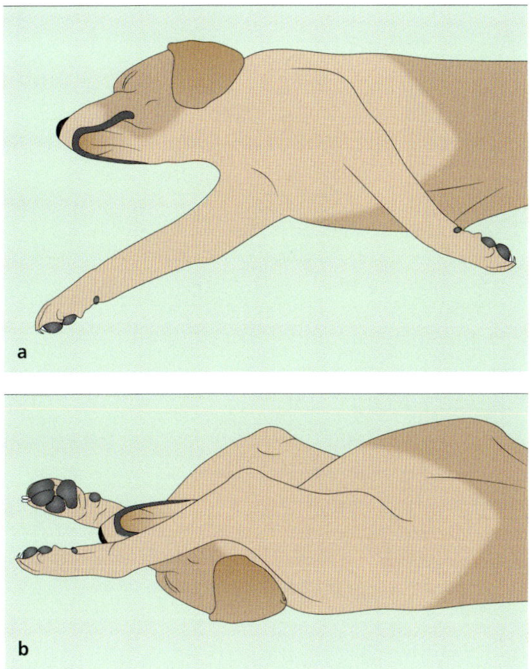

Fig. 15.13 Schematic illustration of patient positioning for a lateral a and a caudocranial b radiograph of the scapula, shoulder joint or humerus.

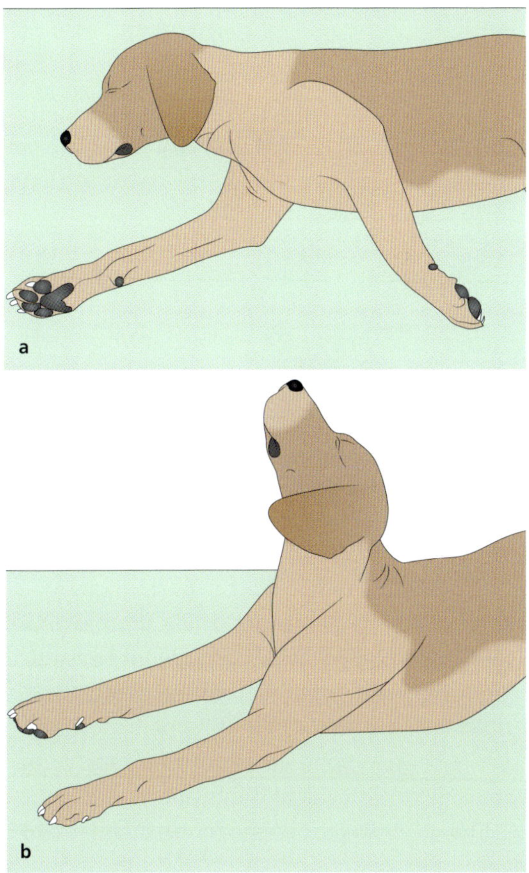

Fig. 15.14 Schematic illustration of patient positioning for a lateral a and a craniocaudal/dorsopalmar b radiograph of the humerus, elbow joint, antebrachium, carpus or manus.

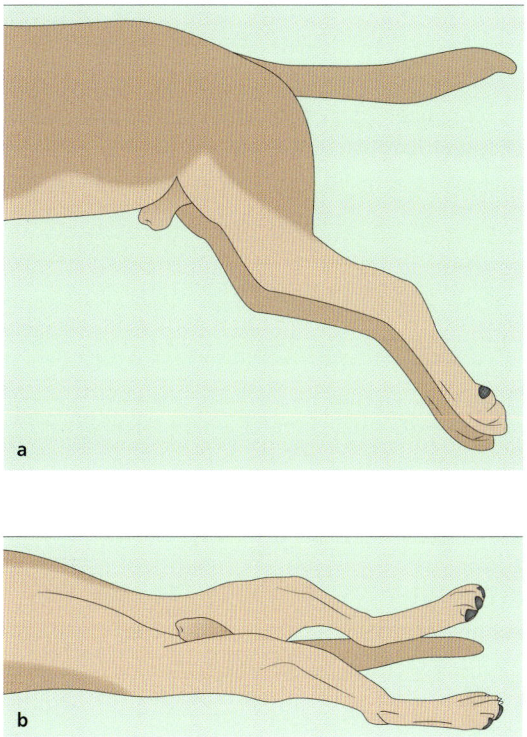

Fig. 15.15 Schematic illustration of patient positioning for a lateral view of the pelvis a and a ventrodorsal view of the pelvis or craniocaudal view of the femur b.

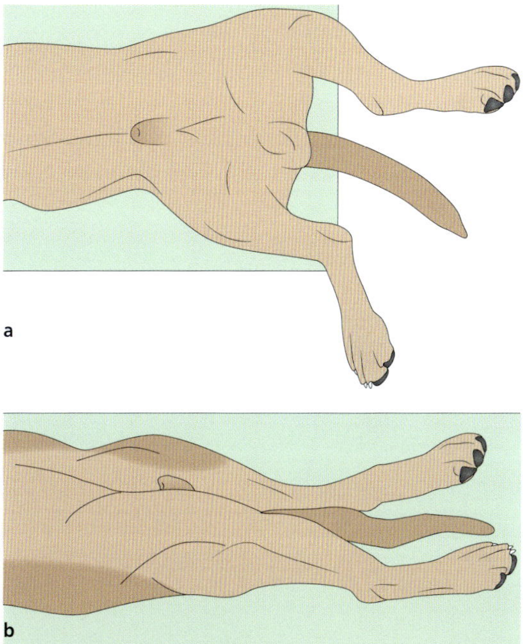

Fig. 15.16 Schematic illustration of patient positioning for a lateral a and a craniocaudal/dorsoplantar b radiograph of the femur, stifle joint, crus, tarsus or pes. For radiographs from the stifle joint distally, caudocranial/plantarodorsal views (in sternal recumbency) are also possible.

and craniocaudal / caudocranial views are obtained for the proximal extremity, and lateral and dorsopalmar / dorsoplantar radiographs are acquired for the distal extremity. As for all radiographic examinations, positioning must be as straight as possible, and the primary beam must be collimated to the area of interest. Survey radiographs including the entire limb are often nondiagnostic.

15.2.2 Special radiographic techniques

To allow evaluation of soft-tissue lesions, structures superimposed with each other and disorders with a dynamic component, specific radiographic techniques may be indicated. Contrast examination of a joint (**arthrography**) is rarely performed in small animals nowadays, and will not be covered in this chapter. An overview of more common special radiographic techniques can be found in Table 15.3.

Oblique views

These may be helpful, for instance in the diagnosis of mildly displaced fractures. Another indication is the evaluation of fracture repair and healing following osteosynthesis if metallic implants overlie the area of interest on the conventional orthogonal views.

Specific radiographs for joint evaluation

Radiographs with flexion or extension of a single joint, or a variable degree of flexion / extension of the metacarpophalangeal / metatarsophalangeal joints, are helpful in the evaluation of structures that are otherwise obscured by superimposition. Examples include radiographs of a flexed elbow joint for evaluation of the anconeal process and medial humeral epicondyle (Fig. 15.17), and radiographs of individual digits for evaluation of interphalangeal joints and phalanges (Fig. 15.18).

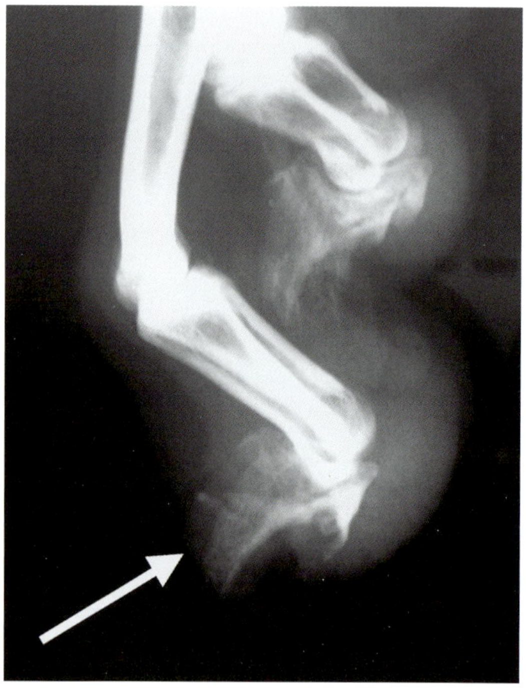

a

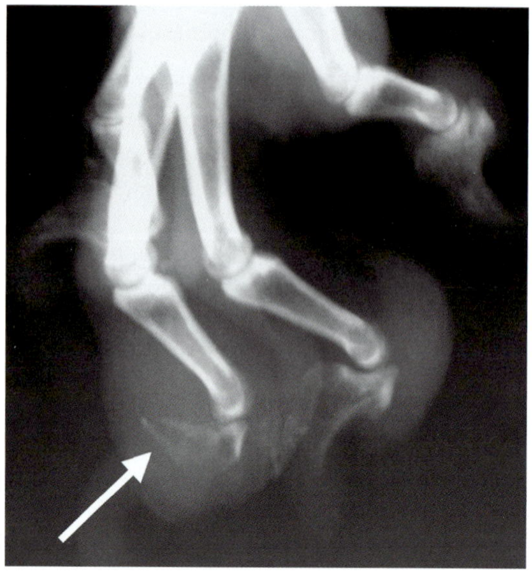

b

Fig. 15.18 Radiographs of the left pes in a 12-year-old Greyhound with swelling of the fourth digit.
a Lateral view: The phalanges of the third and fourth digit are superimposed (arrow) and cannot be evaluated.
b Lateral view with separation of the digits: The digits are individually projected without superimposition. This can easily be accomplished by affixing tape or bandage material to individual digits and spreading them apart. The third phalanx of the fourth digit (arrow) has evidence of extensive lysis. Associated soft-tissue swelling is also evident. The primary differential diagnosis was a lytic bone tumour (such as squamous cell carcinoma or malignant melanoma), and amputation was recommended. Histopathology was consistent with osteomyelitis without evidence of underlying neoplasia.

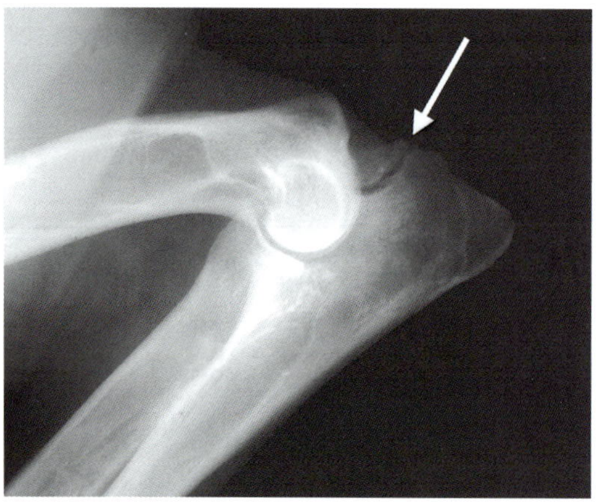

Fig. 15.17 Flexed lateral elbow radiograph in a 1-year-old German Shepherd Dog. The radiolucent line separating the ununited anconeal process from parent bone is clearly visible (arrow).

Table 15.3 Special radiographic techniques to evaluate the appendicular skeleton in small animals.

Body part	Indication	Radiograph	Figure	Commentary
Shoulder	Suspected bicipital tendinopathy/ mineralization	Dorsoventral or ventrodorsal tangential view with shoulder flexion, centred on the bicipital groove		
	Suspected shoulder instability	Stress views		
Elbow	Suspected ununited anconeal process; suspected periarticular new bone formation associated with dorsal anconeal process	Flexed lateral	15.17	
	Suspected medial coronoid process disease	Craniolateral–caudomedial 15° oblique; distomedial–proximolateral 35° oblique	16.4	
	Suspected instability of collateral ligaments	Stress views		
Carpus	Suspected ligamentous instability (lateral, medial, or palmar – hyperextension injury)	Stress views	15.23, 15.24	
Digits	Suspected lesions of individual digits (e.g. fractures or osteolytic changes)	Lateral with toes spread apart; use of high-resolution (dental) film/plate to image individual digits	15.18b	Use of a dental system results in improved detail, but necessitates adjustment of exposure parameters
Coxofemoral joint	Suspected laxity of the coxofemoral joints/hip dysplasia	Ventrodorsal stress/distraction techniques using a wedge	16.12	Technically demanding, may require specific equipment and training (e.g. PennHIP radiographs)
Stifle joint	Suspected patella luxation and/or shallow conformation of femoral trochlea	Tangential/'skyline' views	15.21, 15.22	
	Suspected cranial cruciate ligamentous injury	Mediolateral view while eliciting a 'drawer sign'		
	Suspected collateral ligament instability	Stress views		
Tarsus	Suspected lesion of the lateral trochlear ridge of the talus (osteochondrosis or fracture)	'Skyline' views	15.19, 15.20	
	Suspected ligamentous instability	Stress views		

A special type of radiograph in this category is the tangential/skyline view of a joint. A skyline view of the flexed scapulohumeral joint allows evaluation of the intertubercular groove and biceps tendon. Other examples include a dorsoplantar view of the tarsus under flexion for evaluation of the trochlear ridges of the talus (Fig. 15.19 and 15.20), and a skyline view of the stifle joint for evaluation of the patella and trochlear ridges of the femur (Fig. 15.21 and 15.22).

Functional views

The goal of these techniques is the evaluation of a potential dynamic component of a musculoskeletal disease process, which may not be evident on conventional survey radiographs. The most common indication for functional views of the appendicular skeleton is suspected joint instability.

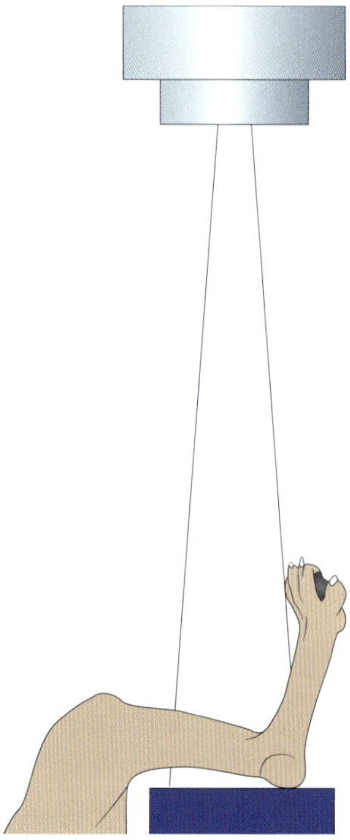

Fig. 15.19 Schematic illustration of positioning for a tangential/skyline view of the tarsocrural joint. The tarsus is flexed to 90°. This can be accomplished by means of sand bags, adhesive tape or bandage material.

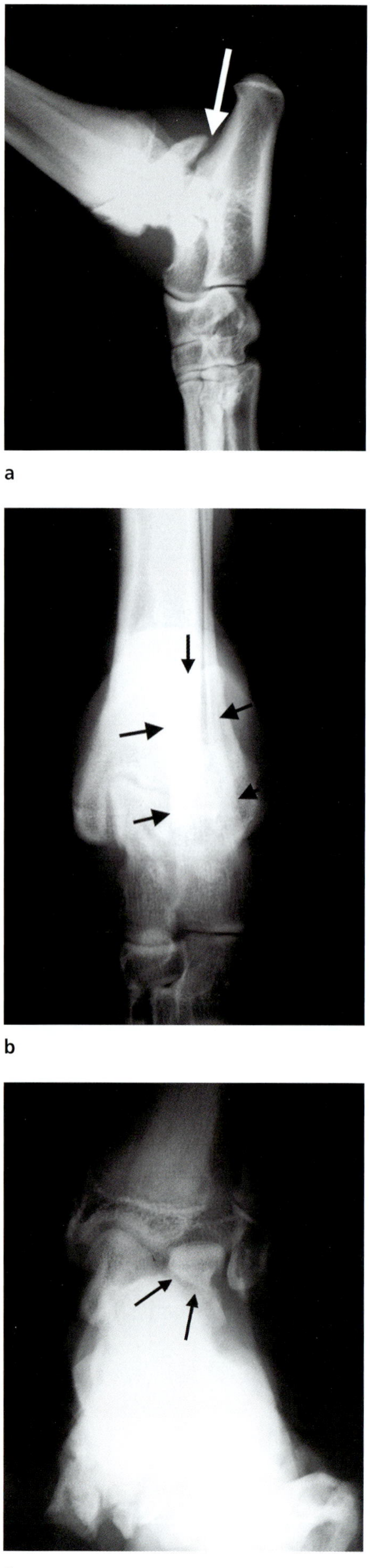

a

b

c

Fig. 15.20 Fracture of the lateral trochlear ridge of the talus in a 1-year-old mixed-breed dog. The fracture line (arrow) is clearly seen on the lateral view a. While the calcaneus (arrows) is superimposed with the lateral trochlear ridge on the dorsoplantar view limiting evaluation b, the fracture (arrows) is easily visualized on the skyline view c.

There are generally two different types of stress views available to the veterinary practitioner.

WEIGHT-BEARING STANDING RADIOGRAPHS

While this technique is commonly used in large animal radiology, it is problematic in small animal imaging for several reasons.

- **Technical requirements:** The examination is performed using a horizontal beam view. This requires the availability of an X-ray tube which can be turned by 90° and lowered to patient level (in dogs, slightly above the floor depending on the area of interest). Additionally, the X-ray suite has to be large enough to accommodate the tilted X-ray tube, examiner, patient, handler and radiographic cassette, while still allowing for adequate focus–object and focus–film distance.
- **Patient cooperation:** Animals have to be awake (or only minimally sedated) for this procedure. Animals in pain are often unable and/or unwilling to bear weight on the injured extremity. Additionally, even if animals are quiet, and even if the owners are present, dogs are often scared of both the equipment and the noise of the rotating anode, making it difficult to position and maintain the X-ray tube and cassette in an appropriate position. These limitations are even more significant in cats.
- **Radiation safety:** The necessity of several people being present in the room (one holding the animal, one operating the X-ray tube and one holding the cassette) in combination with the horizontal beam direction are major disadvantages of this technique from a radiation safety perspective.

Possible applications for radiographic evaluation of the appendicular skeleton in standing small animal patients are as follows.

- Evaluation of complex angular limb deformities, as this technique allows imaging of nearly the entire extremity in its natural position.
- Determination and comparison of exact joint angles for both limbs, for example when planning a surgical arthrodesis.
- Evaluation of actual joint space width, which is commonly overestimated or underestimated in non-weight-bearing radiographs.
- Evaluation of unstable joints.

Joint instability is, however, better evaluated using true 'stress views'.

STRESS VIEWS

For stress views, a certain amount of force is applied to two or more components of the skeletal system to identify any abnormal mobility or laxity (e.g. widening of a joint space in case of ligamentous injury; (Fig. 15.23).

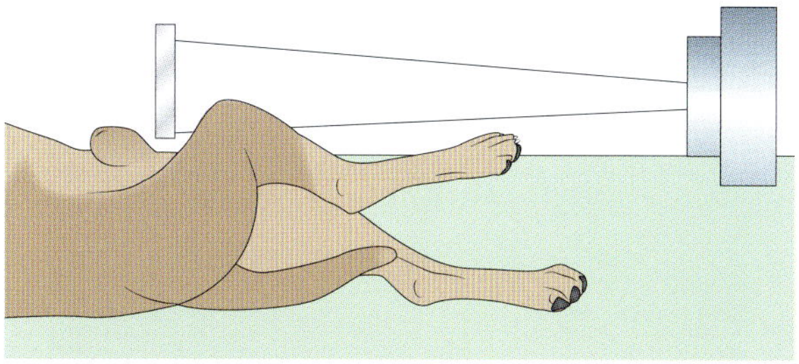

Fig. 15.21 Schematic illustration of patient positioning for a tangential/skyline view of the stifle joint. The stifle joint is flexed to approximately 95–115°. The disadvantages of this technique are the horizontal beam orientation and the need to manually position the cassette, which requires the presence of personnel close to the primary beam (a radiation safety problem!).

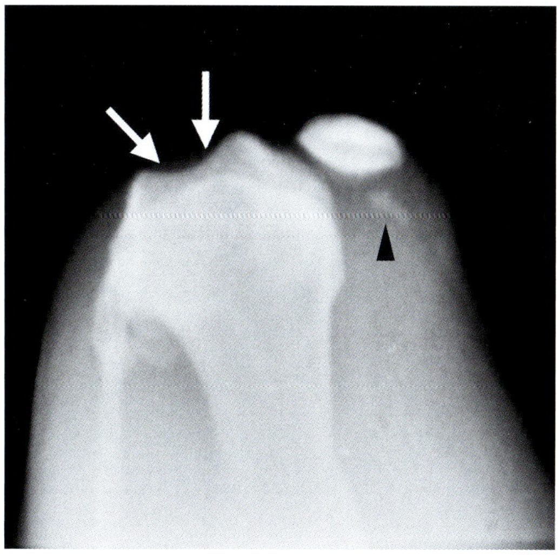

Fig. 15.22 Traumatic patella luxation in a dog. The skyline view demonstrates luxation of the patella as well as a small isolated bone fragment (arrowhead) in close proximity to the sesamoid bone. The femoral trochlea (arrows) appears normal.

The following **forces** can be applied to the appendicular skeleton:

- shearing forces
- wedge forces
- rotational forces
- pull forces.

Stress radiographs in small animal patients require at least deep sedation, but typically **anaesthesia**, as this technique is unpleasant and in case of unstable, traumatized joints, even painful. In addition, conscious animals will resist any test of

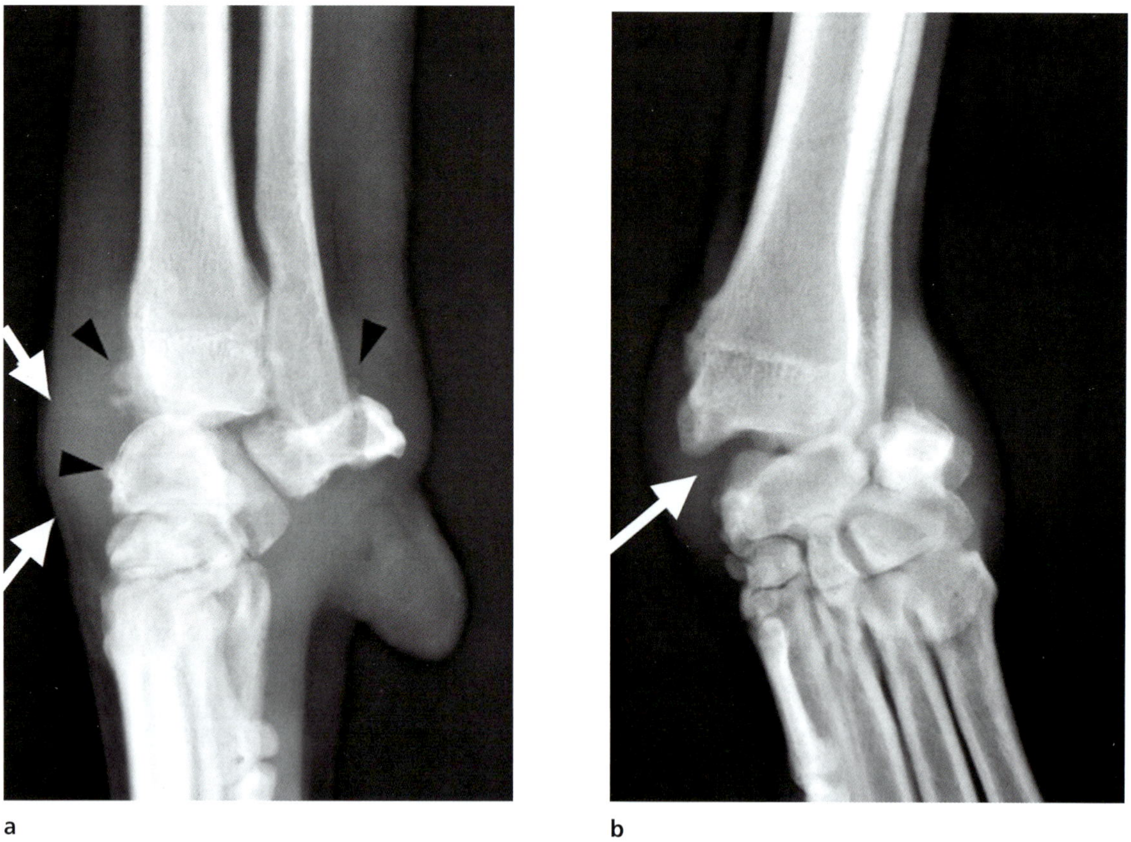

Fig. 15.23 Instability of the carpus in a dog. Radiographic abnormalities on the lateral view a include marked soft-tissue swelling (arrows) and periarticular osteophytosis indicating chronicity (arrowheads). The dorsopalmar stress view b shows medial widening/subluxation of the antebrachiocarpal joint (arrow), consistent with injury to the medial collateral ligaments.

(ligamentous) instability by increasing muscle tone, which may alter the results of the examination. From a radiation safety perspective, another advantage of an examination under general anaesthesia is that the number of personnel within the X-ray room can be minimized.

Stress forces can be applied in different ways.

- **Manual:** The examiner holds the bones adjacent to the joint in question and manually applies the desired force. This technique is commonly used when testing the collateral ligaments of the carpus and tarsus for instability. The major advantage of this technique is the level of control over the degree and direction of the force applied to the joint. A significant disadvantage is the proximity of the examiner's hand to the primary beam. The primary beam must be avoided at all cost, and careful collimation and the wearing of lead gloves are mandatory!
- **Instrumental:** These techniques use a wooden or plastic wedge (a simple kitchen spoon is often sufficient) to apply stress to a joint. The examiner's hands are distant from the primary beam. Unfortunately, this technique cannot be used to apply rotational forces. Even though traction is not commonly used to evaluate the appendicular skeleton, this can easily be achieved by tying a weight to the paw and lowering it over the edge of the table.

An assessment of **stability versus instability** of a joint is often difficult. In addition to differences between dog breeds and between species (when examining the carpal joint in a healthy cat it often appears subjectively unstable), differences between individual patients are also common. Injuries to nearby structures (e.g. proximal metatarsal fractures) may mimic joint injury and instability or may be a confounding problem. When in doubt, comparison stress radiographs of the opposite limb should be obtained (Fig. 15.24).

15.3 Approach to radiographic evaluation

The assessment of small animal musculoskeletal radiographs requires a systematic approach. As for other radiographs, images should be evaluated using specific **view boxes** (conventional film–screen radiology) or adequate **computer monitors** (digital radiology) in a **darkened room**. Use of a **hot lamp and/or a magnifying glass** for conventional films, and judicial use of **manipulation**

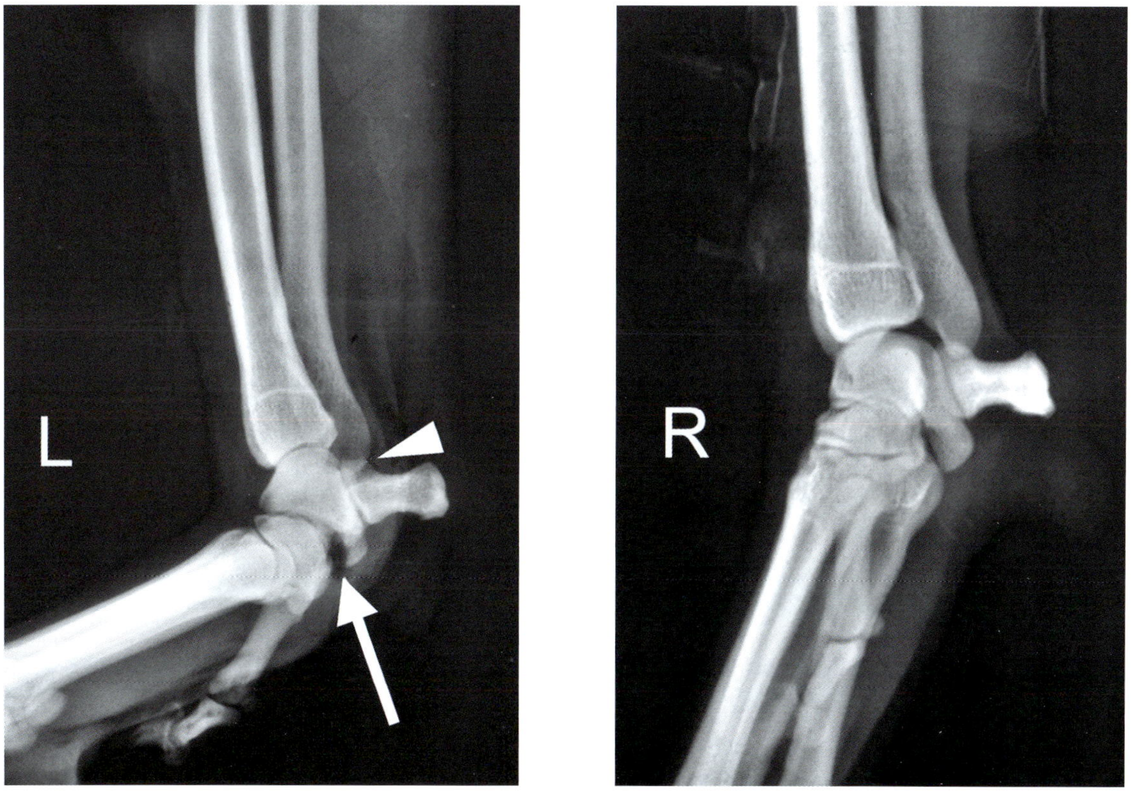

a b

Fig. 15.24 Comparative stress radiographs of both carpi in a dog presented with left forelimb lameness.
a Left carpus: There is marked widening of the palmar aspect of the middle carpal joint (arrow), resulting in overall hyperextension of the carpus. A small fracture fragment originating from the accessory carpal bone is also noted (arrowhead) (L = left).
b Comparison radiograph of the right carpus with a similar degree of stress application. The joint is stable (R = right).

tools in the viewing software, are often needed for evaluation of small and peripheral structures.

The approach to a small animal orthopaedic radiograph varies with the individual investigator's preferences, but should always be systematic. The following list is an example of how a radiograph of the musculoskeletal system may be approached.

1. Verification that patient information, laterality marker(s) and date are correct.
2. Evaluation of image quality for positioning and radiographic technique, including artefacts.
3. Evaluation of soft tissues (swelling, defects, foreign bodies, mineralization, gas).
4. Evaluation of the periosteal and endosteal bone surfaces.
5. Evaluation of the bone (medullary cavity/spongiosa and cortex) for any defects and for regions of increased or decreased opacity.
6. Evaluation of the joint spaces, joint surfaces and attachment sites of the joint capsule.
7. Evaluation of the spatial alignment of bones with each other.
8. In young animals: evaluation of physes.

15.4 Soft-tissue abnormalities

Radiographic soft-tissue anomalies of the extremities include changes in radiographic opacity, and increase or decrease in soft-tissue volume.

15.4.1 Abnormal radiographic opacity

Fat accumulations between fascial planes and soft-tissue structures

Normal fat deposits are less opaque than soft tissues and allow the assessment of the margins of some muscles, tendons/ligaments and joints. The contrast between fat and soft tissues blurs with pathological accumulations of fluid or with soft-tissue swelling (secondary to oedema, haemorrhage, inflammation or neoplasia). A typical example is the obliteration of the infrapatellar fat pad and the fascial fat planes caudal to the stifle joint in the case of intracapsular joint swelling. Conversely, accumulation of an increased amount of fat between soft-tissue structures (such as seen with intermuscular lipomas) increases the visibility of typically indistinguishable soft-tissue margins.

Gas accumulations within soft tissues

These may occur secondary to open wounds or infections with gas-producing bacteria, or they can be iatrogenic, following surgical procedures or injections. Radiographically, they appear as variably sized and shaped regions of gas opacity within soft tissues (Fig. 15.25).

> Regions of decreased opacity caused by gas accumulations within soft tissues should not be confused with normal fat planes and vice versa!

Soft-tissue mineralization

This is characterized by focal, multifocal or generalized increased opacity of soft tissues and can have different aetiologies.

- **Dystrophic mineralization** describes the deposition of calcium salts in necrotic, devitalized or degenerative soft tissues (Fig. 15.26a). Possible causes include trauma, inflammation or vascular compromise (infarct).
- **Metastatic mineralization** refers to systemic mineralization of normal soft tissues due to elevated serum calcium and/or phosphorus levels. Generally, this is due to a sustained increase in circulating levels of serum calcium and phosphorus. Possible underlying disease processes include chronic renal failure, hyperparathyroidism, hypervitaminosis D, etc. Metastatic mineralization can affect abdominal viscera such as the stomach, lung, kidneys and heart, but also other structures including periarticular soft tissues, subcutis and vessel walls (Fig. 15.26b). Affected organs display increased radiographic opacity and are better visible than normal.
- **Idiopathic mineralization:** Occasionally, mineralization of soft tissues is observed without evidence of tissue damage or abnormalities in calcium/phosphorus metabolism.

Mineralization or ossification of a soft-tissue tumour is a special type of soft-tissue mineralization. This can occur secondary to central tumour necrosis followed by dystrophic mineralization, or it can be the result of bone production by the tumour, such as seen with extraskeletal osteosarcoma (Fig. 15.26c). These processes cannot be distinguished radiographically. However, it is important to recognize the soft-tissue mineralization as abnormal, and recommend appropriate follow-up tests (advanced imaging, fine-needle aspiration or biopsy).

> If soft-tissue mineralization associated with an extremity is suspected, it is extremely important to obtain radiographs in at least two orthogonal planes. Dirt on the skin or wet hair artefacts can mimic soft-tissue mineralization and lead to an erroneous diagnosis.

15.4.2 Changes in soft-tissue volume

Increase in soft-tissue mass (swelling)

This can be the result of many different disease processes. Soft-tissue swelling may be extensive and poorly defined (diffuse swelling such as seen with trauma, lymphoedema, diffuse infiltrative neoplasia or cellulitis), or may be limited to specific structures of the musculoskeletal system (e.g. a specific ligament with tendinitis).

For soft-tissue swelling of an extremity it is important to determine if the swelling originates from a joint (intracapsular soft-tissue swelling) or from extracapsular tissues, as this allows ranking of differential diagnoses as well as planning of further diagnostic steps.

Compared to a normal joint (Fig. 15.27a), **intracapsular soft-tissue swelling** is characterized by increased soft-tissue/fluid opacity within the joint capsule (Fig. 15.27b). This may indicate joint effusion and/or synovial proliferation.

Extracapsular soft-tissue swelling is characterized by focal or diffuse soft-tissue swelling located outside the joint space (Fig. 15.27c). This is a nonspecific finding seen with oedema, haemorrhage, inflammation or neoplastic infiltrates.

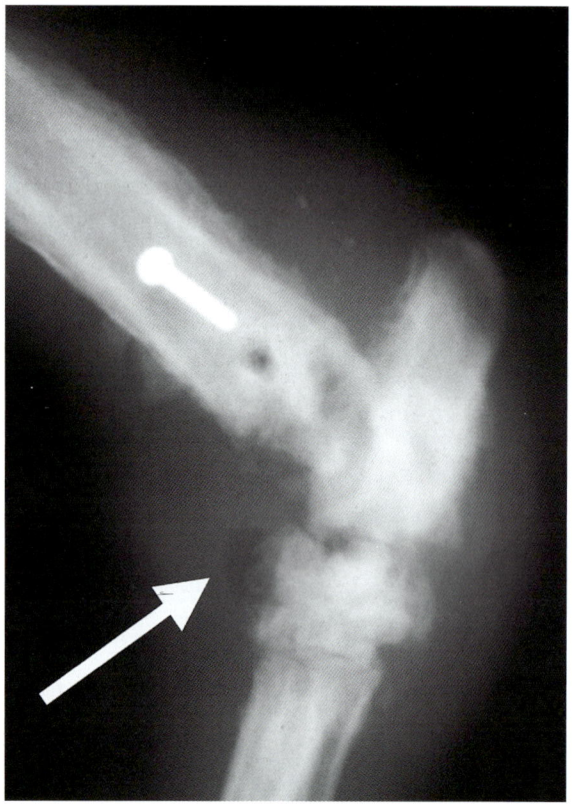

Fig. 15.25 Gas accumulations within soft tissues (arrow) are recognized by the presence of variably sized regions of decreased opacity, which must be distinguished from normal fat planes. The underlying cause in this case was an infection with gas-producing bacteria.

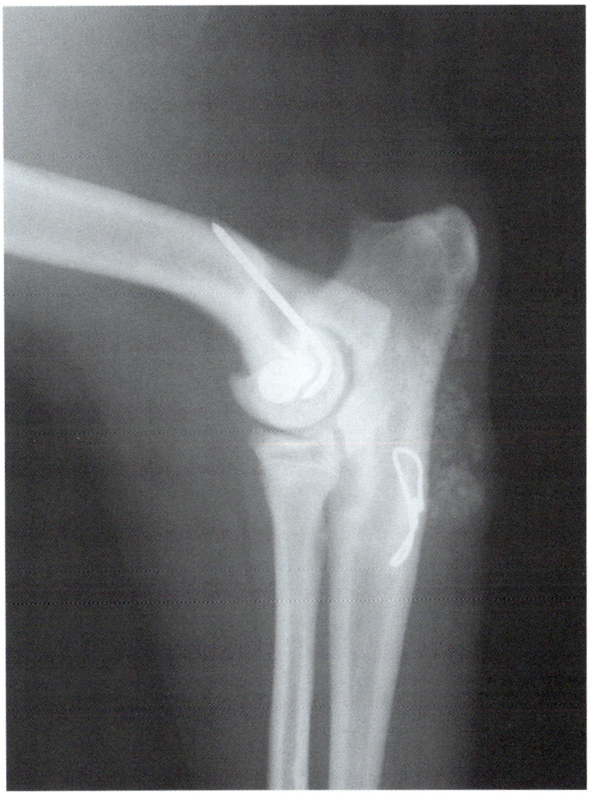
a

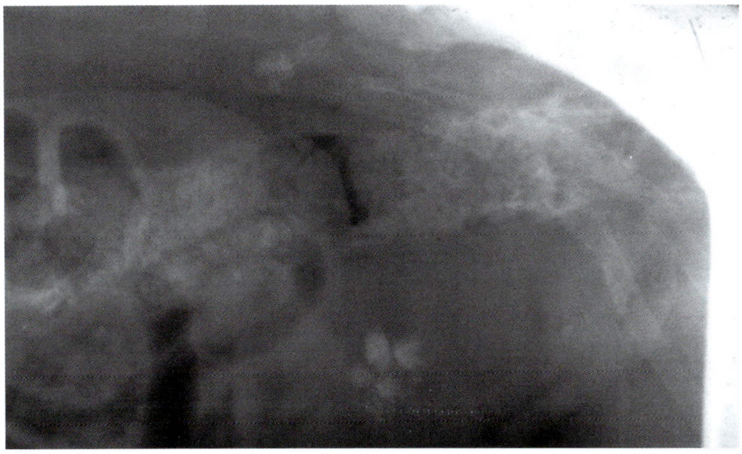
b

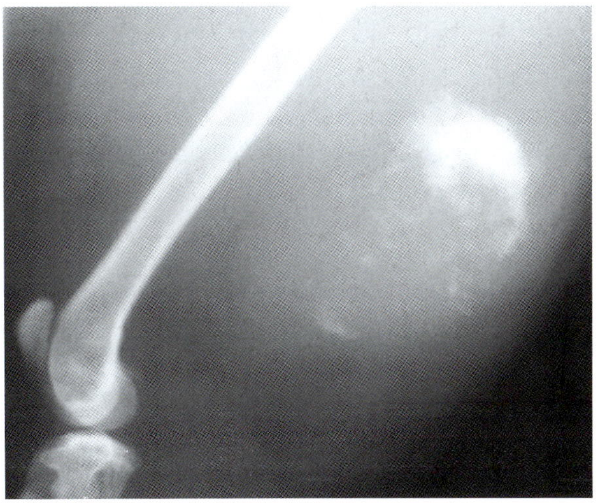
c

Fig. 15.26 Mineralization of soft tissues.

a Dystrophic mineralization occurs secondary to calcium salt deposition in necrotic tissue. The region of faint irregular mineralization within soft tissues caudal to the proximal ulna occurred secondary to prior trauma in this case.

b Metastatic mineralization of the paired external iliac arteries in a dog with chronic calcium/phosphorus imbalances due to renal insufficiency. The arteries appear as mineral opaque tubular structures extending from the retroperitoneal space to the hind limbs. Note that bladder calculi are also present.

c Extraskeletal osteosarcoma of the caudal thigh musculature in a cat. A poorly defined soft-tissue mass with extensive mineralization is seen caudal to the femur. As this cannot be radiographically distinguished from dystrophic mineralization in a haematoma, granuloma or soft-tissue tumour, further diagnostic testing (fine-needle aspiration cytology or biopsy) is indicated.

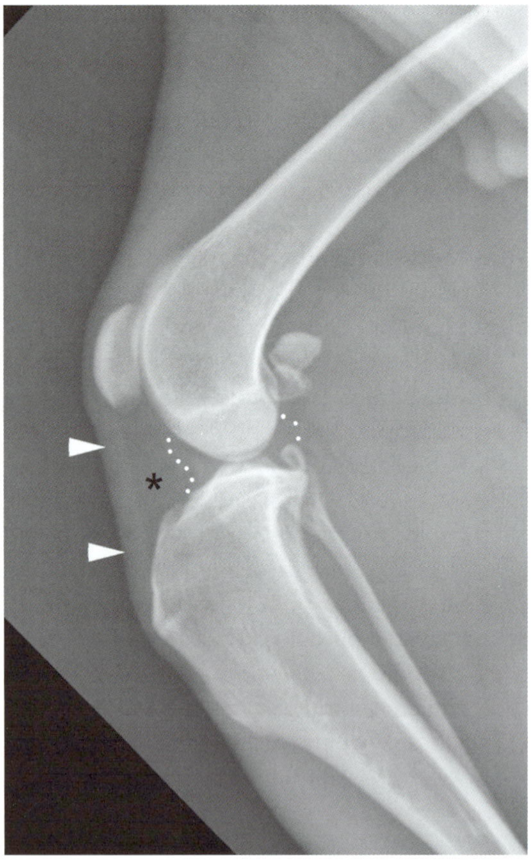

a

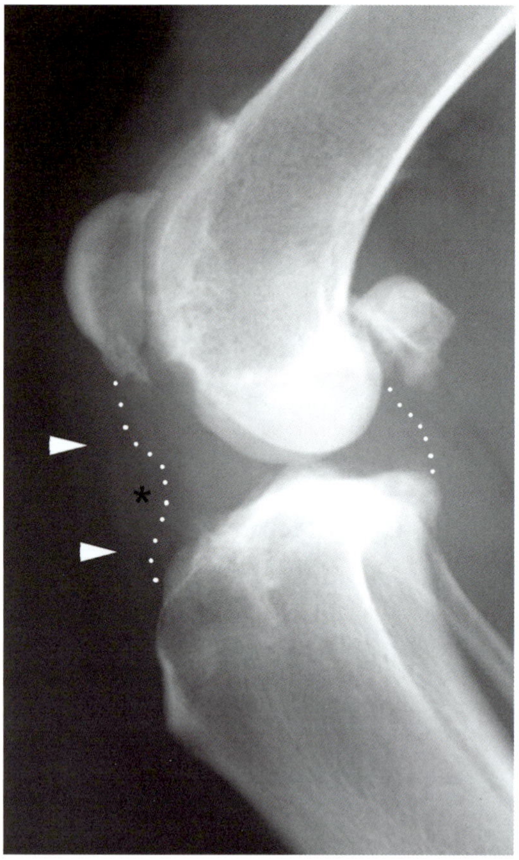

b

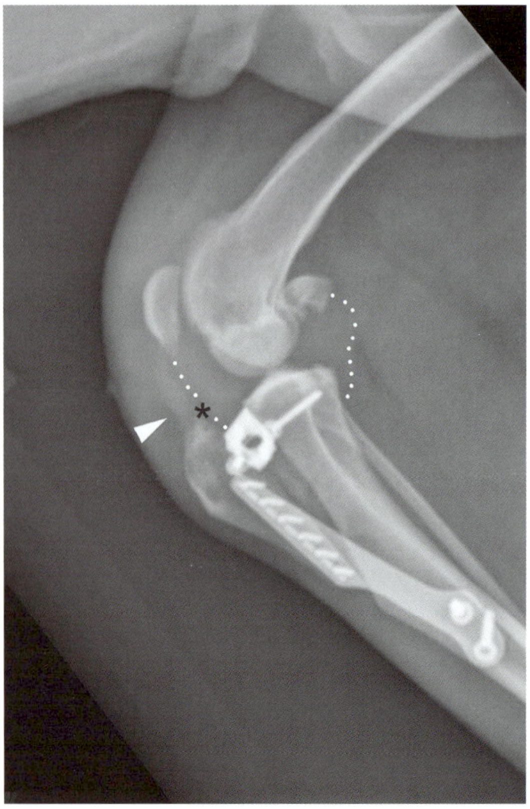

c

Fig. 15.27 Examples of intra- versus extracapsular soft-tissue swelling of the stifle joint in different large-breed dogs.

a Normal stifle joint. The patellar ligament (arrowheads) and the femorotibial joint space (outlined by dotted lines) are separated by a distinct infrapatellar fat pad (*).

b Intracapsular soft-tissue swelling (and severe degenerative joint disease of the stifle joint) in a dog with cranial cruciate ligament rupture. There is increased soft-tissue/fluid opacity associated with the stifle joint (outlined by dotted lines), resulting in displacement of the infrapatellar fat pad (*). Intracapsular soft-tissue swelling in this case is attributed to joint effusion and soft-tissue proliferation of synovial structures. The patellar ligament remains visible (arrowheads).

c Intra-and extracapsular soft-tissue swelling of the stifle joint in a dog with periarticular abscess following surgical correction of cranial cruciate ligament rupture (TTA, tibial tuberosity advancement). The intracapsular soft-tissue swelling is recognized by increased soft-tissue accumulation within the joint capsule (outlined by dotted lines) and displacement of the infrapatellar fat pad (*). Extracapsular swelling is recognized by diffuse swelling of the patellar ligament (arrowhead) and of the soft tissues cranial to the stifle joint. Moderate periarticular osteophytosis is consistent with degenerative joint disease.

Decrease in muscle mass of a limb (atrophy)

This is typically a clinical examination finding. The most common causes are denervation (**neurogenic atrophy**) or decreased weight bearing such as seen in cases of chronic lameness (**disuse atrophy**). Radiographically, the muscle mass of one limb is reduced compared to the opposite side (Fig. 15.28).

> When evaluating for an increase or decrease in muscle mass, it is important that both legs are symmetrically positioned. Oblique positioning or incomplete extension of a leg can easily evoke the impression of muscular asymmetry and thus mimic swelling or atrophy.

15.5 Skeletal abnormalities

15.5.1 Bone response to disease

When evaluating radiographs for evidence of orthopaedic disease, the examiner must be aware of the fact that bone tissue has limited options for response to different diseases:

- bone lysis
- bone production
- combination of bone lysis and production.

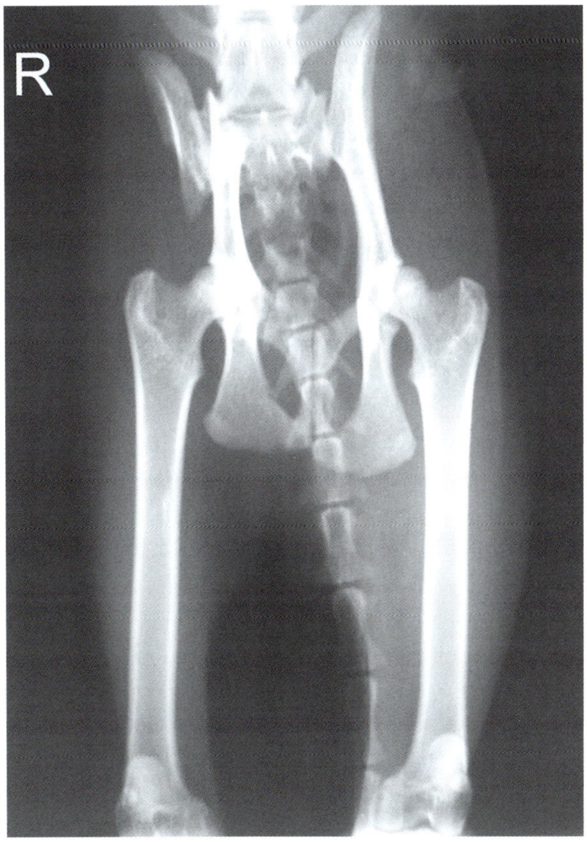

Fig. 15.28 Neurogenic muscle atrophy of the right hind limb in a cat with nerve damage secondary to an ilial fracture. The muscle mass of the right hind limb is significantly reduced compared to the left. Note that a diagnosis of muscle asymmetry requires well-positioned radiographs (R = right).

While the radiographic changes seen in some diseases are essentially pathognomonic, allowing a definitive diagnosis based solely on radiographic findings (e.g. panosteitis, ununited anconeal process, fractures), other bone diseases may appear very similar radiographically due to the limited response of bone tissue to different disease processes. In these cases, it may be difficult or impossible to establish a specific diagnosis based on radiographic findings alone (e.g. neoplasia versus osteomyelitis).

Another factor to take into consideration when evaluating musculoskeletal radiographs is that radiographic changes and clinical presentation may follow different time courses. For example, with osteomyelitis, osteoproliferative changes do not appear until 10–14 days and lytic changes do not appear until 5–7 days following the onset of clinical signs. If initial radiographs in a lame patient are normal but clinical signs persist or worsen, repeat radiographs after one to two weeks may be needed to document bony changes. On the other hand, some lesions (including neoplasia) may be found on radiographs before causing clinical signs such as lameness or pain.

15.5.2 Classification of bone lesions

This section will initially cover the basic principles applied to the classification of bone lesions. Specific details will be discussed later. To establish a reasonable list of differential diagnoses and an appropriate diagnostic and treatment plan for a radiographic bone lesion of unknown aetiology, the following are taken into consideration:

- location and number of lesion(s)
- presence and type of bone lysis
- presence and type of new bone proliferation (especially periosteal reaction)
- cortical disruption
- length and margination of the transition zone from the lesion to normal bone
- change in radiographic appearance over time.

These factors allow classification of a bone lesion as aggressive versus nonaggressive, which in turn allows listing of reasonable differential diagnoses.

A typical **aggressive bone lesion** (e.g. primary bone tumour) is characterized by moth-eaten to permeative lytic regions, irregular periosteal new bone formation, cortical disruption, a long and poorly defined transition zone to normal bone, and/or rapid change of the lesion over a short time period.

A typical **nonaggressive lesion** is characterized by focal (geographic) lysis, smooth and well-defined periosteal reaction, cortical integrity, a short transition zone to normal bone, and minimal to no change over time.

Important considerations for lesion classification as aggressive or nonaggressive

A lesion should always be graded based on the most aggressive feature. In other words, it is sufficient for some or only a few of the above criteria to be met to classify a lesion as aggressive. When in doubt, the clinician should err on the side of caution and initiate appropriate further diagnostic or treatment steps, rather than missing an early and possibly treatable aggressive lesion.

Aggressive is not equivalent with malignant. A 'benign' bone disease such as osteomyelitis can exhibit radiographic features of aggressiveness, and some malignant lesions, such as multiple myeloma, exhibit nonaggressive radiographic features.

If an aggressive bone lesion is suspected, further diagnostic and therapeutic steps such as a bone biopsy should be initiated as quickly as possible to minimize the risk of disease progression, metastasis or pathological fracture. Many nonaggressive lesions may be ignored or treated conservatively. However, even with nonaggressive lesions, appropriate follow-up (recheck radiographs after 2–3 weeks) is indicated, so an atypical aggressive lesion does not go unnoticed.

Location and number

Generalized bone lesions are usually a sign of metabolic, hormonal or nutritional diseases. Only a significant change (30–60%) in skeletal mineral content will result in a radiographic change in opacity. This explains the often marked discrepancy between onset of clinical signs and radiographic changes. Typical examples of generalized bone opacity changes are osteopenia (as seen with hyperparathyroidism) and osteosclerosis.

Focal or multifocal bone lesions are easier to recognize than generalized bone lesions, based on comparison with adjacent normal bone tissue, and they are typically diagnosed at an earlier stage. The location and number of focal lesions may aid in determining the underlying aetiology; however, further diagnostic tests, such as fine-needle aspiration cytology or biopsy, are often needed for a definitive diagnosis.

Typical examples of focal bone lesions with their preferred, albeit not exclusive, locations include the following.

- **Primary bone tumours:** These often originate from the metaphyseal region of long bones. Preferred locations are the proximal humerus, distal radius, proximal tibia and distal femur ('away from the elbow, towards the knee'). However, they can also be found in other regions of the skeletal system. Primary bone tumours are usually solitary and they neither cross joint spaces nor involve adjacent bones.
- **Metastatic bone tumours:** These are typically polyostotic. They are often found in bones of the axial skeleton (ribs, vertebrae and pelvis). Metastases to the long bones of the appendicular skeleton are often located in the diaphysis and metaphysis, in close proximity to the vascular channels.
- **Bacterial osteomyelitis:** Osteomyelitis in juvenile animals typically involves haematogenous spread of infectious agents. The epiphyses and metaphyses are predominantly affected. In adult animals, bone infection typically occurs secondary to a nidus such as an open fracture or an infected surgical implant, and may spread along the entire length of the affected bone. The involvement of additional bones and overall extent of the disease process depends on the underlying cause and secondary spread of infectious agents.
- **Fungal osteomyelitis:** Bone infection with mycotic organisms can occur anywhere and is often found in the metaphyseal regions of long bones, similar to primary bone tumours. However, unlike primary bone tumours, polyostotic lesions are common, and the infection can spread along soft-tissue structures into neighbouring bones, or extend across joint spaces.

Abnormal bone opacity

A change in radiographic opacity of one or more bones can result from a decrease in bone mass (**decreased radiographic opacity**) or from increased bone production (**increased radiographic opacity**). As discussed above, discrepancies between the time of onset of the disease process and the appearance of radiographic changes are common.

DECREASED BONE OPACITY

In normal bone, there is homeostasis between osteoclastic (resorptive) and osteoblastic (productive) activity. Bone undergoes constant adaptive remodelling based on current load. Bone diseases that result in a decrease in radiographic opacity are either characterized by excessive osteoclastic bone resorption, or by decreased new bone formation. Lytic bone changes may also be caused by direct bone destruction (e.g. by tumour cells), or bacterial proteolytic enzyme secretions, or they may be secondary to pressure from adjacent space-occupying lesions.

A **generalized decrease in bone opacity (osteopenia)** may be limited to a single extremity or part of an extremity (e.g. due to decreased vascularization, denervation or chronic lameness; Fig. 15.29) or may affect the entire skeleton (e.g. in the case of metabolic or nutritional diseases; Fig. 15.30; see also Fig. 6.21 and Fig. 7.51). Osteopenia can result from osteoporosis or osteomalacia.

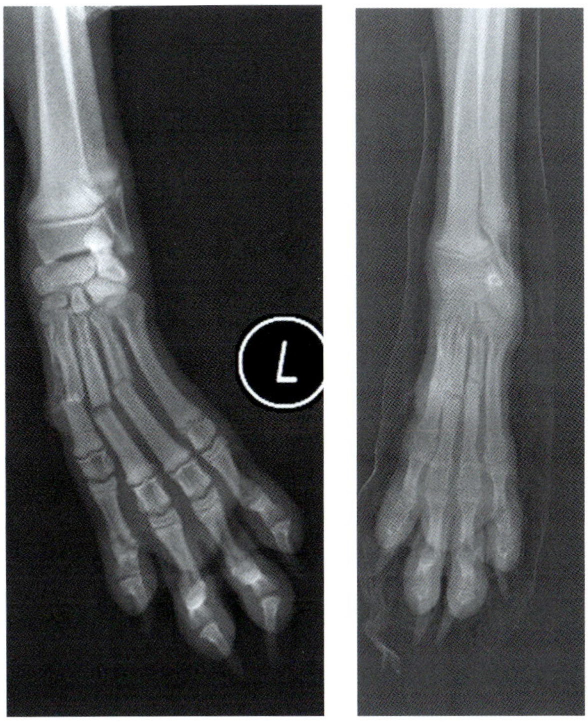

a b

Fig. 15.29 Osteopenia limited to the left forelimb in a young dog with serial metacarpal fractures (metacarpal bones II–IV). When compared to radiographs obtained at initial presentation a, follow-up radiographs obtained after 4 weeks of conservative treatment (bandage) reveal marked cortical thinning, decreased opacity of the skeletal structures, and coarse trabeculation of the long bones b (L = left).

With **osteoporosis**, bone structure is normal, but there is a decrease in bone substance. Typical underlying diseases include:

- osteogenesis imperfecta
- age-related bone involution
- hyperadrenocorticism
- disuse atrophy.

With osteomalacia, there is insufficient mineralization of otherwise normal bone matrix. Typical underlying diseases include:

- hyperparathyroidism
- hypovitaminosis D
- malabsorption
- excessive loss of calcium (lactation, renal disease).

Radiographic findings Regardless of the underlying cause, osteopenic bones are characterized by decreased radiographic opacity, cortical thinning, and a coarse appearance of the trabecula due to endosteal resorption. With rapid bone resorption, intracortical bone resorption, in combination with maintained outer margins, may result in a double cortical line sign. The metaphysis of the long bones and the vertebral endplates often appear relatively increased in opacity. As discussed for radiographic examination of the head (see Chapter 6), loss of the lamina dura will give the impression of free floating teeth. Osteopenic bones are weaker than normal and predisposed to pathological fractures (Fig. 15.31).

A **focal decrease in bone opacity** (**lysis**) initially results in a subtle change in bone texture. As mentioned above, there is a discrepancy between clinical, histological and radiographic changes. A time lapse is expected between the onset of a lytic lesion and its radiographic manifestation.

Other factors also affect the detectability of a lytic lesion: destruction of the cortex is usually easier to identify than a lytic focus within the medullary cavity due to the more pronounced difference in density between normal and abnormal tissue. The margination of the lesion (sharp versus irregular transition to normal bone) also plays a role: a smooth margin is typically easier recognized than an irregular margin.

Depending on the margination of the lytic region, lesions can be categorized as **aggressive** or **nonaggressive**. Unsharp margins, a long or ill-defined transition

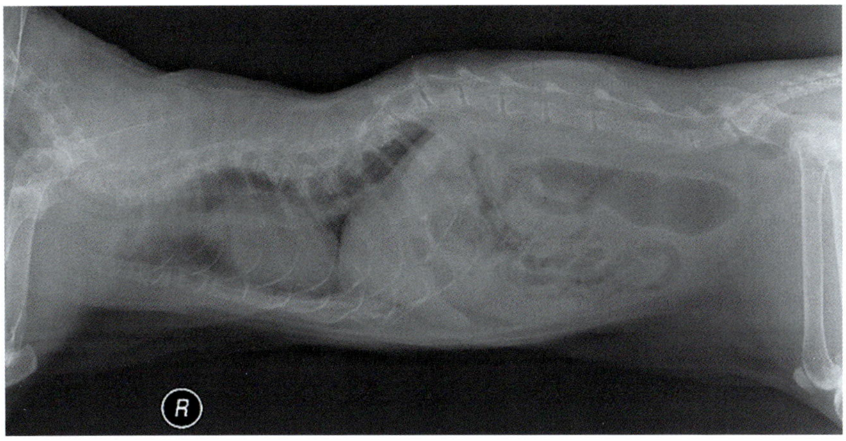

Fig. 15.30 Generalized osteopenia in a cat with secondary renal hyperparathyroidism. Radiographic abnormalities include a generalized decrease in cortical thickness and decreased radiographic opacity of the skeletal structures. Scoliosis of the spine is attributed to pathological (micro)fractures (R = right).

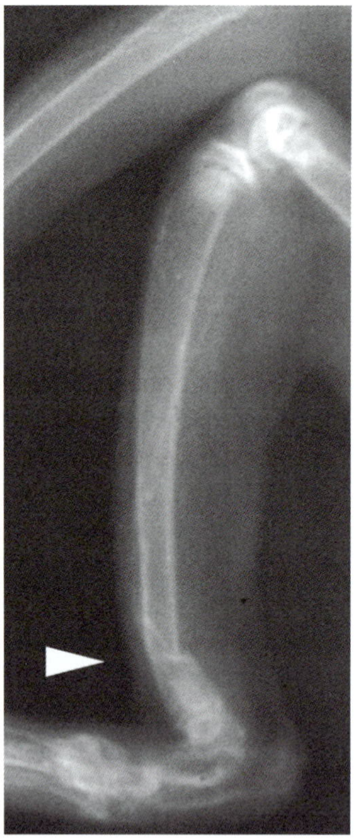

Fig. 15.31 Generalized osteopenia and pathological fracture secondary to nutritional hyperparathyroidism. The long bones are characterized by severe cortical thinning and generally decreased bone opacity. The crus is curved cranially, and a mildly displaced pathological fracture is associated with the distal tibia (arrowhead).

zone from the destructive process to normal bone and cortical destruction are features of aggressiveness (Fig. 15.32a). A typical example is a lytic bone tumour such as an osteosarcoma.

With a nonaggressive process, the body has time to adjust to the osseous changes. The lytic lesion is sharply marginated and may even be surrounded by a sclerotic rim of variable thickness. Instead of causing cortical destruction, these lesions rather result in expansile bone deviation (Fig. 15.32b). A typical example is a bone cyst.

a

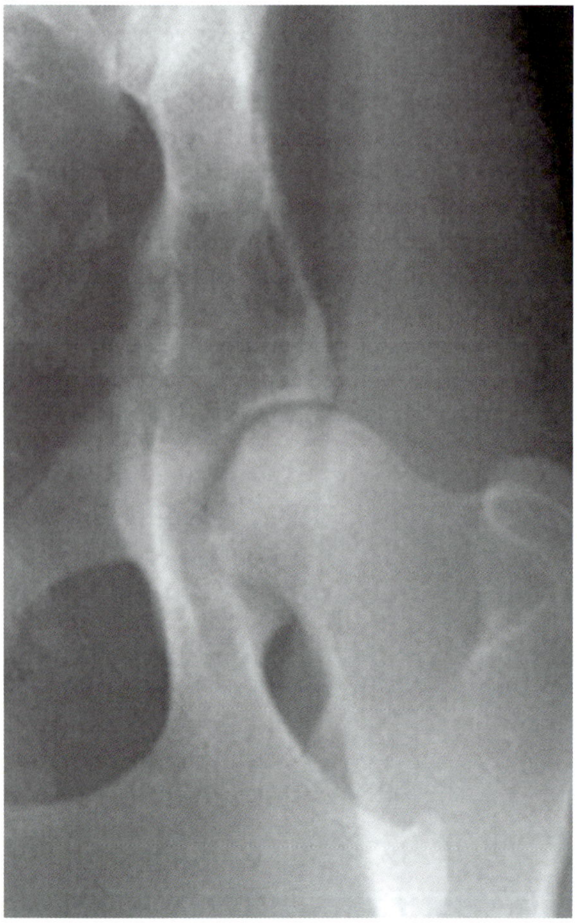

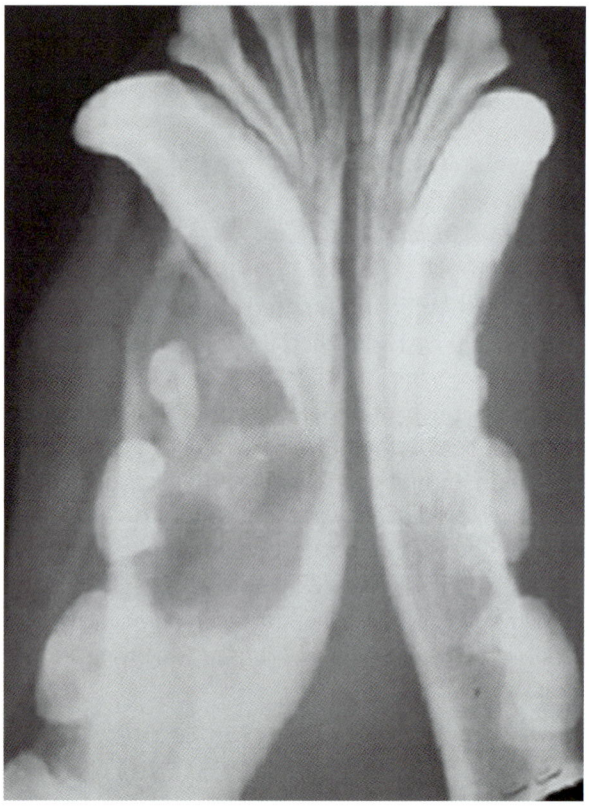

b

Fig. 15.32 Aggressive versus nonaggressive lytic bone changes.

a Aggressive lesion: A focal region of decreased opacity is associated with the left ilium. This lesion is characterized by irregular margins, a long and poorly defined transition zone to normal bone, and cortical disruption particularly along the medial margin of the ilium. There is little evidence of periosteal new bone formation in this patient.

b Nonaggressive lesion: A smoothly marginated radiolucent region is associated with the right rostral mandible. The transition zone to normal bone is sharp and well defined. The mandibular cortex bordering the lytic lesion is displaced but not disrupted. Despite the non-aggressive appearance, a neoplastic process is the most likely differential diagnosis for this lesion.

RADIOGRAPHIC FINDINGS Lytic lesions may have different patterns (Fig. 15.33):

- **Geographic lysis** results in a single, typically larger, lytic region. Depending on the transition zone to normal bone and cortical integrity, this may be seen with aggressive or nonaggressive lesions. However, nonaggressive lesions are rather common in this category.
- **Moth-eaten lysis** is characterized by multiple smaller or medium-sized bone defects which can become confluent and result in larger lytic regions. This is a sign of a regionally aggressive lesion. Lytic regions usually have irregular margins and a long transition zone to normal bone.
- **Permeative lysis** is characterized by numerous small irregularly marginated bone defects which have an indistinct transition zone to adjacent normal osseous tissue. This finding is consistent with an aggressive lesion.

INCREASED BONE OPACITY

A **generalized increase in skeletal opacity** is significantly less common than osteopenia in small animal patients. **Osteopetrosis** is uncommon in dogs and cats and results from decreased or absent osteoclastic activity. Several reports describe cases of acquired 'osteopetrosis' in cats (e.g. secondary to a feline leukaemia virus [FeLV] infection, myeloproliferative diseases, lupus erythematosus and lymphosarcoma). However, as the pathophysiology of these conditions is different from osteopetrosis in humans, '**osteosclerosis**' should be the preferred term.

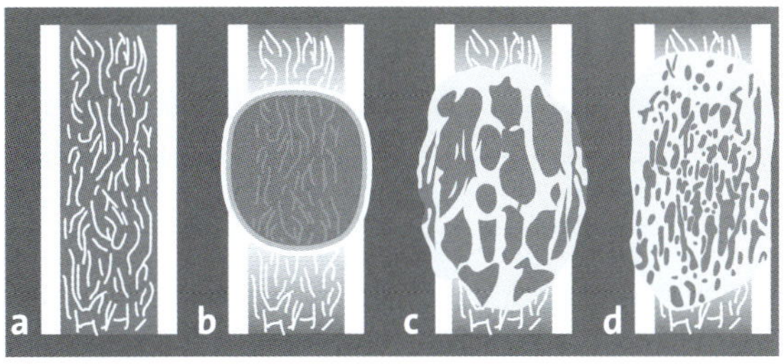

Fig. 15.33 Schematic illustration of different types of bone lysis.
a Normal bone.
b Geographic lysis is characterized by presence of a single, often large, lytic lesion. Even though this is more common with benign lesions, both aggressive and nonaggressive processes may be geographic. Other factors such as the transition zone to normal bone, cortical destruction, etc., must be taken into consideration when deciding if the lesion is aggressive or nonaggressive.
c Moth-eaten lysis is characterized by numerous small to medium-sized bone defects which may become confluent to form larger lytic regions. This is typically a sign of a regionally invasive and aggressive lesion.
d Permeative lysis is characterized by numerous small irregularly marginated bone defects with an indistinct transition zone to adjacent normal bone. This is characteristic of an aggressive lesion.

RADIOGRAPHIC FINDINGS With both osteopetrosis and osteosclerosis, there is a general increase in opacity of the medullary cavities, and possibly cortical thickening of skeletal structures (Fig. 15.34).

Focal or multifocal regions of increased radiographic opacity typically result from endosteal new bone production, sclerotic or fibrotic changes. Possible causes include bone infarcts (e.g. seen in association with metallic implants such as total hip arthroplasty, or secondary to neoplastic processes), panosteitis, enostosis and metastatic lesions. Regions of increased opacity associated with the medullary cavity are also commonly seen following trauma (e.g. secondary to fracture healing); however, these typically disappear over time due to physiological bone remodelling.

RADIOGRAPHIC FINDINGS Focal hyperostotic lesions manifest as more or less well-defined regions of increased opacity associated with the medullary cavity (Fig. 15.35).

> Periosteal reaction may be projected over the medullary cavity and give the impression of intramedullary hyperostotic lesions. Radiographs in at least two planes are needed to localize and distinguish these processes.

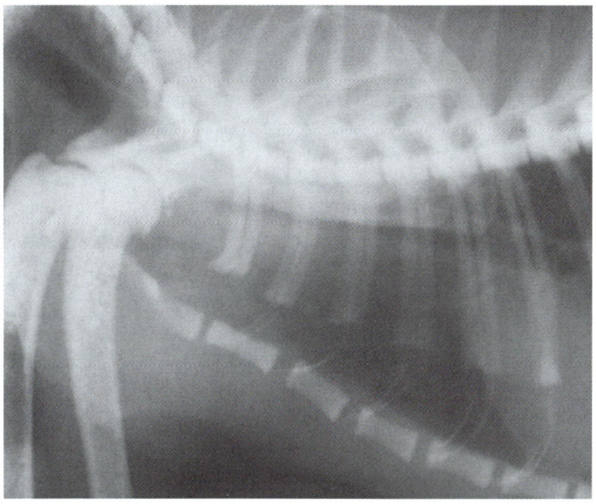

Fig. 15.34 Generalized osteosclerosis in a cat. Radiographic abnormalities include a generalized increase in radiographic opacity of the appendicular and axial skeleton. (From Hanel et al. 2004; with permission)

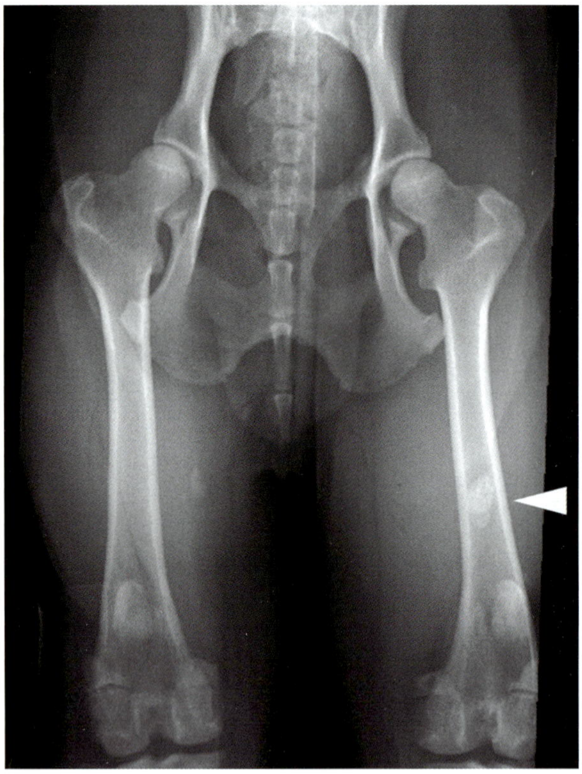

Fig. 15.35 Focal, sharply marginated region of increased opacity at the level of the mid diaphysis of the left femur (arrowhead). This was an incidental finding in a dog presented for cranial cruciate ligament rupture. Differential diagnoses for this lesion include a bone infarct, enostosis or metastatic disease.

Periosteal reactions

Periosteal new bone formation occurs when the periosteum is elevated from the underlying cortex. This can be caused by an accumulation of fluid or cells (haemorrhage, inflammatory products, oedema, neoplastic or granulomatous infiltrates) between the periosteum and cortex, or by mechanical separation (trauma, surgery).

Periosteal reactions can be categorized in light of their aggressiveness, activity and chronicity. The evaluation is sometimes straightforward; however, in other cases, periosteal changes may have a different appearance in one area of the lesion compared to another, and a definitive classification is more difficult.

> For detailed evaluation of a periosteal reaction on conventional and digital radiographs, respectively, a hot lamp or change in window setting, and a magnifying glass or post processing tools to enlarge the area of interest are often needed.

Periosteal new bone formation is evaluated with regards to organization (regularity, continuity and homogeneity), margination, surface and radiographic opacity (Fig. 15.36).

- **Aggressiveness:** The categorization of a periosteal reaction as aggressive or nonaggressive is based on the appearance of new bone formation. The less organized (i.e. the more irregularly marginated) the periosteal reaction, the more aggressive the disease process (Fig. 15.36 and 15.37). Spiculated and lamellar periosteal new bone formation, and periosteal elevation in close proximity to an aggressive lesion with new bone formation in the resulting gap ('Codman triangle'), are also indicators of an aggressive lesion.
- **Activity:** The categorization into active and inactive periosteal reaction is based on the sharpness of its margins and surface. Active periosteal reaction is characterized by an ill-defined ('fuzzy') surface, while inactive periosteal reaction has a smooth and well-defined surface (Fig. 15.36 and 15.38).
- **Chronicity:** The assessment of periosteal reaction as immature versus chronic is based on its radiographic opacity: with long-standing processes, more bone is formed, and the lesion increases in opacity (Fig. 15.36 and 15.39).

Fig. 15.37 Aggressive versus nonaggressive periosteal reaction. →

a Aggressive periosteal reaction is characterized by irregular and ill-defined regions of new bone formation. In this case, spiculated new bone formation and a Codman triangle (arrow) seen at the proximal aspect of the lesion are additional indicators of an aggressive lesion.

b Nonaggressive periosteal reaction is characterized by the organized and homogeneous appearance of periosteal new bone.

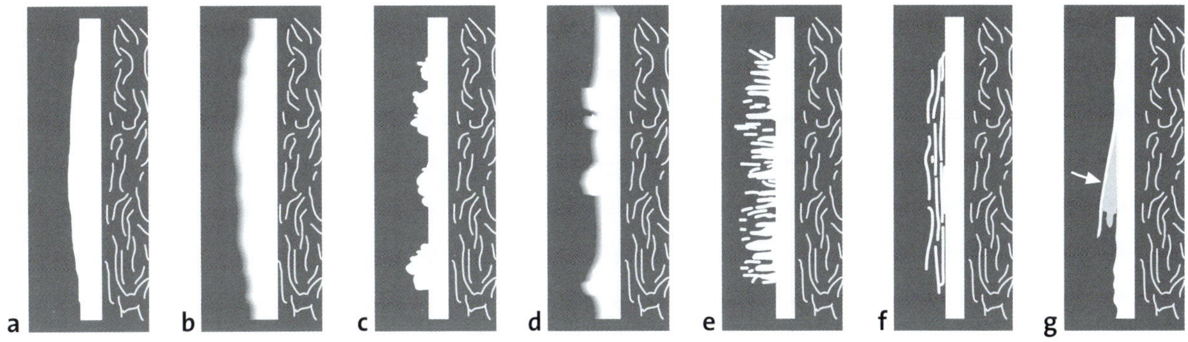

Fig. 15.36 Schematic illustration of different types of periosteal reaction.

a Continuous, smooth, well-defined periosteal reaction. The periosteal new bone formation is very opaque and homogeneous. This indicates a nonaggressive, inactive and chronic process which can be seen, for example, secondary to prior trauma (organized subperiosteal haematoma).

b Continuous lesion with a poorly defined ('fuzzy') surface. This also indicates a nonaggressive lesion which, unlike the lesion shown in a, is active at this point.

c Discontinuous, irregular periosteal reaction with a well-defined surface. Even though this change is indicative of an aggressive process, the lesion appears inactive at this point. Due to the bone production occurring in columns perpendicular to the bone surface, the terms 'columnar' or 'palisading' are commonly used to describe this finding. A possible differential diagnosis is chronic inactive osteomyelitis.

d Discontinuous, irregular periosteal reaction with a poorly defined surface. This change indicates an active aggressive process such as osteomyelitis. Even though this type of periosteal reaction is atypical for a neoplastic process, an underlying tumour cannot be excluded.

e Spiculated periosteal reaction: Discontinuous, markedly irregular and poorly defined periosteal reaction with linear hairline projections. This indicates an active aggressive process and is a common periosteal reaction seen with primary bone tumours.

f Lamellar periosteal reaction: Discontinuous, irregular and often poorly defined periosteal reaction with onion-skin-like layers of new bone. This indicates a cyclical or intermittent aggressive process and is also commonly seen with malignant bone lesions.

g Codman triangle: If a fast-growing aggressive lesion results in peripheral periosteal elevation from underlying bone, new bone fills the resulting gap. Even though the triangle itself is relatively smoothly marginated, it is an additional indicator of malignancy.

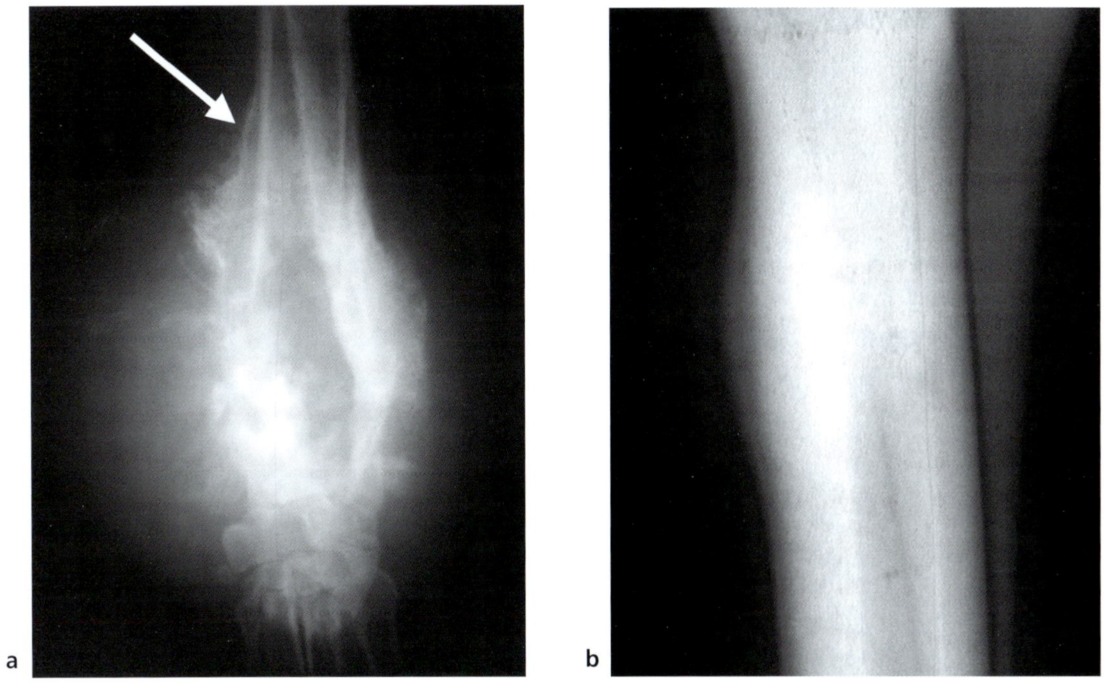

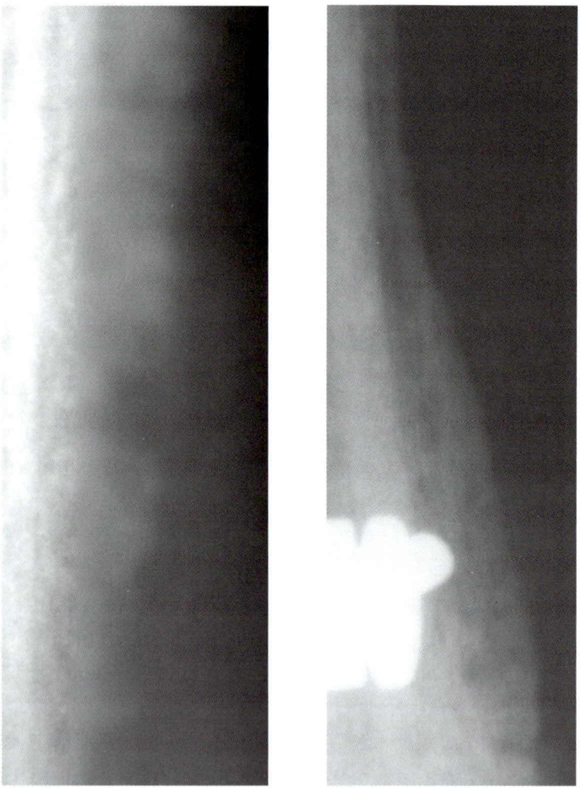

a b

Fig. 15.38 Active versus inactive periosteal reaction (magnified images).
a Active periosteal reaction is characterized by an indistinct ('fuzzy') surface.
b Inactive periosteal reaction is characterized by a well-defined surface.

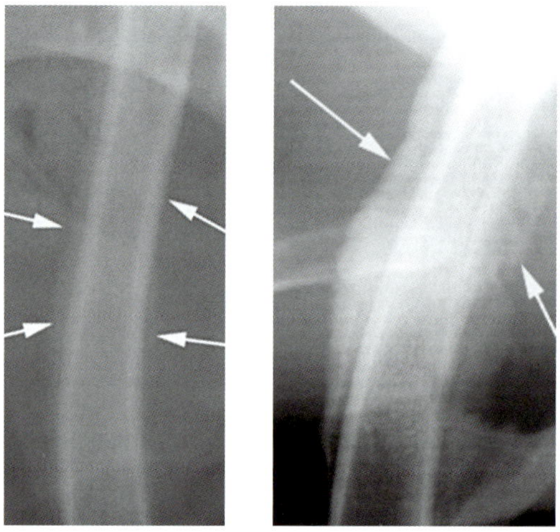

a b

Fig. 15.39 'Young/immature' versus chronic periosteal reaction in a dog with bacterial osteomyelitis.
a Immature periosteal reaction is characterized by decreased opacity compared to underlying cortex (arrows).
b With chronic periosteal reaction, new bone formation has a similar radiographic opacity to the underlying cortex (arrows).

References and further reading

Chapman WL. Appearance of ossification centers and epiphyseal closures as determined by radiographic techniques. J Am Vet Med Assoc 1965; 147: 138–41.

de Lahunta A, Habel RE. Applied Veterinary Anatomy. Philadelphia: WB Saunders 1986.

De Rooster H, van Bree H. Use of compression stress radiography for the detection of partial tears of the canine cranial cruciate ligament. J Small Anim Pract 1999; 40: 573–6.

Dyce KM, Sack WO, Wensing CJG. Textbook of Veterinary Anatomy, 3rd edn. Philadelphia: Saunders 2002.

Farrow CS. Stress radiography: Applications in small animal practice. J Am Vet Med Assoc 1982; 181: 777–84.

Flückiger MA, Friedrich GA. Hüftgelenksdysplasie (HD) beim Hund – Eine neue Röntgentechnik zur Erkennung lockerer Hüftgelenke. Schweiz Arch Tierheilk 1997; 139: 183–5.

Fritz RM. Zur Luxatio patellae des Hundes – klinisches und röntgenologisches Spätergebnis nach Transposition der Tuberositas tibiae und/oder Vertiefung der Trochlea ossis femoris. Dissertation Med Vet, München 1989.

Hanel RM, Graham JP, Levy JK, Buergelt CD, Creamer J. Generalized osteosclerosis in a cat. Vet Radiol Ultrasound 2004; 45: 318–324.

Hare WCD. The age at which epiphyseal union takes place in the limb bones of the dog. Wien Tierärztl Monat 1972; 9: 224–45.

Hecht S. Für Studium und Praxis. Spezielle Techniken der Röntgenuntersuchung der Gliedmassen beim Kleintier. Tierärztl Prax 2003; 31: 261–7.

Horvath A. Röntgenanatomische Untersuchungen zur postnatalen Entwicklung des Hintergliedmassenskelettes der Hauskatze (*Felis cattus*). Dissertation Vet Med München, 1983.

Horvath I. Röntgenanatomische Untersuchungen zur postnatalen Entwicklung des Vordergliedmassenskelettes der Hauskatze (*Felis cattus*). Dissertation Vet Med München, 1983.

Miyabayashi T, Biller DS, Manley PA, Matushek KJ. Use of a flexed dorsoplantar radiographic view of the talocrural joint to evaluate lameness in two dogs. J Am Vet Med Assoc 1991; 199: 598–600.

Morgan JP. Radiology of Veterinary Orthopedics, 2nd edn. Napa, CA: Venture Press 1999.

Nickel R, Schummer A, Seiferle E. Lehrbuch der Anatomie der Haustiere. Vol 1: Bewegungsapparat, 5th edn. Berlin: Paul Parey 1984.

Owens JM, Biery DN. Radiographic Interpretation for the Small Animal Clinician, 2nd edn. Baltimore: Williams & Wilkins 1999.

Pomriaskynski-Kobozieff N, Kobozieff, N. Etude radiologique de l'aspect du squelette normal de la main du chien aux divers stades de son évolution de la naissance à l'âge adult. Rec Med Vet 1954; 130: 617–46.

Smith GK, Biery DN, Gregor TP. New concepts of coxofemoral joint stability and the development of a clinical stress-radiographic method for quantitating hip joint laxity in the dog. J Am Vet Med Assoc 1990; 196: 59–70.

Smith RN, Allcock J. Epiphyseal fusion in the Greyhound. Vet Rec 1960; 72: 75–9.

Smith RN. Fusion of ossification centers in the cat. J Small Anim Pract 1969; 10: 523– 30.

Sumner-Smith G. Observations on the epiphyseal fusion of the canine appendicular skeleton. J Small Anim Pract 1966; 7: 303–11.

Sumner-Smith G. Bone in Clinical Orthopedics, 2nd edn. Stuttgart: Thieme 2002.

Thrall DE. Textbook of Veterinary Diagnostic Radiology, 6th edn. St. Louis: Elsevier Saunders 2013.

Thrall DE, Robertson ID. Normal Radiographic Anatomy and Anatomic Variants in the Dog and Cat. St. Louis: Elsevier Saunders 2011.

Ticer JW. Radiographic Technique in Small Animal Practice. Philadelphia: WB Saunders 1975; 101.

Van Sickle D. The relationship of ossification to elbow dysplasia. Anim Hosp 1966; 2: 24–31.

Waibl H, Mayrhofer E, Matis U, Brunnberg L, Köstlin R (eds). Atlas der Röntgenanatomie der Katze (founded by Schebitz H, Wilkens H). Stuttgart: Parey 2004.

Waibl H, Mayrhofer E, Matis U, Brunnberg L, Köstlin R (eds). Atlas der Röntgenanatomie des Hundes (founded by Schebitz H, Wilkens H), 2nd edn. Stuttgart: Parey 2005.

Congenital and developmental bone and joint diseases

16

Federica Morandi, Silke Hecht and Gregory B. Daniel

A definitive categorization of bone and joint diseases is difficult, as different disorders may result in similar radiographic abnormalities, some diseases may occur in young and older animals, and some conditions may be already present in young animals but may not result in clinical problems until later in life. This chapter covers important bone and joint diseases in young animals, while subsequent chapters discuss acquired and traumatic conditions. Some overlap between chapters is unavoidable. Select diseases of the musculoskeletal system are also described in Chapters 6, 7 and 9.

16.1 Joint diseases

Osteochondrosis (OC) and osteochondritis dissecans (OCD)

Osteochondrosis is a disease of joint cartilage predominantly seen in young large- and giant-breed dogs. The underlying problem is a failure of endochondral ossification, which results in thickening of the joint cartilage, decreased supply of the thickened cartilage with synovial nutrients, and subsequent death of the cartilage. Joint motion and strain on the cartilage surface results in cartilage fissures and, ultimately, formation of a cartilage flap (osteochondritis dissecans). The disease can affect various joints (shoulder, elbow, stifle joint, tarsus, etc.) and is often bilateral, frequently necessitating comparison radiographs of the opposite leg.

RADIOGRAPHIC FINDINGS OC and OCD are characterized by flattening of the affected joint surface, with (OCD) or without (OC) a visible isolated mineralized flap adjacent to the defect. Secondary degenerative joint disease is common.

OC/OCD (if applicable) and other (specific) diseases will be discussed for individual joints below.

16.1.1 Diseases of the shoulder joint

OC and OCD

Osteochondrosis and osteochondritis dissecans are among the most important differential diagnoses for forelimb lameness in young dogs. Large-breed dogs are most commonly affected and typically present between 5 and 10 months of age. However, clinical signs may not become apparent until later in life. Male dogs are more commonly affected than female dogs.

RADIOGRAPHIC FINDINGS OC is characterized by flattening or a concave defect associated with the caudal aspect of the humeral head, with adjacent subchondral sclerosis. These changes are best seen on a lateral view of the shoulder joint. With OCD, the isolated cartilage flap becomes mineralized and thus radiographically visible (Fig. 16.1). If an isolated cartilage flap is suspected but not confirmed on survey radiographs, the shoulder joint can be further evaluated by means of **arthrography** (Fig. 16.2), advanced imaging or arthroscopy. With increasing age, affected patients typically develop secondary degenerative joint disease, which is often associated with free intra-articular bone fragments ('joint mice'). Periarticular new bone formation is predominantly associated with the caudal margin of the glenoid cavity, the caudal aspect of the humeral head, and the bicipital grove.

Shoulder dysplasia and (sub)luxation

Shoulder dysplasia is most commonly seen in Dachshunds, but may occasionally be diagnosed in other dog breeds and cats. Shoulder (sub)luxation in young animals may be secondary to shoulder dysplasia or may have a different (typically traumatic) aetiology.

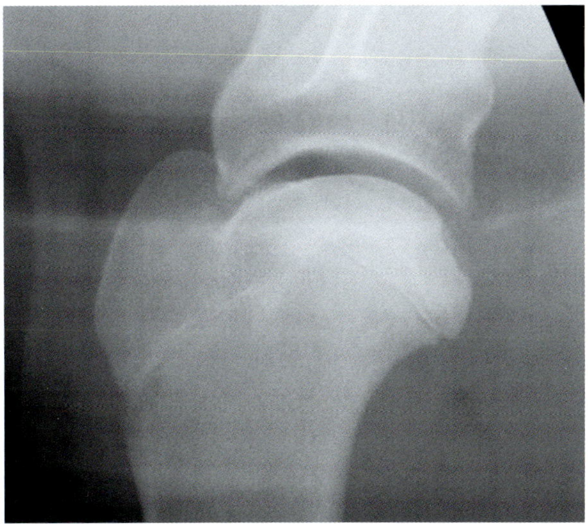

Fig. 16.1 Osteochondritis dissecans (OCD) of the shoulder joint in a young dog. Radiographic findings include an irregularly marginated defect associated with the caudal humeral head, with an isolated mineralized flap and adjacent subchondral sclerosis.

RADIOGRAPHIC FINDINGS Shoulder dysplasia is characterized by hypoplasia of the joint surfaces, flattening of the glenoid cavity of the scapula, incomplete ossification of the distal scapula, and flattening and deformation of the humeral head. Secondary abnormalities include joint incongruity, subluxation or even complete luxation of the shoulder joint. Secondary degenerative joint disease is common and usually present even at a young age.

16.1.2 Diseases of the elbow joint

Elbow dysplasia

Several different developmental diseases of the elbow joint are summarized under the term 'elbow dysplasia':

- osteochondrosis (OC) and osteochondritis dissecans (OCD)
- fragmentation of the medial coronoid process of the ulna (FCP)
- ununited anconeal process (UAP).

A radiographic evaluation of the elbow for elbow dysplasia is certainly important not only in the diagnostic workup of a lame patient, but also in the context of reproduction programmes, certification and pre-purchase examinations.

OC AND OCD

As for other joints, OC / OCD predominantly affects young, large-breed dog. Labradors and other retriever breeds are predisposed.

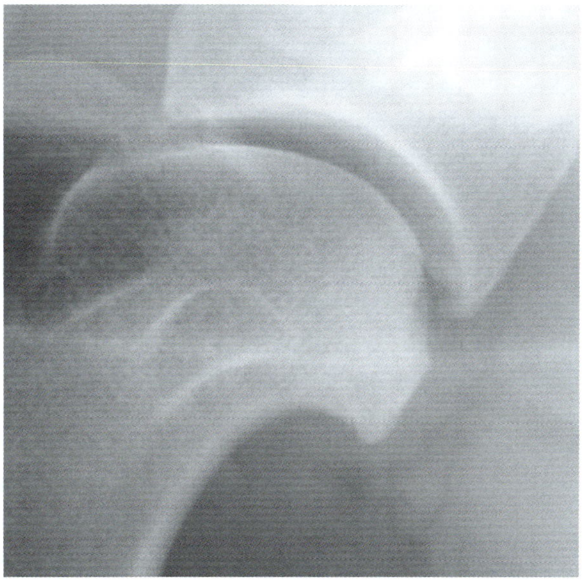

a

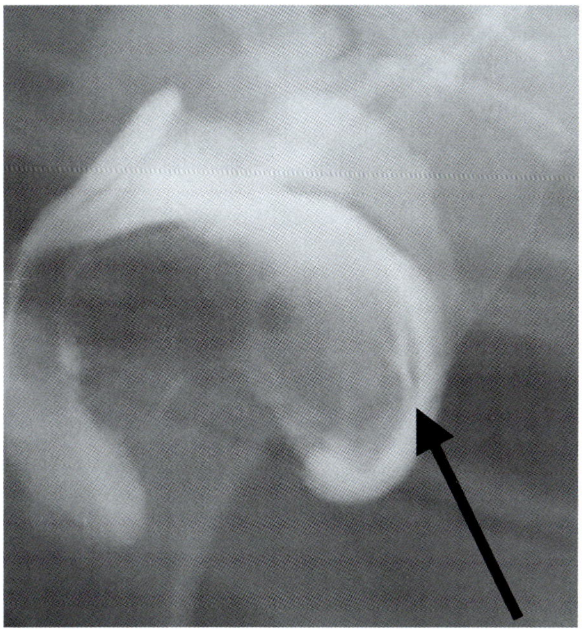

b

Fig. 16.2 OCD of the shoulder joint.
a As the isolated cartilage flap is not mineralized, it is not visible on this survey radiograph.
b During arthrography, positive contrast medium enters the gap between the cartilage flap and the humeral head (arrow), which allows a diagnosis of OCD.

RADIOGRAPHIC FINDINGS A concave defect is present at the medial aspect of the distal humeral condyle, commonly associated with subchondral sclerosis (Fig. 16.3). This is usually seen on a craniocaudal view of the elbow joint, but may be highlighted by obtaining a radiograph with slight rotation of the elbow joint (craniolateral–caudomedial oblique view) (Fig. 16.4). In contrast to shoulder OC / OCD, an isolated mineralized flap is usually absent.

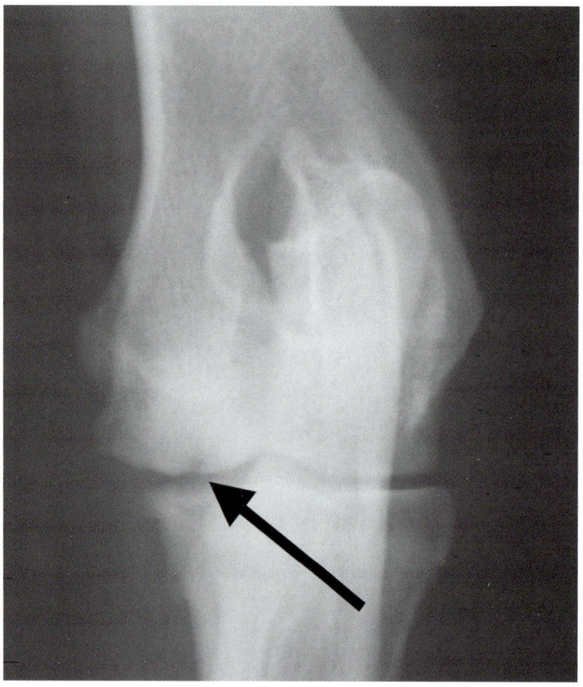

Fig. 16.3 OC of the elbow joint. On this craniocaudal view there is a concave defect with adjacent subchondral sclerosis associated with the distal aspect of the medial part of the humeral condyle (arrow). Periarticular osteophytosis is consistent with degenerative joint disease.

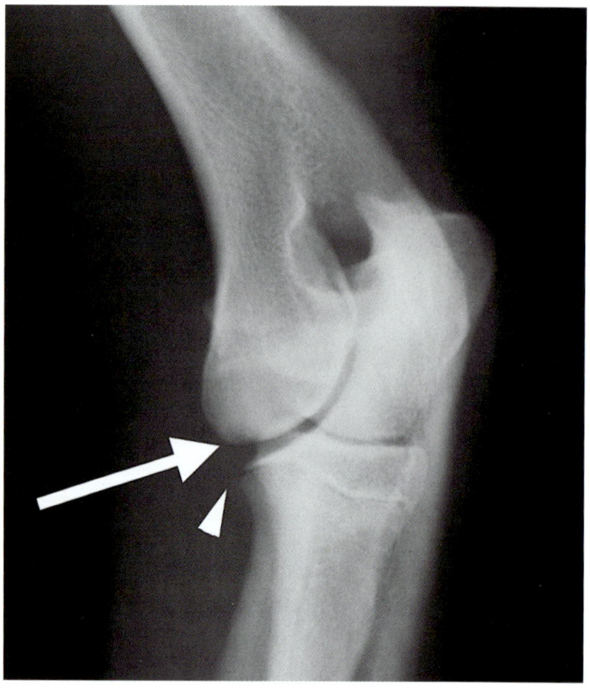

Fig. 16.4 OC of the elbow joint. Even though the medial humeral condylar lesion is usually visible on a craniocaudal view, it can be accentuated by obtaining a radiograph with slight external rotation of the elbow joint (i.e. a craniolateral–caudomedial projection; arrow). This radiographic view also results in excellent visualization of the medial coronoid process (arrowhead).

Secondary degenerative joint disease usually develops early, and is characterized by periarticular new bone formation at the radial head, along the dorsal aspect of the anconeal process and along the trochlear notch of the ulna. Fragmentation of the medial coronoid process (see below) may cause a secondary defect of the medial aspect of the humeral condyle, which may be indistinguishable from a true OC lesion.

FCP

This is a disease of large-breed dogs (Labradors and other retriever breeds, German Shepherd Dogs, Rottweilers, Bernese Mountain Dogs, etc.). Affected animals typically present between 5 and 12 months of age; however, radiographic abnormalities may not become apparent until the dog reaches 7 or 8 months in age.

Radiographic findings A definitive radiographic diagnosis may be difficult. The most important indicators of FCP are elbow joint incongruity with relative shortening of the radius compared to the ulna, sclerosis of the ulnar trochlear notch, blunting of the medial coronoid process and periarticular new bone formation associated with the dorsal aspect of the anconeal process, the distal humerus, the head of the radius and the medial coronoid process (Fig. 16.5). An isolated bone fragment is rarely visible (Fig. 16.6).

FCP may occur concurrently with OC/OCD of the elbow joint, or the isolated bone fragment may come in contact with the medial aspect of the humeral condyle and damage its surface ('kissing lesion'). It is usually impossible to determine if a dog has a true OC/OCD lesion of the medial aspect of the humeral condyle in conjunction with FCP, or a 'kissing lesion' secondary to FCP.

UAP

This disease is most common in large dogs (especially German Shepherd Dogs, less commonly St. Bernard, Labradors and other retriever breeds) but has occasionally been reported in chondrodystrophic breeds (Bassett Hound, Bulldog and Dachshund). Physiologically, the anconeal process is formed from a separate centre of ossification and fuses to the proximal ulna before the age of 5 months. Failure of osseous union results in elbow joint instability and secondary degenerative joint disease.

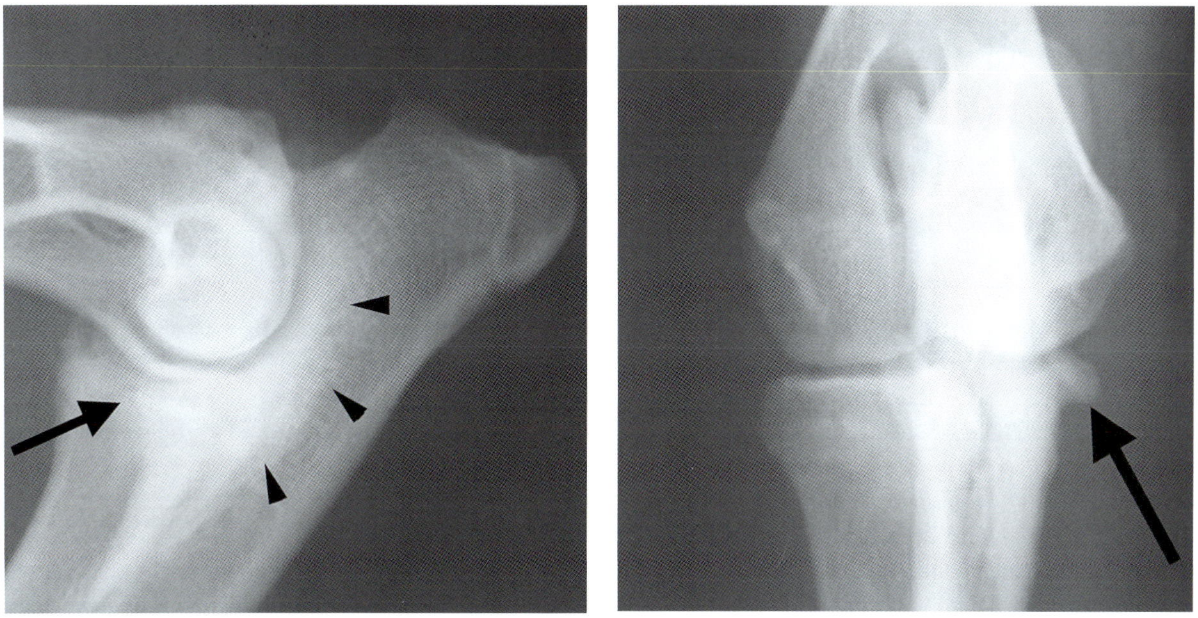

a b

Fig. 16.5 Lateral a and craniocaudal b radiographs of the elbow joint in a dog with fragmentation of the medial coronoid process (FCP). There is incongruity of the elbow joint, the medial coronoid process (arrow) is blunted, and on the lateral view there is sclerosis along the ulnar trochlear notch (arrowheads). Periarticular new bone formation is associated with the dorsal aspect of the anconeal process, the distal humerus and the cranial aspect of the radial head.

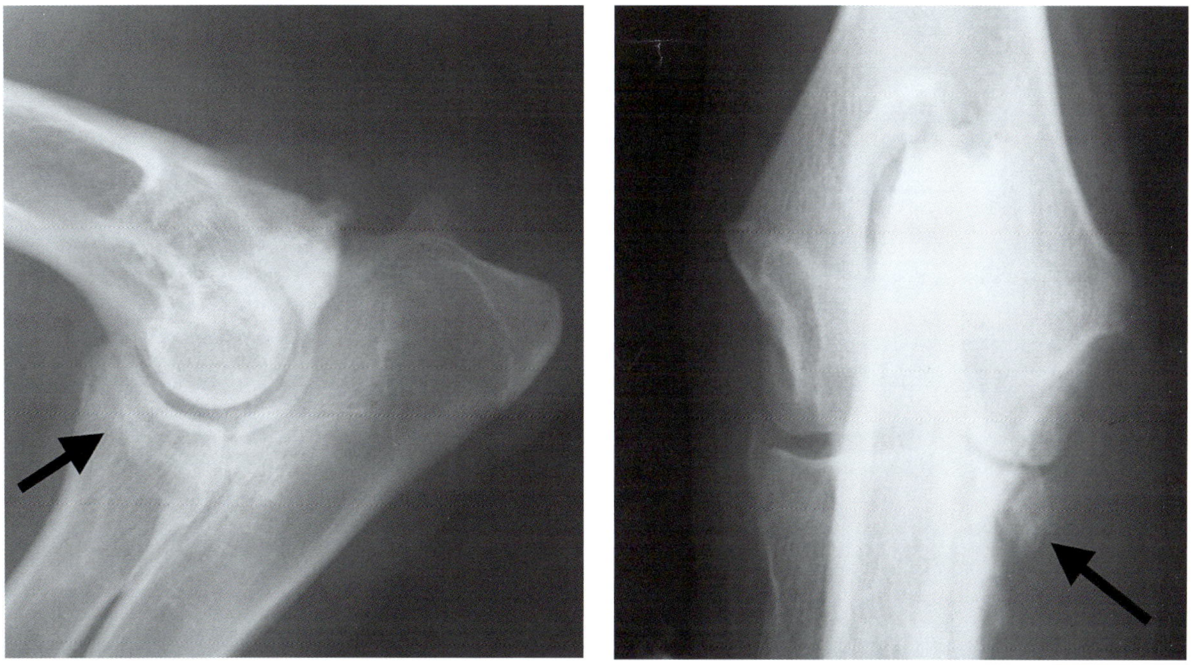

a b

Fig. 16.6 Lateral a and craniocaudal b views of the elbow joint in a dog with fragmentation of the medial coronoid process (FCP). The isolated bone fragment is distinctly visible (arrows). Additional findings include marked incongruity of the elbow joint with shortening of the radius in comparison to the ulna, sclerosis of the ulnar trochlear notch, and periarticular osteophytosis of the elbow joint.

Radiographic findings A radiographic diagnosis of ununited anconeal process is easiest on a (flexed) lateral view, which demonstrates a persistent linear lucent line separating the anconeal process from the parent bone (Fig. 16.7). The bone fragment may remain in position or may be displaced. Common secondary findings include sclerosis of the fragment and parent bone as well as elbow degenerative joint disease.

Incomplete ossification of the humeral condyle

This developmental anomaly has only been reported fairly recently in the veterinary literature. It is characterized by failure, or incomplete closure, of the physis between the two ossification centres of the humeral condyle. Cocker Spaniels and certain hunting breeds appear predisposed, but the disease has also been reported in several other breeds. Affected animals may present at a young age with lameness, or the condition may be silent for many years. Affected older animals commonly present with unilateral or bilateral articular distal humeral fractures following minor trauma.

Radiographic findings A radiolucent line between the lateral and medial aspect of the humeral condyle persists beyond the expected time of physeal closure (variable according to the literature, and ranging from 2 to 5 months) (Fig. 16.8). A secondary fracture is typically intercondylar and results in separation of both components of the humeral condyle from the humeral shaft ('T or Y fracture'). Isolated fractures of either the medial or the lateral aspect of the humeral condyle are also possible (Fig. 16.9).

As this condition is commonly bilateral, comparison radiographs of the opposite elbow are always indicated in dogs with an acute intercondylar distal humeral fracture after minor trauma. However, the radiographic diagnosis of incomplete ossification of the humeral condyle is often difficult, as the physis is usually thin and obscured by superimposition of the olecranon. Computed tomography (CT) should be considered for full assessment in questionable cases, and to establish a definitive diagnosis.

Distractio cubiti

This term describes a growth abnormality of the antebrachium in young chondrodystrophic dogs such as Dachshunds. The anomaly is characterized by typically bilateral asynchronous growth of the radius and ulna, with shortening of the ulna compared to the radius. This results in a cranial bowing of the radius ('radius curvus'), elbow joint incongruity and valgus deformity of the carpus (Fig. 16.10). If left untreated, the deformity will result in severe degenerative joint disease of the elbow joint and carpus.

Traumatic premature closure of the distal ulnar physis and other diseases affecting the growth of the ulna (e.g.

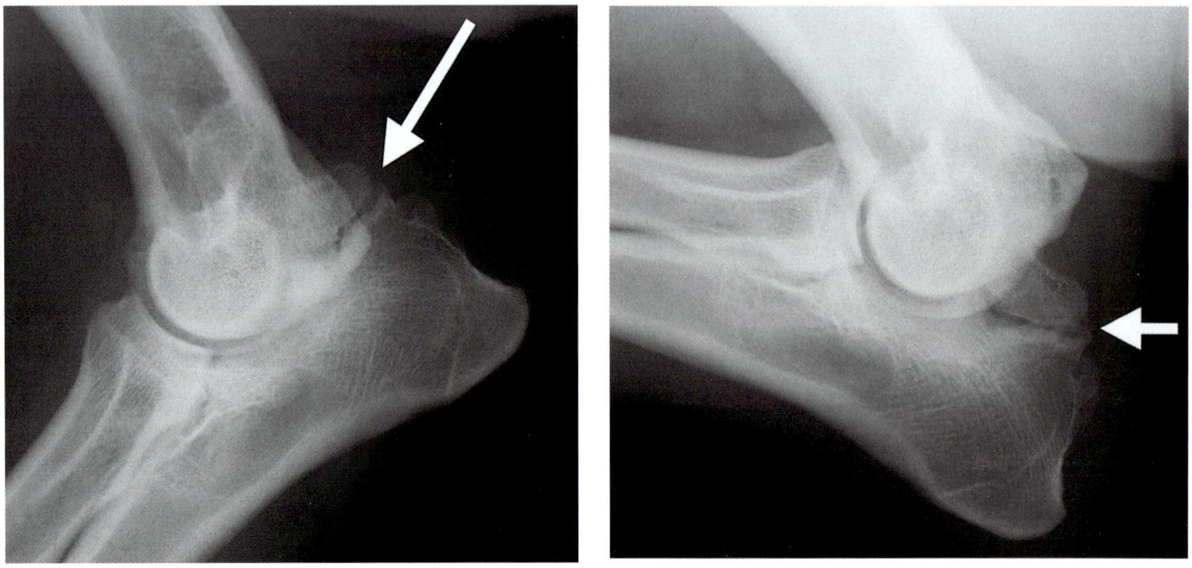

a b

Fig. 16.7 Ununited anconeal process. The diagnosis is possible on the lateral a and flexed lateral b view of the elbow joint. The physis of the anconeal process (arrows) remains visible beyond its expected closure time, and is recognized as a linear lucent line separating the anconeal process from the parent bone. The adjacent region of the ulna is diffusely increased in opacity (sclerosis) and the joint is incongruous.

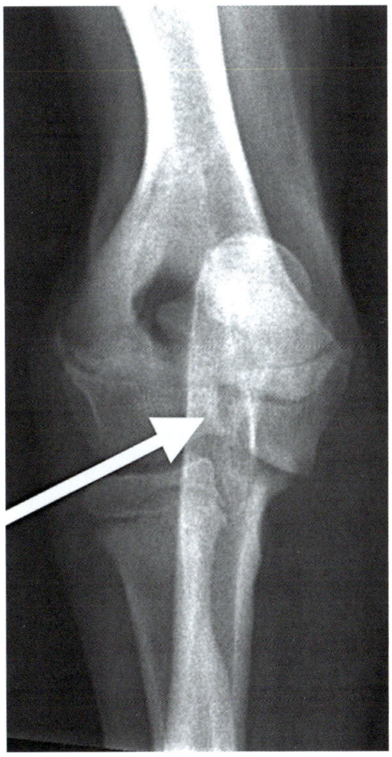

Fig. 16.8 Incomplete ossification of the humeral condyle (IOHC) in a 3.5-month-old dog presented with lameness. The physis between the separate centres of ossification of the humeral condyle (arrow) is wide and irregularly marginated. Note that this region is often difficult to evaluate due to superimposition with the olecranon.

Fig. 16.9 Salter-Harris type IV fracture of the lateral aspect of the humeral condyle (capitulum) in a 4-month-old dog secondary to incomplete ossification of the humeral condyle (IOHC).→

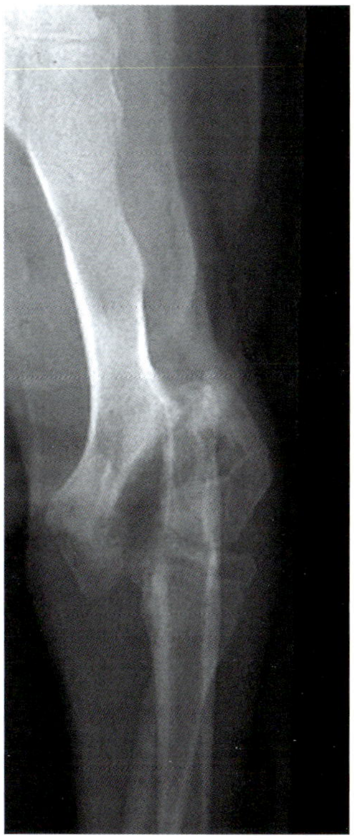

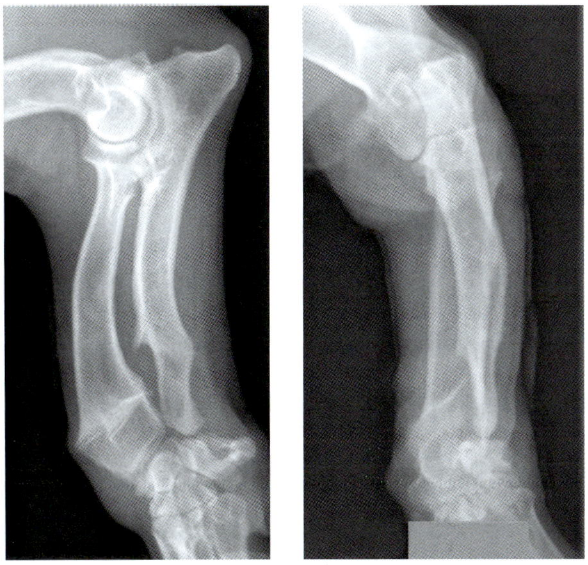

a b

Fig. 16.10 Lateral a and craniocaudal b radiographs of the antebrachium in a 10-month-old Bassett Hound with distractio cubiti. The ulna is shortened compared to the radius. This results in a cranial convex bowing of the radius (radius curvus), incongruity and varus deformity of the elbow joint, as well as valgus deformity of the carpus. Despite the young age of the patient, early degenerative joint disease of the elbow and carpus are evident.

retained cartilage core) result in similar changes of the antebrachium, but are more common in large-breed dogs.

Congenital elbow luxation

This is an occasional diagnosis in young animals (typically dogs between 1 and 6 months of age). To the authors' knowledge, neither a sex nor a breed predisposition has been identified. The disease can be unilateral or bilateral. Three types are possible:

- type I: luxation of the radius
- type II: luxation of the ulna
- type III: luxation of both radius and ulna, typically with 90° rotation of the antebrachium in relation to the humerus.

A distinction between a true congenital luxation and an injury sustained in utero or at very young age may be difficult or impossible.

16.1.3 Diseases of the carpus

An **angular limb deformity** of the carpus (**valgus** is more common than **varus** deformity) secondary to asynchronous growth of the antebrachium is probably the most common and most important disease of the carpus in young animals (see also 'Distractio cubiti' in section 16.1.2).

Incomplete or **failed fusion of the separate centres of ossification of the intermedioradial carpal bone** is occasionally encountered (Fig. 16.11). In the authors' experience this is usually an incidental finding; however, it is conceivable that these patients may be predisposed to fracture after minor trauma, as has been described for incomplete ossification of the distal humeral condyle.

16.1.4 Diseases of the coxofemoral joint

Hip dysplasia

Hip dysplasia is a congenital disease of tremendous importance in small animal orthopaedics due to its common occurrence and the wide range of diagnostic and therapeutic opportunities. Even though large and fast-growing dog breeds such as German Shepherd Dogs, Labradors and other retriever breeds are predominantly affected, the disease may also be seen in other dog breeds and even in cats. In addition to genetic predisposition, other factors such as nutrition are believed to play a role in disease manifestation.

The disease is characterized by a variable degree of laxity of the coxofemoral joint and shallow conformation of the acetabulum, with resultant subluxation, malformation of the femoral head and neck, and development of secondary degenerative joint disease. Depending on severity and individual factors, affected animals may present at young age (3–12 months) with joint instability, or later in life due to degenerative joint disease. A radiographic evaluation of the pelvis for hip dysplasia is certainly important not only in the diagnostic workup of a lame patient, but also in the context of reproduction programmes, certification and pre-purchase examinations.

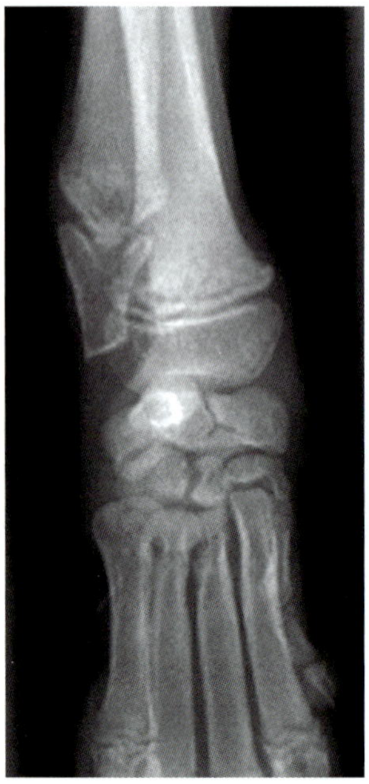

Fig. 16.11 Incomplete fusion of the separate centres of ossification of the intermedioradial carpal bone seen as an incidental finding in a young dog presented with metaphyseal osteopathy. The border between the ossification centres of the radial carpal bone and the intermediate carpal bone is recognized as a near-sagittal linear lucent line. The changes in the distal antebrachium (linear lucent lines parallel to the distal physes of radius and ulna) are characteristic of metaphyseal osteopathy.

RADIOGRAPHIC FINDINGS Radiographic indicators of hip dysplasia are best identified on a ventrodorsal (VD) view, and include unilateral or bilateral subluxation or incongruity of the coxofemoral joint, shallow conformation of the acetabulum with inadequate femoral head coverage, and deformity of the femoral head and neck (Fig. 16.12a). Utilization of a distraction wedge between the stifle joints during the radiographic examination can aid in demonstrating coxofemoral joint laxity in questionable cases, and should be considered if initial radiographs are normal despite clinical suspicion of hip dysplasia (Fig. 16.12b). With increasing age, affected animals develop degenerative joint disease of varying severity, which manifests as periarticular osteophytosis along the margin of the acetabulum, the femoral head and the femoral neck (Fig. 16.13).

A detailed discussion of screening methods and classification schemes used in different countries in the evaluation of dogs for hip dysplasia (e.g. Orthopedic Foundation for Animals [OFA] evaluation in the US) is beyond the scope of this chapter. To assign a dog to a category ranging from normal/excellent to severe hip dysplasia, the following criteria are typically taken into consideration.

- Femoral head coverage (may be assigned an objective number by measurement of the 'Norberg angle' between two imaginary lines, one connecting the centres of both femoral heads and one connecting the centre of a femoral head and the cranial margin of the acetabulum on the same side, on a VD view).
- Shape of the cranial lateral margin of the acetabulum.
- Subchondral bone opacity of the cranial acetabular margin.
- Femoral head and neck conformation.
- Presence of degenerative joint disease including early indicators ('Morgan line').

Quantitative measurements of hip joint laxity using distraction techniques may also be utilized (e.g. the 'PennHIP' examination technique).

For further descriptions of hip dysplasia screening methods the reader is referred to specific literature.

Legg–Calvé–Perthes disease (avascular necrosis of the femoral head)

This is a condition affecting young (4–11 months) small-breed dogs (<20kg, commonly Poodle or terrier breeds).

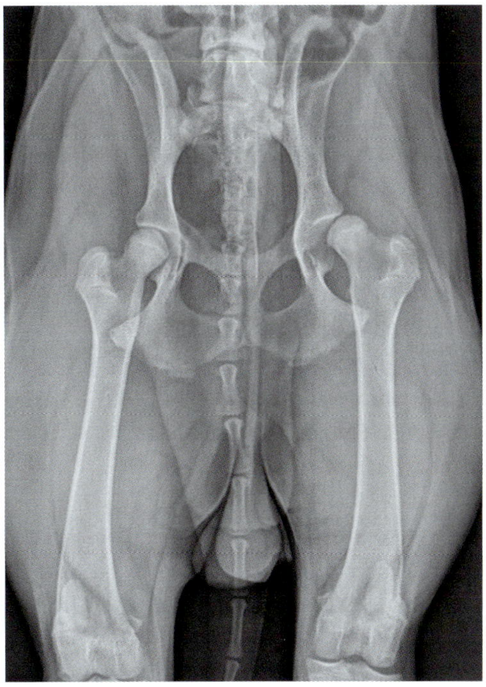

a

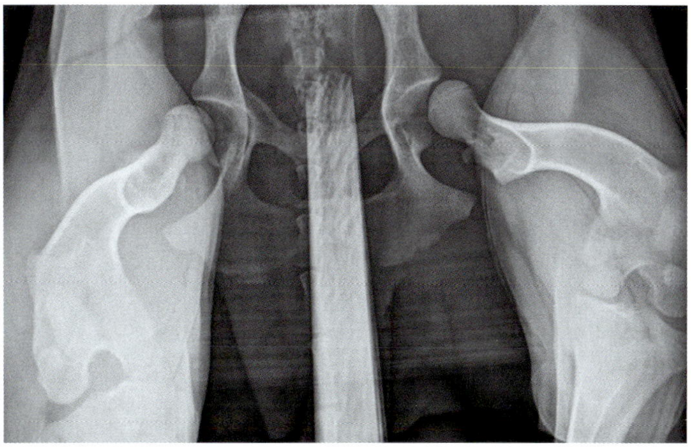

b

Fig. 16.12 Hip dysplasia in a dog.

a The ventrodorsal (VD) view shows subluxation of the left coxofemoral joint with inadequate femoral head coverage and square conformation of the femoral head. The right coxofemoral joint appears relatively normal. Note the lumbosacral transitional vertebra.

b Repeat radiograph following placement of a wedge between the stifle joints and application of stress demonstrates laxity of both coxofemoral joints. (Note that positioning on the initial VD view is suboptimal for hip dysplasia evaluation. It is possible that a diagnosis of bilateral hip dysplasia would have been possible on a well-positioned VD view without a wedge technique in this patient.)

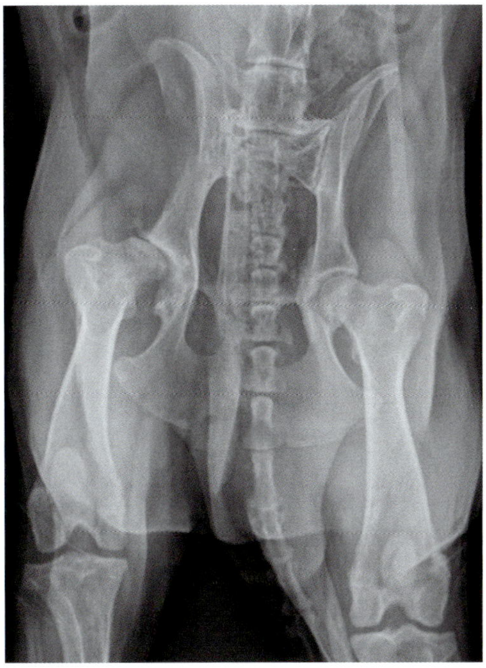

Fig. 16.13 Severe degenerative joint disease of the right coxofemoral joint secondary to chronic joint incongruity (hip dysplasia). Extensive periarticular osteophytosis is associated with the acetabulum, the femoral head and the femoral neck. Additional findings include joint incongruity, inadequate femoral head coverage and deformity of the femoral head and neck. Mild degenerative joint disease of the left coxofemoral joint is characterized by a curvilinear region of increased opacity along the femoral neck ('caudal curvilinear osteophytosis' or 'Morgan line').

It is commonly limited to one coxofemoral joint, but may be bilateral. Even though multiple possible inciting factors (infection, trauma, metabolic, hormonal, vascular and genetic causes) have been discussed, the aetiology of this disease remains uncertain. Decreased blood supply to the proximal femoral epiphysis (i.e. the femoral head) by epiphyseal vessels leads to ischaemia and subsequently necrosis of the femoral head. The subchondral bone collapses, the femoral head loses its normal shape, and the patient ultimately develops degenerative joint disease.

Radiographic findings Legg–Calvé–Perthes disease results in widening of the joint space of the coxofemoral joint, irregular regions of increased and decreased radiographic opacity of the femoral head due to trabecular collapse and ingrowth of granulation tissue, and ultimately in collapse and deformation of the femoral head and degenerative joint disease (Fig. 16.14).

Femoral head and neck osteopathy

This condition was originally reported in cats and manifests as spontaneous unilateral or bilateral femoral capital physeal fracture(s) ('slipped physis'). Young (approximately 2-year-old) overweight male castrated cats are most commonly affected. A comparable atraumatic separation of the proximal femoral epiphysis from the metaphysis may on occasion also be seen in dogs. The cause is unknown. A radiographic distinction between this condition and a traumatic capital physeal fracture may be difficult or impossible.

Radiographic findings Affected patients have unilateral or bilateral capital physeal fracture(s) which may be acute or chronic. In some cases (especially in dogs), the epiphysis may be only minimally displaced without a visible gap between epiphysis and metaphysis, and pelvic radiographs with extended legs may be normal. In such instances, additional radiographs with the legs flexed forwards ('frog position') are indicated (similar to cases of traumatic capital physeal fractures), as these allow improved visualization of the isolated bone fragment (see Chapter 18, Fig. 18.1). This is important, as surgical stabilization of an acute capital physeal separation should be performed as quickly as possible to avoid resorption of the femoral neck (see Chapter 18, Fig. 18.10).

16.1.5 Diseases of the stifle joint

OC/OCD

OC/OCD of the stifle joint predominantly affects large-breed dogs (German Shepherd Dogs and Great Danes are predisposed) at the age of 5–11 months.

Radiographic findings A concave defect is associated with the distal aspect of the lateral (or less commonly medial) femoral condyle, often associated with subchondral sclerosis (Fig. 16.15). While this abnormality is best seen on a craniocaudal or caudocranial radiograph, the lateral view is superior for identification of concurrent, often substantial, intracapsular soft-tissue swelling (joint effusion). An isolated mineralized cartilage flap is only rarely visible. OC/OCD of the stifle joint is commonly bilateral, and radiographs of the contralateral joint are indicated in affected patients.

With increasing age, development of secondary degenerative joint disease is common, and is characterized by periarticular new bone formation associated with the femoral trochlea, femoral condyles, the periphery of the tibial condyle, the patella and the fabellae.

Care must be taken to not confuse the normal extensor fossa (origin of the long digital extensor tendon) with an OC/OCD lesion (Fig. 16.16). The extensor fossa does not result in a defect of the joint surface on a craniocaudal/caudocranial view, and on a lateral view it is located further cranially and proximally compared to an OC/OCD lesion.

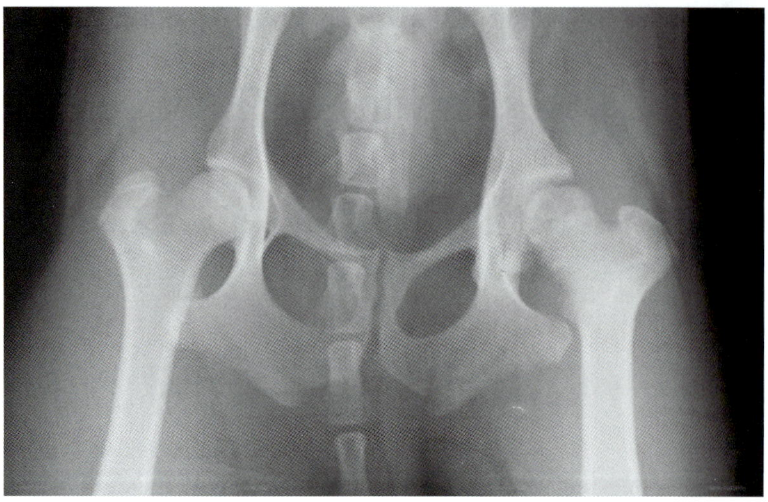

Fig. 16.14 Legg–Calvé–Perthes disease in a dog. The joint space of the left coxofemoral joint is widened, and irregular regions of increased and decreased bone opacity are noted associated with the deformed femoral head. Periarticular osteophytosis associated with acetabulum and femoral neck are consistent with degenerative joint disease.

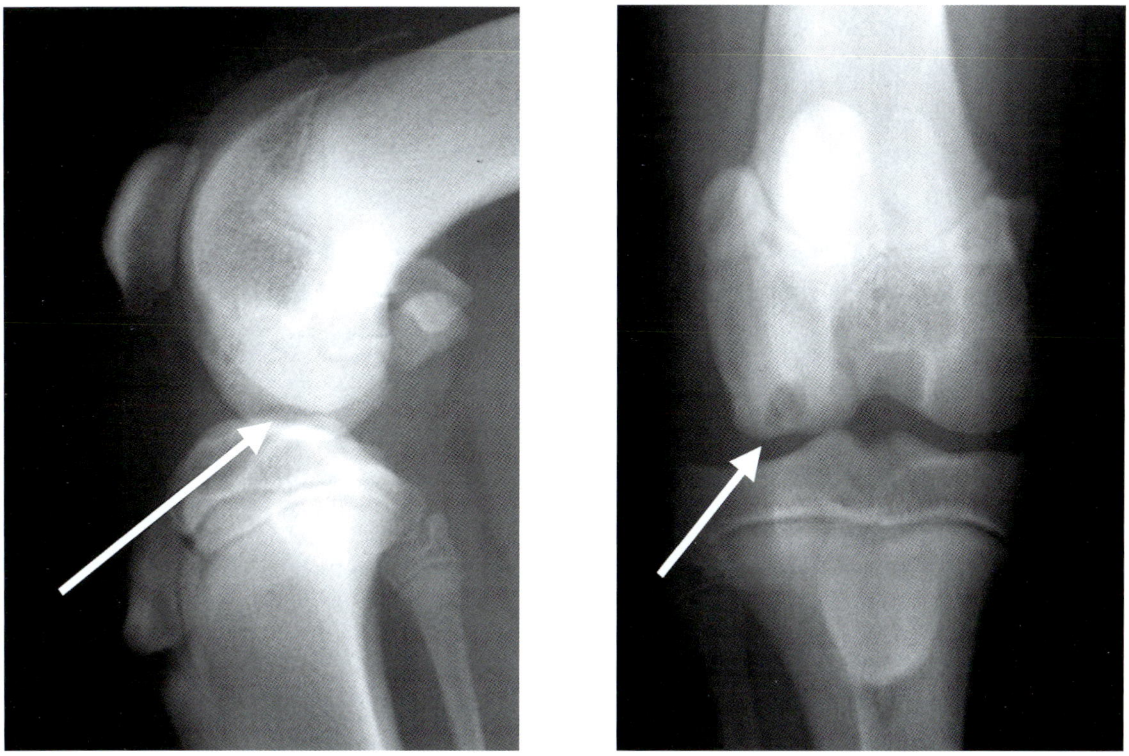

a b

Fig. 16.15 OCD of the stifle joint in a dog. A concave defect with adjacent sclerosis is associated with the lateral femoral condyle (arrows). This is not easily seen on the lateral view a but is obvious on the craniocaudal view b. An isolated flap is not distinctly visible but was diagnosed by means of arthroscopy. Note secondary intracapsular soft-tissue swelling (joint effusion).

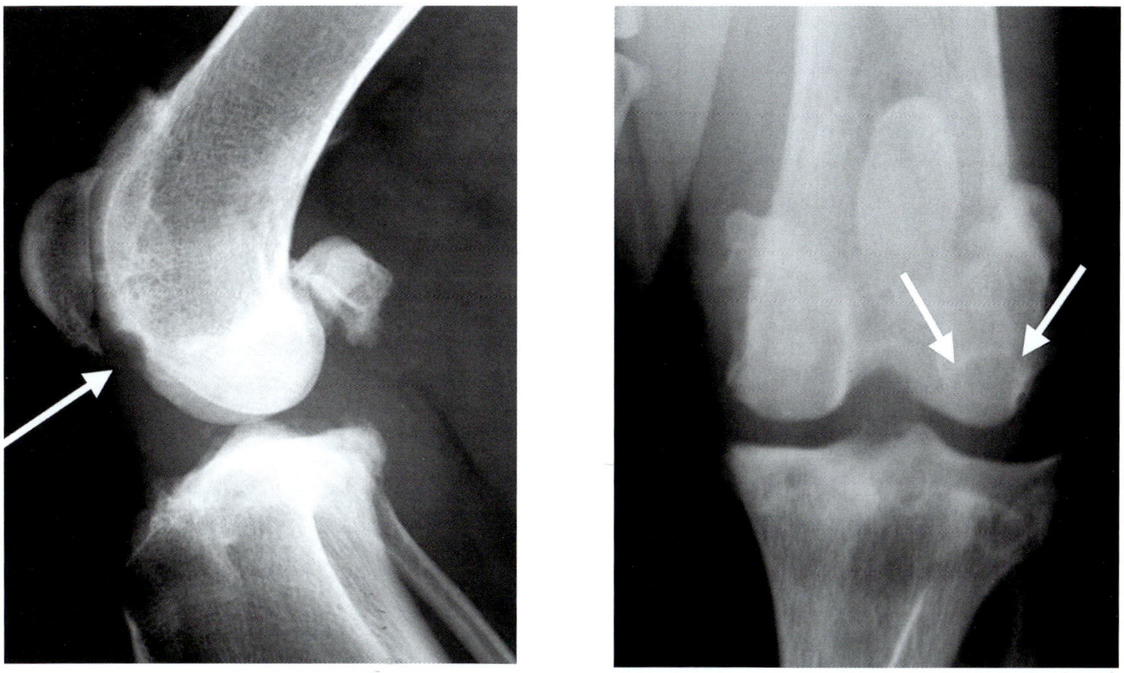

a b

Fig. 16.16 Comparison radiographs to aid in differentiation of the normal extensor fossa (arrows) from an OC/OCD lesion in a dog with intracapsular soft-tissue swelling and degenerative joint disease of the stifle joint secondary to cranial cruciate ligament rupture. On the lateral view a the extensor fossa is located further cranially and proximally, and on the craniocaudal view b it appears as a region of decreased opacity of the lateral femoral condyle without causing a defect of the articular surface (compare to Fig. 16.15).

Patellar luxation

In this disease there is temporary or permanent displacement of the patella from its normal position in the femoral trochlea. The **congenital form** may be diagnosed at a young age; however, clinical signs are often mild, and a diagnosis may not be made until later in life. Small-breed dogs are predisposed, but large-breed dogs (and occasionally cats) may be affected. An interesting difference between small- and large-breed dogs lies in the direction of patellar displacement. Small-breed dogs are typically affected by medial patellar luxation, while lateral patellar luxation is more common in large-breed dogs.

Patellar luxation can be subdivided into four grades.

- **Grade 1:** Intermittent patellar luxation. The patella can be dislodged from the femoral trochlea if the stifle joint is completely extended, but returns to its physiological position following manipulation. A radiographic examination of the stifle joint is normal in these cases.
- **Grade 2:** Patellar luxation is more common and easier to accomplish than with grade 1. The patella typically spontaneously returns to its normal position. The tibial tuberosity may be deviated from midline (up to 30°) on radiographs.
- **Grade 3:** There is permanent luxation of the patella with notable torsion of the tibia and deviation of the tibial tuberosity from midline (30–60°). The femoral trochlea appears shallow.
- **Grade 4:** There is permanent luxation of the patella, and the tibial tuberosity deviates 60–90° from midline. The femoral trochlea is flat and may, in extreme cases, even be convex.

Patellar luxation may also result from **trauma** and can effect animals of any age or breed. This condition differs pathophysiologically and radiographically from the congenital form.

Radiographic findings These are variable and depend on the type and severity of the disease. For simplicity, this description will be limited to the most common type (medial patellar luxation in small-breed dogs) (Fig. 16.17). The most obvious finding is displacement of the patella medially from its normal position in the femoral trochlea. There is often lateral bowing of the distal femur, medial bowing of the proximal tibia and medial deviation of the tibial tuberosity. The femoral trochlea is usually abnormal and/or hypoplastic, which is best evaluated by means of skyline radiographs or advanced imaging. In contrast to other diseases of the stifle joint, stifle joint effusion and secondary degenerative joint disease are often comparatively mild in patellar luxation. However, concurrent rupture of the cranial cruciate

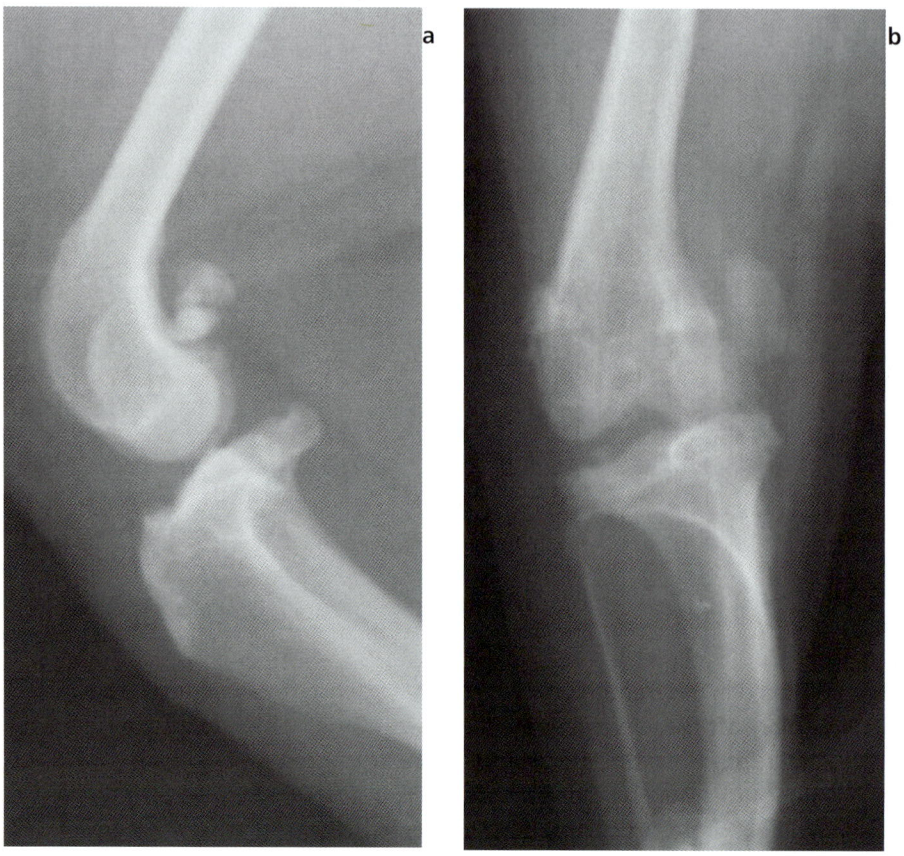

Fig. 16.17 Lateral a and craniocaudal b radiographs of the stifle joint in a small-breed dog with medial patellar luxation. The patella is located medial to the femoral trochlea. The distal femur is bent laterally and the proximal tibia medially, and the tibial tuberosity is more medially located than normal. Additional findings include mild intracapsular soft-tissue swelling and stifle degenerative joint disease.

ligament is a relatively common problem in dogs with this condition, and will result in intracapsular soft-tissue swelling and periarticular osteophytosis (see section 17.1 and Fig. 17.1).

Osgood–Schlatter disease

This disease is well documented in the human orthopaedic literature, and describes a developmental anomaly of the tibial tuberosity or tibial crest resulting in unilateral or bilateral pathological fracture (avulsion) of the tibial tuberosity in children and adolescents. A similar condition is occasionally seen in dogs. Affected animals present at a young age with lameness and swelling of one or both stifle joints.

RADIOGRAPHIC FINDINGS The tibial tuberosity or tibial crest are partially or completely separated from the tibia, resulting in proximal displacement of the fragment along with the patellar ligament and patella (Fig. 16.18). This is associated with extracapsular soft-tissue swelling, and may be unilateral or bilateral.

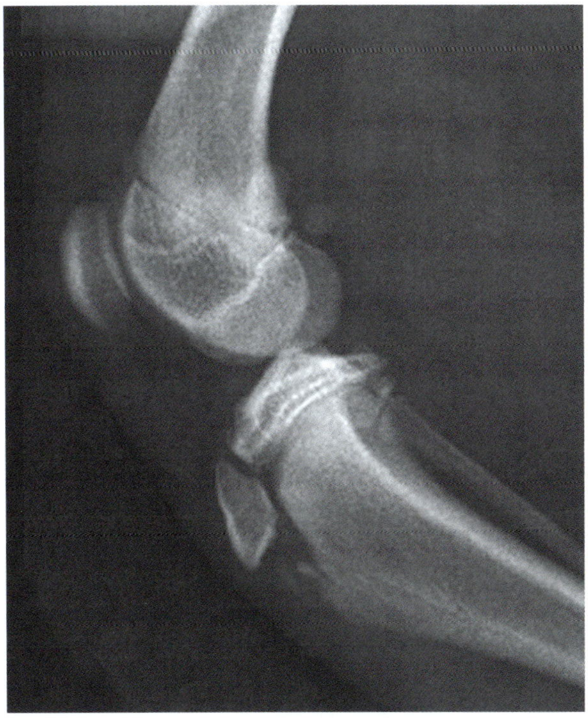

Fig. 16.18 Developmental anomaly of the tibial tuberosity and crest with secondary pathological fracture in a young dog (comparable with Osgood–Schlatter syndrome in human medicine). This patient presented with bilateral stifle lameness and without history of trauma. Similar radiographic findings were seen in both stifle joints. The tibial tuberosity is mildly displaced proximally. Associated swelling of the patellar ligament is difficult to appreciate on this overexposed radiograph.

A radiographic distinction between this developmental condition and a traumatic avulsion fracture of the tibial tuberosity is not possible.

16.1.6 Diseases of the tarsus

OC/OCD

OC/OCD is the most important disease of the tarsus in young animals. Large-breed dogs (Rottweilers, Labrador Retrievers, Golden Retrievers and others) are predominantly affected, and typically present at the age of 6 to 12 months.

RADIOGRAPHIC FINDINGS Radiographic abnormalities include flattening of the medial (or lateral) trochlear ridge of the talus, widening of the tarsocrural joint space, and intracapsular soft-tissue swelling of the tarsocrural joint (joint effusion). In the case of OCD, an isolated mineralized cartilage flap is visible adjacent to the defect (Fig. 16.19).

Secondary degenerative joint disease develops with increasing age, and is typically severe. If there is clinical suspicion of OC/OCD of the tarsus but standard radiographs are inconclusive, flexed dorsoplantar views, which allow evaluation of the trochlear ridges without superimposition of the calcaneus (see Chapter 15), or advanced imaging (CT), may aid in further evaluation of the joint.

As the disease is commonly bilateral, radiographs of the contralateral tarsus are usually indicated.

16.2 Bone diseases

This chapter will cover some select, interesting diseases and anomalies of the appendicular skeleton, some of which are common and some less so. Additional bone diseases of young animals affecting the spine and head are covered in Chapters 6 and 7.

16.2.1 Congenital dysostoses

There are multiple malformations in this category which may affect individual bones or entire extremities.

Polydactyly

With this condition, an extremity has more toes than normal. These are normally found at the medial aspect of the distal fore or hind limbs ('dewclaws'), are often bilaterally symmetric, and are not usually associated with clinical signs.

Syndactyly

The congenital fusion of two or more toes is also usually an incidental finding. However, if the abnormal conformation results in abnormal weight bearing, affected animals may present with lameness.

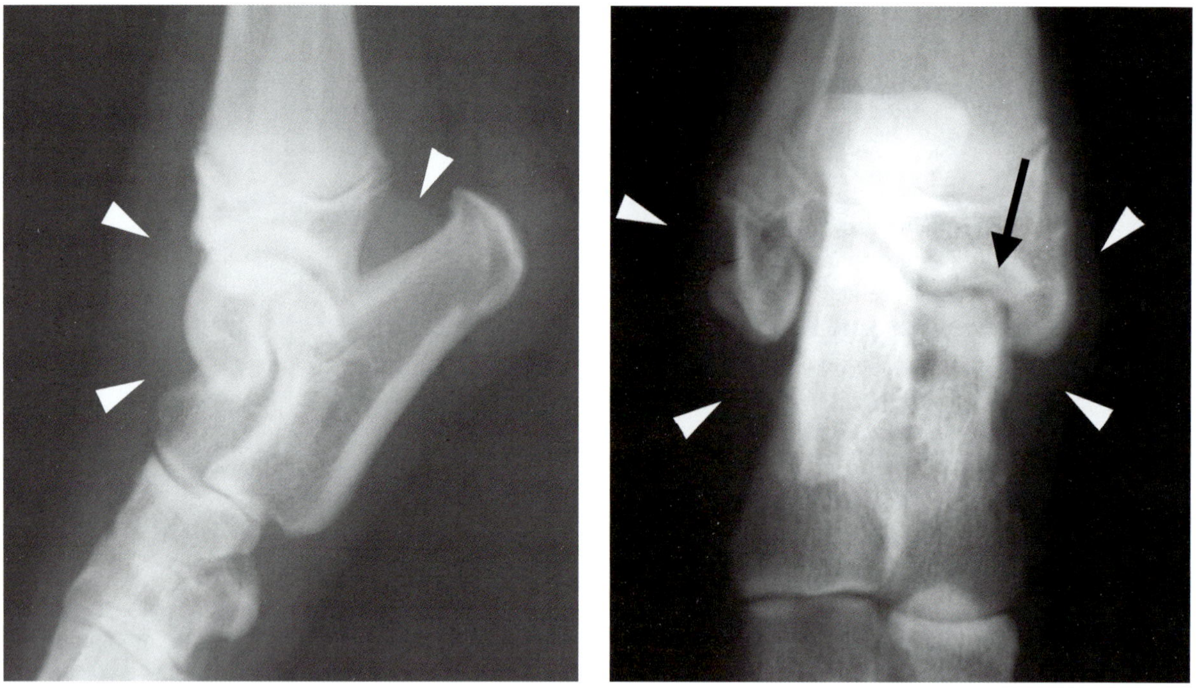

a b

Fig. 16.19 Lateral a and dorsoplantar b radiographs of the tarsus in a dog with OCD. The medial trochlear ridge of the talus is irregularly flattened, resulting in focal widening of the tarsocrural joint. A mineralized bone flap is visible (arrow). Intracapsular soft-tissue swelling is compatible with joint effusion (arrowheads).

Amelia, hemimelia and phocomelia

These conditions describe an absence of osseous structures from the appendicular skeleton.

Amelia is the complete congenital absence of one or more extremities, which must be distinguished from traumatic amputation or injury in utero.

With **phocomelia**, an intercalary segment of a limb is missing, while proximal and distal segments are developed. In extreme cases, the paw is attached directly to the trunk, comparable to a flipper. This condition gained notoriety in the 1950s and 60s when approximately 10,000 children were born with severe malformations after their mothers had taken the drug thalidomide during pregnancy. The disease is rarely reported in veterinary patients.

With **hemimelia**, part of a limb is absent. With **longitudinal hemimelia**, one portion of corresponding extremity segments located at the same level is missing. Radial agenesis is the most common type of longitudinal hemimelia in small animals; it may be unilateral or bilateral, and may result in angular limb deformity (Fig. 16.20). With **transverse hemimelia**, the distal part of an extremity is completely absent.

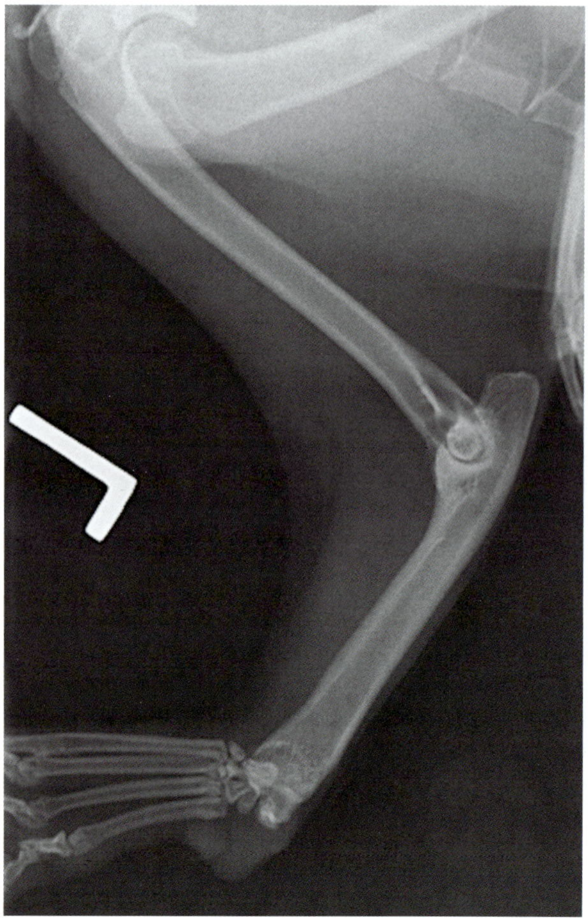

Fig. 16.20 Radiograph of the left forelimb of a cat with congenital agenesis of the radius. The ulna is thickened and shortened secondary to abnormal weight bearing. There is malangulation and soft-tissue swelling of the carpus. Both legs were affected in this patient (L = left).

Ectrodactyly

This anomaly is occasionally seen in small animals and is also termed 'split hand deformity' or 'lobster claw deformity'. The skeleton of the distal antebrachium, carpus and manus develops embryologically from three longitudinal 'rays' which fuse in certain predetermined ways during skeletal development. With ectrodactyly, fusion of the rays does not occur at all, or remains incomplete, resulting in more or less severe splitting of the distal extremity (Fig. 16.21). The carpal bones and digits may be absent or abnormal.

16.2.2 Anomalies in cartilage and bone development

Numerous hereditary, congenital, hormonal, nutritional and developmental anomalies of the skeletal system have been reported in small animals. The most important disorders are briefly covered in this chapter.

Mucopolysaccharidoses (MPS)

This is a group of genetic lysosomal storage diseases which predominantly affect the head and spine. Different subtypes result in musculoskeletal lesions of varying severity.

> RADIOGRAPHIC FINDINGS Depending on the subtype, affected animals may show facial deformities and signs of generalized epiphyseal dysplasia, resulting in growth disturbances and skeletal deformities. Osteopenia, vertebral fusion and spinal cord compression secondary to vertebral remodelling and new bone formation are also possible.

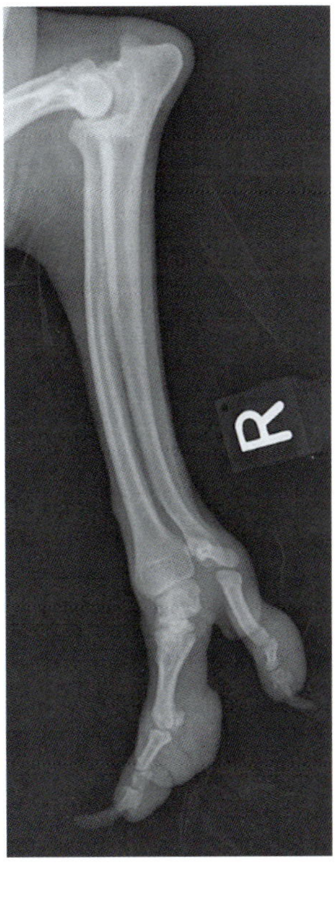

Fig. 16.21 Lateral radiograph of the right distal forelimb in a dog with ectrodactyly. Only a few carpal bones and two digits are present and are abnormal. The two metacarpal bones are separate, resulting in a 'lobster claw' appearance of the distal extremity. Secondary changes include abnormal thickening of the ulna and incongruity and degenerative joint disease of the elbow joint (R = right).

Pituitary dwarfism

This disorder is caused by lack of hypophyseal growth hormone. German Shepherd Dogs are predisposed; however, this disorder is also found in other dog breeds and cats. Affected animals are small, but skeletal anatomy is normal ('proportional dwarfism').

> RADIOGRAPHIC FINDINGS The bones, especially those of the appendicular skeleton, are short. Delayed physeal closure and incomplete ossification of the epiphyses are also possible.

Congenital hypothyroidism

Congenital hypothyroidism is rare but may occur in dogs and cats. Affected animals display disproportionate dwarfism.

> RADIOGRAPHIC FINDINGS In addition to abnormalities of the long bones, incomplete and delayed ossification of the vertebral epiphyses, with shortened and widened vertebral bodies, are also noted (see Chapter 7, Fig. 7.50).

Rickets

This disease of the skeletal system in growing animals results in insufficient mineralization of newly formed osteoid, and is typically caused by nutritional vitamin D deficiency. Other causes include congenital abnormalities of vitamin D metabolism and nutritional calcium/phosphorus imbalances or deficiencies. In older animals this disease is referred to as osteomalacia. Rickets is rare today.

> RADIOGRAPHIC FINDINGS The long bones are osteopenic and show flaring and cupping of the metaphyseal edges ('rachitic rosary'). Secondary angular limb deformities are common.

Nutritional secondary hyperparathyroidism

This disease is also covered in Chapter 7. It occurs in young animals secondary to nutritional excess of phosphorus and/or deficiency in calcium (e.g. with a pure meat diet) causing an increased production of parathyroid hormone and resultant excessive bone resorption.

> RADIOGRAPHIC FINDINGS Affected animals show diffuse osteopenia with cortical thinning (see Chapter 7, Fig. 7.51). Secondary multifocal pathological fractures are common.

Osteogenesis imperfecta

This cover term describes a group of hereditary diseases characterized by a defect in bone production and resultant severe bone fragility. This is rare in small animals, and is radiographically characterized by generalized osteopenia with numerous pathological fractures.

Hereditary osteochondral dysplasias

These are fairly common disorders in dogs and cats characterized by abnormal development of cartilage and/or bone. Examples include epiphyseal dysplasia in Beagles and osteochondrodysplasia in Scottish Fold cats. As numerous different diseases are included in this category, radiographic findings are variable.

Multiple cartilaginous exostoses

These were already discussed in Chapter 7. They are benign proliferative bone lesions of unknown aetiology which may affect vertebrae and/or other bones. They occur in young dogs and cats and are characterized by an initial rapid increase in size. Growth of these lesions ceases with skeletal maturity. Exostoses originate in the metaphyseal region of bones formed by endochondral ossification, but may 'migrate' to the diaphyseal region with progressive bone growth.

Radiographic findings Exostoses appear as rounded or cauliflower-like regions of bone proliferation surrounded by a smooth, thin cortical shell (Fig. 16.22; see also Fig. 7.49).

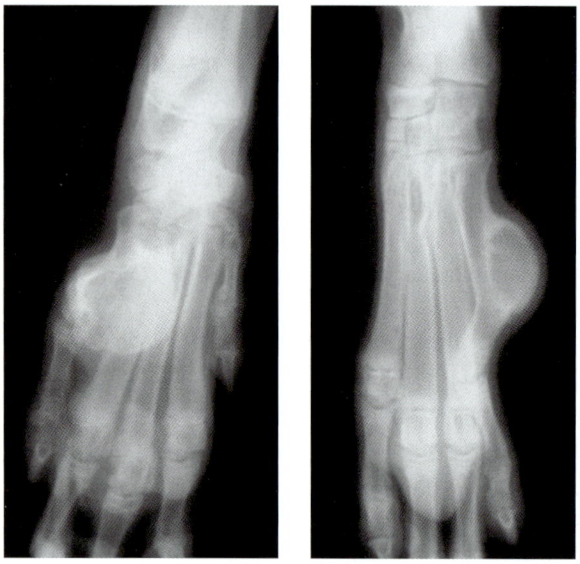

a b

Fig. 16.22 Multiple cartilaginous exostoses in a young dog.

a On the dorsopalmar view of the right carpus and manus a large, smoothly marginated, bony proliferative lesion is noted originating from and deforming the fifth metacarpal bone.

b On the dorsoplantar view of the right tarsus and pes an oval, smoothly marginated, bone opaque mass with a thin shell is associated with the diaphysis of the fifth metatarsus and results in marked deformity of this bone.

Retained cartilaginous core of the distal ulna

This is an occasional finding in young large-breed dogs such as Saint Bernards and Great Danes. The aetiology of this disease is uncertain, but it is believed to be a form of osteochondrosis with a defect in ossification of the distal ulnar physis. This results in a typically cone-shaped cartilaginous region in the distal ulna, which extends from the distal physis into the distal metaphysis.

Radiographic findings The cartilaginous region is less opaque compared with surrounding bone (Fig. 16.23). This anomaly may be an incidental radiographic finding, but may also impair physeal growth and result in angular limb deformity (Fig. 16.24).

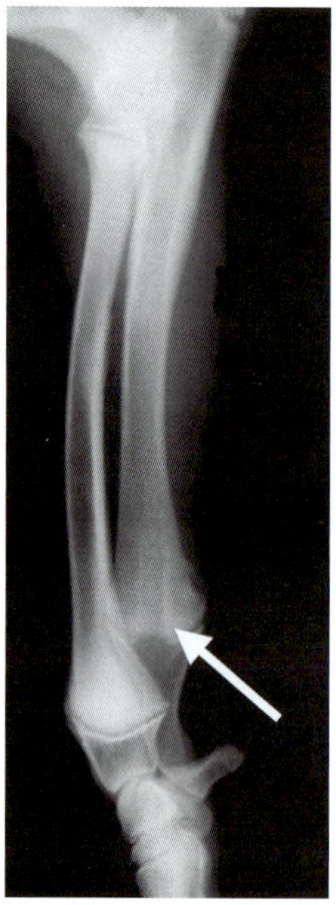

Fig. 16.23 Retained cartilaginous core of the distal ulna in a young dog (incidental finding). This lateral view of the antebrachium shows a cone-shaped region of decreased opacity extending from the distal ulnar physis proximally into the metaphysis (arrow).

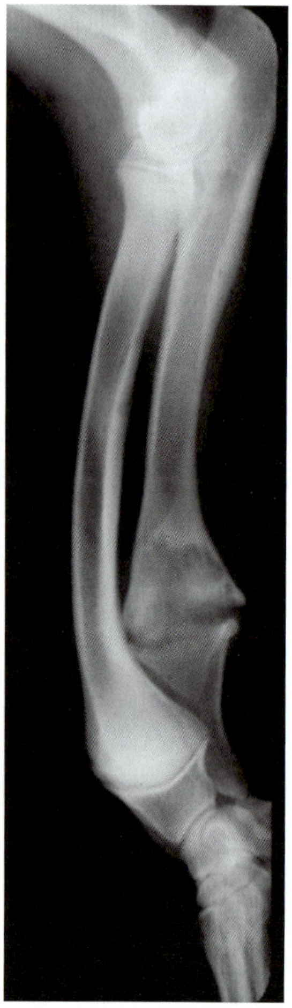

Fig. 16.24 Retained cartilaginous core in the distal ulna in a young dog presented with lameness. The lateral view of the antebrachium shows an extensive, irregularly marginated, radiolucent region in the distal ulna. The ulna is shortened, and there is cranial convex bowing of the radius, indicative of premature physeal closure of the distal ulnar physis secondary to the abnormal cartilaginous area in the distal ulnar metaphysis.

16.2.3 Other bone diseases

(Eosinophilic) panosteitis

This disease is predominantly seen in young dogs (5–18 months), but may occasionally be encountered in older patients. Male medium-sized to large dogs are predominantly affected, with a presumed predisposition in German Shepherd Dogs. Affected animals typically present with shifting lameness and pain upon palpation of the long bones. The disease is usually polyostotic.

RADIOGRAPHIC FINDINGS Initial radiographs may be normal or may show poorly marginated regions of increased opacity associated with the medullary cavities of long bones, mostly associated with the mid diaphysis and resulting in loss of the normal trabecular pattern (Fig. 16.25). Over time, the bone lesions increase in size and opacity and become more sharply delineated, resulting in a patchy appearance of the medullary cavities of affected bones (Fig. 16.26). Smooth periosteal reactions may also be observed in this later stage.

Metaphyseal osteopathy (hypertrophic osteodystrophy, HOD)

This is a disorder of large, fast-growing dogs which usually occurs at 3–5 months of age. Affected animals present with fever, reluctance to move and swollen, painful metaphyses of the long bones. The disease is usually polyostotic.

RADIOGRAPHIC FINDINGS Radiographic abnormalities with this disease are usually bilaterally symmetric. At initial patient presentation radiographs may be normal, but a linear region of decreased opacity, proximal and parallel to the physis of the affected bone ('double physis'), associated with increased opacity (sclerosis) of the adjacent region of the metaphysis, will soon develop (Fig. 16.27; see also Fig. 16.11). In later stages, a cuff or sleeve of periosteal new bone develops adjacent to the metaphyseal cortex, and is separated from the cortex by a thin radiolucent zone. Over time this periosteal sleeve fuses to the cortex, resulting in bony widening of the metaphysis (Fig. 16.28). Soft-tissue swelling adjacent to the abnormal metaphysis is commonly seen. Even though metaphyseal osteopathy is self-limiting, the metaphyseal new bone formation may interfere with normal growth of the adjacent physis, and therefore may result in premature physeal closure and angular limb deformity.

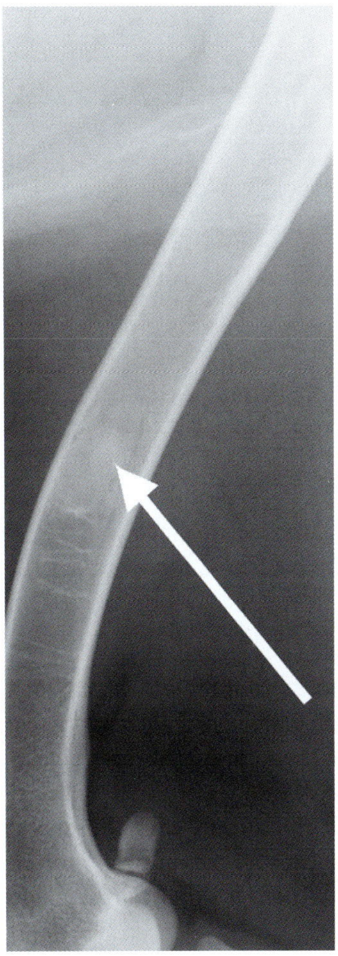

Fig. 16.25 Lateral radiograph of the femur in a dog with panosteitis (early stage). A small, irregularly marginated region of increased opacity is associated with the medullary cavity, in close proximity to the vascular channel (arrow).

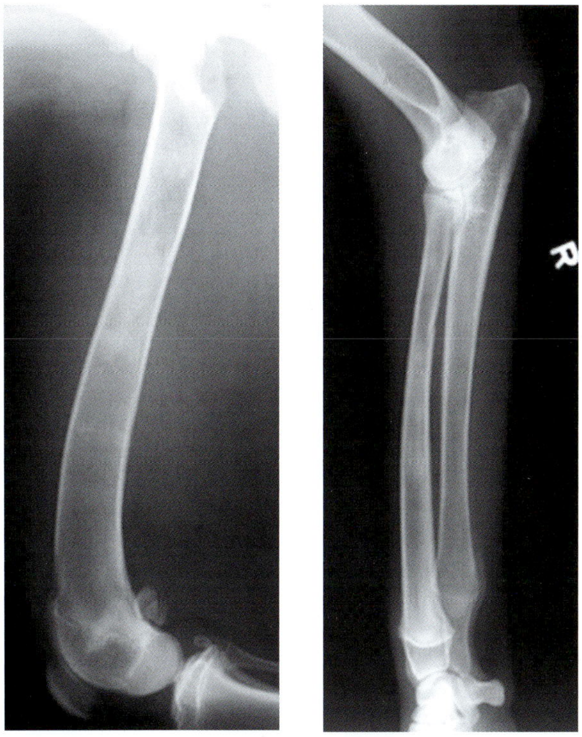

a b

Fig. 16.26 Lateral radiographs of the femur a and antebrachium b in a dog with panosteitis (later stage). There are extensive, sharply marginated regions of increased bone opacity associated with the medullary cavities of the femur and radius (R = right).

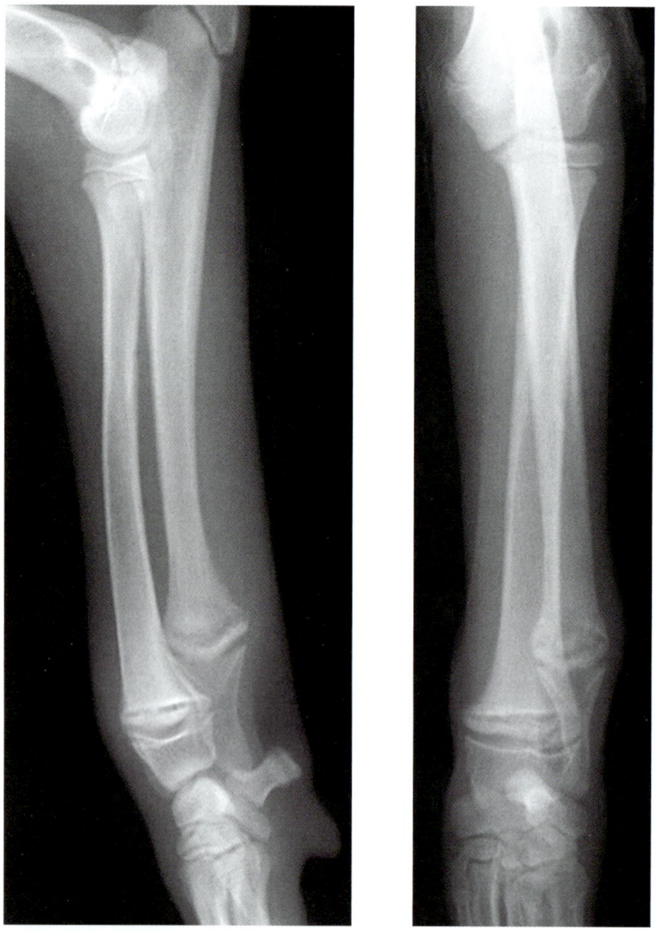

a b

Fig. 16.27 Lateral a and craniocaudal b radiographs of the antebrachium in a young dog with metaphyseal osteopathy (early stage). A metaphyseal linear lucent line with adjacent sclerosis is visible proximal to the distal physis of the radius and ulna ('double physis').

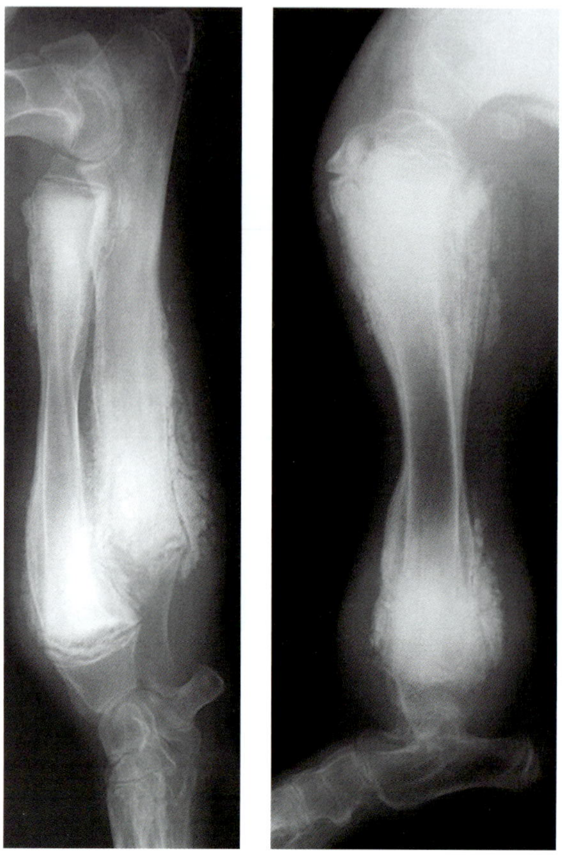

a b

Fig. 16.28 Lateral radiographs of the antebrachium a and crus b in a young dog with advanced metaphyseal osteopathy. There is marked periosteal reaction surrounding the metaphyseal regions of the long bones in a sleeve-like fashion. Thin lucent lines are seen in some areas separating the periosteal proliferation from underlying cortex. There is significant swelling of adjacent soft tissues.

Suggested reading

Craig LE. Physeal dysplasia with slipped capital femoral epiphysis in 13 cats. Vet Pathol 2001; 38: 92–7.

Demko J, McLaughlin R. Developmental orthopedic disease. Vet Clin North Am Small Anim Pract 2005; 35: 1111–35.

Johnson KA, Watson ADJ. Skeletal diseases. In: Ettinger SJ, Feldman EC (eds). Textbook of Veterinary Internal Medicine. Philadelphia: WB Saunders 2000; 1887–916.

Kene ROC, Lee R, Bennett D. The radiological features of congenital elbow luxation/subluxation in the dog. J Small Anim Pract 1982; 23: 621–30.

LaFond E, Breur GJ, Austin CC. Breed susceptibility for developmental orthopedic diseases in dogs. J Am Anim Hosp Assoc 2002; 38(5): 467–77.

Linnmann S. Die Hüftgelenksdysplasie des Hundes. Berlin: Parey 1998.

Mayrhofer E, Koppel E. Schultergelenkdysplasie beim Dachshund. I. Klinik und Röntgenbefunde. Zentralblatt für Veterinärmedizin A 1985; 32: 202–13.

Moores AP, Owen MR, Fews D, Coe RJ, Brown PJ, Butterworth SJ. Slipped capital femoral epiphysis in dogs. J Small Anim Pract 2004; 45: 602–8.

Morgan JP. Radiology of Veterinary Orthopedics. Napa, CA: Venture Press 1999.

Morgan JP, Wind A, Davidson AP. Hereditary Bone and Joint Diseases in the Dog. Hannover: Schlütersche 2000.

Owens JM, Biery DN. Radiographic Interpretation for the Small Animal Clinician. Baltimore: Williams & Wilkins 1999.

Pedersen NC, Morgan JP, Vasseur PB. Joint diseases of dogs and cats. In: Ettinger SJ, Feldman EC (eds). Textbook of Veterinary Internal Medicine. Philadelphia: WB Saunders 2000; 1862–86.

Piermattei DL, Flo GL (eds). Handbook of Small Animal Orthopedics and Fracture Repair. Philadelphia: WB Saunders 1997.

Wisner ER, Pollard RE. Orthopedic diseases of young and growing dogs and cats. In: Thrall DE (ed). Textbook of Veterinary Diagnostic Radiology, 5th edn. Philadelphia: WB Saunders 2007; 268–83.

17

Acquired bone and joint diseases

Federica Morandi, Silke Hecht and Gregory B. Daniel

17.1 Degenerative joint disease

Degenerative disease of synovial joints is characterized by damage to the joint cartilage, followed by a complex process of destructive and restorative mechanisms within the cartilage, the adjacent bone and the joint capsule. This condition is also referred to as 'arthrosis'. Even though the term 'arthritis' is frequently applied to degenerative changes of a joint, it is better avoided due to possible confusion with inflammatory and infectious disease processes. Degenerative joint disease affecting one or multiple joints is extremely common in small animals. Even though animals of any breed and age may be affected, older and large-breed patients are predisposed. Degenerative joint disease may occur as a primary problem as part of the physiological ageing process; however, in most cases it develops secondary to other factors such as trauma, joint instability or inflammation.

RADIOGRAPHIC FINDINGS Changes vary with the duration and severity of the disease process.

- **Intracapsular soft-tissue swelling** is the predominant radiographic feature during the acute stage (Fig. 17.1). In severe cases, joint effusion may even result in joint space widening. With increasing duration of the disease process, the joint space becomes narrowed or may even collapse secondary to destruction of the joint cartilage (Fig. 17.2). Intracapsular soft-tissue swelling persists with chronic degenerative joint disease due to persistent joint effusion and synovial proliferation (see Fig. 15.27b).
- The attempted repair processes result in **excessive cartilage proliferation** in non-weight-bearing areas of the joint, i.e. especially at the periphery of the joint surface. This newly formed cartilage outgrows its nutritional supply and dies off, followed by metaplastic ossification of cartilage fragments. This results in radiographically visible periarticular new bone formation (**osteophytosis**; Fig. 17.3). Osteophytes also frequently develop at the insertion site of the joint capsule.
- The subchondral bone plate of joints affected by degenerative joint disease undergoes hypertrophy of the trabecular bone, resulting in more or less extensive regions of increased bone opacity (**subchondral sclerosis, eburnation**). This is most severe in regions of the joint where extensive cartilage loss results in direct bone-to-bone contact. Irregular lucent regions within the subchondral bone plate may occur secondary to bone necrosis. Subchondral lucent regions may also be caused by ingrowth of proliferative synovium into the subchondral bone plate. These lesions typically have smooth margins and resemble bone cysts. They are frequently referred to as 'subchondral bone cysts', or better as **'osseous cyst-like lesions'**.
- The chronic disease process may result in **dystrophic mineralization of the joint capsule and ligaments**. New bone formation at the insertion site of joint capsule and ligaments (**enthesophytosis**) is common.
- Free bone fragments within the joint space are often referred to as **'joint mice'**. These may represent isolated osteophytes, fragmented mineralized cartilage segments, small fracture fragments or osteochondritis dissecans (OCD) lesions.

17.2 Inflammatory bone and joint diseases

17.2.1 Inflammatory bone diseases

Bone infection (osteomyelitis) can be caused by different pathogens including bacteria and, in endemic areas, fungal organisms.

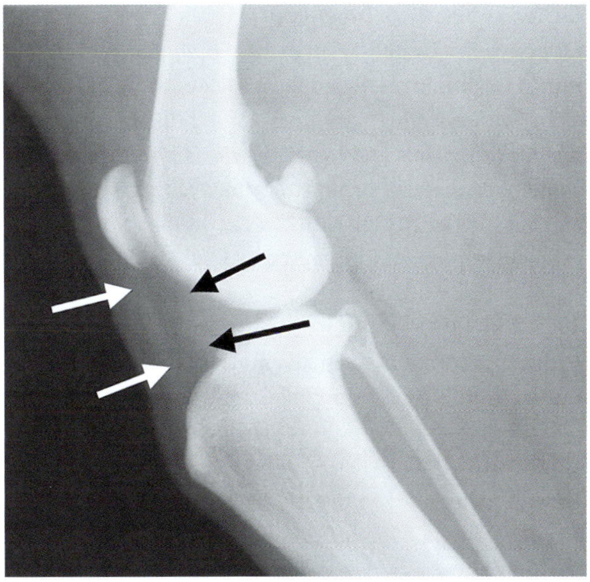

Fig. 17.1 Intracapsular soft-tissue swelling in a dog with rupture of the cranial cruciate ligament. The infrapatellar fat pad, bordered by the patellar ligament cranially (white arrows) and the margin of the femorotibial joint caudally (black arrows), is cranially displaced due to joint effusion and/or synovial thickening. Soft-tissue swelling predominates in the early stages of degenerative joint disease; osseous changes develop later.

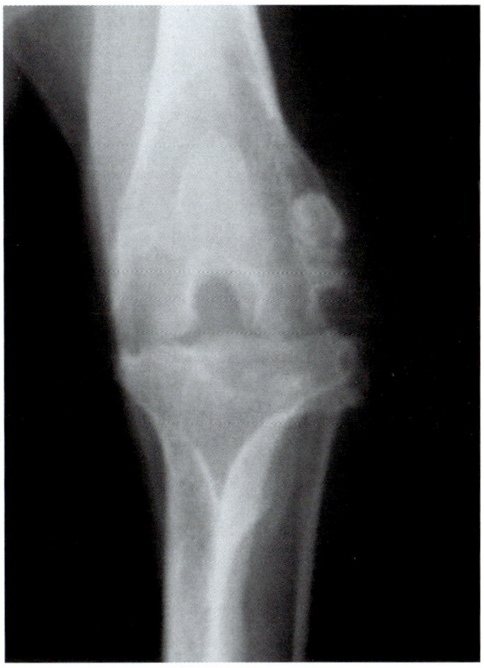

Fig. 17.2 Joint space collapse in a dog due to extensive cartilage erosion. This radiographic diagnosis is often difficult as extremity radiographs in small animals are typically non-weight-bearing (i.e. not obtained in standing animals). Additionally, oblique positioning can mimic joint space narrowing.

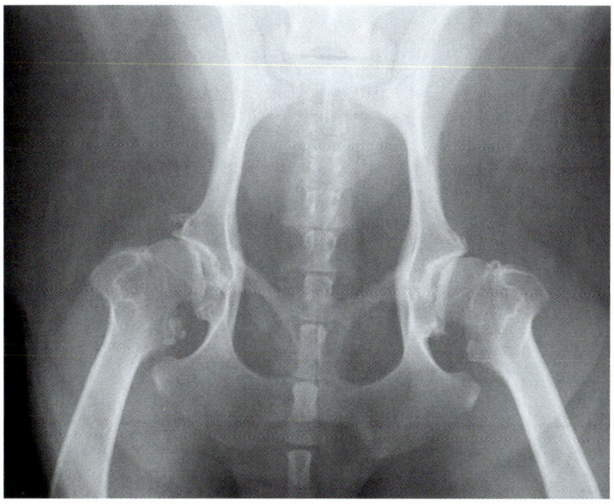

Fig. 17.3 Severe bilateral degenerative joint disease of the coxofemoral joints in a dog. Extensive periarticular osteophytosis is noted along the periphery of the femoral heads, along the femoral necks and along the acetabular margins. Note also inadequate femoral head coverage due to shallow conformation of the acetabulum.

Bacterial osteomyelitis

A bacterial bone infection can affect animals of any age and breed. Haematogenous osteomyelitis is most common in young and immunocompromised patients and is often polyostotic. Infection in older animals typically occurs via direct extension from contaminated wounds or wounds with foreign body inclusions, via open fractures, or following surgical procedures. Multiple aetiological agents are possible, and often more than one organism is involved in the process. *Staphylococcus*, *Streptococcus* and gram-negative bacteria such as *Escherichia coli*, *Pseudomonas* or *Klebsiella* are examples of bacteria commonly involved in osteomyelitis in small animals. *Actinomyces*, *Brucella* and *Nocardia* are examples of less common causative agents of bacterial osteomyelitis.

RADIOGRAPHIC FINDINGS The predominant finding in the early stages of the disease is soft-tissue swelling adjacent to the affected bone. Bony changes develop over time. Infection with gas-producing bacteria may result in gas opaque foci in the soft tissues (see Chapter 15, Fig. 15.25).

After 7–14 days, periosteal reaction develops, which in the case of an underlying fracture may be difficult to distinguish from bony callus. However, in contrast to physiological callus, periosteal reaction due to osteomyelitis will rapidly progress and extend beyond the margin of the fracture or implant, often involving the entire circumference and/or length of the affected bone (Fig. 17.4; see also Fig. 15.39). The infection often remains limited to one bone, unless extensive soft-tissue infection results in spread. If metallic implants are present there is often evidence of implant failure / loosening, with areas of radiolucency surrounding the devices. In addition to early periosteal proliferation, more or less extensive bone lysis may develop over time.

A possible sequela of bacterial osteomyelitis is a compromised blood supply to the outer cortex, which may result in loss of viability of a bone fragment. This **sequestrum** appears as a sharply marginated bone fragment within a corresponding lucent defect in the adjacent cortex (**involucrum**). A sequestrum is most commonly seen secondary to an injury with extensive soft-tissue damage, resulting in a compromised vascular supply to the underlying bone.

Haematogenous osteomyelitis is most commonly seen in young animals, predominantly affects the metaphyseal regions of long bones, and is polyostotic.

Mycotic osteomyelitis

This condition is rare in Europe but common in other regions of the world (especially the US) and may be seen anywhere in imported animals, or animals with a travel history. Young dogs and middle-aged dogs are most commonly affected. Mycotic osteomyelitis can be caused by a variety of agents, with *Coccidioides*, *Blastomyces* and *Cryptococcus* playing the most important roles. Mycotic osteomyelitis occurs secondary to a systemic infection and is often polyostotic due to haematogenous spread. The metaphyses of long bones are most commonly affected, but infection of any area is possible. Extension into joints or adjacent bones is also possible.

RADIOGRAPHIC FINDINGS The appearance of mycotic osteomyelitis is variable. Typical findings include mixed osteolytic / osteoproliferative semi-aggressive to aggressive lesions which may resemble bone tumours (Fig. 17.5).

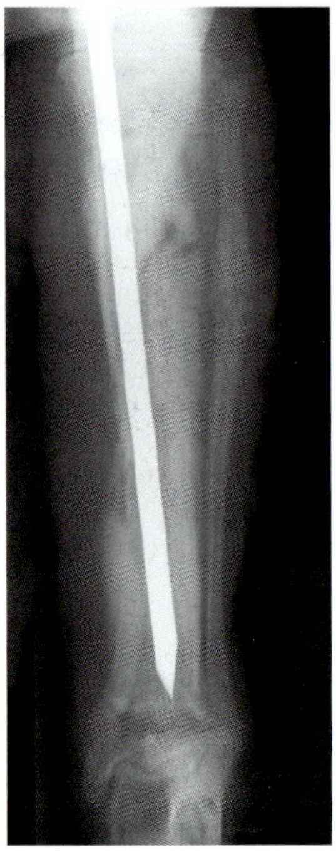

Fig. 17.4 Bacterial osteomyelitis following surgical repair of a diaphyseal tibia and fibula fracture. The predominant radiographic finding is extensive irregular periosteal proliferation extending well beyond the region of the fracture and involving nearly the entire length of the affected bone. The fracture line is clearly recognized.

Other types of osteomyelitis

Osteomyelitis caused by other aetiological agents is rather rare in small animals. Examples of protozoal agents which, along with systemic signs, may cause bone inflammation include *Leishmania* and *Hepatozoon*. It is hypothesized that some bone diseases of undetermined aetiology in young animals such as metaphyseal osteopathy (aka hypertrophic osteodystrophy) may be caused by viral infections.

17.2.2 Inflammatory joint diseases

Arthritis is common in small animal patients and may be caused by infectious or noninfectious causes.

Infectious arthritis

As with bacterial osteomyelitis, **bacterial or septic** arthritis can develop via haematogenous spread and infection of (possibly already damaged) joints, or via direct contamination (penetrating wound, iatrogenic). Depending on the underlying cause, the infection may be limited to one joint or be multifocal.

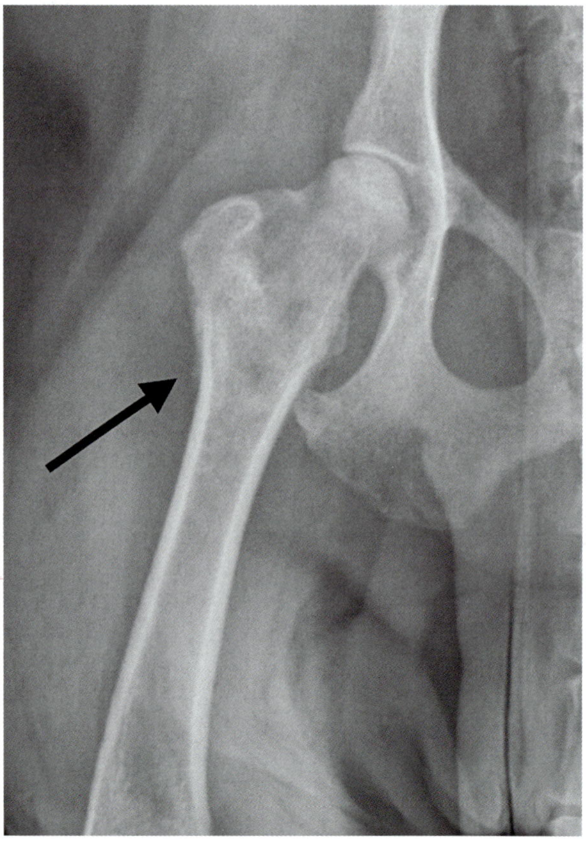

Fig. 17.5 Mycotic osteomyelitis (blastomycosis) in a dog. The proximal femur has a mixed lytic/proliferative lesion (arrow) which cannot be radiographically distinguished from a primary bone tumour.

Radiographic findings Intracapsular soft-tissue swelling predominates initially and may be accompanied by intra-articular gas accumulations. Subsequent bone changes are predominantly lytic and affect all adjacent joint surfaces (Fig. 17.6). Even though the bony changes may initially resemble abnormalities seen with degenerative joint disease, the subchondral bone erosions are more severe and rapidly progressive in cases of septic arthritis. In chronic cases, periosteal reaction and osteophytosis develop, consistent with degenerative joint disease.

Mycotic arthritis is comparatively rare and usually develops secondary to the extension of adjacent osteomyelitis.

Radiographic findings Fungal infection of a joint results in an extremely aggressive, destructive process with complete or near-complete lysis of bony structures (Fig. 17.7).

Other agents which may result in infectious arthritis in small animals include *Borrelia*, *Mycoplasma*, *Rickettsia*, *Ehrlichia*, protozoa and possibly viruses. Radiographic abnormalities seen in these diseases are poorly documented, and a diagnosis is usually established by other means.

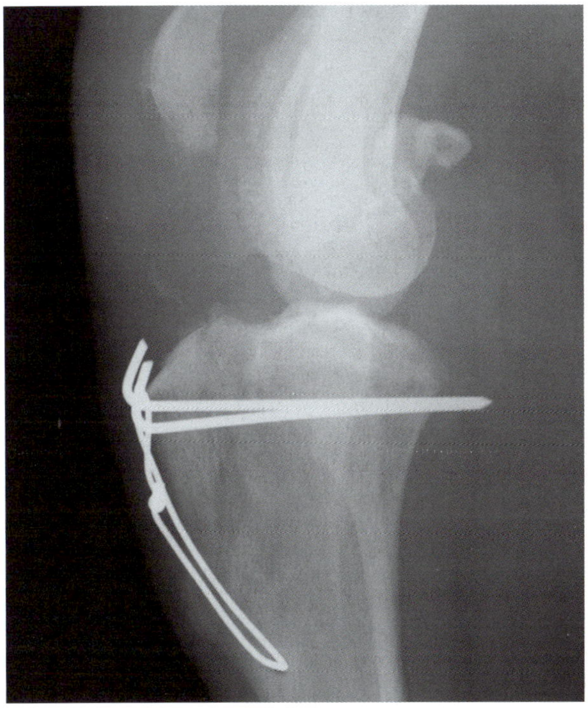

Fig. 17.6 Septic (bacterial) arthritis of the stifle joint in a dog following surgical correction of patellar luxation. Radiographic findings include severe intra- and extracapsular soft-tissue swelling, multifocal lytic regions associated with the patella and femoral trochlea, and irregular faint periosteal reaction associated with the patella. The orthopaedic implants appear stable at this point.

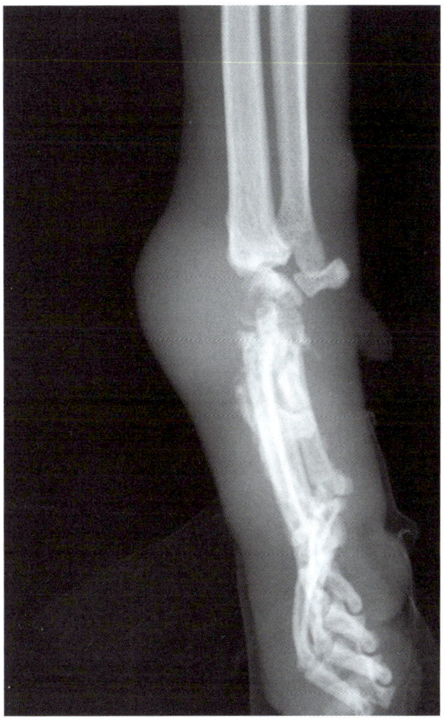

a

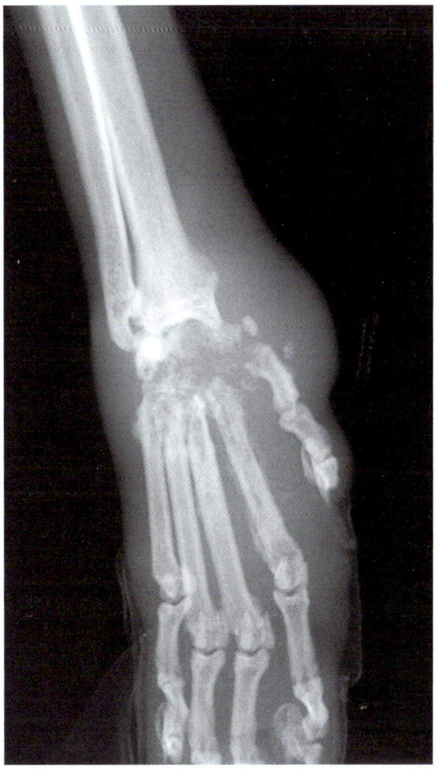

b

Fig. 17.7 Mycotic arthritis (blastomycosis) in a cat. The lateral a and dorsopalmar b views show severe intra- and extracapsular soft-tissue swelling as well as advanced destruction of multiple carpal bones and the proximal metacarpals. Note superimposed bandage material used for positioning.

Noninfectious arthritis

While immune-mediated arthritis plays an important role in veterinary medicine, other noninfectious joint diseases commonly seen in humans (e.g. gout) are not a factor in small animal medicine. Many types of immune-mediated arthritis are reported in small animals.

NONEROSIVE ARTHRITIS

Nonerosive arthritis can occur in dogs and cats and is characterized by lack of osseous changes, even in chronic cases. It may be associated with infectious diseases (such as endocarditis or discospondylitis) or other immune-mediated diseases such as lupus erythematosus; it may be a side effect of specific medications (e.g. trimethoprim–sulphonamide, penicillin and other antibiotics); or it may be idiopathic. Nonerosive arthritis may be limited to one joint or manifest as oligoarthritis or polyarthritis.

RADIOGRAPHIC FINDINGS Intracapsular soft-tissue swelling is usually the only radiographic abnormality, and a diagnosis must be established by other means.

Periosteal proliferative arthritis has been reported in cats as a subtype of the feline chronic progressive polyarthritides. This disease affects male cats between 1.5 and 4.5 years old and is believed to be associated with infection with feline syncytia-forming virus (FeSFV). This disease primarily affects carpal and tarsal joints.

RADIOGRAPHIC FINDINGS Affected joints are initially characterized by osteopenia followed by extensive periosteal new bone production, which may result in complete joint ankylosis. Carpal and/or tarsal subluxation is also possible.

EROSIVE ARTHRITIS

These joint diseases are characterized by destruction of the articular surfaces of affected joints. The most important type of erosive arthritis in dogs is probably **rheumatoid arthritis**, which is predominantly seen in small-breed dogs ranging from 1 to 9 years of age (average age 4–5 years). Poodles and Shelties are predisposed. The carpal and tarsal joints are predominantly affected; however, the disease can involve any joint.

RADIOGRAPHIC FINDINGS As abnormalities are usually bilaterally symmetric, radiographs of both carpi and tarsi, as well as other affected joints, are usually indicated if rheumatoid polyarthritis is suspected. The initial predominant radiographic finding is intracapsular soft-tissue swelling. Bone changes do not develop until later in the disease process. Thus, in the early stages, rheumatoid arthritis cannot be distinguished radiographically from other arthritides. With increasing chronicity, cyst-like subchondral regions develop along the attachment sites of the joint capsule and along joint surfaces. These focal lytic regions become confluent to form extensive erosive regions, with progressive destruction of the joint surfaces. Loss of the joint cartilage results in joint space collapse. With destruction of ligaments, subluxation or even luxation of joints may be noted (Fig. 17.8).

An erosive polyarthritis has been reported in cats as a rare variant of the aforementioned feline chronic progressive polyarthritis.

17.3 Neoplastic bone and joint diseases

Numerous types of neoplasia affecting the skeletal system have been reported in small animals. These include

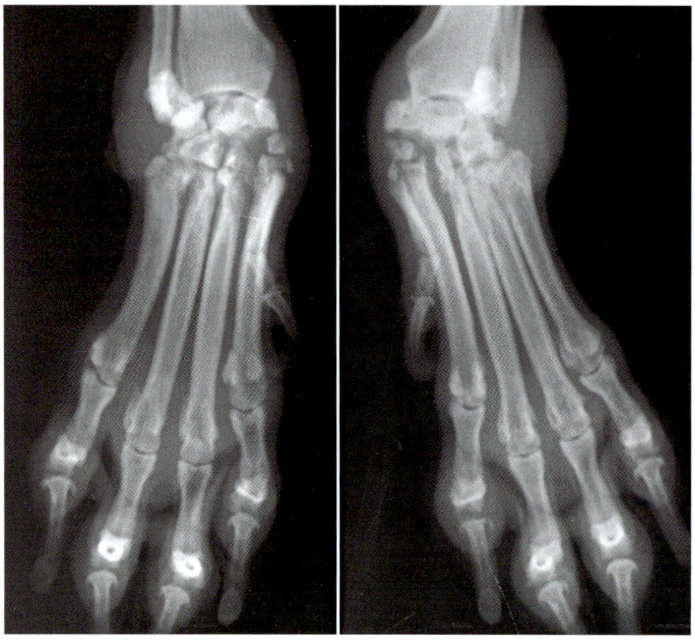

Fig. 17.8 Erosive (rheumatoid) polyarthritis in a dog. The dorsopalmar views of both carpal joints show bilaterally symmetric severe extra- and intracapsular soft-tissue swelling and multifocal irregularly marginated lytic lesions extending from the joint spaces into adjacent carpal and metacarpal bones. There is secondary subluxation and valgus deformity of the carpus bilaterally.

tumours originating primarily from bones or joints and tumours extending into bone from adjacent tissues. Neoplastic bone and joint diseases are more common in dogs, but cats may also be affected. This chapter will cover the most important and common tumour types.

17.3.1 Primary bone tumours

Osteosarcoma

This is the most common primary bone tumour. Older large- and giant-breed dogs are most commonly affected; however, these tumours may also be found in other dog breeds, cats and younger animals.

RADIOGRAPHIC FINDINGS Osteosarcoma generally manifests as a solitary, aggressive bone lesion which predominantly affects the metaphysis of long bones (proximal humerus, distal radius, proximal tibia, distal femur etc.) (Fig. 17.9; see also Fig. 15.37a).

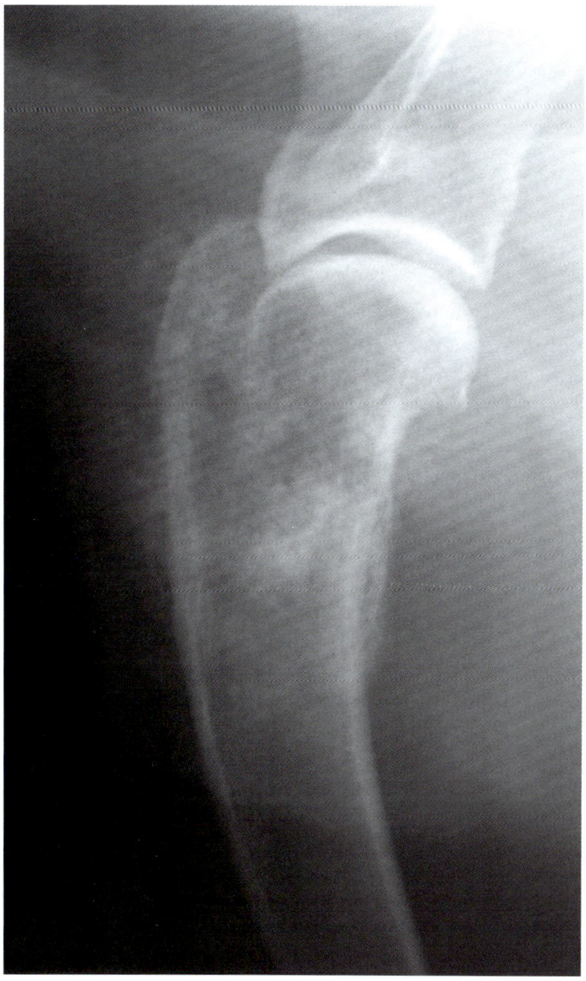

Fig. 17.9 Primary bone tumour (osteosarcoma). An extensive, aggressive, mixed osteolytic and osteoproliferative lesion is associated with the proximal humerus.

Osteosarcomas are most commonly spontaneous tumours. In rare cases, prior surgical intervention may cause development of a bone tumour, typically 5–7 years following the procedure (**implant-associated sarcoma**; Fig. 17.10). A primary bone tumour may be primarily osteoblastic, osteoclastic or mixed. In contrast to other aggressive bone lesions, osteosarcomas remain limited to the bone of origin and do not cross either joint spaces or open physes in young animals. Adjacent soft-tissue swelling is common. Affected bones are predisposed to pathological fractures (Fig. 17.11).

Note: If an older animal presents with a spontaneous fracture without trauma history, or following minor trauma, the radiograph should be carefully evaluated to determine if an underlying aggressive bone lesion is present.

Parosteal osteosarcomas are a special type of osteosarcoma rarely seen in small animals. These tumours originate from the bone surface rather than the medullary cavity and appear radiographically rather benign, with homogeneous radiographic opacity and a rounded or lobulated surface.

Other primary bone tumours

Chondrosarcoma, **haemangiosarcoma** and **fibrosarcoma** cause similar radiographic changes to an osteosarcoma and cannot be distinguished radiographically, requiring bone biopsy and histopathology for definitive diagnosis. **Squamous cell carcinoma** and **melanoma** are relatively common tumours of the phalanges and are characterized by very aggressive behaviour.

17.3.2 Secondary bone tumours

Bone metastases may occur secondary to numerous neoplastic diseases. Epithelial tumours (**carcinomas**) tend to metastasize to bone more commonly than mesenchymal neoplasms (**sarcomas**). Some tumours have a predilection for metastasizing to adjacent osseous structures (e.g. prostatic carcinoma or transitional cell carcinoma of the urinary bladder with metastasis to the caudal lumbar vertebrae, sacrum and pelvis; see Chapter 7, Fig. 7.47), while other tumours may spread haematogenously throughout the entire skeletal system.

RADIOGRAPHIC FINDINGS Multifocal lytic, proliferative and/or mixed lytic and proliferative lesions are found associated with skeletal structures. These lesions are usually small and less conspicuous than primary bone tumours at the time of diagnosis (Fig. 17.12). When affecting long bones, metastases are predominantly found in the region of the vascular channels. A special type of bone metastasis is seen secondary to bronchogenic carcinomas in cats, which metastasize predominantly to the phalanges ('lung digit syndrome').

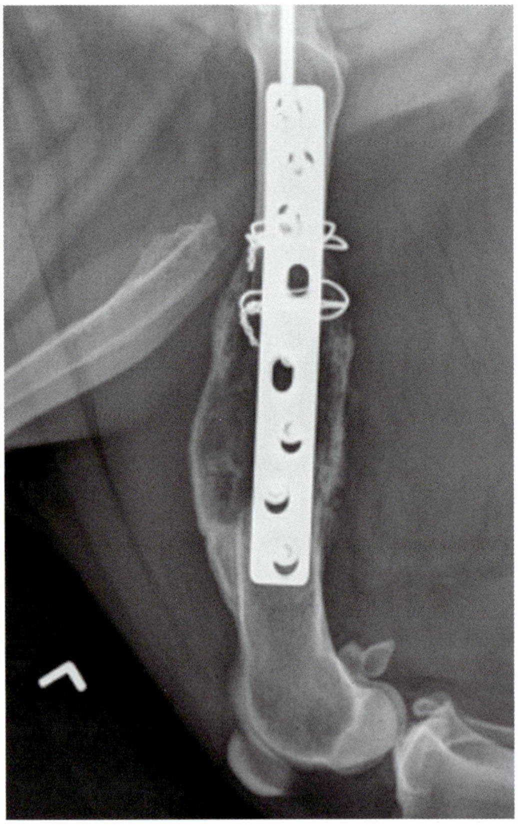

Fig. 17.10 Implant-associated sarcoma following surgical repair of a diaphyseal femoral fracture. The aggressive lesion involves nearly two-thirds of the length of the femur (L = left).

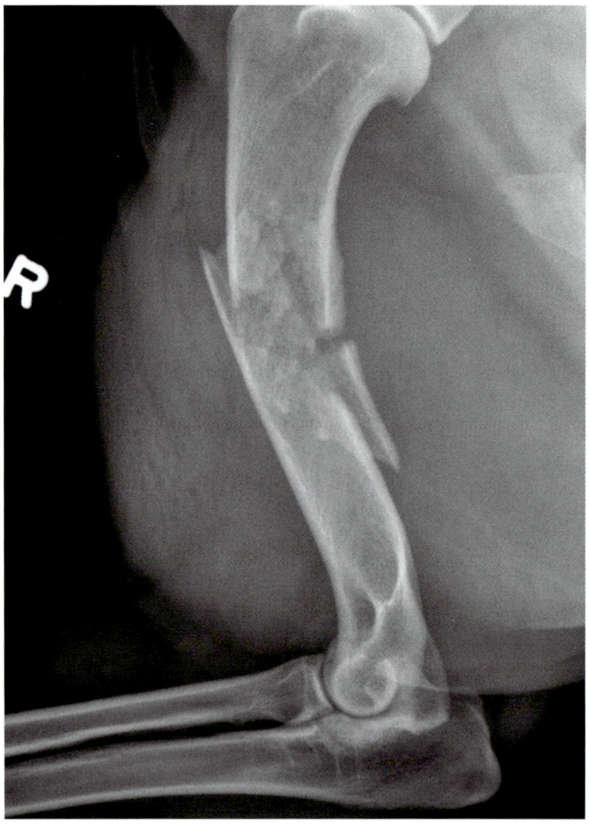

Fig. 17.11 Pathological fracture of the mid-diaphysis of the humerus secondary to an underlying aggressive bone lesion (osteosarcoma). Radiographic findings in addition to the comminuted fracture include heterogeneity of the medullary cavity and faint irregular periosteal new bone formation. The adjacent soft tissues are severely swollen.

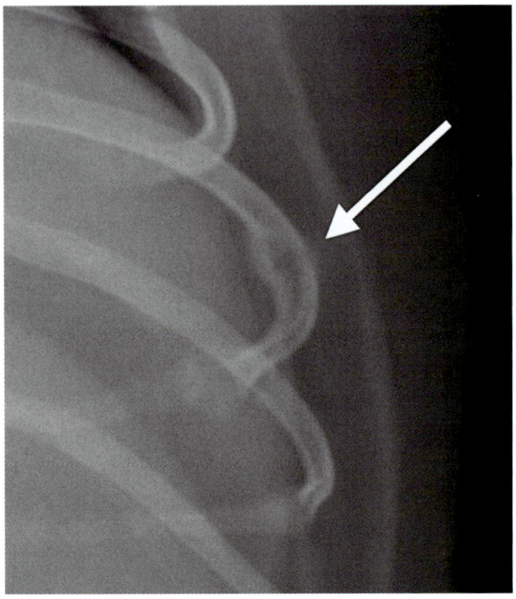

Fig. 17.12 Bone metastasis in a rib of a dog with prostatic carcinoma. There is a small, mixed lytic and proliferative lesion associated with the affected rib (arrow). This dog also had metastases to lumbar vertebrae and the pelvis.

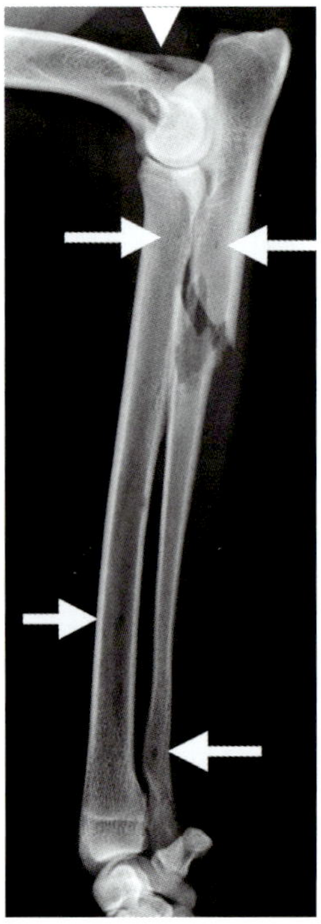

Fig. 17.13 Multiple myeloma and pathological ulnar fracture in a dog. In addition to the oval, smoothly marginated and relatively large lytic lesion in the proximal ulnar diaphysis with pathological fracture, numerous small punctate lytic lesions are found in humerus, radius and ulna (arrows).

17.3.3 Other tumours and tumour-like lesions

Multilobular tumour of bone (multilobular osteochondrosarcoma)

This rare tumour of the skull is characterized by osteoproliferative behaviour. It is of coarse, granular bone opacity and has relatively smooth margins (see Chapter 6, Fig. 6.27).

Round cell neoplasms

These are relatively rare causes of aggressive bone lesions in small animals. Osseous **lymphoma** is predominantly diagnosed in young animals. Radiographic changes include multifocal lytic regions (often permeative), as a result of direct neoplastic infiltration of bone marrow and/or secretion of bone resorbing factors (e.g. parathyroid hormone-related protein, PTHrp). **Disseminated histiocytic sarcoma** can also occasionally result in aggressive bone lesions. Plasma cell tumours may result in solitary (**solitary plasmacytoma**) or multiple lytic bone lesions (**multiple myeloma**; Fig. 17.13).

Benign bone tumours

These are rare in small animals. **Osteomas** appear as well-circumscribed bony proliferative lesions of fairly homogeneous bone opacity.

Multiple cartilaginous exostoses

These are benign proliferative bone lesions of unknown aetiology, which may affect vertebrae and/or other osseous structures. These occur in young dogs and cats and are characterized by initial rapid growth. Growth ceases with skeletal maturity. Exostoses originate in the metaphysis of bones formed by endochondral ossification, but may become located in the diaphyseal region with longitudinal bone growth.

RADIOGRAPHIC FINDINGS Multiple cartilaginous exostoses appear as rounded or cauliflower-like bony proliferative lesions which are surrounded by a smooth, thin cortical shell (see Fig. 7.49 and Fig. 16.22).

Tumours originating from neighbouring structures

Fibrosarcoma, **haemangiosarcoma** and other soft-tissue tumours can involve adjacent bones. In most cases the majority of the lesion/mass is located in soft tissues, and bony changes are seen associated with osseous structures bordering the lesion. In contrast to primary bone tumours, multiple bones may be affected. A typical example is feline vaccine-associated sarcoma in the subcutaneous tissues of the craniodorsal thorax, which may affect multiple adjacent thoracic vertebrae.

Bone cysts

These are rare benign lesions in small animals which are of clinical importance as they may mimic aggressive lytic processes.

RADIOGRAPHIC FINDINGS Bone cysts appear as well-circumscribed, usually round regions of radiolucency, which may be surrounded by a sclerotic rim. **Aneurysmal bone cysts** are a special type. These lesions manifest as sponge-like multicavitary regions of lucency within the affected bone, are filled with blood, and are believed to potentially represent arteriovenous malformations. Even though these lesions are benign, malignant transformation is possible.

17.3.4 Joint-associated tumours

Joint tumours are rare in dogs and almost never seen in cats. Despite information perpetuated throughout many textbooks, **synovial cell sarcomas** only constitute a relatively small percentage of joint tumours in dogs. The most common tumour type is **histiocytic sarcoma** followed by benign **myxomas**. As with many other diseases of the musculoskeletal system, a definitive diagnosis requires biopsy and histopathology.

RADIOGRAPHIC FINDINGS In the early stages, intracapsular soft-tissue swelling of the affected joint is the predominant radiographic finding. With increasing size of the neoplastic lesion, swelling extends beyond the normal dimensions of the joint cavity, and the tumour results in extensive multifocal lysis of the osseous joint surfaces (Fig. 17.14).

17.4 Fractures and luxations

17.4.1 Fractures

Fractures can be categorized in different ways. Important criteria when evaluating a fracture and planning therapeutic intervention include the following.

- **Aetiology**: Trauma, stress fracture, pathological fracture.
- **Location**: Affected bone(s) and affected bone region (diaphysis, metaphysis, physis, epiphysis, apophysis), joint involvement (articular or nonarticular fracture), physeal involvement in young animals (Salter–Harris classification).
- **Degree**: Complete or partial (e.g. greenstick fracture, fissure).
- **Communication with the external environment**: Open or closed fracture.
- **Type**: Simple (transverse, oblique or spiral fracture) or complex (comminuted fracture, segmental fracture); special types: compression fracture, avulsion fracture.
- **Presence** and **degree of dislocation**.
- **Chronicity**: Acute versus chronic fracture.

Details of fracture diagnosis, evaluation of fracture healing and complications are covered in Chapter 18.

17.4.2 Luxations

The dislocation of bones forming a joint is described as **subluxation** (decreased contact of joint surfaces) or **luxation** (complete loss of normal articulation of adjacent joint surfaces). This can be a congenital or developmental condition (joint incongruity such as seen with hip dysplasia or elbow dysplasia; see Chapter 16), or may be traumatic in aetiology. Possible concurrent findings with traumatic (sub)luxation include (bony) avulsion of adjacent ligamentous structures and associated fractures (e.g. fracture of the acetabular margin with luxation of the coxofemoral joint).

Chronic luxation of a joint can result in the formation of a new articulation (**'pseudoarthrosis'**). Chronic subluxation typically results in the development of significant secondary degenerative joint disease.

17.5 Other acquired conditions of the musculoskeletal system

17.5.1 Hypertrophic osteopathy

This is an interesting and unusual disease seen predominantly in older animals, which occurs secondary to intrathoracic and less commonly intra-abdominal (space-occupying) disease processes. It has been reported in association with primary and secondary lung tumours, megaoesophagus and right–left shunt, among other disorders. The aetiology remains undetermined. Possible factors include hormonal imbalances (hyperoestrogenism), neural causes and hypoxia.

RADIOGRAPHIC FINDINGS Affected animals present with bilaterally symmetric periosteal new bone formation, typically affecting both fore and hind limbs. New bone formation is seen along the abaxial margins of digits and metacarpal/metatarsal bones, and successively progresses proximally. The diaphyses are predominantly affected, and the periosteal reaction has a classic pali-

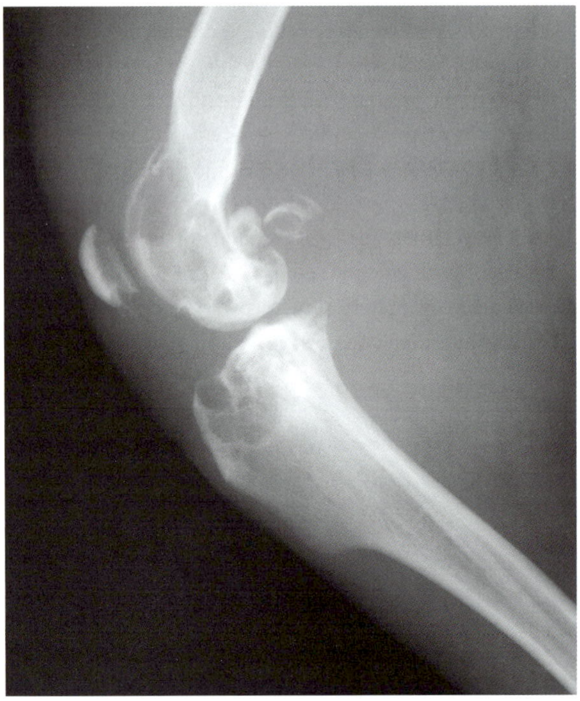

Fig. 17.14 Tumour of the stifle joint in a dog. Severe swelling of the joint extends beyond the margins of the normal joint capsule. Multiple regions of moth-eaten lysis are found in the adjacent bones (femur, tibia, patella and at least one of the sesamoid bones of the gastrocnemius muscle). Surgical biopsy and histopathology yielded a diagnosis of synovial cell sarcoma.

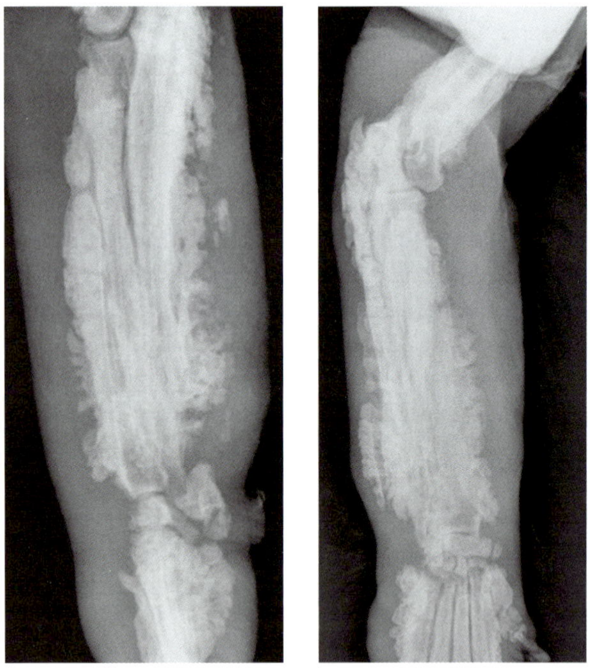

a b

Fig. 17.15 Lateral a and craniocaudal/dorsopalmar b radiographs of the right distal forelimb in a dog with advanced hypertrophic osteopathy. There is polyostotic palisading/columnar periosteal new bone formation and severe associated soft-tissue swelling. Note primary involvement of the diaphyseal regions and sparing of the small carpal bones. All four legs were similarly affected in this dog, and periosteal reaction was documented to extend proximally to the scapula and femur, respectively. Subsequent thoracic radiographs showed numerous pulmonary nodules (metastases).

sading/columnar appearance, with osseous columns forming perpendicularly to the underlying cortices (Fig. 17.15). The small carpal and tarsal bones are usually spared. Bony destruction and medullary changes are not seen with this condition.

17.5.2 Diseases of soft tissues

A radiographic examination often plays only a minor role in the evaluation of soft-tissue lesions of the musculoskeletal system, as advanced imaging techniques (CT, MRI and ultrasound) are superior for soft-tissue evaluation. However, especially with traumatic and chronic processes, radiographs can provide important information. For example, osseous fragments may be visible in cases of **traumatic ligament avulsion**, and a diagnosis of joint instability is possible by means of stress radiography (see Chapter 15, Fig. 15.23 and 15.24).

Cranial cruciate ligament injury/rupture

In contrast to small dogs and cats with this injury, rupture of the cranial cruciate ligament in large-breed dogs is typically a chronic process rather than the result of acute trauma. Predominant radiographic findings thus include degenerative changes of the stifle joint (intracapsular soft-tissue swelling due to joint effusion and/or synovial hypertrophy as well as degenerative joint disease; see Fig. 17.1 and Fig. 15.27). With complete rupture of the ligament, cranial subluxation of the tibia may be evident.

Tendinopathies

Conditions of the shoulder joint affecting the biceps, supraspinatus and infraspinatus tendons are relatively common in large-breed dogs. In chronic cases, degenerative changes such as dystrophic soft-tissue mineralization, sclerosis of the bicipital groove, osteophytes and degenerative joint disease of the shoulder joint may be evident.

Other abnormalities of soft tissues

Radiographs may also aid in the diagnosis of radiopaque foreign bodies within soft tissues and intralesional gas, for example with open wounds or infection with gas-producing bacteria.

References and further reading

Allen GS. Radiographic features of feline joint diseases. Vet Clin North Am Small Anim Pract 2000; 30: 281–302.

Barnhart MD. Malignant transformation of an aneurysmal bone cyst in a dog. Vet Surg 2002; 31: 519–24.

Craig LE, Julian ME, Ferracone JD. The diagnosis and prognosis of synovial tumors in dogs: 35 cases. Vet Pathol 2002; 39: 66–73.

Farrow CS, Newton CD. Ligamentous injury (sprain). In: Newton CD, Nunamaker DM (eds). Textbook of Small Animal Orthopedics. Ithaca: International Veterinary Information Service 1985.

Johnson KA, Watson ADJ. Skeletal diseases. In: Ettinger SJ, Feldman EC (eds). Textbook of Veterinary Internal Medicine. Philadelphia: WB Saunders 2000; 1887–916.

Mahoney PN, Lamb CR. Articular, periarticular and juxtaarticular calcified bodies in the dog and cat: A radiological review. Vet Radiol Ultrasound 1996; 37: 3–19.

Owens JM, Biery DN. Radiographic Interpretation for the Small Animal Clinician. Baltimore: Williams & Wilkins 1998.

Piermattei DL, Flo GL. Handbook of Small Animal Orthopedics and Fracture Repair. Philadelphia: WB Saunders 1997.

Straw RC. Tumors of the skeletal system. In: Withrow SJ, MacEwen E (eds). Small Animal Clinical Oncology. Philadelphia: WB Saunders 1996.

Thomas HL, Pressler BM, Robertson ID. Radiographic Diagnosis – Polyostotic Lymphoma in a 5 month old dog. Vet Radiol Ultrasound 2001; 42: 521–3.

Thrall DE. Textbook of Veterinary Diagnostic Radiology, 5th edn. Philadelphia: WB Saunders 2007.

Weisbrode SE, Doige CE. Bone and joints. In: McGavin MD, Carlton WW, Zachary JF (eds). Thomson's Special Veterinary Pathology. St. Louis: Mosby 2001.

Wrigley RH. Malignant versus nonmalignant bone disease. Vet Clin North Am Small Anim Pract 2000; 30: 315–47.

Fractures

18

Silke Hecht, Federica Morandi and Gregory B. Daniel

18.1 Fracture diagnosis and classification

Diagnosis and full evaluation of a fracture require radiographs of adequate quality. To be able to fully assess the extent, any displacement and potential joint involvement, well-positioned radiographs in at least two planes are needed, and the joints both proximal and distal to the fracture site must be included in the area of collimation. Following assessment of these initial radiographs, additional views (e.g. oblique or tangential) may be requested as needed.

The predominant radiographic finding in most fractures is a **disruption/discontinuity of the cortex**. It is important to note that nondisplaced or minimally displaced fractures may not be visible even on good quality radiographs. In cases where a fracture is suspected clinically but not documented radiographically, additional radiographs with a change in patient position or beam direction, repeat radiographs at a later time point or advanced imaging techniques (CT or MRI, bone scintigraphy) may be needed to establish a diagnosis and initiate appropriate treatment (Fig. 18.1).

As described in Chapter 17, aetiology, location, degree, communication with the external environment, type, dislocation, chronicity of the fracture, joint involvement and, in young animals, physeal involvement are important factors that must be evaluated for any fracture and taken into consideration for therapy planning.

18.1.1 Aetiology

With a **traumatic fracture,** a sudden single impact on healthy bone results in disruption of bone continuity. This may be the result of direct trauma (e.g. bite wound, hit or ballistic injury; Fig. 18.2) or indirect force (e.g. bending or shearing injury). Traumatic fractures are the most common type seen in small animal practice.

A **pathological fracture** occurs secondary to an underlying disease process causing weakening of the affected bone (e.g. bone tumour or osteomyelitis). In these cases a minor impact (which would be tolerated by a healthy bone) causes the abnormal bone to fracture. Examples include jumping off a bed or even running (see Chapter 17, Fig. 17.11 and Fig. 17.13).

A **stress fracture** occurs without external force in bones that have been chronically damaged by repetitive microtrauma. In veterinary medicine, this is most commonly seen in race horses and racing dogs in training. This type of fracture has been well documented in the carpus and tarsus of racing Greyhounds and must be distinguished from pathological fractures in regards to aetiology, therapy and prognosis.

18.1.2 Location

Description of fracture location should include not only the **affected bone**, but also the **bone region** (diaphysis, metaphysis, physis, epiphysis, apophysis). If a fracture line extends into an adjacent joint the fracture is called **'articular'**. Articular fractures usually present a surgical indication to re-establish joint congruity and minimize the risk of later complications (degenerative joint disease).

Fractures involving the **physis** in young animals are categorized according to the **Salter–Harris classification** (Fig. 18.3).

- **Type I:** The fracture results in separation of metaphysis and epiphysis along the physis. A typical example is a capital physeal fracture, which is common in young dogs and cats (Fig. 18.1).
- **Type II:** The fracture involves the physis and extends into the metaphysis.
- **Type III:** The fracture involves the physis, extends into the epiphysis and is usually articular. A typical example is a T-type fracture of the distal humeral condyle.
- **Type IV:** This fracture involves the physis, metaphysis and epiphysis and is usually articular. A typical example is a Y-type fracture of the distal humeral condyle.

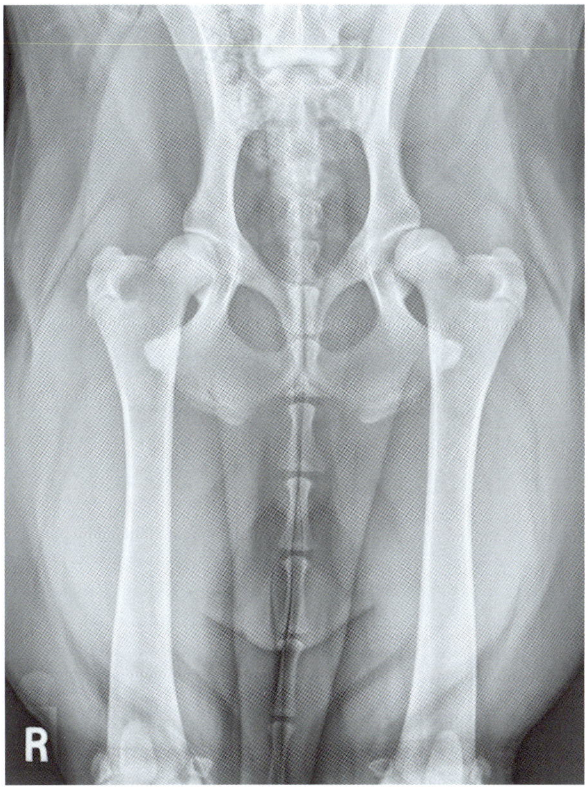

a

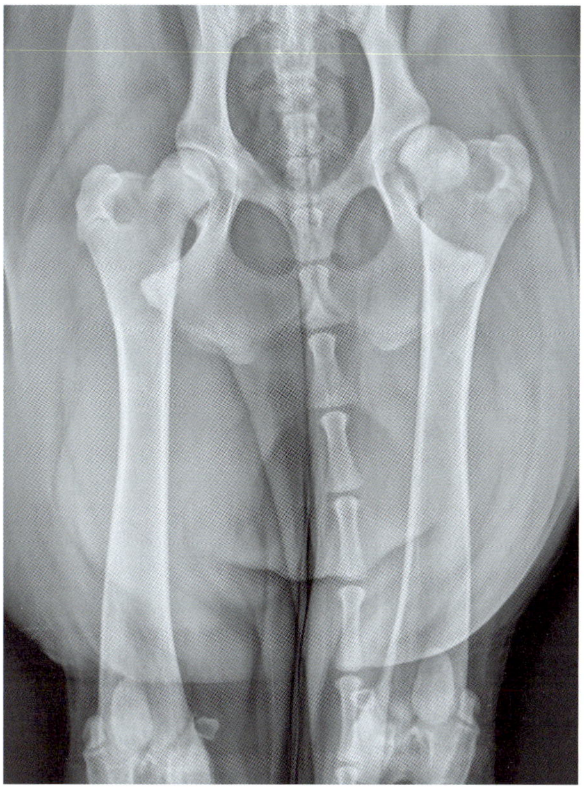

b

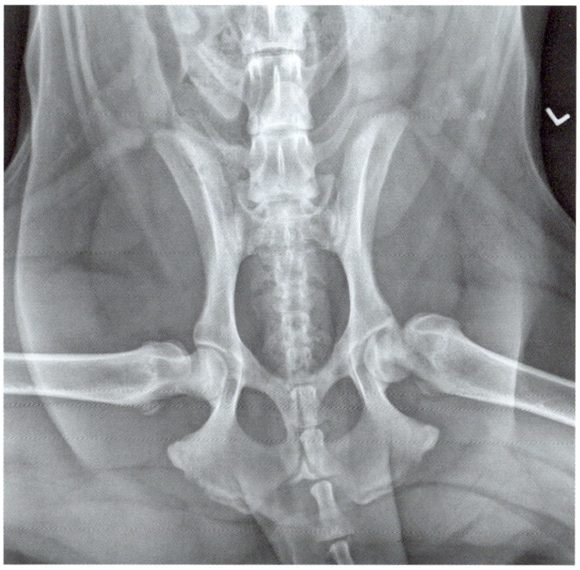

c

Fig. 18.1 Radiographic series of the pelvis demonstrating the necessity for additional views in a dog with traumatic femoral capital physeal fracture.

a On the ventrodorsal view of the pelvis obtained few hours after a road traffic accident, the joint space of the left coxofemoral joint is mildly widened, but there is no evidence of an osseous lesion. No other radiographs were obtained at this point in time (R = right).

b On the repeat ventrodorsal view obtained 2 weeks later, the left femoral head has an unusual contour, but a distinct fracture line is not recognized.

c An additional radiograph with altered positioning was obtained at this point. The 'frog view' with flexion of the coxofemoral joints allows diagnosis of a left proximal capital physeal fracture (L = left).

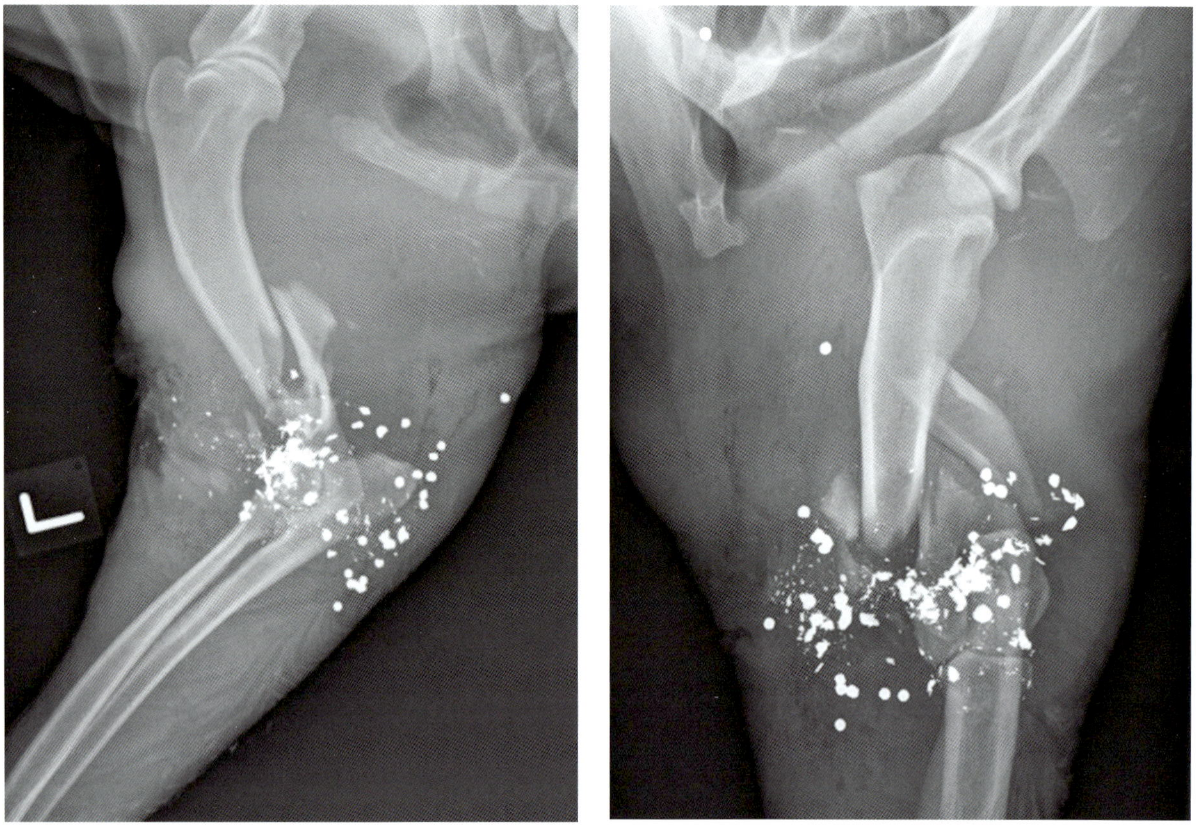

a b

Fig. 18.2 Traumatic fracture in a dog following direct trauma (ballistic injury). The lateral a and craniocaudal b radiographs of the left humerus show an open comminuted fracture with numerous metal opaque fragments associated with the bone and surrounding soft tissues (L = left).

- **Type V:** With this type of trauma there is compression of the physis without associated discontinuity or dislocation of the epiphysis. This type of physeal trauma is problematic, as it is often not recognized on initial radiographs and commonly results in partial or complete premature closure of the physis. The resultant shortening of the affected bone may be clinically insignificant, for example when involving an unpaired bone such as the femur or humerus in an almost skeletally mature animal. However, in cases of premature physeal closure of a paired bone and continued growth of the partner, shortening of the traumatized bone, bowing of the partner bone and incongruity of adjacent joints are common sequelae. Salter–Harris type V injuries commonly involve the distal physis of the ulna and result in radius curvus, carpus valgus and elbow joint incongruity.

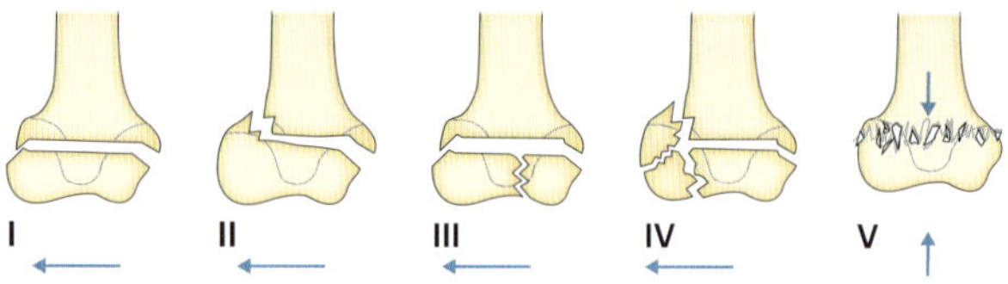

Fig. 18.3 Schematic illustration of different types of physeal injuries in young animals (Salter–Harris classification). Type I: The fracture separates metaphysis and epiphysis along the physis. Type II: The fracture involves the physis and metaphysis. Type III: The fracture involves the physis and epiphysis and extends into the joint. Type IV: The fracture involves the physis, metaphysis and epiphysis and extends into the joint. Type V: Compression injury of the physis without dislocation.

18.1.3 Degree

Complete fractures are characterized by complete loss of bone continuity. With **incomplete fractures** part of the bone and overlying periosteum remain intact. Examples for incomplete fractures include greenstick fractures in young animals (unicortical fractures secondary to bending of a bone) and bone fissures (small gaps in the cortex which may extend peripherally from a complete fracture, for example).

18.1.4 Communication with the external environment

A **closed fracture** is covered by overlying soft tissues and skin and thus protected from infection.

With **open fractures** there is more or less extensive communication between bone fragments and the external environment. Open fractures are subdivided into three (or four) grades of severity depending on the degree of soft-tissue damage and bone exposure.

- **Grade 1**: A sharp fracture fragment temporarily perforates the skin from the inside but then withdraws again into the soft tissues. There is only minor soft-tissue damage. This type of fracture is not usually recognized as an open fracture based on radiographs.
- **Grade 2:** With these injuries there is damage to the skin and soft tissues from the outside with exposure of underlying bone. A soft-tissue defect is visible adjacent to the fracture site on radiographs.
- **Grade 3:** There is extensive damage to skin, subcutaneous tissues and muscles, often associated with nerve and/or vascular damage. The affected bone(s) are usually shattered into numerous fragments. These injuries are typically the result of high-velocity trauma, such as shearing or ballistic injuries (see Fig. 18.2). A traumatic complete or partial amputation of an extremity can be grouped into this category or can be categorized separately as **grade 4**.

With open fractures there is a significant risk of infection of soft tissues and bone, which increases with the severity grade of the fracture. Osteomyelitis is a typical sequela of an open fracture and negatively impacts implant stability and bone healing. Thus, open fractures (especially of higher grade) often have a worse prognosis than closed fractures. The radiographic appearance of osteomyelitis is covered in Chapter 17 (see Fig. 17.4 and also Fig. 15.39).

18.1.5 Type

Fractures can be categorized based on the number of fracture fragments, direction of the fracture lines and other criteria (Fig. 18.4).

- **Simple fractures:** These are 'smooth' fractures which are categorized as **transverse**, **oblique** or **spiral fractures** based on orientation of the fracture line with respect to the long axis of the bone (Fig. 18.4a, b).
- **Complex fractures:** With these fractures there are more than two fracture fragments. **Comminuted fractures** are characterized by the presence of numerous, variably sized bone fragments and communication of individual fracture lines (Fig. 18.2 and Fig. 18.4c). With **segmental fractures** the bone is broken in at least two separate places without communication of the fracture lines ('à deux étages'; Fig. 18.4d).
- **Avulsion fractures:** These result from separation of a tendon or ligament with an embedded piece of bone from their site of origin or insertion (Fig. 18.4e). An **apophyseal fracture** in young animals is a type of avulsion fracture.
- **Compression fractures:** These result in foreshortening and increased opacity of the affected bone. This type of bone trauma is most commonly seen affecting the spine following blunt trauma (e.g. fall from a window). The Salter–Harris type V fractures in young animals discussed in section 18.1.2 are a special type of compression fracture.

18.1.6 Dislocation

In most fractures, some degree of displacement of fracture fragments is noted. The direction of fracture dislocation is by convention described based on the position of the distal fracture fragment compared to the proximal fracture fragment. Possible types of dislocation of fracture fragments include abnormal long axis alignment of bone fragments, lateral displacement of fragments, separation of fracture ends in the longitudinal direction, foreshortening of the bone due to lateral displacement and overlap of fragments, and rotational malalignment.

18.1.7 Chronicity

Most small animal patients with fractures are seen in the acute stage. However, a complete history may not be available in some cases (e.g. in animals that have been found or recently adopted), or bony changes may be seen as a secondary finding, for example on thoracic or abdominal radiographs. Determination of the chronicity of a fracture is important for therapy planning and prognostication.

- **Acute fractures:** The fracture margins are sharply marginated, and there is no evidence of healing (i.e. findings such as callus formation or bridging of the fracture gap by new bone are absent). Concurrent soft-tissue changes such as swelling or gas inclusions are common.
- **Chronic fractures:** These may be completely healed or in the healing process at the time of presentation. Complications of fracture healing may also be observed (see section 18.2.5). In any case, the fracture margins are more rounded/less sharp than with acute fractures, periosteal reaction is usually evident due to callus formation and/or osteomyelitis, and muscle atrophy is common due to reduced weight bearing of the affected limb.

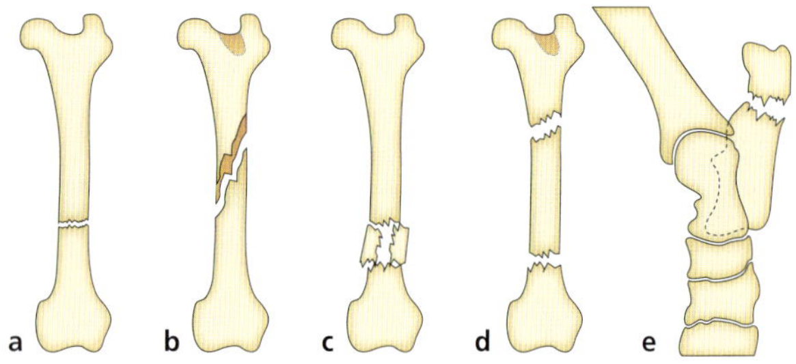

Fig. 18.4 Schematic (simplified) illustration of different fracture types: a transverse fracture; b spiral fracture; c comminuted fracture; d segmental fracture ('à deux étages'); e avulsion fracture.

18.2 Fracture healing

The two basic types of fracture healing are called primary and secondary healing.

18.2.1 Primary or direct healing

Fracture healing occurs directly via internal osseous remodelling and without formation of a fracture callus. This type of healing occurs in fractures with a very small fracture gap (<0.1 mm) and stable apposition, such as can be achieved following internal fracture fixation utilizing a dynamic compression plate. The fracture gap is bridged by remodelling of the Haversian system with extension of osteons across the fracture gap into the opposite fracture fragment.

Radiographic findings This type of fracture healing is characterized by the absence of periosteal callus, gradual decrease in bone opacity of the fracture margins, and progressive disappearance of the fracture line (Fig. 18.5).

18.2.2 Secondary healing

Secondary fracture healing occurs in all fractures which cannot be perfectly reduced or in which perfect stability cannot be achieved. This type of fracture healing is much more common than direct healing. The process involves numerous successive steps during which the fracture is stabilized by material of increasing strength (from granulation tissue to fibrous tissue to bone). Briefly, haemorrhage into the fracture gap initially results in the formation of a blood clot which initiates an inflammatory process, which in turn results in proliferation of mesenchymal stem cells. These are pluripotent, may differentiate into osteoblasts, fibroblasts or chondroblasts, and are instrumental in forming callus tissue which stabilizes and bridges the fracture gap. Increasing ossification results in osseous fracture healing, and bony remodelling over time re-establishes cortical integrity.

Radiographic findings Secondary fracture healing is initially characterized by loss of visibility of the sharp fracture margins and demineralization of the fracture ends. After 10–20 days (in adult animals) an endosteal and periosteal callus develops, which increases in radiographic opacity over time due to progressive ossification. The fracture gap increasingly narrows and is less well visualized. Ultimately (after approximately 3 months) remodelling at the fracture site results in re-establishment of the cortex and medullary cavity, possibly with near-complete resorption of the initial stabilizing callus (Fig. 18.6). Following complete and uncomplicated fracture healing, and assuming adequate re-establishment of the original shape of the fractured bone, a prior fracture may be difficult to identify radiographically once healed.

Resorption of the fracture margins during the early stage of secondary fracture healing is physiological and should not be confused with a pathological process (osteomyelitis or atrophy of the fracture ends).

18.2.3 Factors influencing fracture healing

Numerous factors may impact healing of a given fracture.

- **Age of the patient:** Fractures in young animals heal faster than in older animals. While an uncomplicated diaphyseal fracture in a puppy may clinically heal and achieve stability in a few weeks, healing of a similar fracture in an adult dog may take several months to complete.
- **Fracture location:** Some fractures (e.g. fractures of the distal antebrachium in toy-breed dogs) have a markedly worse chance of healing than others.
- **Alignment of the fracture fragments:** The better the apposition of fracture fragments, i.e. the smaller the fracture gap, the faster fracture healing will occur. A large bone defect with soft tissues extending into the fracture gap and complicated comminuted fractures with numerous displaced fracture fragments heal more slowly and have more complications than nondisplaced or minimally displaced uncomplicated fractures.
- **Vascularization:** Any compromise in vascular supply to the affected bone (e.g. soft-tissue trauma, periosteal injury or presence of surgical implants) may impair fracture healing.
- **Stability:** Instability results in delayed fracture healing or even nonunion. Affected animals often develop exuberant callus adjacent to the fracture site but have no tendency to bridge the fracture gap. Mobility at the fracture site and implant loosening are often closely associated.
- **Infection:** Osteomyelitis, for example secondary to open fractures or postoperative infection, significantly interferes with bone healing.

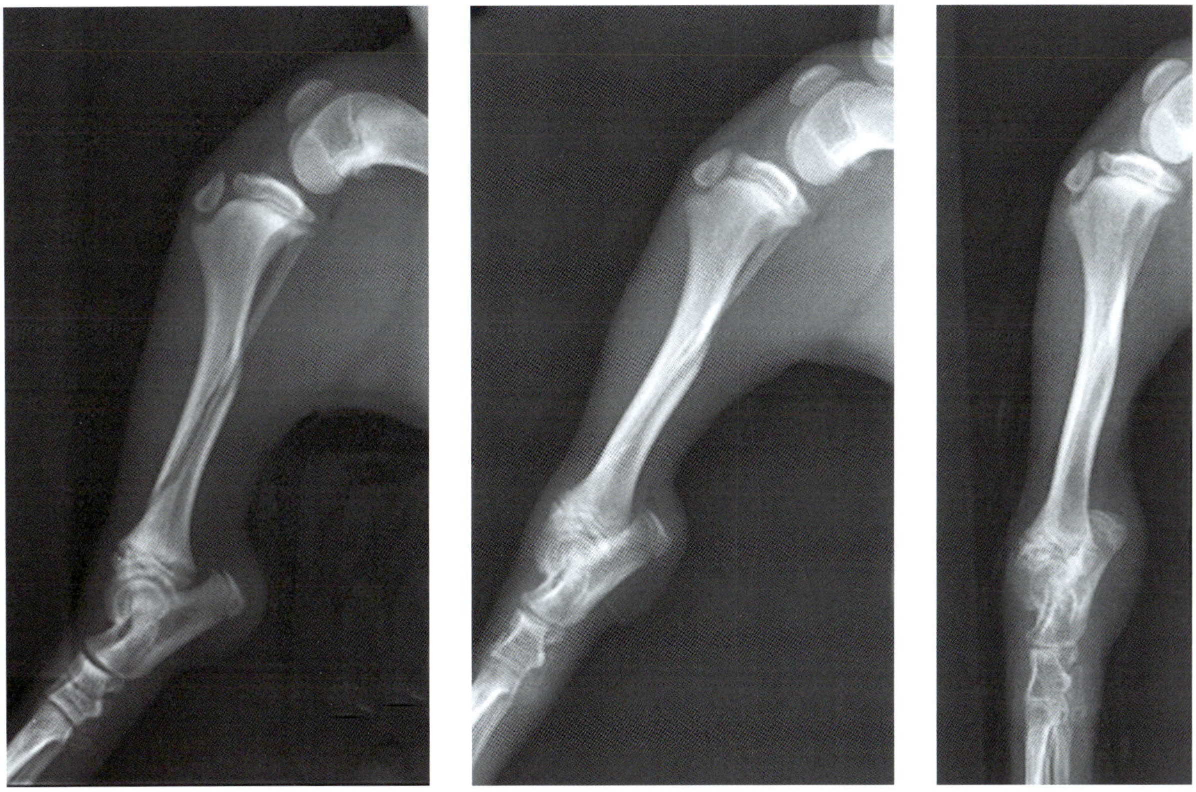

a b c

Fig. 18.5 Primary healing of a diaphyseal fracture of the tibia in a puppy.

a The lateral view at initial presentation shows a minimally displaced tibial fracture.

b Recheck radiograph after only 8 days of conservative treatment with a stabilizing bandage. The fracture line is barely visible. There is no evidence of periosteal callus formation.

c After 3 weeks the fracture is completely healed. Note the marked hyperextension of the tarsus secondary to bandaging. Primary fracture healing is rarely achieved with conservative management and is attributed to perfect apposition of the fracture fragments and excellent fracture stabilization in this case.

a b c

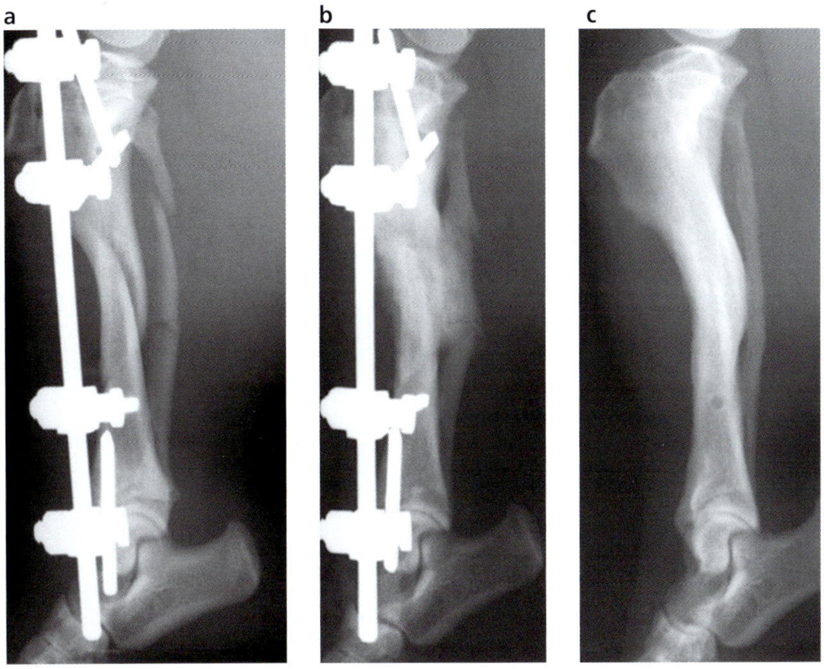

Fig. 18.6 Secondary healing of diaphyseal fractures of the tibia and fibula in a young dog.

a Following stabilization of the tibial fracture by means of an external fixator, there is mild to moderate displacement of the tibial and fibular fracture fragments.

b After 6 weeks there is extensive bony periosteal callus formation, resulting in osseous bridging of the fracture gaps of tibia and fibula.

c Recheck radiographs after another 4 weeks show remodelling of most of the callus. The fractures are no longer visible. Note mild malformation of the tibia at the former fracture site with cranial concave bowing.

- **Others:** Depending on the underlying bone lesion, pathological fractures have little to no chance of healing. Some disorders or conditions independent from the fracture, and certain medications (e.g. corticosteroids), may also negatively impact fracture healing.

18.2.4 Radiographic evaluation

Accurate assessment of fracture healing may not be easy as this may be influenced by all of the above factors and has to be judged on a case-by-case basis.

Immediately following stabilization of a fracture by means of a bandage/cast or orthopaedic implants, radiographs in at least two planes should be acquired to ascertain anatomically correct re-establishment of the bone axis, adequate apposition of fracture fragments and adequate implant position (if applicable).

The time and frequency of follow-up radiographs depend on the age of the patient, the type of treatment (conservative versus surgical) and any complications. For example, recheck radiographs in a young dog with a simple nondisplaced fracture that is conservatively treated are usually obtained after 7–10 days. In adult animals in which a surgical fracture repair is performed by means of internal fixation, recheck radiographs are typically obtained after approximately 6 weeks, unless complications develop.

Radiographic assessment of fracture healing includes evaluation of apposition of the fracture fragments, implant stability, evidence of the beginning of fracture healing (early callus formation, width and bridging of the fracture gap), and the adjacent soft tissues. Clinical healing of an uncomplicated diaphyseal fracture following repair with a bone plate will take approximately 1–3 months in a 3-month-old dog and 5–8 months in an adult dog.

18.2.5 Complications

As already indicated in section 18.2.3, numerous factors may impact the normal healing process.

Implant failure (bending or breaking, loosening and migration)

These complications may occur secondary to technical errors during surgery (choice of inappropriate implants, screws placed in close proximity to or within the fracture gap, etc.), excessive weight bearing on the affected limb before adequate stability has been reached, or infection.

RADIOGRAPHIC FINDINGS A broken implant or an implant that has migrated is easily recognized. Implant loosening is characterized by linear lucent regions along the affected implants.

A digital radiography artefact occasionally seen adjacent to metallic structures (**Überschwinger artefact**; see Chapter 3, Fig. 3.27) may mimic implant loosening.

Osteomyelitis

Infection of the fracture site may occur during the actual trauma (open fractures and fractures secondary to perforating injuries), during surgical repair, or later secondary to haematogenous spread of bacteria in case of systemic infection.

RADIOGRAPHIC FINDINGS Osteomyelitis manifests as an aggressive, mixed osteolytic and osteoproliferative bone lesion which typically extends well beyond the actual fracture margins, and often involves the entire length of the affected bone (see Fig. 17.4 and Fig. 15.39). Secondary implant failure and delayed or absent fracture healing are common.

Malunion

Bone healing with abnormal alignment of the fracture fragments is a relatively common complication. Depending on the location and degree of malalignment and the presence or absence of joint involvement, animals may be asymptomatic or show lameness of varying severity.

RADIOGRAPHIC FINDINGS The affected bone has an abnormal contour or malangulation. The underlying fracture is healed and no longer visible (Fig. 18.7).

Delayed union

A delay in fracture healing may be caused by a variety of problems including extensive soft-tissue damage, decreased vascularization, osteomyelitis, etc. (see above). In contrast to nonunion fractures, healing does occur eventually, even though later than expected.

Nonunion

This is caused by a failure in fracture healing and subsequent development of a pseudo joint (sometimes called pseudarthrosis) at the fracture site. This can be caused by multiple problems including instability, large bone defects with soft tissues present in the fracture gap, infection and vascular compromise. Depending on the cause and appearance of the fracture site, the following types can be distinguished.

- **Hypertrophic nonunion** is characterized by excessive callus formation without evidence of healing. This is also called 'elephant foot' or 'horse foot' nonunion (Fig. 18.8).
- **Oligotrophic nonunion** is characterized by the persistent and nearly unchanged appearance of the original fracture site (Fig. 18.8).
- **Atrophic nonunion** is characterized by resorption of the fracture ends with no tendency to heal (Fig. 18.9).

Resorption of the femoral neck following femoral capital physeal fracture

This is a special type of a fracture healing complication seen following traumatic or spontaneous proximal capital physeal fracture. It is most common in a case of a failure to diagnose and stabilize an acute capital physeal fracture, but it may also sometimes be seen following surgical correction.

RADIOGRAPHIC FINDINGS The femoral neck becomes progressively circumferentially narrowed and assumes the appearance of an 'apple core' (Fig. 18.10).

This complication, unique to the proximal femur, was previously attributed to excessive formation of vascular plexus and secondary pressure atrophy on adjacent bone. The current belief is that damage to regional vessels (circumflex femoral artery, caudal gluteal arteries) results in aseptic necrosis of the femoral neck.

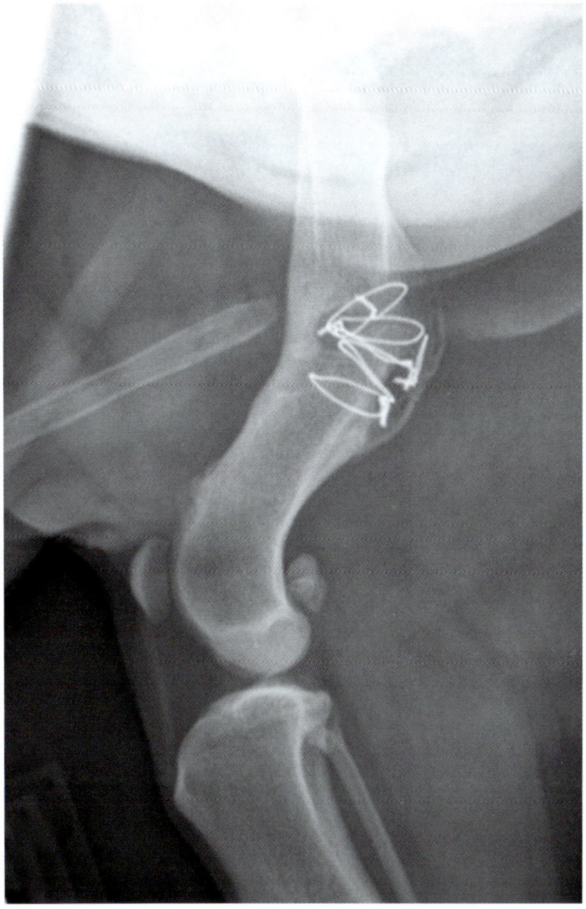

Fig. 18.7 Malunion fracture of the femur in a young dog. There is abnormal angulation of the femur at the prior fracture site; the fracture itself is healed. Multiple cerclage wires are still present. A focal round lucent region surrounding the proximal implants raises concern for (chronic) osteomyelitis.

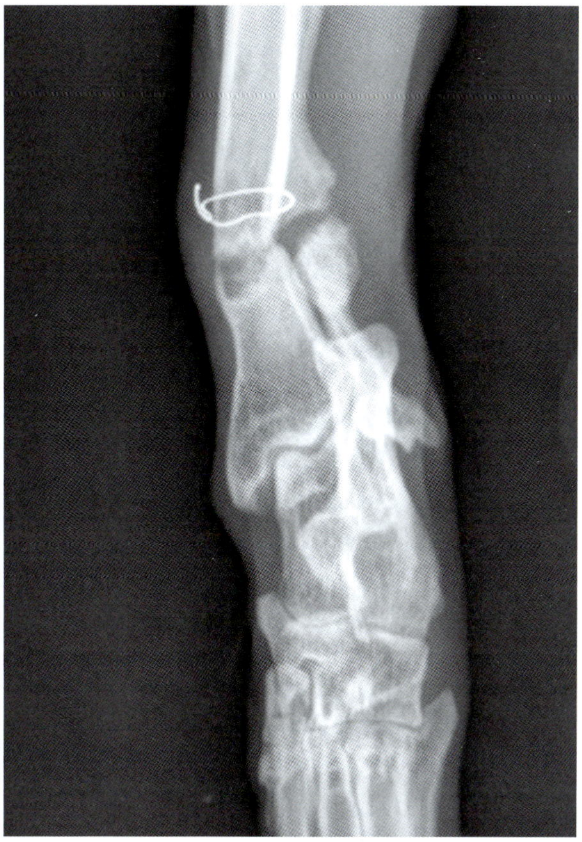

Fig. 18.8 Hypertrophic and oligotrophic nonunion of distal tibial and fibular fractures following an unsuccessful attempt at surgical fixation and persistent mobility at the fracture site. The fibular fracture is characterized by excessive callus formation with no evidence of osseous bridging (hypertrophic pseudarthrosis). There is no evidence of new bone formation at the site of the tibial fracture (oligotrophic nonunion).

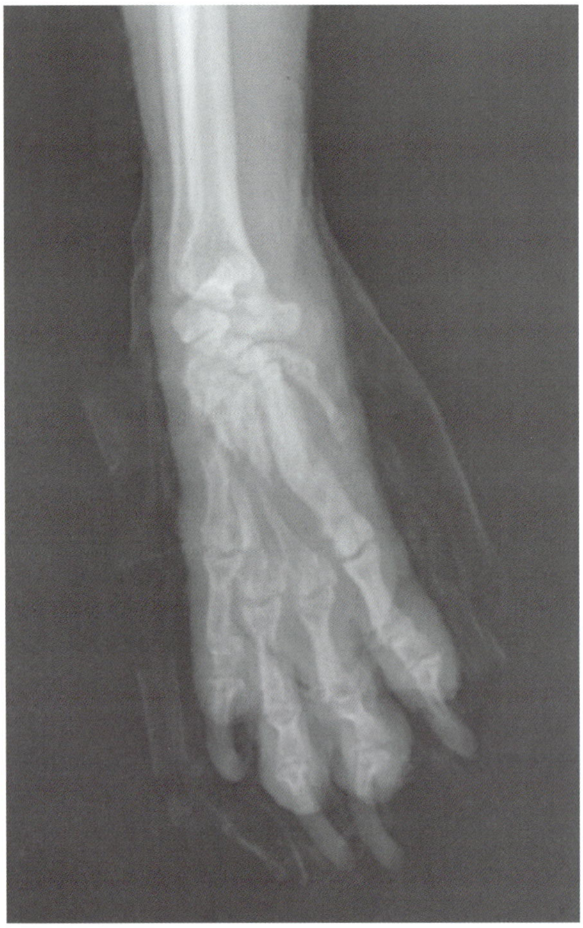

Fig. 18.9 Atrophic nonunion of the third through fifth metacarpal bones secondary to extensive bone defects and decreased vascularization of the fracture site. The bone ends are resorbed with no evidence of callus formation or fracture healing. Note adequate fracture healing of the second metacarpal bone and generalized bone atrophy secondary to long-standing immobilization.

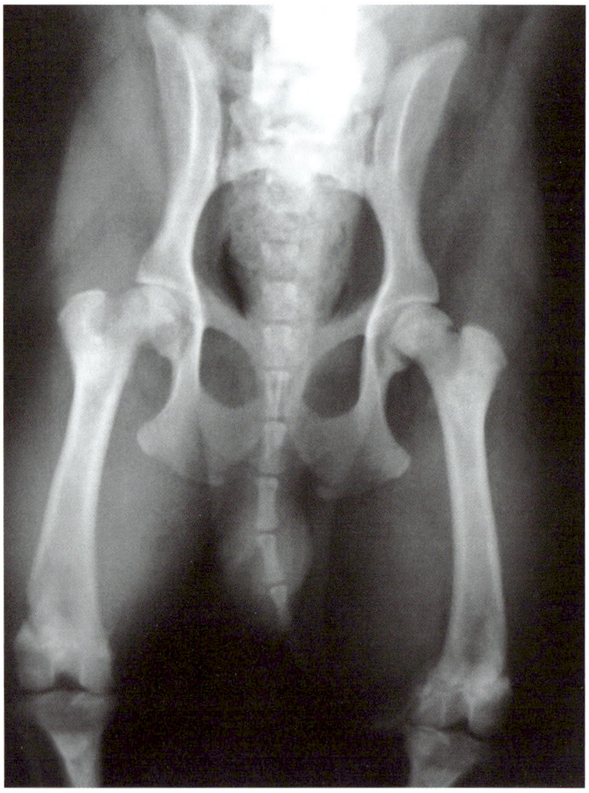

a

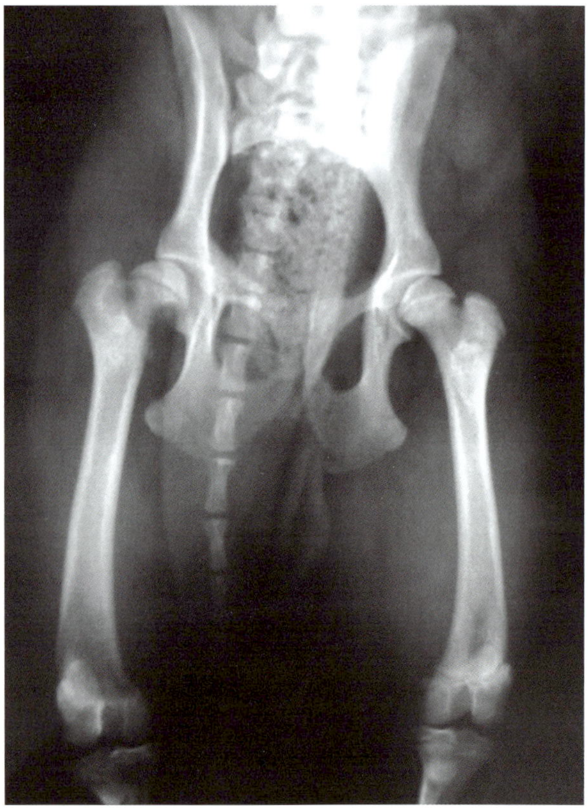

b

Fig. 18.10 Resorption of the femoral neck following undiagnosed proximal femoral capital physeal fracture.

a At initial patient presentation, an acute right capital physeal fracture was missed, as a 'frog view' was not obtained. The patient was treated conservatively.

b Repeat radiographs 12 days later show widening of the right proximal femoral physis and marked thinning (resorption) of the femoral neck, which has assumed an 'apple core' appearance. Note also marked muscle atrophy of the right hind limb at this point.

Suggested reading

Beale B. Orthopedic clinical techniques femur fracture repair. Clin Tech Small Anim Pract 2004; 19: 134–50.

Boudrieau RJ, Dee JF, Dee LG. Central tarsal bone fractures in the racing Greyhound: a review of 114 cases. J Am Vet Med Assoc 1984; 184: 1486–91.

Boulay JP, Wallace LJ, Lipowitz AJ. Pathological fracture of long bones in the dog. J Am Anim Hosp Assoc 1987; 23: 297–303.

Braden TD, Brinker WO. Radiological and gross anatomic evaluation of bone healing in the dog. J Am Vet Med Assoc 1991; 169: 1318–23.

Henry GA. Fracture healing and complications. In: Thrall DE (ed.). Textbook of Veterinary Diagnostic Radiology, 5th edn. Philadelphia: WB Saunders 2007; 284–305.

Johnson KA. Accessory carpal bone fractures in the racing greyhound. Classification and pathology. Vet Surg 1987; 16: 60–4.

Marquardt SA, Rochat MC. What is your diagnosis? Capital physeal fracture. J Am Vet Med Assoc 2008; 232: 1637–8.

Morgan JP. Radiology of Veterinary Orthopedics. Napa, CA: Venture Press 1999.

Muir P. Distal antebrachial fractures in toy-breed dogs. Compendium 1997; 137–45.

Piermattei DL, Flo GL. Handbook of Small Animal Orthopedics and Fracture Repair. Philadelphia: WB Saunders 1997.

Schelling SH. Secondary (classical) bone healing. Semin Vet Med Surg 1991; 6: 16–20.

Sumner-Smith G. Bone in Clinical Orthopedics. Stuttgart: Thieme 2002.

Birds

19

Marcy Souza and Jürgen Schumacher

Avian medicine has evolved into an important component in small animal and exotics practice, and at this point, specialty hospitals focused on the diagnosis and treatment of diseases in birds exist in the academic as well as the private sector. A radiographic examination can be helpful in the diagnosis of various diseases in avian patients. It is especially useful in assessment of the musculoskeletal system as well as the respiratory, gastrointestinal (GI) and reproductive tracts. Advanced diagnostic imaging procedures such as ultrasound, computed tomography (CT) and magnetic resonance imaging (MRI) are increasingly used but are often limited to specialty practices.

Due to the large number of avian species, and often marked anatomic and physiological differences, it is important to be familiar with the anatomy and physiology of the individual avian patient. When evaluating avian radiographs it may be useful to have an atlas or article on hand showing examples of normal radiographs in the respective species (see 'Suggested reading' at the end of the chapter). Alternatively, obtaining radiographs of a healthy comparison bird of the same species may be helpful.

This chapter covers normal anatomy, indications for radiographic examination, radiographic abnormalities seen with various diseases, and further diagnostic tests.

19.1 Anatomy and indications

19.1.1 Anatomy

As mentioned above, marked anatomic differences exist not only between mammals and birds but also between different avian species. This chapter will only cover basic avian anatomy important for basic radiographic interpretation. The reader is referred to advanced literature for specific anatomic descriptions of different species. Schematic drawings of normal avian anatomy and normal radiographs are shown in Fig. 19.1 to 19.3.

Musculoskeletal system

Both the axial as well as the appendicular skeleton in birds differ significantly from mammals.

SKULL

The anatomy of the skull markedly differs between bird species. The skull is very mobile in all birds, and in contrast to mammals many species are able to move the **upper jaw** (upper beak) independently. The unpaired **occipital condyle** articulates with the atlas and allows 180° rotation of the neck. Birds have large **sinuses** and often have diverticula associated with their facial bones.

SHOULDER GIRDLE

The shoulder girdle consists of the paired **scapulae**, the paired **coracoid bones** and the **furcula** formed by the fused **clavicles**.

SPINE

The number of **cervical vertebrae** is inconsistent and varies between species. The **thoracic vertebrae** are closely connected with the **ribs**. Most cranial thoracic vertebrae are fused into a unified bone (**notarium**). In many bird species, this is followed by only a single **free thoracic vertebra**. The caudal thoracic, lumbar and sacral vertebrae are again fused to form a second larger bone (**synsacrum**). Caudal to the synsacrum, the spine continues with a variable number of **free caudal vertebrae** and terminates with a last single bone (**pygostyle**) resulting from fusion of the last caudal vertebrae.

RIBS AND STERNUM

The ribs can have variable shape. **Complete ribs** consist of a dorsal (vertebral) and a ventral (sternal) part which connect via a cartilaginous joint. **Incomplete ribs** only have a vertebral part and end freely in the body wall. The first two pairs of ribs are typically incomplete.

The **sternum** is characterized by a large keel (**carina**) which serves as an attachment point for the flight muscles.

PELVIC GIRDLE

The **ilium**, **ischium** and **pubis** are not only connected with each other, but also firmly attached to the contralateral side dorsally via the synsacrum.

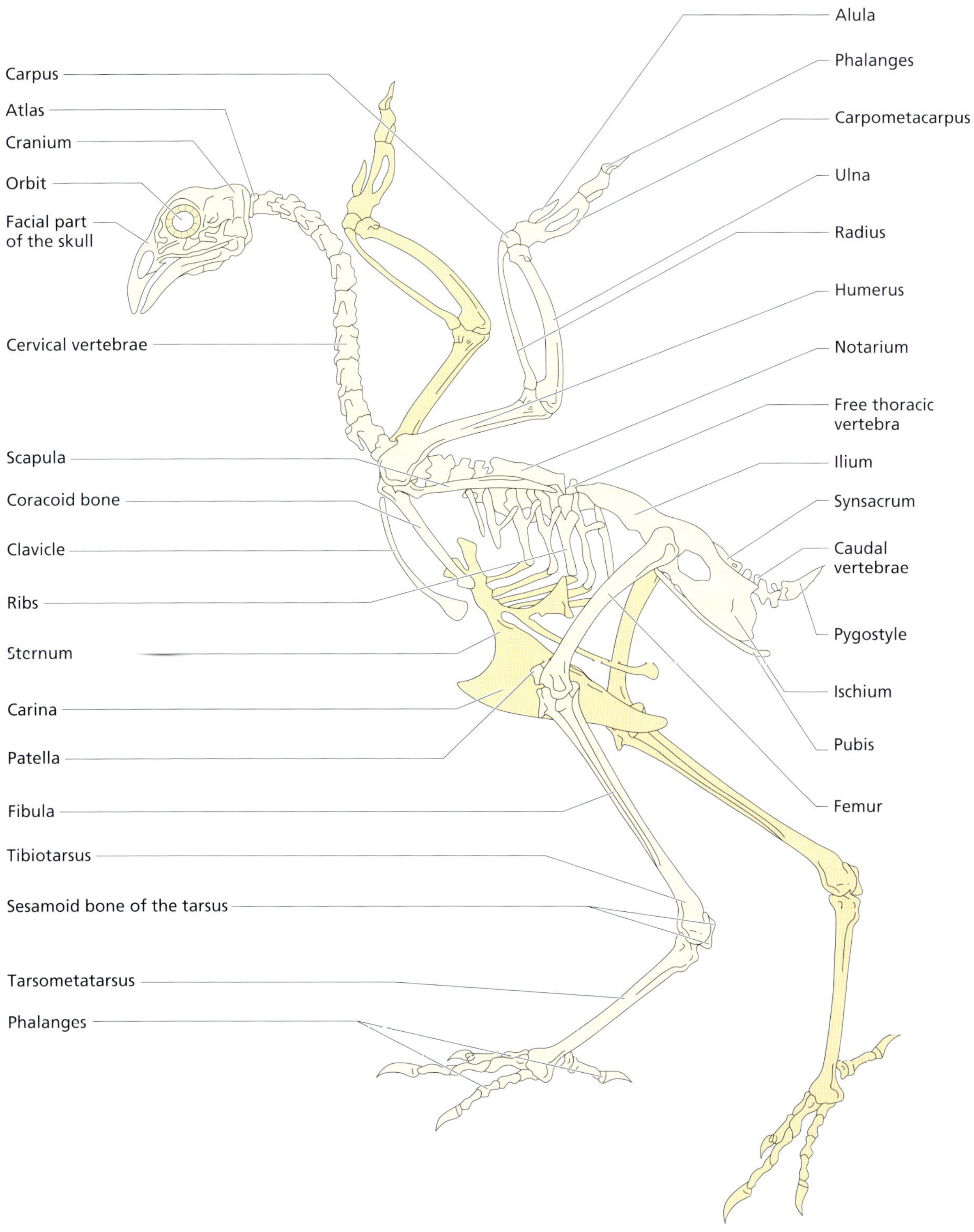

Fig. 19.1 Schematic illustration of the skeleton of a bird.

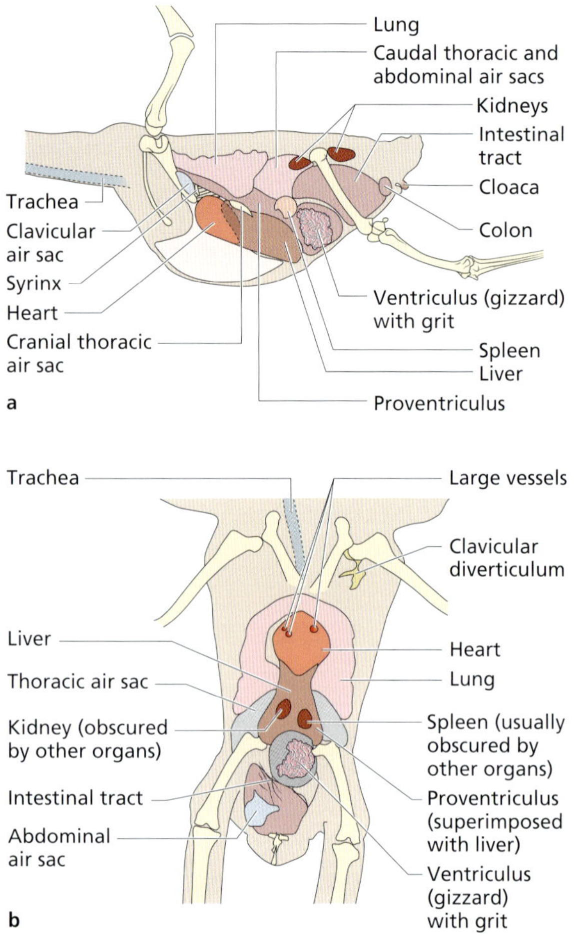

Fig. 19.2 Schematic illustration of the coelomic organs in a bird: lateral a and ventral view b.

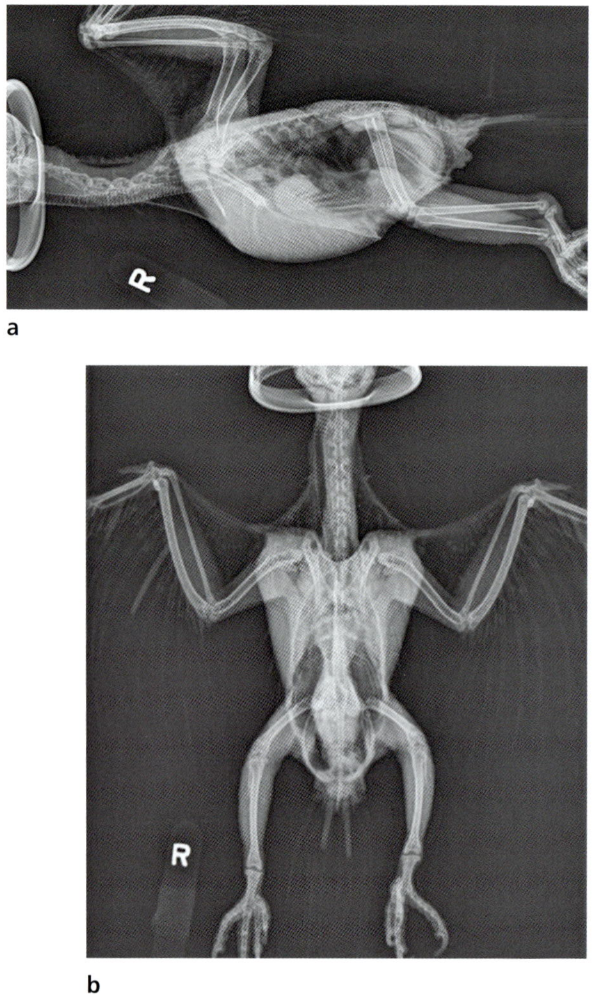

Fig. 19.3 Lateral a and ventrodorsal b radiographs of a normal Amazon parrot. Note the hourglass shape of the heart and liver on the VD view (R = right).

WINGS

The appendicular skeleton of the front extremities reflects the ability to fly in most avian species. The **humerus** articulates with the shoulder girdle. The **antebrachium** is formed by the **radius** and **ulna**, but in contrast to mammals the ulna is larger than the radius.

The connection from the antebrachium to the distal extremity occurs via only two **carpal bones** (radial carpal bone and ulnar carpal bone). The middle and distal carpal row and the metacarpal bones are fused to form the **carpometacarpus** which consists of a major and a minor metacarpal bone.

The **manus** differs between bird species. Generally, the **alular digit** and the **minor digit** each have one phalanx while the **major digit** has two phalanges. From proximal to distal the following joints are associated with the wing:

- shoulder (humeral) joint
- elbow (cubital) joint
- carpal joint
- metacarpophalangeal and interphalangeal joints.

HIND LIMBS

The femur is the strongest bone of the hind extremity. The major part of the distal limb is formed by the tibiotarsus consisting of the fused tibia and proximal tarsal bones. The fibula is rudimentary.

The distal tarsal bones are fused with the second through fourth metatarsal bones to form the tarsometatarsus. The first metatarsal bone is separate and carries the first digit.

The first through fourth digits generally have two, three, four and five phalanges, respectively.

The joints of the hind limb from proximal to distal are:

- hip (coxofemoral) joint
- stifle joint (with a cranial sesamoid bone = patella)
- intertarsal joint (with a plantar sesamoid bone = intertarsal sesamoid bone)
- metatarsophalangeal and interphalangeal joints.

Most birds presented in small animal practice are flighted species and have undergone evolutionary anatomic modifications to decrease weight. One important anatomic feature is the communication of air sacs and bones resulting in pneumatized bones. The cervical vertebrae are connected to the cervical air sacs, the thoracic vertebrae, ribs and humeri are connected to the clavicular air sac, and the synsacrum and femora are connected to the abdominal air sacs. In addition, avian bones are characterized by a thin cortex compared to mammalian bones.

Inner organs

In contrast to mammals, there is no diaphragm separating the thoracic and abdominal cavity, and birds therefore have a single body cavity (pleuroperitoneal cavity, coelom).

TRACHEA AND SYRINX

The trachea is easily recognized as an air-filled tubular structure with distinct cartilaginous rings and, depending on the species, may have a straight or curved course. The syrinx is located dorsal to the heart in most avian species.

LUNGS

These are located in the dorsolateral aspect of the coelom and are best evaluated on a lateral view. The pulmonary parenchyma is air-filled and of low opacity but has a characteristic reticular or honeycomb pattern which results from an end-on view of the tertiary bronchial walls and should not be confused with a pathological bronchial pattern seen in mammals. In small birds, it may be difficult to differentiate the bronchial walls radiographically. The volume of the lung does not change between inspiration and expiration.

AIR SACS

These are a special feature of the avian respiratory tract. They occupy large areas of the coelomic cavity, physiologically contain air and are thus radiolucent, and are in intimate association with the skeletal system as described above. They are best evaluated on a ventrodorsal view.

Most bird species have nine air sacs. The **cervical air sacs** are paired and located in the region of the neck, the **cranial thoracic air sacs** are paired and occupy the cranial part of the coelom, and the unpaired **clavicular air sac** is located in the region of the cranial coelom and axillary region. The paired **caudal thoracic air sacs** and the paired **abdominal air sacs** overlap, are located lateral to the viscera and (in contrast to the lungs) change size during respiration. The abdominal air sacs extend caudally to the cloaca, with the right air sac often reaching further caudally than the left.

The margins between individual air sacs are not physiologically visible. Because the air sacs are in close proximity to inner organs, coelomic detail in many birds is very good.

HEART

The heart is located in the cranioventral coelomic cavity (second through sixth sternal ribs) and appears subjectively large compared to the mammalian heart. In parrot species, the length of the heart is approximately 40% of the length of the sternum and the width approximately 50–60% of the width of the coelomic cavity on a ventrodorsal view.

The cardiac and hepatic silhouette form a characteristic **hourglass** shape on the ventrodorsal view. Depending on the orientation and beam angle, the **large vessels** appear as punctate or linear structures.

GASTROINTESTINAL TRACT

Radiographically relevant components are the oesophagus (with associated crop in many species), proventriculus, ventriculus and intestinal tract.

The **oesophagus** connects the pharynx with the proventriculus and, with the exception of the crop, which is located at the thoracic inlet, is not normally radiographically visible. The **crop** can be very large, especially in seed-eating species, and its contents vary depending on the last time of feeding and the type of food (Fig. 19.4 and 19.5). On a ventrodorsal view, the crop is located mostly to the right of midline but can expand to the left depending on its size.

The **proventriculus** is a tubular structure of variable size in the mid aspect of the coelomic cavity on a lateral view and to the left of midline and superimposed with the cardiohepatic silhouette on a ventrodorsal view. The **ventriculus** (gizzard) is usually recognized as a distinct, round, soft-tissue opaque structure (often with mineral

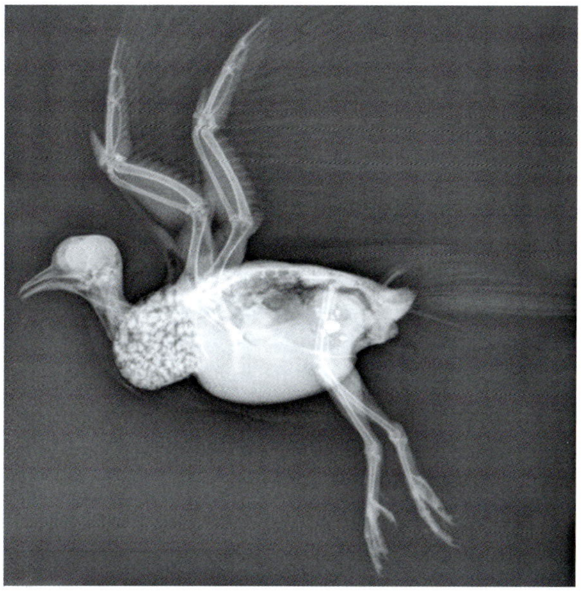

Fig. 19.4 Lateral radiograph of a normal dove. Note the distention of the crop with ingesta and numerous small stones (grit) within the ventriculus.

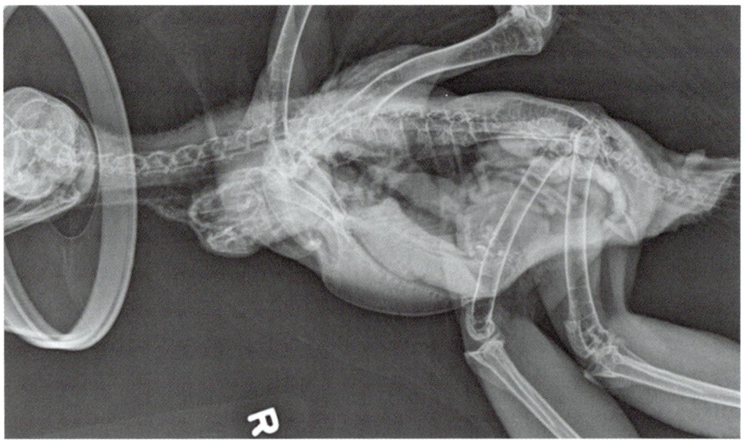

Fig. 19.5 Lateral radiograph of a falcon initially presented for inappetence. A nearly intact small mammal is present within the crop. Following a request for further information it was revealed that the bird had ignored its supper overnight but had accepted a mouse for breakfast immediately before the radiographic examination (R = right).

opaque intraluminal grit particles) within the caudal coelomic cavity. On a ventrodorsal view, the ventriculus is located to the left of midline approximately at the level of the coxofemoral joints, and on a lateral view, it is located in the ventral aspect of the coelomic cavity. The ventriculus is mobile, and intracoelomic mass lesions may result in displacement of this organ. The **small intestine** and paired **caeca** occupy the caudal coelom and are usually not distinguished radiographically. The gastrointestinal tract in birds usually does not contain air; however, a small amount of air may be present within the **cloaca**.

LIVER

The liver is located in the ventral coelomic cavity and forms an hourglass-shaped silhouette with the heart as described above. The lateral liver margins are usually well seen on a ventrodorsal view due to the adjacent air sacs. On a lateral view, the liver should not extend beyond the sternum and on a ventrodorsal view not beyond the acetabula.

SPLEEN AND PANCREAS

The spleen is often not clearly visible on radiographs but becomes increasingly visible with enlargement. On a lateral view, the spleen is located in the mid coelom dorsal to the margin between the proventriculus and ventriculus. The pancreas is not radiographically visible.

KIDNEYS

The kidneys are located in the caudodorsal coelom ventral to the synsacrum. They are mostly obscured by the overlying pelvis. The cranial poles extend into the coelomic cavity and appear as rounded soft-tissue opaque structures ventral to the spine which are bordered by air within the air sacs.

REPRODUCTIVE ORGANS

The testicles or single left ovary are located ventral to the cranial poles of the kidneys and immediately caudal to the adrenal glands, which are not radiographically visible. The size depends on hormonal influences and undergoes cyclic variations.

INTRA-ABDOMINAL FAT

Most birds only have a small amount of fat within the coelomic cavity, and visibility of inner organ margins mostly depends on adjacent air sacs. It is interesting to note that based on the authors' experience, coelomic detail in thin birds is often better than in fat animals (Fig. 19.6), which is in contrast to radiographic examination in mammals.

19.1.2 Indications

The radiographic examination is an important part of the diagnostic workup of an avian patient. It may be advisable to obtain baseline radiographs even in healthy birds presented for their annual physical examination because these can serve as a comparison if the patient presents with a medical problem later on. A radiographic examination is imperative in any ill bird to be able to evaluate morphology and pathological changes of coelomic organs. Indications for the radiographic examination of the avian patient include trauma, respiratory diseases, suspected diseases of specific inner organs and nonspecific signs such as anorexia or depression.

19.2 Radiographic technique and positioning

19.2.1 Preparation, positioning and technique

In most avian species seen in small animal practice, whole body radiographs are feasible. In species with long legs or a long neck, separate radiographs of these areas are typically obtained.

Awake (standing) radiographs

Radiographs of a standing patient can be considered in emergency cases where anaesthesia is considered an unacceptable risk, and may be helpful for some specific

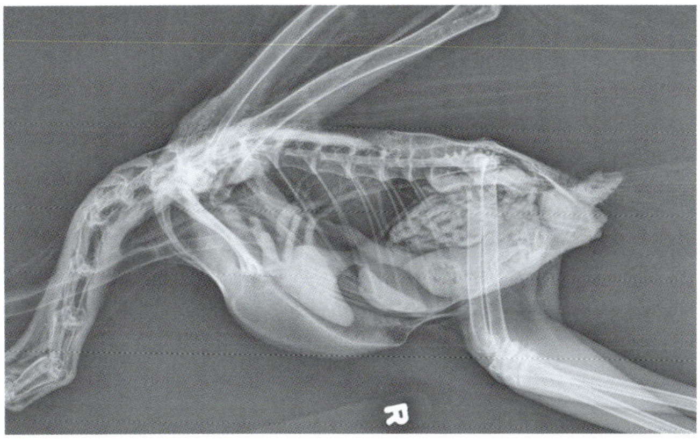

a

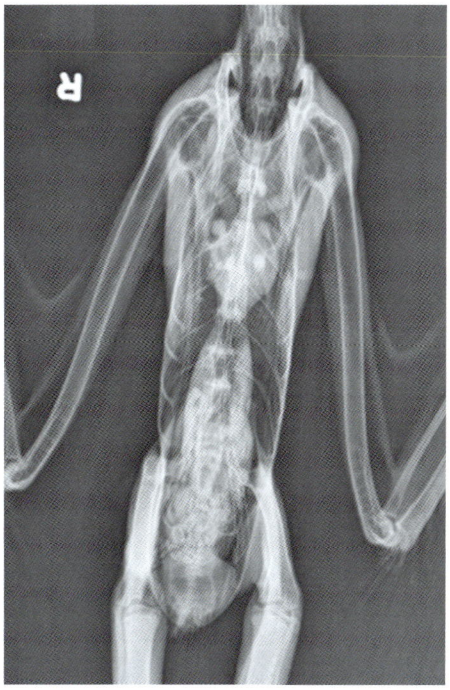

b

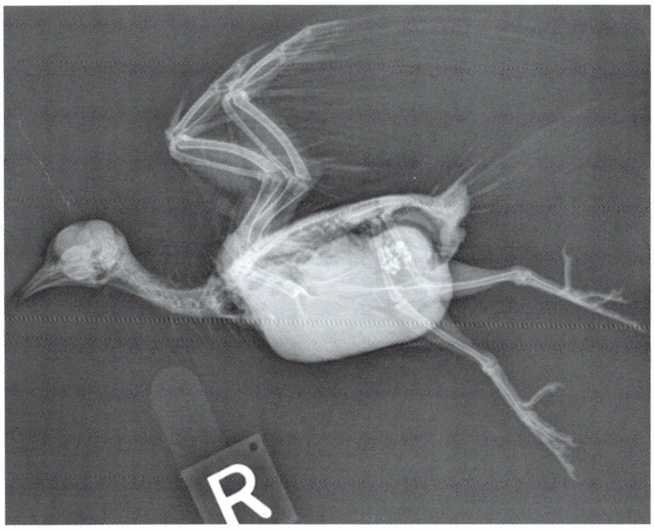

c

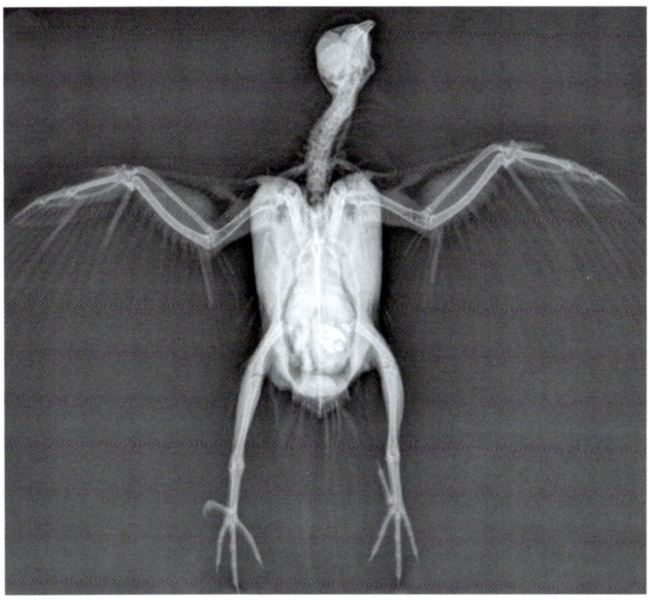

d

Fig. 19.6 Lateral a and ventrodorsal b radiographs of a very emaciated heron, and lateral c and ventrodorsal d radiographs of an obese dove. It is interesting to note that the abdominal detail is much better in the thin than in the overweight bird (probably due to the immediate proximity of the air sacs to the coelomic organs). The coelomic cavity including all organs was determined to be normal on subsequent necropsy in both birds (R = right).

indications. However, it is important to note that these radiographs are typically of limited diagnostic quality. Standing radiographs of the awake avian patient can be helpful in the diagnosis of metallic foreign material (e.g. lead, zinc), determine the presence of an egg, aid in the diagnosis of some fractures, and monitor contrast medium passage during an upper GI contrast study (Fig. 19.7). The bird is placed in a container (typically a cardboard box) during the procedure. A standing dorsoventral view is usually less informative than a lateral view obtained with a horizontal beam technique.

Radiographs under general anaesthesia

Most avian radiographs are obtained under general anaesthesia, which not only improves the diagnostic quality of the radiographs but also reduces stress and possibly the risk of injury to the patient. To facilitate rapid anaesthesia induction and recovery, isoflurane inhalation is the method of choice. If possible, the bird should be intubated to keep the airway open and support respiration.

The bird is positioned directly (without a grid) on the cassette. Radiographs are obtained in at least two planes.

- **Lateral views:** The patient is positioned in right lateral recumbency and both wings are pulled dorsally and affixed to the cassette by means of adhesive tape. The legs are pulled caudally and spread (Fig. 19.8a).
- **Ventrodorsal views:** The bird is positioned on the cassette in dorsal recumbency. The wings are spread laterally and affixed to the cassette by means of adhesive tape. The legs are pulled caudally and also affixed with adhesive tape (Fig. 19.8b).

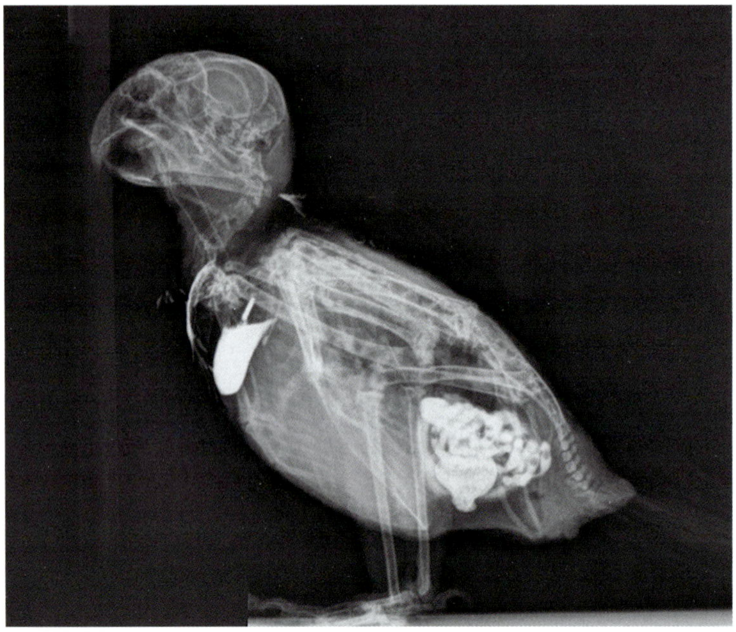

Fig. 19.7 Lateral radiograph of an awake (standing) bird to check for progression of positive contrast medium (barium sulphate suspension) through the gastrointestinal tract. Note that only a limited evaluation of the skeletal system and coelomic organs is possible on this view.

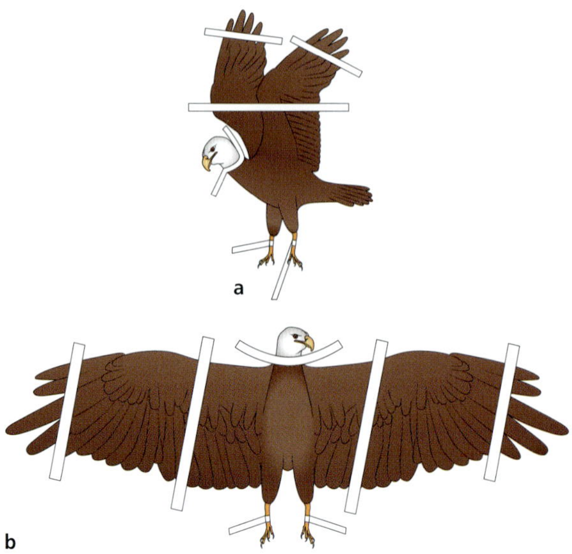

Fig. 19.8 Schematic illustration of positioning of an avian patient for a lateral a and ventrodorsal b radiographic projection. Note spreading of the wings and legs on the lateral view to avoid superimposition.

High-detail film or film–screen combinations are advisable to optimize resolution for the evaluation of small birds, as well as of the head and extremities.

19.2.2 Contrast studies

Contrast studies of the gastrointestinal tract

These are an important part of the diagnostic workup of avian patients. Even though contrast studies are routine procedures, some security measures are indicated to perform these studies effectively and safely. If the patient is dehydrated, supportive therapy including fluid administration is indicated before contrast medium is given. Additionally, it is advisable to administer the contrast medium to the awake bird directly into the crop by means of a tube, as anaesthetised patients are at risk of contrast medium aspiration. As with mammals, survey radiographs are obtained as a baseline prior to contrast medium administration.

INDICATIONS

- Regurgitation, vomiting or diarrhoea.
- Abnormal findings on palpation of the crop or coelom.
- Dilated intestinal segments.
- History of foreign body ingestion.
- Coelomic mass lesions of undetermined aetiology.

CONTRAST MEDIUM In most cases, barium sulphate suspension is used (10–20 ml/kg). If the primary indication for the examination is evaluation of the crop, additional insufflation of air may be performed to achieve a double contrast study (see below). If gastrointestinal tract perforation is of concern, nonionic iodinated contrast medium (e.g. iohexol) is preferred.

RADIOGRAPHS These are obtained immediately after contrast medium administration into the crop or distal oesophagus and after 15, 30, 60, 120, 240 and 480 minutes. Normal transit time depends on the bird species, and in parrots usually ranges from 2 to 4 hours.

PATHOLOGICAL FINDINGS

- Generalized or focal infiltrative changes of the wall of the gastrointestinal tract.
- Gastrointestinal dilatation.
- Obstruction.
- Mass lesions of adjacent structures with resultant displacement of gastrointestinal tract segments.

A pathological increase in gastrointestinal transit time can be caused by various infectious and noninfectious diseases resulting in intestinal luminal narrowing or obstruction. Foreign bodies, strictures or neoplastic lesions of the gastrointestinal tract should be ruled out. Additionally, chronic lead or zinc toxicity, as well as a variety of infectious organisms (viruses, bacteria, fungi) may result in an increased gastrointestinal transit time.

Double contrast study of the cloaca

This study may aid in the evaluation of cloacal abnormalities. Barium sulphate suspension (10 ml/kg) is administered into the cloaca, followed by air (10 ml/kg). This technique can aid in the diagnosis of various pathological changes such as papillomas, neoplasms and ulcerations.

Urography

This contrast study is helpful in the evaluation of kidneys, ureters and cloaca. (Nonionic) iodinated contrast medium (700–800 mg I/kg) is administered intravenously, and radiographs are obtained after 10 seconds, 60 seconds and 2 minutes. Possible pathological findings include enlargement or mass lesions of the kidneys and cloacal changes.

Other contrast procedures such as myelography have been described for birds but are rarely used in practice and are not further discussed at this place.

19.3 Disorders of the head

Diseases of the head are common in birds. A radiographic diagnosis requires perfect positioning (under anaesthesia) and acquisition of radiographs in multiple planes. With the increasing availability of computed tomography, radiographs of the head are less commonly performed in birds nowadays, as is also the case in mammals.

Obvious traumatic changes such as fractures of the beak or the skull are the most common indications for a radiographic evaluation of the head. In animals held in captivity, these may be related to inappropriate husbandry, and in wild birds they are usually caused by vehicular accidents or collisions during flight (e.g. with windows). On occasion, radiographs can be helpful in the evaluation of upper airway disease and sinusitis and may demonstrate regions of increased opacity in the paranasal sinuses.

19.4 Disorders of the cardiovascular system

Diseases of the heart and great vessels are often congenital or caused by infectious processes. As in mammals, the radiographic examination is only of limited value in the evaluation of the cardiovascular system, and echocardiography is necessary for further assessment.

RADIOGRAPHIC FINDINGS Enlargement of the cardiac silhouette beyond the normal reference range, abnormal shape of the cardiac silhouette, as well as signs of cardiac decompensation (enlarged vessels, lung infiltrates or coelomic effusion) are possible findings in avian patients with cardiac disease. Enlargement of the cardiac silhouette can be caused by pericardial abnormalities or can be due to true cardiomegaly.

Pericardial effusion can be caused by a variety of infectious organisms (e.g. polyomavirus, chlamydia or mycobacteria). On radiographs, symmetric globoid enlargement of the cardiac silhouette will be evident.

True cardiomegaly is most often the result of cardiomyopathy, which may be caused by chronic anaemia, endocarditis or viral infections.

Mineralization of the large vessels can be seen in patients with imbalances in calcium metabolism. Arteriosclerosis may result in similar changes in old psittacine birds.

19.5 Disorders of the respiratory tract

A radiographic examination generally allows a good assessment of the complex respiratory tract of birds. In birds with long necks, the trachea is easily recognized and a (presumptive) diagnosis of abnormalities such as strictures, foreign bodies and granulomas is straightforward. For a definitive diagnosis, endoscopy (tracheoscopy) is often necessary. Similarly, recognition of abnormalities affecting the normally air-filled lungs and air sacs is often relatively straightforward.

RADIOGRAPHIC FINDINGS Diseases of the lower respiratory tract may result in pulmonary infiltrates with loss of the normal reticular pulmonary pattern, soft-tissue opaque material within the air sacs, subcutaneous emphysema, gas dilatation of the gastrointestinal tract due to aerophagia and discrete mass lesions.

Mycotic and bacterial **pneumonia** results in irregular regions of increased opacity within the pulmonary parenchyma with loss of the normal honeycomb pattern and often marked thickening of the bronchial walls. Granulomas, abscesses and neoplasia appear as relatively well-circumscribed soft-tissue opaque masses which are often visible on both views.

An infection of the air sacs (**air sacculitis**) results in thickening of the air sac walls which then become radiographically visible. Accumulations of secretions or masses within the air sacs appear as focal soft-tissue opacity lesions. Abnormal air sacs with a thickened wall are less pliable than normal air sacs and barely change in size during the respiratory cycle. Granulomatous masses within the air sacs commonly indicate a fungal infection (**aspergillosis**) (Fig. 19.9). An endoscopic evaluation is usually needed for a definitive diagnosis and allows assessment of the extent of the abnormalities and diagnostic sampling for cytological, bacteriological and mycotic examinations.

During radiographic evaluation, it is important to pay attention to the symmetry of the air sacs. Overdistention of an air sac is most commonly related to an **obstructive process** (e.g. foreign body or mass lesion such as a granuloma), and the contralateral air sac is often collapsed in these cases.

Air sac rupture is usually related to trauma and may result in gas accumulations within the coelomic cavity or extensive subcutaneous emphysema (Fig. 19.10).

Due to the intimate association between the respiratory and the musculoskeletal systems, respiratory tract infections may result in **osteomyelitis** of the pneumatized bones or vice versa.

19.6 Disorders of the coelomic cavity, liver and spleen

19.6.1 Coelomic cavity

When evaluating an avian patient for coelomic anomalies, the following are taken into consideration: abnormal size, shape, position or opacity of one or more organs, loss of abdominal detail as an indicator of coelomic effusion, and presence of any mass lesions.

In the case of an inconclusive radiographic examination, advanced imaging procedures such as contrast medium studies or ultrasound (as well as possibly fine-needle aspiration or biopsy) may be necessary to establish a diagnosis.

19.6.2 Liver

Hepatomegaly is a relatively common and nonspecific finding. Possible differential diagnoses include inflammatory/infectious diseases (viruses, bacteria, chlamydia, mycobacteria, fungi and parasites), neoplasia and metabolic disorders such as haemochromatosis, lipidosis, fat deposition and visceral gout.

RADIOGRAPHIC FINDINGS On the lateral view, the enlarged liver results in dorsal displacement of the ventriculus and diffuse increased opacity of the coelom (Fig. 19.11a). On the ventrodorsal view, the liver extends laterally beyond the coxofemoral joints and may obliterate the abdominal air sacs (Fig. 19.11b). An **irregular hepatic contour** indicates infiltrative processes (granulomas, neoplasia). A **decrease in size of the hepatic silhouette** is rare but may indicate atrophy.

19.6.3 Spleen

An enlarged spleen is seen on a lateral radiograph as a rounded to ovoid soft-tissue opaque structure dorsal to the border between the proventriculus and ventriculus (Fig. 19.12). As in mammals, **splenomegaly** can be caused by many diseases. Possible underlying causes include infectious disorders (viruses, bacteria, chlamydia, mycobacteria), neoplasia and metabolic diseases (lipidosis, haemochromatosis). Concurrent abnormalities of other organs (liver, kidneys, air sacs) are common. For example, patients with psittacosis usually have inflammatory changes in the lungs and air sacs in addition to severe splenic enlargement.

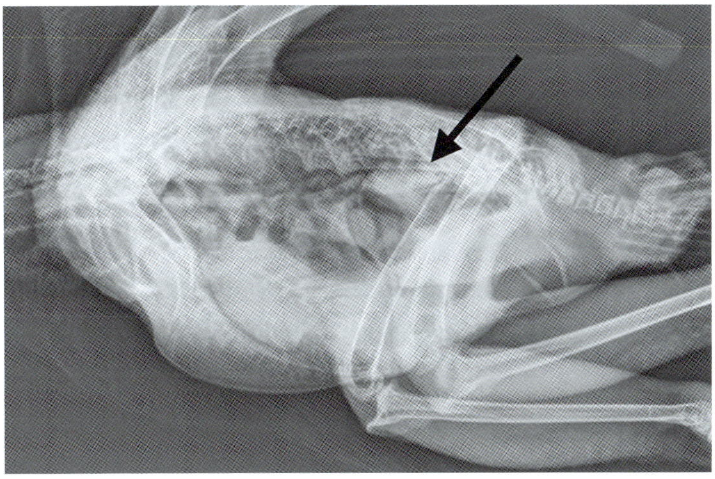

a

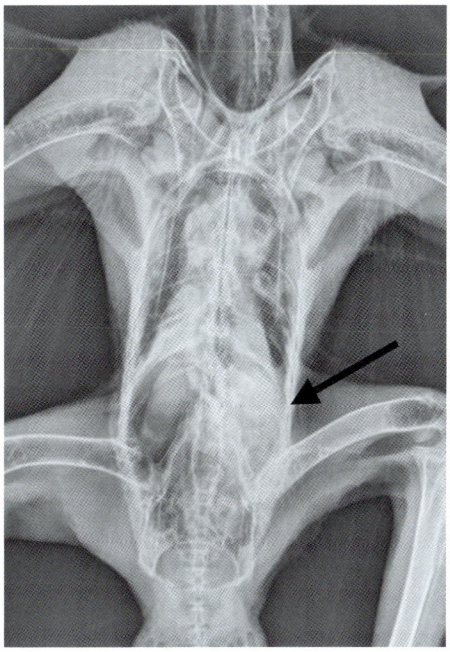

b

Fig. 19.9 Aspergillosis in an eagle. The lateral a and ventrodorsal b radiographs demonstrate a large granuloma in the left abdominal air sac (arrow).

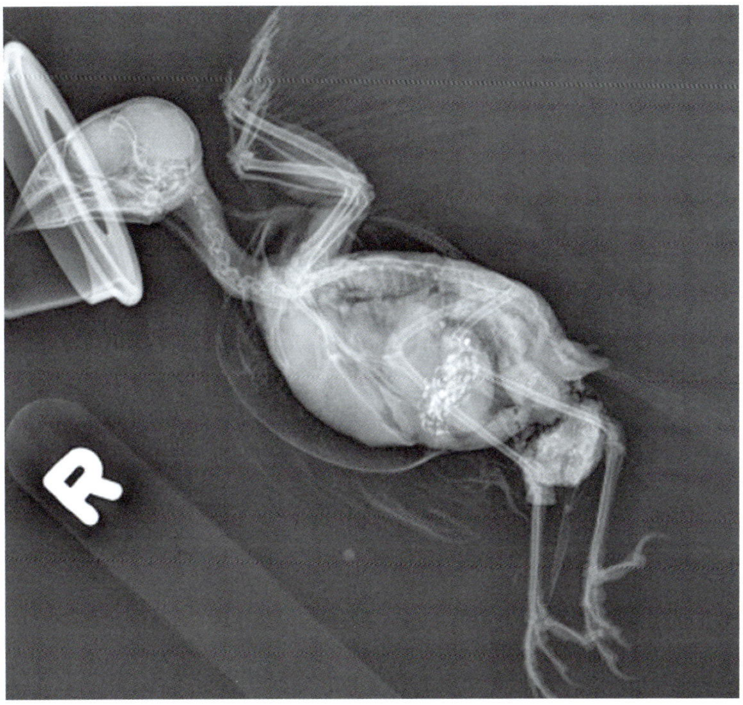

Fig. 19.10 Traumatic air sac rupture in a songbird characterized by extensive subcutaneous emphysema. Note also the soft-tissue opaque mass lesion caudoventral to the coelom consistent with cloacal prolapse (R = right).

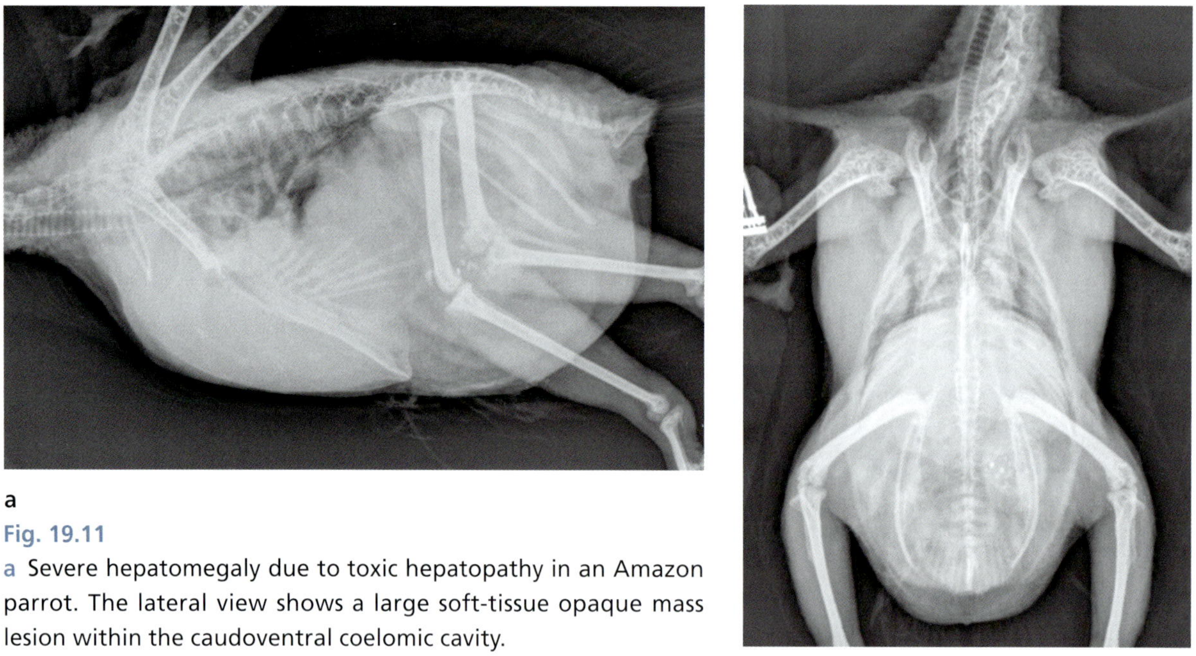

a

b

Fig. 19.11
a Severe hepatomegaly due to toxic hepatopathy in an Amazon parrot. The lateral view shows a large soft-tissue opaque mass lesion within the caudoventral coelomic cavity.
b On the ventrodorsal view, the hepatic silhouette extends laterally well beyond the level of the coxofemoral joints and the abdominal air sacs are greatly decreased in size.

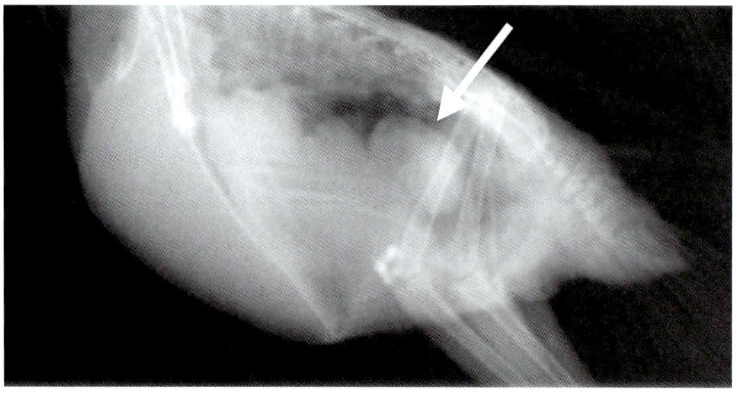

Fig. 19.12 Severe splenomegaly in a budgerigar. The enlarged spleen appears as an ovoid soft-tissue opaque mass dorsal to the margin between proventriculus and ventriculus (arrow). The primary differential diagnosis was an infectious or neoplastic disease process; further tests were declined by the owner.

19.7 Disorders of the gastrointestinal tract

As in mammals, survey radiographs are of limited value in the evaluation of the gastrointestinal tract, and an upper GI contrast study may be necessary, particularly for the diagnosis of infiltrative wall changes.

19.7.1 Impaction

Radiopaque foreign material or ingesta within the gastrointestinal tract (e.g. bone pieces or lead particles) are easily seen radiographically and can be diagnosed on survey radiographs without the need for further imaging (Fig. 19.13 and 19.14).

19.7.2 Dilatation

Crop

Pathological dilatation of the crop can occur secondary to thyroid disease, lead poisoning, infectious diseases or ileus. A diagnosis may be difficult as the crop is physiologically highly distensible and may be dilated in normal animals (see Fig. 19.4).

Proventriculus

In psittacines and some other species, dilatation of the proventriculus is a radiographic indicator of proventricular dilatation disease (PDD; 'macaw wasting disease'). The enlarged gas- and fluid-filled proventriculus is clearly visible especially on a lateral view (Fig. 19.15). Other possible causes of proventricular dilatation include bacterial and fungal infections as well as small intestinal ileus.

Intestinal tract

Dilatation of the intestine can have many underlying causes. **Mechanical ileus** (due to foreign bodies, massive parasite infestation, granulomatous or neoplastic mass

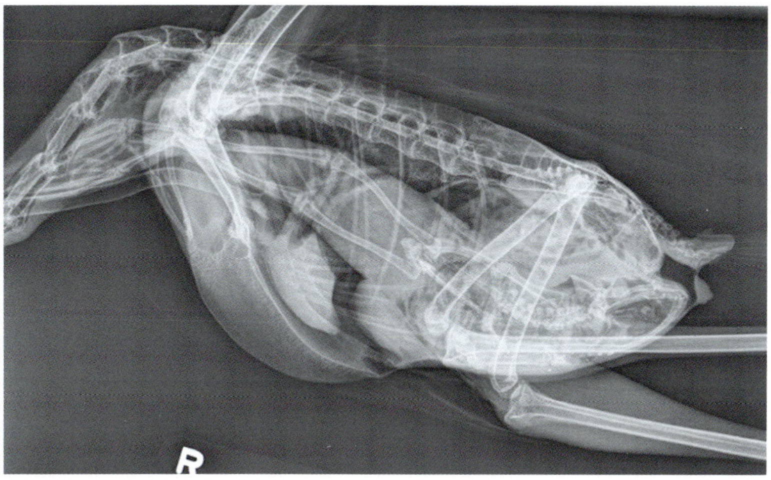

Fig. 19.13 Lateral radiograph of a heron found at the border of a pond and apparently 'retching'. An intact skeleton (frog, recognizable by the long legs) extends from the cervical oesophagus to the ventriculus. The bird proverbially has a 'frog in the throat'. Interestingly, the patient was able to digest the majority of its prey (the frog's feet were regurgitated) and was released back into the wild.

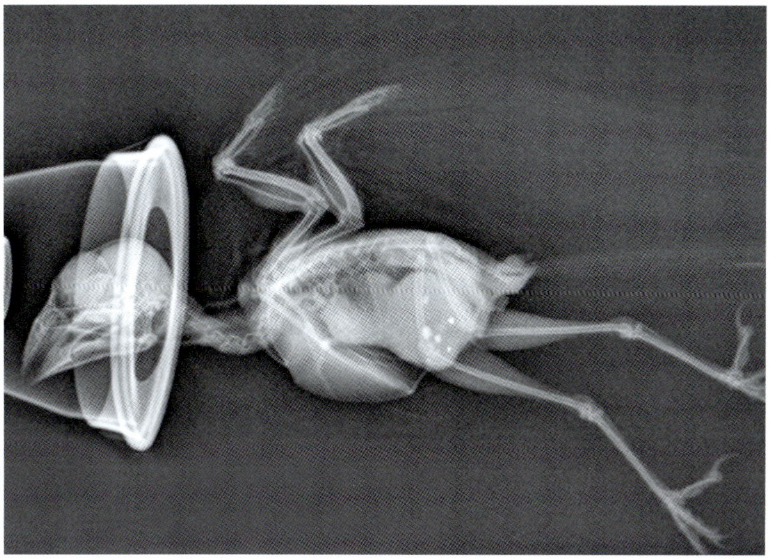

Fig. 19.14 Lateral radiograph of a cardinal with lead poisoning. Numerous small metal opaque fragments are present within the ventriculus.

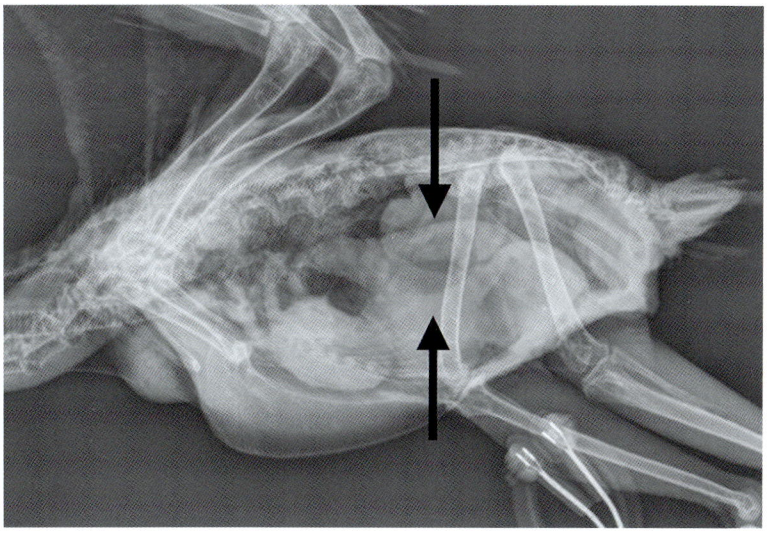

Fig. 19.15 Lateral radiograph of a parrot with proventricular dilatation disease ('macaw wasting disease'). The proventriculus (arrows) is dilated with gas and fluid.

lesions or strictures) typically results in intestinal distension proximal to the obstructive lesion. **Paralytic ileus** results in dilatation of the entire intestinal tract and may be caused by infectious diseases, toxicity (lead), parasites or peritonitis (e.g. secondary to rupture of an egg).

Cloaca

Gas dilatation of an **atonic** cloaca can occur secondary to spinal trauma or neoplastic infiltration of the sacral nerves (e.g. with renal neoplasia). **Obstruction** of the cloaca due to mass lesions (e.g. papillomas) can also lead to dilatation. Gas accumulation within the cloaca with concurrent **increased opacity of the cloacal wall** can on occasion be seen with cloacal or rectal infection or neoplasia. Laying hens physiologically have a wide cloaca, which should not be mistaken for a pathological process.

19.7.3 Other findings

- **Generalized increase in opacity of the gastrointestinal wall:** Along with increased opacity of other organs, this can be a radiographic finding with visceral gout. As previously mentioned, imaging diagnosis of infiltrative disorders of the intestinal wall usually requires an upper GI contrast study.
- **Excessive amount of grit:** An increased amount of small stones within the ventriculus and intestinal tract may indicate inappropriate nutrition or diseases of the crop, stomach or intestinal tract.
- **Heavy metal toxicity:** The metallic particles (lead, zinc) are usually located within the ventriculus. Generalized dilatation of the intestinal tract (paralytic ileus) is a common concurrent finding in affected animals.
- **Thickening and irregular mucosal contour of the oesophagus and crop:** This can be seen subsequent to a fungal infection (**candidiasis**). Vitamin A deficiency is another reported cause for this radiographic abnormality.
- **Filling defects:** Even though they are rare in birds, these may indicate granulomatous or neoplastic diseases of the gastrointestinal tract (Fig. 19.16).

19.8 Disorders of the urogenital tract

19.8.1 Diseases of the kidneys

Enlargement of one or both kidneys (**renomegaly**) can be caused by infectious agents (bacteria, chlamydia), neoplasia (adenocarcinoma, embryonal nephroma), metabolic disorders (renal gout, dehydration, lipidosis), cystic changes or toxicity. A renal biopsy is necessary for definitive diagnosis in many cases. Enlarged kidneys may appear as soft-tissue opacity masses ventral to the synsacrum and cranial to the pelvic inlet and are best seen on a lateral view (Fig. 19.17).

In birds, there is an intimate association between the kidneys, the **pelvic nerve** and the **sacral nerves**. Neoplastic renal diseases may involve these nerves, and affected animals may present with lameness, muscle or bone atrophy, or cloacal dilatation.

Increased radiopacity of the kidneys can be caused by renal gout, dehydration or nephrocalcinosis.

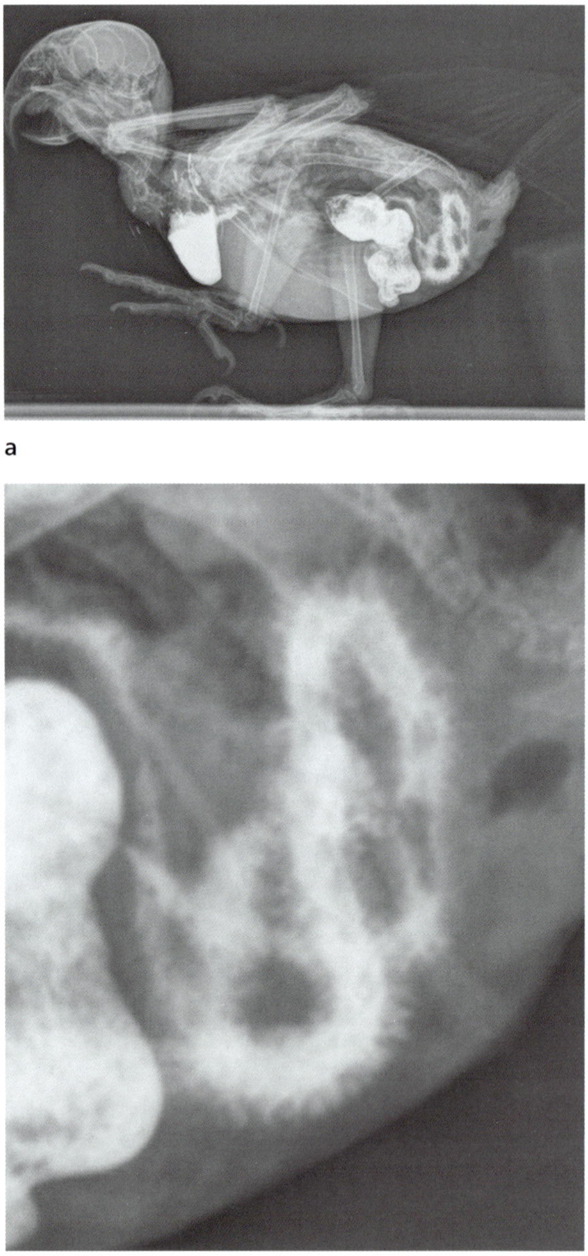

a

b

Fig. 19.16 Intestinal neoplasia in a parrot. The upper GI contrast study shows decreased transit time of the contrast medium through the GI tract, proventricular dilatation and markedly irregular margination of the small intestinal luminal surface. a Lateral view immediately following contrast medium administration and b magnified area of a. Histological examination of intestinal biopsies was consistent with diffuse lymphoma.

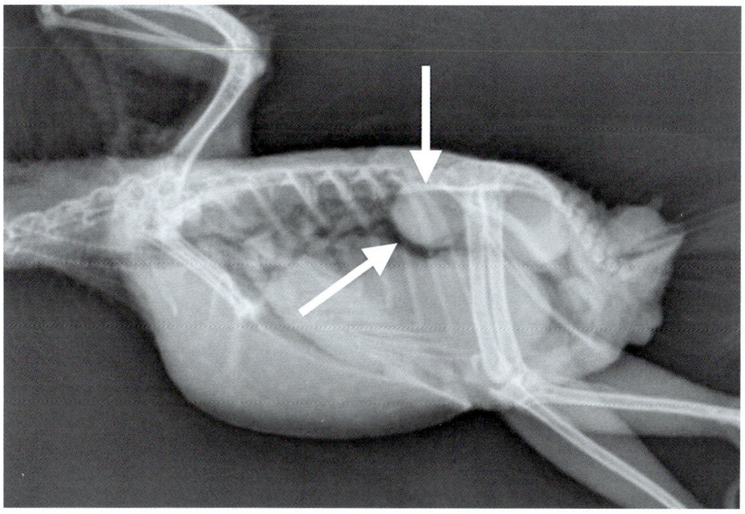

Fig. 19.17 Renomegaly in a lory with gout. The enlarged kidneys extend far cranially and ventrally into the coelomic cavity (arrows).

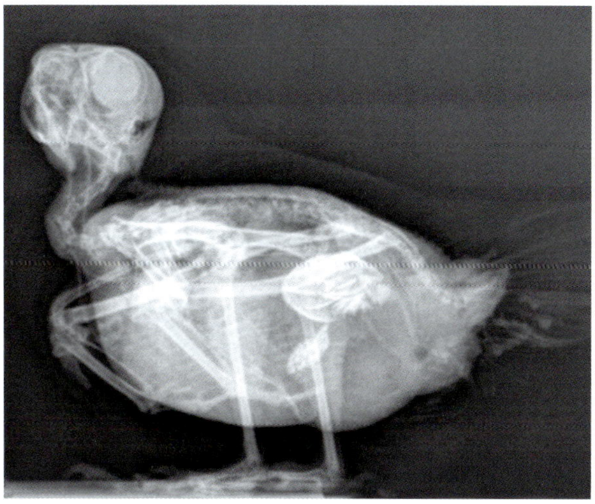

Fig. 19.18 Fractured egg and yolk coelomitis in a small parrot. The standing radiograph shows the abnormal egg and extensive loss of detail within the coelomic cavity.

19.8.2 Diseases of the gonads

The appearance of the reproductive organs depends on the reproductive status of the bird. During the breeding season, the testicles and ovaries increase in size. Inactive testicles and ovaries are not usually visible radiographically except when pathological processes such as neoplasia are present. **Enlargement of testicles or ovaries** (both physiological and pathological) manifests as soft-tissue opaque mass lesion(s) cranioventral to the kidneys. However, depending on their size and concurrent anomalies, the gonads may be difficult to distinguish from the kidneys and other coelomic structures.

Egg binding

This is a relatively common problem in birds. A radiographic examination allows assessment of size, integrity and position of the egg or eggs, consistency of the shell, and possible concurrent pathological abnormalities of the coelom such as mass lesions or loss of detail (**coelomitis**) (Fig. 19.18).

Polyostotic hyperostosis

Multifocal regions of increased opacity in the medullary cavity of the long bones are observed under the influence of oestrogen. This may be a normal finding in egg laying birds or may indicate a hormone producing ovarian or testicular tumour.

19.9 Disorders of the musculoskeletal system

Pathology of the musculoskeletal system is one of the most common indications for radiographic evaluation of captive and wild birds.

19.9.1 Fractures and luxations

Traumatic bone fractures or luxations are common. Fractures of the wings and legs are most commonly observed, and radiographic documentation of the fracture in at least two planes is necessary for planning successful surgical repair (Fig. 19.19). Spinal fractures are also most commonly traumatic in nature, but in many cases are difficult to diagnose on survey radiographs.

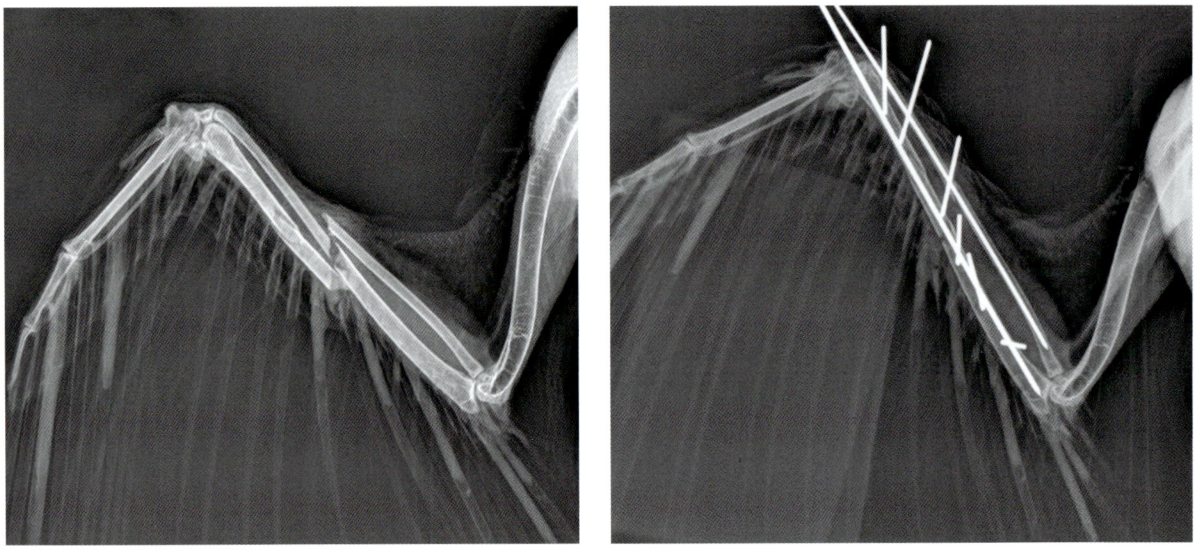

a b

Fig. 19.19 Mid-diaphyseal fractures of radius and ulna before a and after b osteosynthesis by means of intramedullary pins and an external fixator. An orthogonal view (not shown here) is essential, as for orthopaedic radiographs in mammals.

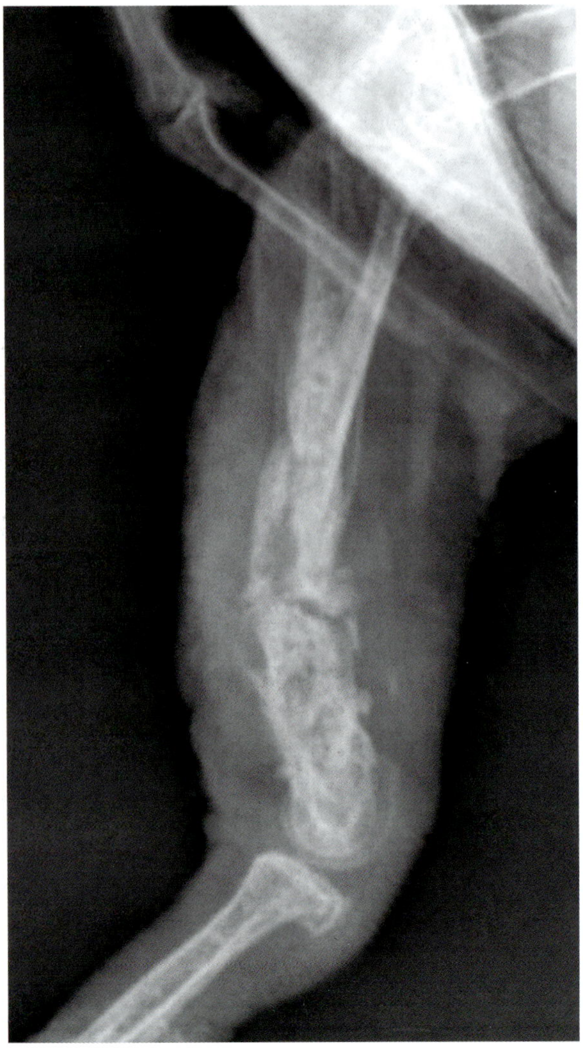

Fig. 19.20 Osteomyelitis (Actinomyces pyogenes) and delayed fracture healing of the tibiotarsus in a parrot. The implants originally placed for fracture repair have been removed, but the fracture is still visible. The bone has an irregular blistered appearance with numerous lytic foci as well as mild periosteal reaction. Concurrent soft-tissue swelling is present.

19.9.2 Osteomyelitis

Bone infection can result from a variety of infectious agents including fungi and bacteria (e.g. *Mycobacterium*). Radiographically, osteomyelitis in birds differs from mammals because periosteal reaction is usually negligible. Instead, caseous abscesses in the medullary cavity result in deformation of the affected bone, which may appear blistered or lytic (Fig. 19.20). **Mycobacterial infection** can result in multifocal lytic lesions with adjacent sclerosis in the long bones.

19.9.3 Bone tumours

These are rare in birds and typically result in monostotic aggressive bone lesions. Because bone tumours may be difficult to distinguish from inflammatory changes, a biopsy is often necessary to establish a definitive diagnosis for an aggressive bone lesion and obtain samples for culture and sensitivity to rule out osteomyelitis.

19.9.4 Arthritis and degenerative joint disease

Septic arthritis initially results in intracapsular and later extracapsular soft-tissue swelling, widening of the joint space, and erosive changes of the articular surfaces (Fig. 19.21). Degenerative joint disease is common, especially in older birds, and appears similar to mammals.

19.9.5 Other diseases

Inflammatory diseases of the plantar surface of the foot ('bumble foot') are especially common in birds of prey, may be limited to the soft tissues of the foot, or may result in osteomyelitis of individual or multiple phalanges.

Metabolic bone diseases are usually nutritional in aetiology and result in generalized osteopenia, often with deformation and pathological fractures of the long bones (Fig. 19.22).

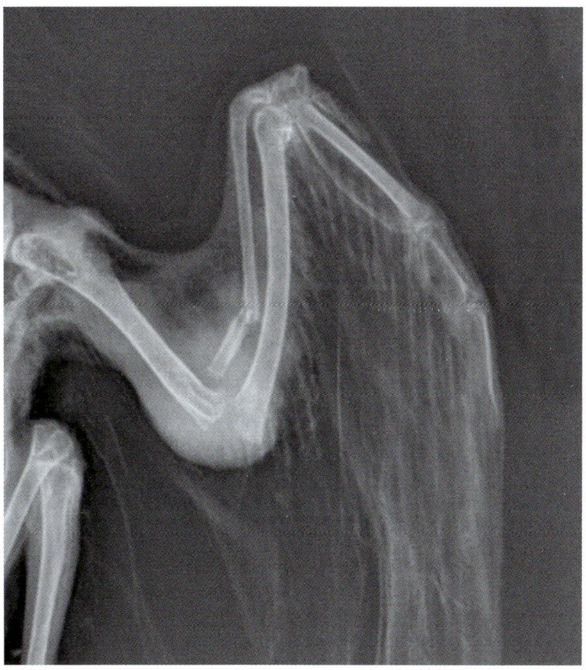

Fig. 19.21 Septic arthritis of the elbow joint and chronic fracture of the radius in a dove. There is severe intracapsular soft-tissue swelling of the joint, the joint space is widened, and the joint surfaces have irregular erosive lesions.

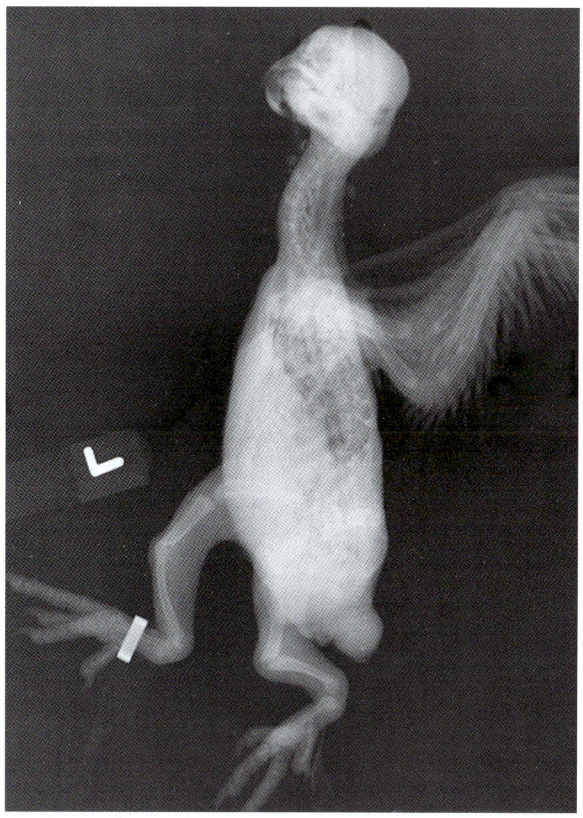

Fig. 19.22 Metabolic bone disease in a juvenile grey parrot. Generalized osteopenia as well as multiple pathological fractures are noted (L = left).

Suggested reading

Beregi A, Molnár V, Felkai F, Bíró F, Szentgáli Z. Diagnostic radiology of pet and wild birds: a review. I. Radiographic techniques and radiographs of healthy birds. Acta Vet Hung 1999; 47: 291–302.

Freeman KP, Hahn KA, Jones MP, Toal RL. Right leg muscle atrophy and osteopenia caused by renal adenocarcinoma in a cockatiel (*Melopsittacus undulates*). Vet Radiol Ultrasound 1999; 40: 144–7.

Gumpenberger M, Scope A. Diagnosis of abdominal diseases in birds by combined radiography and ultrasonography. Eur J Companion Anim Pract 2002; 12: 153–62.

Harcourt-Brown NH. Diagnostic imaging. In: Harcourt-Brown NH, Chitty J (eds). BSAVA Manual of Psittacine Birds, 2nd edn. Gloucester: BSAVA 2005.

Harr KE, Kollias GV, Rendano V, DeLahunta A. A myelographic technique for avian species. Vet Radiol Ultrasound 1997; 38: 187–92.

Kostka V. Röntgenologische Untersuchungen am Rumpf- und Gliedmaßenskelett von Zier- und Wildvögeln. Anatomische, physiologische und pathologische Befunde. Dissertation Vet Med, Justus-Liebig-Universität Gießen 1992.

Krautwald ME, Tellhelm B, Hummel G. Atlas zur Röntgenanatomie und Röntgendiagnostik der Ziervögel. Berlin: Parey 1992.

Krautwald-Junghanns ME, Schumacher F, Tellhelm B. Evaluation of the lower respiratory tract in psittacines using radiology and computed tomography. Vet Radiol Ultrasound 1993; 34: 382–90.

McMillan MC. Radiology of avian respiratory diseases. Compend Contin Educ Pract Vet 1986; 8: 551–8.

McMillan MC. Radiographic diagnosis of avian abdominal disorders. Compend Contin Educ Pract Vet 1986; 8: 616–32.

McMillan MC. Avian gastrointestinal radiography. Compend Contin Educ Pract Vet 1983; 5: 273–8.

Naldo J. Radiology. In: Samour J (ed.). Avian Medicine. Philadelphia: Elsevier 2000; 50–60.

Nickel R, Schummer A, Seiferle E. Lehrbuch der Anatomie der Haustiere. Vol V: Vögel, 2nd edn. Berlin: Parey 1992.

Paul-Murphy JR, Koblik PD, Stein G, Penninck DG. Psittacine skull radiography. Anatomy, radiographic technique and patient application. Vet Radiol 1990; 31: 125–31.

Pees M, Straub J, Schumacher J, Gompf R, Krautwald-Junghanns ME. Pilotstudie zu echokardiographischen Untersuchungen mittels Farb- und pulsed-wave-Spektraldoppler an Blaukronenamazonen (*Amazona ventralis*) und Blaustirnamazonen (*Amazona a. aestiva*). Deutsche Tierärztliche Wochenschrift 2005; 112: 39–43.

Rübel GA, Isenbügel E, Wolvekamp P. Atlas der Röntgendiagnostik bei Heimtieren. Hannover: Schlütersche 1991.

Samour J, Naldo JL. Anatomical and Clinical Radiology of Birds of Prey: Including Interactive Advanced Anatomical Imaging. Philadelphia: WB Saunders 2007.

Smith BJ, Smith SA, Flammer K, Spaulding KA, Smallwood JE. The normal xeroradiographic and radiographic anatomy of the orangewinged Amazon parrot (*Amazona amazonica amazonica*). Vet Radiol 1990; 31: 114–24.

Smith BJ, Smith SA, Spaulding KA, Flammer K, Smallwood JE. The normal xeroradiographic and radiographic anatomy of the cockatiel (*Nymphicus hollandis*). Vet Radiol 1990; 31: 226–34.

Smith SA, Smith BJ. The normal xeroradiographic and radiographic anatomy of the red-tailed hawk (*Buteo jamacencis*). Vet Radiol 1990; 31: 301–12.

Smith BJ, Smith SA. Normal xeroradiographic and radiographic anatomy of the bobwhite quail (*Colinus virginianus*) with reference to other galliform species. Vet Radiol 1991; 32: 127–34.

Smith SA, Smith BJ. Atlas of Avian Radiographic Anatomy. Philadelphia: Saunders 1992.

Straub J, Pees M, Krautwald-Junghanns ME. Measurement of the cardiac silhouette in psittacines. J Am Vet Med Assoc 2002; 221: 76–9.

Vink-Nooteboom M, Lumeij JT, Wolvekamp WT. Radiography and image-intensified fluoroscopy of barium passage through the gastrointestinal tract in six healthy Amazon parrots (*Amazona aestiva*). Vet Radiol Ultrasound 2003; 44: 546–52.

Walsh MT. Radiology. In: Harrison GJ, Harrison LR (eds). Clinical Avian Medicine and Surgery. Philadelphia: WB Saunders 1986; 201–33.

Williams J. Orthopedic radiography in exotic animal practice. Vet Clin North Am Exot Anim Pract 2002; 5: 1–22.

Small mammals

20

Michaela Gumpenberger, Jasmin Hassan and Alexandra Böhler

This chapter will cover the most common diseases of **rabbits, guinea pigs, chinchillas, rats, mice, degus, hamsters** and **ferrets** which can be diagnosed radiographically.

20.1 Anatomy

The radiographic anatomy of small mammals is similar to dogs and cats in many regards. Anatomic variations in different species, as far as they are relevant for radiographic diagnostics, will be discussed under individual diseases.

20.1.1 Head

Teeth

There are important anatomic differences in dental anatomy between species. An overview of dental formulas in small mammals can be found in Table 20.1.

DECIDUOUS TEETH

In ferrets, deciduous teeth have erupted by 20 to 28 days of age and permanent teeth by 50 to 74 days. Rabbits have 16 deciduous teeth. The large incisors are already present at birth and are permanent. The small upper incisors are exfoliated with development of the permanent dentition. Most rodents do not have deciduous teeth (monophyodont) or lose them before birth.

INCISIVE (AND CANINE) TEETH

Rabbits belong to the order Lagomorpha and have two pairs of incisors associated with the upper jaw. The secondary upper incisors ('peg teeth') are located immediately caudal to the primary upper incisors, which form a semicircle. With normal occlusion, the lower incisors are located at the lingual surface of the distal quarter of the upper incisors.

In **guinea pigs**, the upper and lower incisors are not in contact during physiological mouth closure.

Hamsters have four incisors, one on each side of the upper and lower jaw, respectively.

The incisors in **hamsters**, **gerbils**, **mice** and **rats** grow continuously, and the lower incisors are approximately three times as long as the upper incisors. It is interesting to note that rodent teeth can grow as much as 5 to 7 centimetres per year.

The dentition of **ferrets** is typical for carnivores, with three incisors and one canine tooth per quadrant.

CHEEK TEETH

The **rabbit** has six maxillary and five mandibular cheek teeth bilaterally, with the last maxillary molar being very small and often barely discernible. The caudal mandibular cheek teeth may be slightly curved rostrally. Even though rabbit teeth are aradicular, their intra-alveolar component is referred to as 'tooth root' throughout this chapter to facilitate radiographic description.

Chinchillas, **degus** and **guinea pigs** have four and **hamsters**, **gerbils**, **mice** and **rats** only three cheek teeth in each quadrant. With a closed mouth, the mandibular cheek teeth are located slightly medial to the maxillary cheek teeth. The dentition of **ferrets** is typical for carnivores, with three premolar and two molar teeth per quadrant.

Table 20.1 Dental formulas in small mammals.

	Ferret	Rabbit	Chinchilla, guinea pig, degu	Rat, mouse, hamster
Upper arcade	3-1-3-1	2-0-3-3	1-0-1-3	1-0-0-3
Lower arcade	3-1-3-2	1-0-2-3	1-0-1-3	1-0-0-3

RADIOGRAPHIC FINDINGS In general, cheek teeth should be parallel, the tooth roots and occlusal surfaces should be located at the same level, and they should be smoothly marginated. The lamina dura should be visible.

On dorsoventral views, the lamina dura can only be assessed around the rostral cheek tooth; it should be smooth and sharply marginated. A faint, less opaque rim around the roots represents germinal tissue and is a physiological finding.

While the normal occlusal surfaces on lateral views with closed mouth appear as an undulating contour in rabbits and guinea pigs, they form a straight line in chinchillas and rats. The borders, as well as the centre of each cheek tooth, should be marked by distinct opaque lines representing dental enamel. The ventral mandibular contour is smooth, with a distinct cortical margin.

OTHER ANATOMIC PARTICULARITIES

The **tympanic bulla** is thin-walled, notably large and traversed by radiating bony septa especially in chinchillas (Fig. 20.1). The **parietal bones** in rabbits are physiologically porous or spongy in appearance.

20.1.2 Axial skeleton

Ribs and sternum

In **rabbits**, the first seven pairs of ribs connect to the sternum while the eighth and ninth pairs are confluent with the seventh. Ferrets have up to 15 pairs of ribs, and the first 10 pairs are connected to the sternum.

Spine

The vertebral formulas of select small mammals are listed in Table 20.2. The lumbar vertebrae in rabbits are characterized by especially long transverse processes.

20.1.3 Appendicular skeleton

Even though the bones of the appendicular skeleton in most small mammals are slender, the **apophyses** (especially of the hind limbs) are very prominent in rabbits as well as mice and rats.

Shoulder girdle

The **clavicle** develops as a long and slightly curved bone in mice, rats, chinchillas, hamsters and rabbits, while it is small and rudimentary, respectively, in guinea pigs and ferrets.

Pelvic girdle

The pelvis has the shape of a lyre in hamsters, chinchillas, guinea pigs and rabbits, while it is straight (similar to cats) in mice, rats and ferrets.

Digits

In guinea pigs, the first digit is absent in the forelimbs and rudimentary in the hind limbs. The fifth digit is completely absent in the hind limbs, so only three digits are fully developed.

The hind limbs in rabbits lack a first digit. In chinchillas, the first digit of the hind limbs is rudimentary and the fifth shortened.

20.1.4 Inner organs

Thorax

Generally, the thorax in rabbits and rodents is comparatively small in relation to the abdomen, with a cranially located and relatively large **heart**. Ferrets, on the other hand, have a slender thoracic shape, similar to cats, with a centrally positioned heart (sixth through eighth intercostal space; Fig. 20.2).

The **lungs** in ferrets have a total of six lobes, cranial and caudal on the left and cranial, middle, caudal and accessory on the right. The left cranial lung lobe is subdivided in rabbits and guinea pigs. Rats and mice only have one large left lung lobe without subdivision. The right-sided anatomy is the same as in the ferrets.

Mineralization of the **tracheal cartilages** is common and physiological.

Abdomen

ABDOMINAL FAT

The visibility of abdominal organs is predominantly determined by the presence of intra-abdominal fat. Many small mammals kept as pets are obese, which, especially in rab-

Table 20.2 Vertebral formulas in small mammals.

	Cervical vertebrae	Thoracic vertebrae	Lumbar vertebrae	Sacral vertebrae
Rabbit	7	12–13	6–8	4
Guinea pig	7	13–14	6	2–3
Rat	7	13	7	3
Hamster	7	13	7	4
Chinchilla	7	14	6	2
Ferret	7	14–15	5–7	3

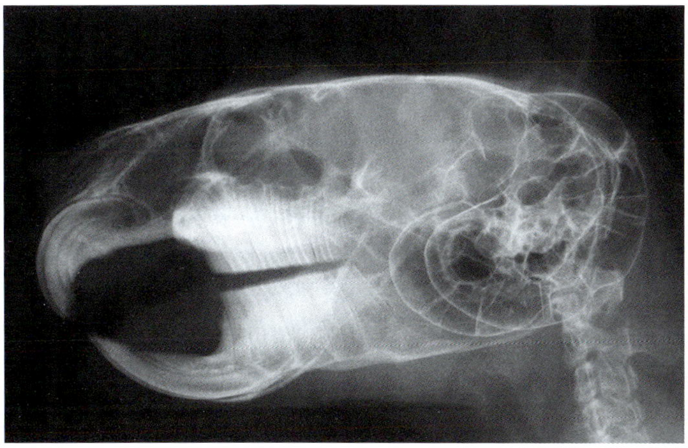

a

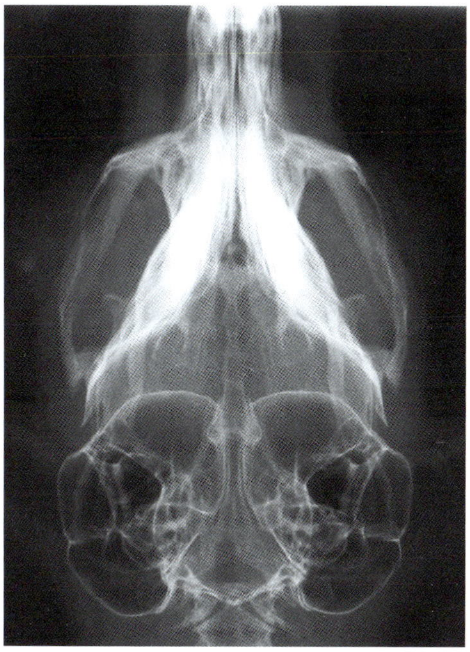

b

Fig. 20.1 Lateral a and dorsoventral b radiographs of the head in a chinchilla showing the normal tympanic bullae and teeth.

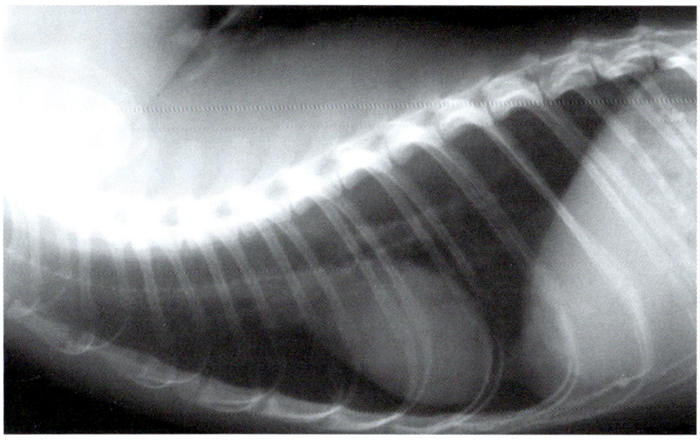

a

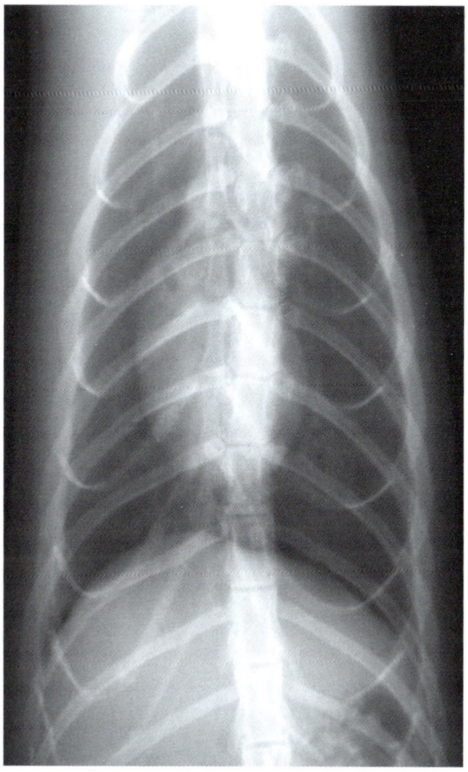

b

Fig. 20.2 Lateral a and dorsoventral b thoracic radiographs in a normal ferret.

bits, results in displacement of most organs cranioventrally (Fig. 20.3). The colon, which courses obliquely in a cranioventral–caudodorsal direction, and the urinary bladder are usually the only visible structures in the caudal abdomen. The kidneys are typically located in the mid abdomen in obese animals, and the lumbar musculature is conspicuous. Overweight older rabbits develop fat deposits in the mid to caudal abdomen, which may lead to misinterpretation as an abdominal mass on radiographs.

GASTROINTESTINAL TRACT

The **stomach** in rabbits has a single compartment, is thin-walled and should always contain ingesta. The stomach in hamsters has two compartments, a nonglandular part (forestomach) and a glandular main compartment. While rabbits and many rodents have a voluminous **caecum** to allow digestion of cellulose, it is completely absent in carnivorous ferrets. Ferrets generally have a rather short gastrointestinal tract with passage times of only few hours.

LIVER, SPLEEN, PANCREAS AND ADRENAL GLANDS

The appearance of the liver in small mammals is similar to that in dogs and cats. While the spleen is large and easily recognized in ferrets, it is often not visible in other small mammals. Pancreas and adrenal glands are not usually visible radiographically.

URINARY TRACT

The **kidneys** are often only partially visible on survey radiographs in thin rabbits. Superimposition of a full gastrointestinal tract further hampers identification. The **urinary bladder** is usually visible and may be soft-tissue opaque or almost the opacity of contrast medium because of the high calcium carbonate content in urinary sediment (see section 20.6.3). The kidneys and urinary bladder are usually visible in ferrets, while their visibility in other species is significantly affected by the contents of adjacent gastrointestinal segments.

REPRODUCTIVE TRACT

On average, rabbits give birth to five to eight, guinea pigs two to five, rats four to twelve, ferrets two to ten, and chinchillas one to five young. Guinea pigs, degus and chinchillas are precocial. After a long pregnancy (guinea pigs 68 days, degus 90 days, chinchillas 111 days) they give birth to young that are relatively large in comparison to the mother's size.

The normal **ovaries** and **uterus** are not usually visible on survey radiographs. However, in obese animals, the uterus may be visible as a tubular soft-tissue opaque structure between the colon and urinary bladder.

Testicles appear as large structures with homogeneous soft-tissue opacity, especially in mice, rats, hamsters, chinchillas and guinea pigs.

The **male accessory glands** are not usually visible radiographically.

An anatomic particularity is the **os penis**, which is short and slightly ventrally convex in guinea pigs and rats, and long with a dorsal cranial hook in ferrets.

20.2 Radiographic technique and positioning

Positioning for the evaluation of individual body regions is performed as described for the dog and cat unless noted otherwise. Severe abnormalities such as obviously dis-

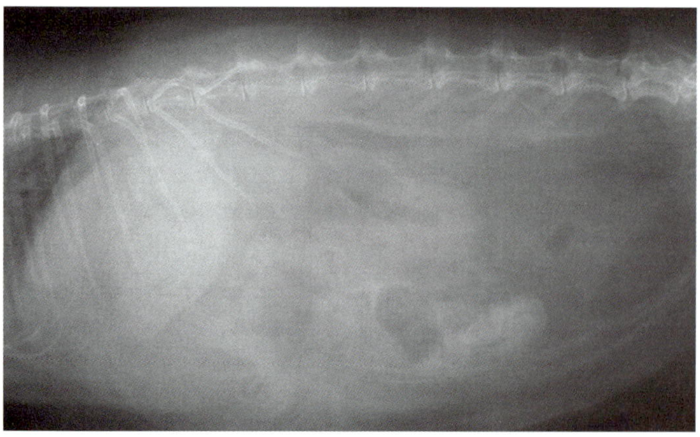

a

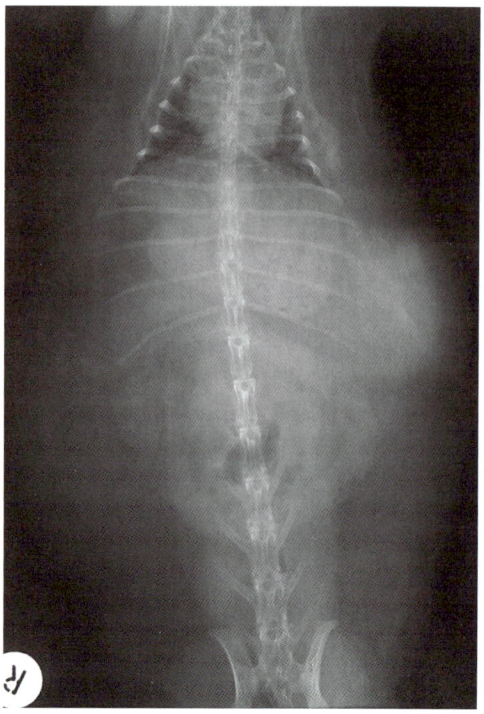

b

Fig. 20.3 Abdominal radiographs in an obese rabbit. a The lateral radiograph demonstrates cranial displacement of abdominal organs due to intra-abdominal fat deposits. b On the ventrodorsal view, a neoplastic lesion of a rib (11th left rib) is noted, which is obscured by gastrointestinal tract segments on the lateral view (R = right).

placed vertebral fractures or pleural effusion can usually be diagnosed on a single view and, depending on the circumstances, an orthogonal view may not be obtained to minimize patient distress. If sedation is prohibited by poor patient condition, survey radiographs with the patient awake and placed in a **radiolucent box** may be obtained in select cases. However, it is important to recognize that even significant lesions may be missed in these cases due to suboptimal patient positioning. If needed, ropes or adhesive strips may be used as positioning aids.

Due to the small size of most small mammals, **whole body radiographs** are commonly acquired. However, as described for dogs and cats, exposure parameters should be chosen to optimize imaging of the region of interest. Most radiographs can be obtained without the use of a grid. Particularly for dental radiographs, high-detail film–screen systems (e.g. mammography film) are recommended.

Even where only one view is shown to illustrate disease features in this chapter, orthogonal projections were obtained in all patients.

20.2.1 Teeth

A diagnosis of dental disease requires symmetric lateral and dorsoventral radiographs. While intraoral views are usually difficult to accomplish due to the small size of the mouth, tangential views are helpful in evaluation of the tooth roots. Rostrocaudal views can only be acquired under general anaesthesia and are helpful in the evaluation of dental curvatures, tooth tips and bridging, although these are usually readily assessed during the clinical examination. A definitive diagnosis of dental disease is often only possible by means of computed tomography.

Diseases of the **tympanic bulla** are more easily diagnosed on dorsoventral or tangential than on lateral radiographs.

20.2.2 Musculoskeletal system

Radiographic examination of the musculoskeletal structures in small mammals is performed as described for dogs and cats (see Chapter 15).

20.2.3 Thorax and abdomen

As in the dog, the forelimbs should be extended cranially to allow adequate assessment of the thorax. To avoid patient rotation on lateral views, the extremities have to be held or affixed parallel to each other. To avoid superimposition in the pelvic region, the hind limbs should be extended caudally on abdominal radiographs.

20.3 Disorders of the head and upper neck region

20.3.1 Dental diseases

These are amongst the most common diseases for most small mammal species included here.

Incisive (and canine) teeth

Malocclusion in rabbits is usually characterized by overly long mandibular incisors which are located rostral to the upper incisive teeth (Fig. 20.4). The mandibular incisors may

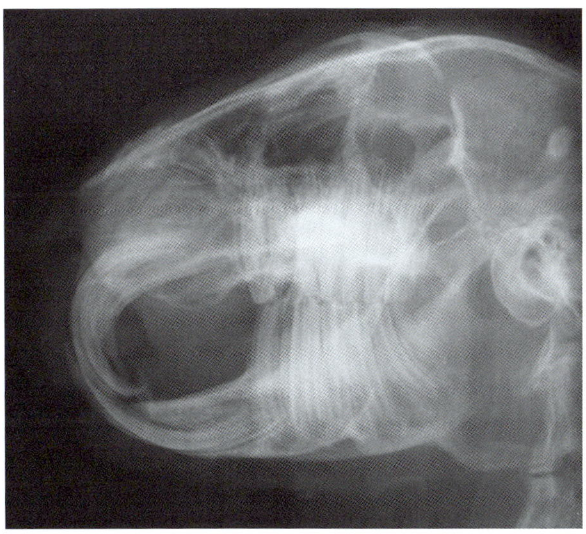

a

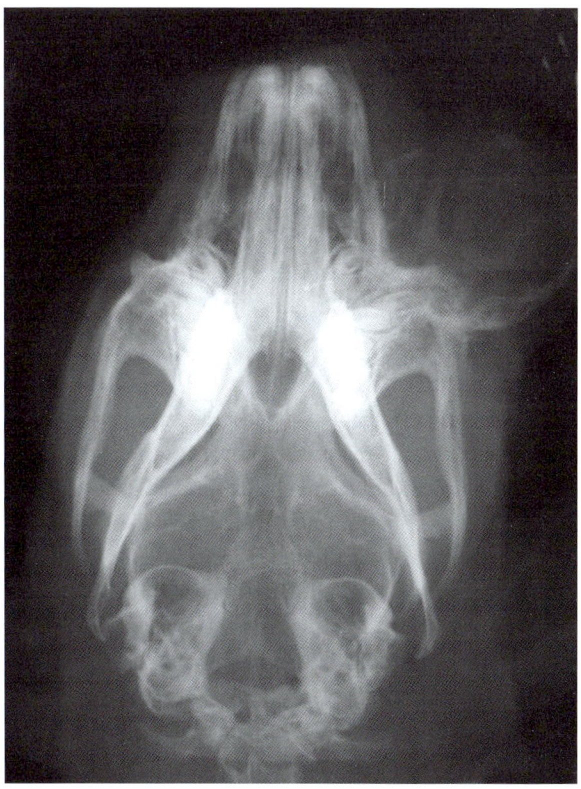

b

Fig. 20.4 Radiographs of the head in a rabbit with an abscess originating from the upper jaw. On the lateral view a, globoid expansion of the palatine bone is evident. On the dorsoventral view b, a bony shell is noted around the abscess. The upper incisors are abnormally curved, and the lower incisors extend too far rostrally.

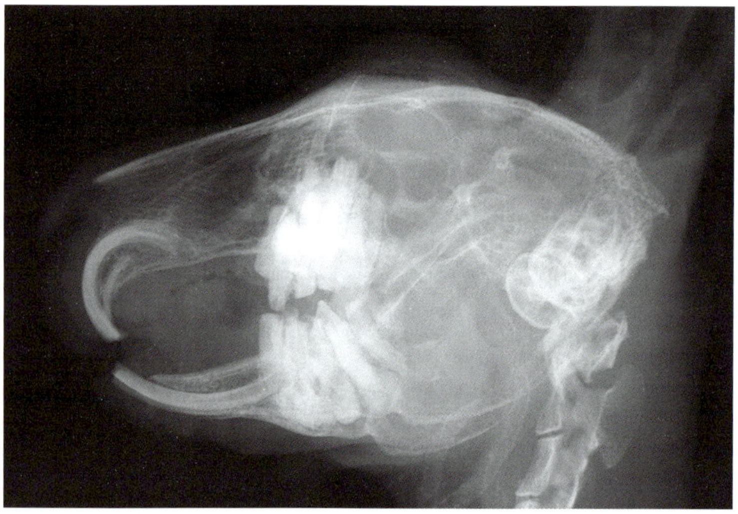

Fig. 20.5 Malocclusion in a rabbit. Radiographic abnormalities include abnormal curvature of the upper incisors and retrograde overgrowth of the maxillary and mandibular cheek teeth with loss of their normal parallel alignment. Additionally, mineralization of the vessels of the neck is evident. The rabbit also had renal mineralization (see Fig. 20.29).

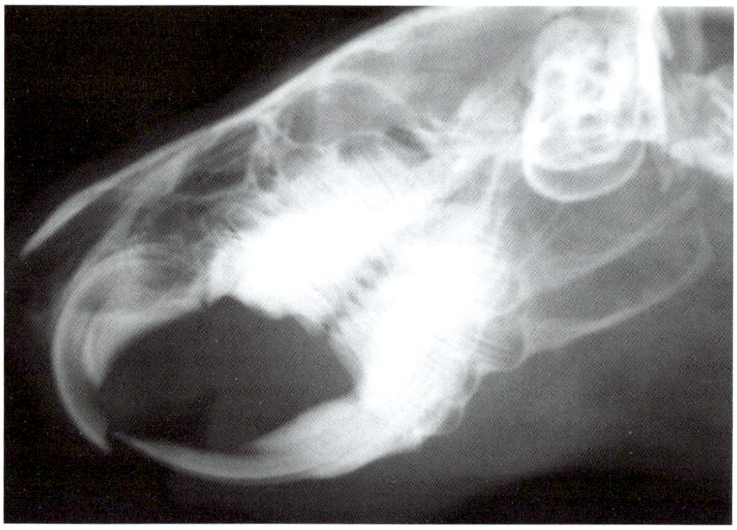

Fig. 20.6 Dental disease in a guinea pig. There is mild retrograde elongation of the tooth roots of the mandibular cheek teeth with a thinning and bumpy contour of the mandibular cortex.

also grow in a straight direction, while the upper incisors grow in a semicircular course towards and into the hard palate due to lack of wear. Direct contact between the tips of the upper and lower incisors in rabbits and rodents is pathological. **Dental (crown) fractures**, especially of the canine teeth, are not uncommon in ferrets due to their playful nature and tendency to chew on inappropriate materials.

Cheek teeth

Loss of the normal parallel alignment of the cheek teeth, differing length and excessive curvature of the teeth, especially of the rostral cheek teeth, are pathological findings. Differing tooth length results in a **wave mouth**.

Excessive length of the tooth roots ('teeth with retrograde elongation', 'extraoral tooth overgrowth'; Fig. 20.5) may result in retrobulbar swelling and exophthalmos, and bullous enlargement of the mandibular body, respectively, when upper or lower jaw are affected (Fig. 20.6).

Severe mandibular changes result in polymorphous and often massive **abscesses** with variable degree of bone involvement (Fig. 20.4 and 20.7) which may resemble neoplasia. Gas inclusions within the soft-tissue swelling are occasionally observed (Fig. 20.8). Other pathological findings include **retained root fragments**, an irregular **rough tooth contour** (e.g. secondary to tooth decay) and sometimes **aberrant** (Fig. 20.9) or **giant** teeth. **Tooth (crown) fractures** have already been discussed.

20.3.2 Other diseases

With **otitis media**, there is thickening of the bulla wall and increased opacity to the lumen (Fig. 20.10). Unilateral is almost as common as bilateral disease. In rare cases, lysis of the bulla wall may occur (Fig. 20.11).

Salivary mucoceles are occasionally seen in ferrets and manifest as soft-tissue swelling in the region of the upper neck. These can be further evaluated by means of ultrasonographic examination. An important differential diagnosis is **abscess** formation secondary to external or oesophageal foreign body penetration (Fig. 20.12).

Inflammation or displacement of the **nasolacrimal**

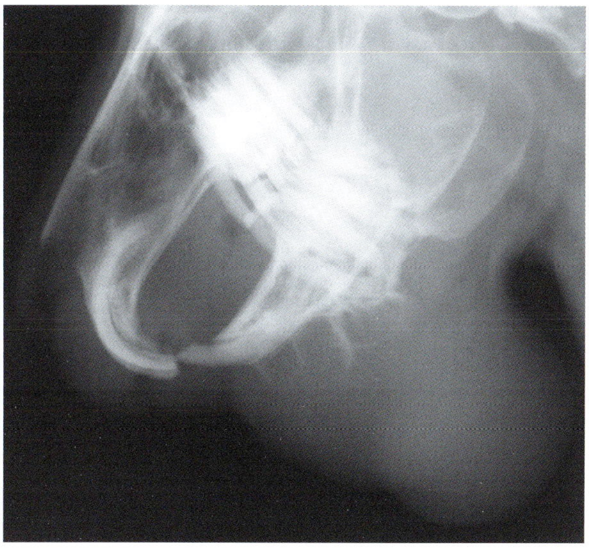

Fig. 20.7 Dental disease and abscess in a rabbit. The lateral view shows irregular alignment of the mandibular cheek teeth with retrograde overgrowth and an abscess ventral to the mandible, which causes severe soft-tissue swelling and is associated with a mineralized shell and finger-like mineral projections.

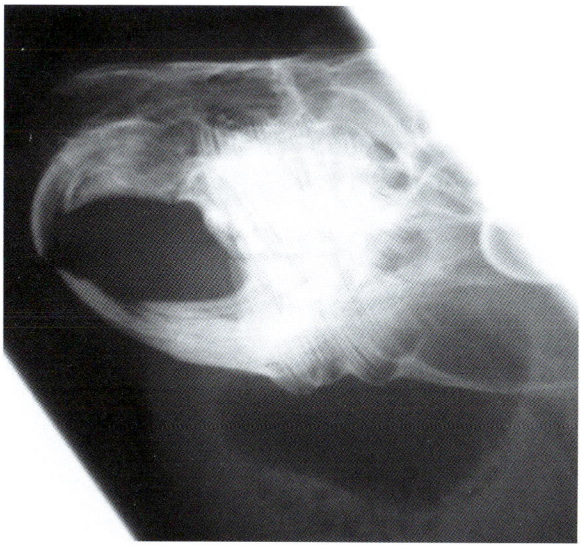

Fig. 20.8 Dental disease and abscess in a guinea pig. In addition to retrograde overgrowth of the mandibular cheek teeth, a large abscess with gas inclusions is noted.

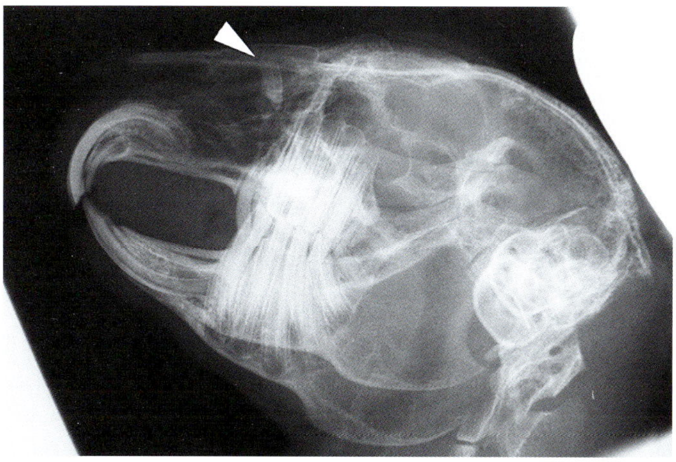

a

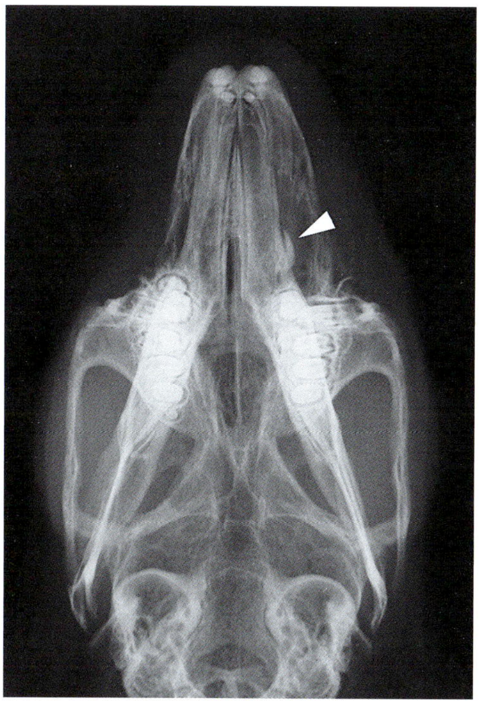

b

Fig. 20.9 Lateral a and dorsoventral b radiographs of the head in a rabbit with an aberrant tooth located in the left nasal cavity (arrowhead). The porous appearance of the frontal and parietal bones is physiological in rabbits.

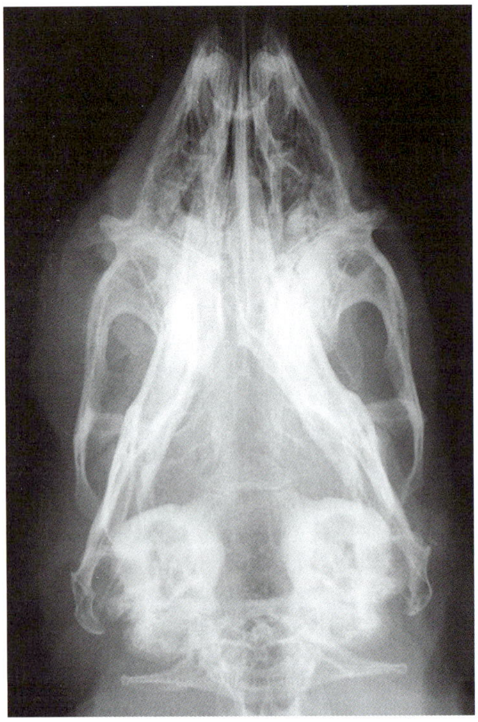

a

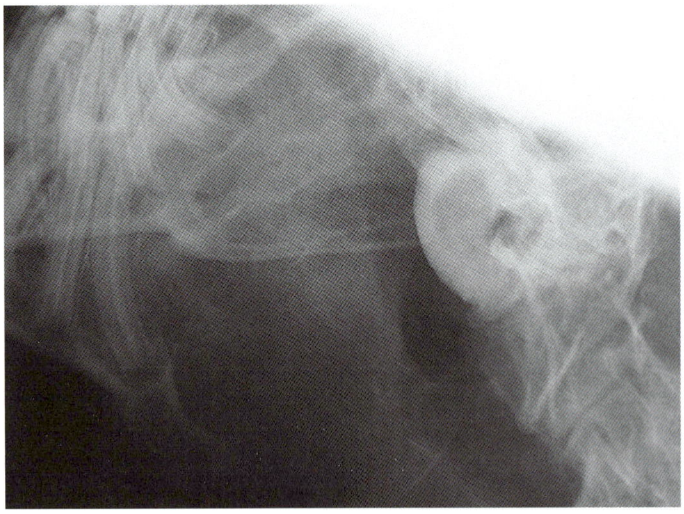

b

Fig. 20.10 Severe bilateral otitis media in a rabbit. The dorsoventral view a demonstrates increased opacity of both tympanic bullae. The tangential view b allows better assessment of wall thickening in the individual bulla.

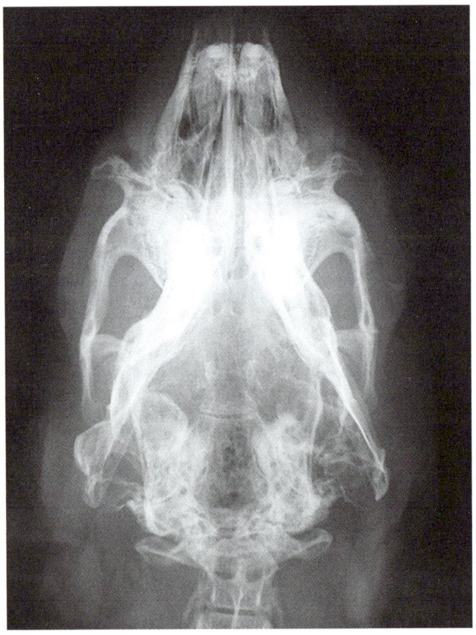

Fig. 20.11 Atypical otitis media and externa in a rabbit. Both tympanic bullae are enlarged, and the wall of the left tympanic bulla shows extensive regions of lysis.

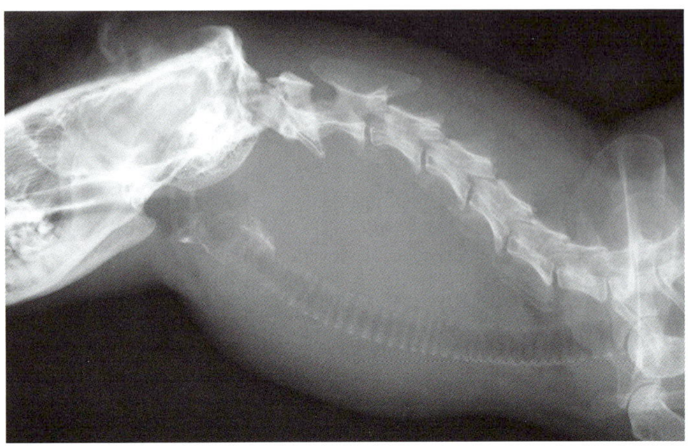

Fig. 20.12 Large cervical abscess caused by a penetrating foreign body in a ferret. Soft-tissue swelling results in ventral displacement of the trachea.

duct may occasionally be seen in rabbits and can be diagnosed by means of contrast medium administration into the lacrimal punctum (dacryocystorhinography).

Foreign bodies associated with the mouth or head region are seen in isolated cases.

20.4 Disorders of the locomotor apparatus

20.4.1 Spinal diseases

Fractures and luxations

These are the most common abnormalities of the spine in small mammals. **Compression fractures** especially in the lumbar spine are especially common in rabbits and may be caused by excessive kicking during restraint attempts. Compression fractures are often only recognized as foreshortening of the affected vertebral body (Fig. 20.13). This may in some instances be better visible on ventrodorsal than on lateral views. Subtle lesions such as subluxations or vertebral endplate fractures require high-quality radiographs for diagnosis.

Other findings

Spondylosis deformans is commonly seen in larger rabbits. With **secondary hyperparathyroidism**, decreased opacity of the skeletal structures, cortical thinning and vertebral deformities develop secondary to loss of bone mineralization as in dogs and cats (Fig. 20.14; see also sections 7.3, 15.5 and 16.2).

20.4.2 Diseases of the extremities

Fractures and luxations

Fractures (especially of the femur, tibia and fibula but also the radius and ulna) and luxations (especially of the elbow and coxofemoral joints caused by jumping from a height) are common in animals allowed to roam freely within the house or apartment (Fig. 20.15 and 20.16). According to Lorinson (1998), lesions of the hind limbs are more common than lesions of the forelimbs in dwarf rabbits (65% vs. 35%). Fracture healing in rabbits usually occurs in 5–8 weeks. Complications include nonunion fractures ('pseudarthrosis'; especially with conservative treatment of fractures close to a joint) and osteomyelitis. An untreated femur luxation can also result in formation of an articulation resembling a new joint (pseudarthrosis or nearthrosis).

Degenerative joint disease

Degenerative joint disease, especially of the stifle joint (Fig. 20.16), is common in rabbits. Periarticular new bone formation can develop on the patella but also on the distal femur and proximal tibia. Mineralization of the collateral ligaments close to their sites of origin and insertion is common.

Ligamentous lesions

These usually require stress views (flexion and extension) and comparison with the contralateral limb for diagnosis (see section 15.2.2). An abnormal widening of the joint space is indicative of a ligamentous injury (Fig. 20.17).

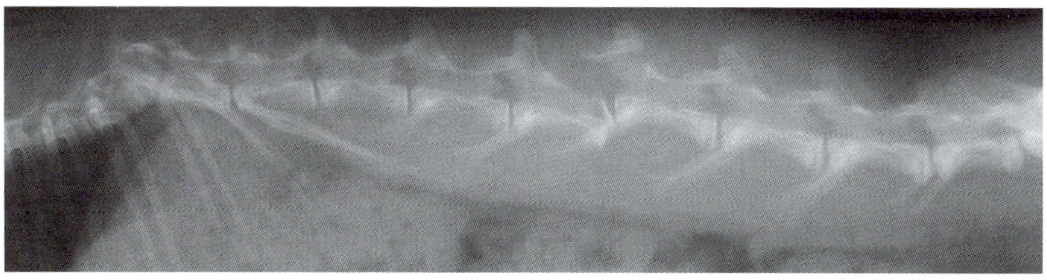

Fig. 20.13 Lateral radiograph of the spine in a rabbit with compression fracture of the 12th thoracic vertebra and fracture and luxation of the third lumbar vertebra (vertebral endplate and lamina).

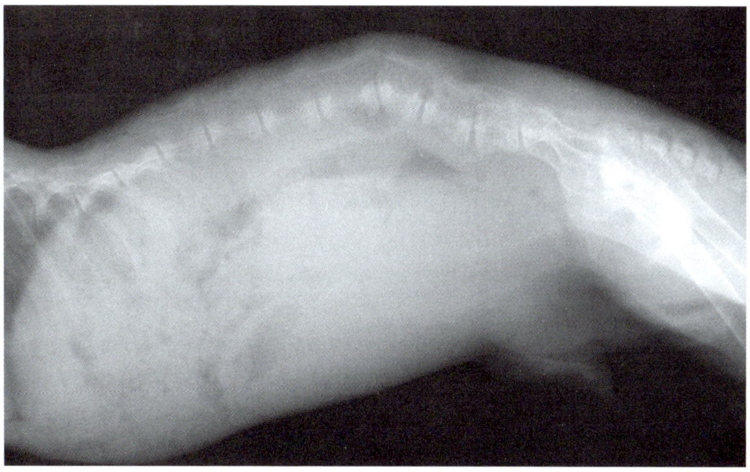

Fig. 20.14 Secondary hyperparathyroidism in a young squirrel. As is seen in cats, convex malformation of the pelvis, osteopenia and pathological fractures are noted. There is also a compression fracture of the fifth lumbar vertebra.

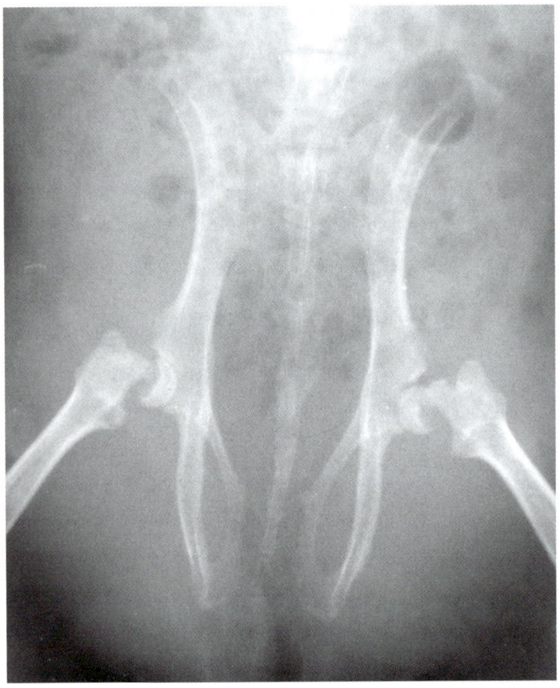

Fig. 20.15 Ventrodorsal radiograph of the pelvis in a guinea pig with bilateral femoral capital physeal fractures.

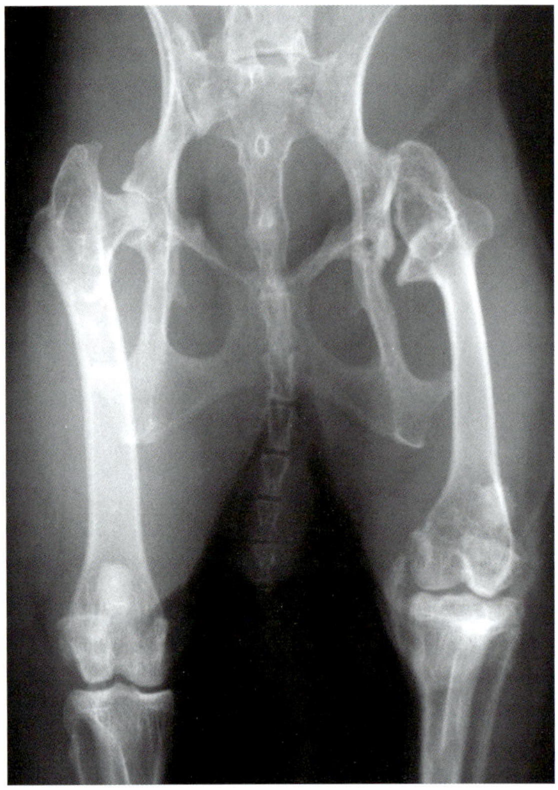

Fig. 20.16 Ventrodorsal radiograph of the pelvis in a rabbit with chronic luxation of the left femur, resulting in pseudarthrosis/nearthrosis. Degenerative joint disease of the left stifle is also noted.

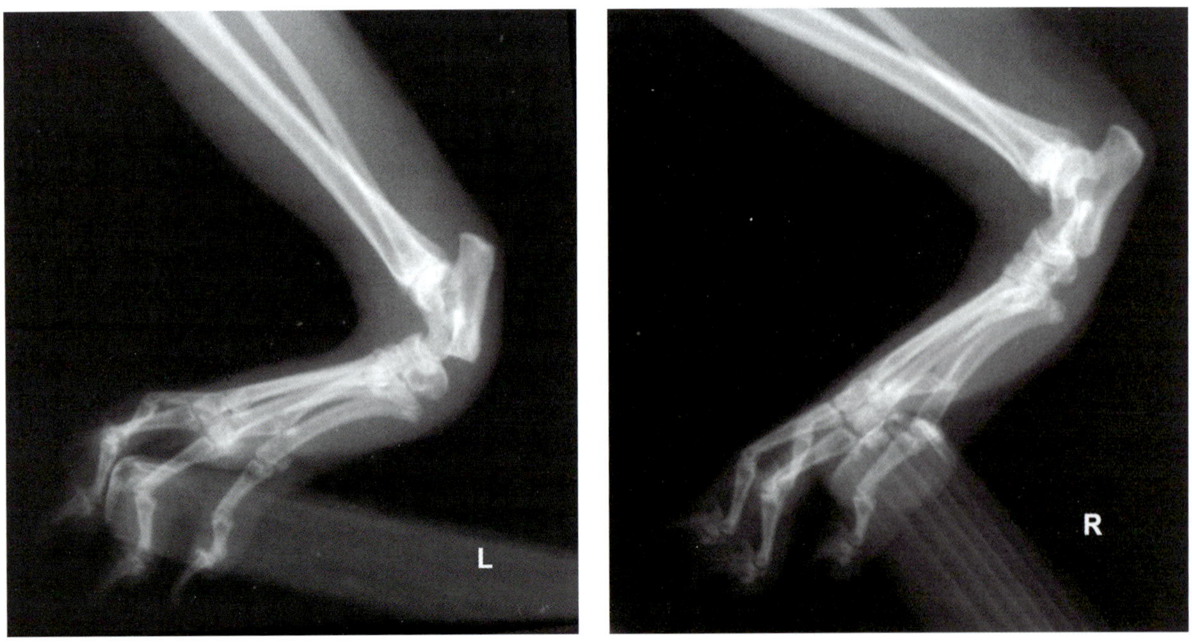

a b

Fig. 20.17 Plantar instability of the left tarsal joint in a ferret due to ligamentous damage. A stress radiograph performed using a fulcrum demonstrates widening of the left intertarsal joint a, while the right tarsus remains stable during a similar application of stress b (L = left, R = right).

Osteodystrophy

Osteodystrophy occurs in hamsters and satin guinea pigs and results in porous to 'moth-eaten' bone loss. The disease affects the entire skeleton but is most pronounced in the extremities and the head (Fig. 20.18).

Bone neoplasia

These are significantly less common than in dogs and cats (see Fig. 20.3b). Tumours are predominantly osteoblastic and result in spiculated or lobulated infiltration into surrounding soft tissues. They are sometimes found in the head region in rabbits. In rabbits and guinea pigs, the caudal spine and femur may also be affected.

20.5 Disorders of the thorax

20.5.1 Heart diseases

The most common heart disease in ferrets is **dilated cardiomyopathy (DCM)**. Affected animals show tachycardia and nonspecific clinical symptoms such as weight loss, anorexia or weakness. Concurrent findings may include pleural effusion, pulmonary oedema, ascites, hepatomegaly or splenomegaly. **Hypertrophic cardiomyopathy (HCM)** is occasionally seen in this species but is rare. In endemic areas, ferrets may be affected by **heartworm disease**.

In rabbits, **AV valve insufficiency** is most common; **DCM** is rare.

In guinea pigs, **HCM** is most common.

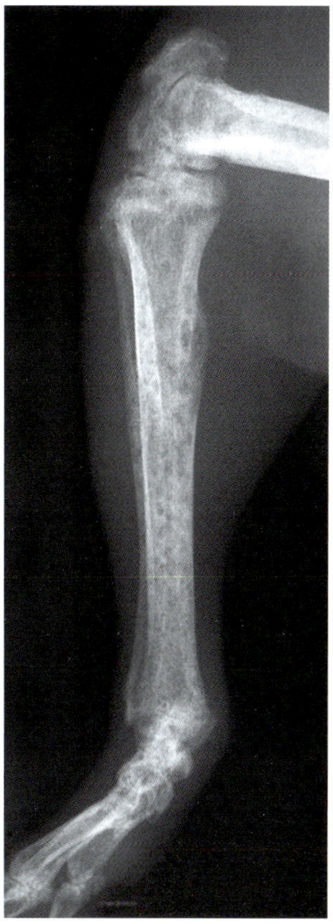

Fig. 20.18 Generalized fibrous osteodystrophy in a guinea pig. The appendicular skeleton and head are characterized by numerous punctate lucencies. Severe degenerative joint disease of the stifle is also noted in this patient.

Echocardiography is indicated in any case of radiographic cardiomegaly.

RADIOGRAPHIC FINDINGS Cardiomyopathies result in enlargement of the cardiac silhouette which, especially in ferrets, is commonly associated with pleural effusion. Concurrent pulmonary oedema is possible, which results in increased opacity of the lung or diffuse infiltrates. Pericardial effusion is rare and, in small mammals, cannot be distinguished from true cardiomegaly (Fig. 20.19 and 20.20).

20.5.2 Lung diseases

Rabbits may develop **bronchopneumonia** secondary to upper respiratory infections. Lung abscesses are a possible complication but are not always visible radiographically. However, radiographs are recommended to evaluate the severity of disease and confirm lung involvement. Bronchopneumonia is very common in guinea pigs, gerbils and degus. In rats, pneumonia and neoplastic lesions are similarly common.

RADIOGRAPHIC FINDINGS Patients presenting at an advanced stage of disease often have opacification of the lung to a degree that the cardiac silhouette may not be visible. In some cases, abnormalities are more focal and may result in consolidation of individual lung lobes (Fig. 20.21 and 20.22).

20.5.3 Thoracic neoplasia

Primary neoplasms of the thorax are rare. **Pulmonary metastases** in rabbits may be seen secondary to uterine adenocarcinoma and less commonly secondary to testicular neoplasia. Lung metastases in guinea pigs are most common secondary to mammary tumours and osteosarcoma. **Lymphoma** is common in ferrets and may result in widening of the cranial mediastinum due to thymic enlargement. Clinical signs are similar to a cardiomyopathy, and concurrent pleural effusion may be present.

RADIOGRAPHIC FINDINGS As in dogs and cats, most lung metastases appear on radiographs as variably sized, round, homogeneously soft-tissue opaque nodules (Fig. 20.23). Cranial mediastinal mass lesions result in dorsal and lateral displacement of the trachea.

20.5.4 Other thoracic diseases

Dog or cat induced **bite wounds** are regularly seen, especially in ferrets. **Foreign bodies** penetrating or obstructing the oesophagus are also common in ferrets and may result in gas dilatation of the oesophagus proximal to the lesion and possibly in pulmonary infiltrates (**aspiration pneumonia**). As in other animals, any kind of thoracic trauma may lead to **pulmonary haemorrhage**, **pneumomediastinum**, **pneumothorax** and **fractures**.

Megaoesophagus has been reported in ferrets and a few rat breeding lines.

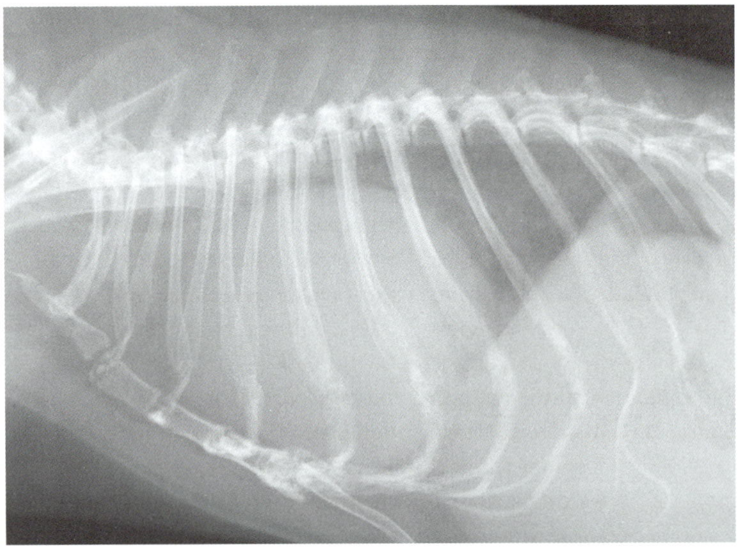

Fig. 20.19 Severe enlargement of the cardiac silhouette in a guinea pig due to pericardial effusion.

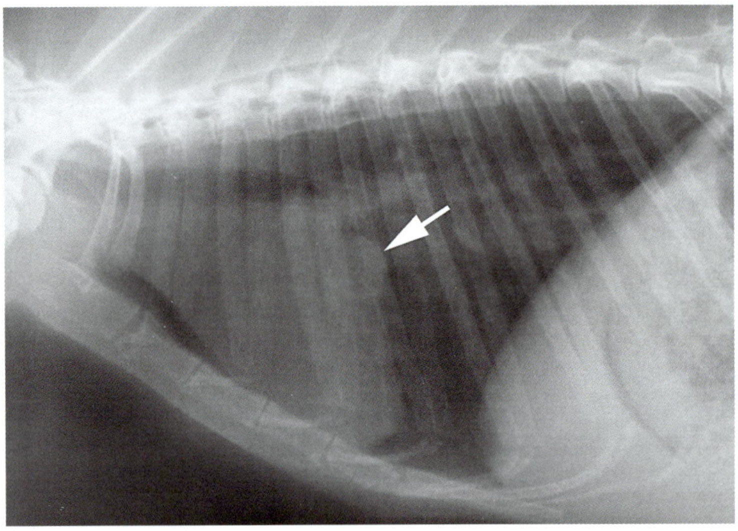

Fig. 20.20 Mitral insufficiency in a rabbit. The lateral thoracic radiograph demonstrates focal enlargement of the left atrium (arrow).

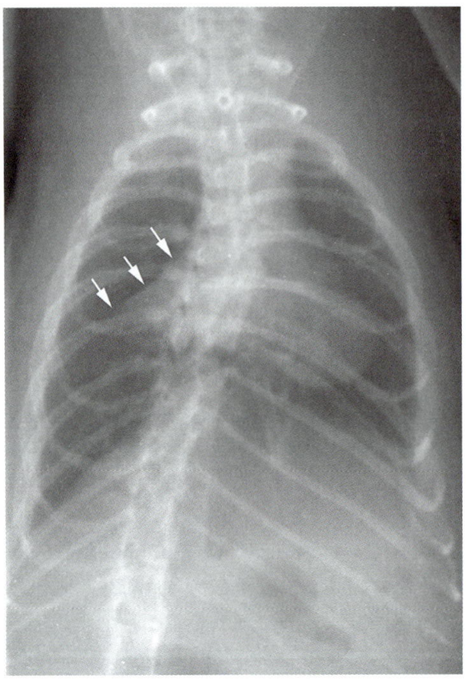

Fig. 20.21 Pneumonia in a rabbit. A right-sided, focal, sharply marginated alveolar pulmonary pattern indicative of consolidation is noted (arrows).

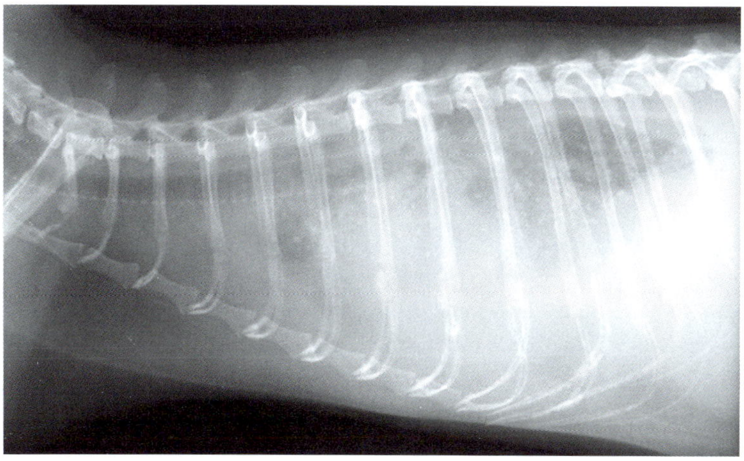

Fig. 20.22 Pleural effusion in a ferret. Homogeneous soft-tissue opacity is associated with the ventral thorax, silhouetting with the heart and diaphragm and resulting in retraction of the lung lobes. Additionally, multiple small, almost mineral opaque foci are disseminated throughout the lung fields, which raise suspicion of metastatic disease.

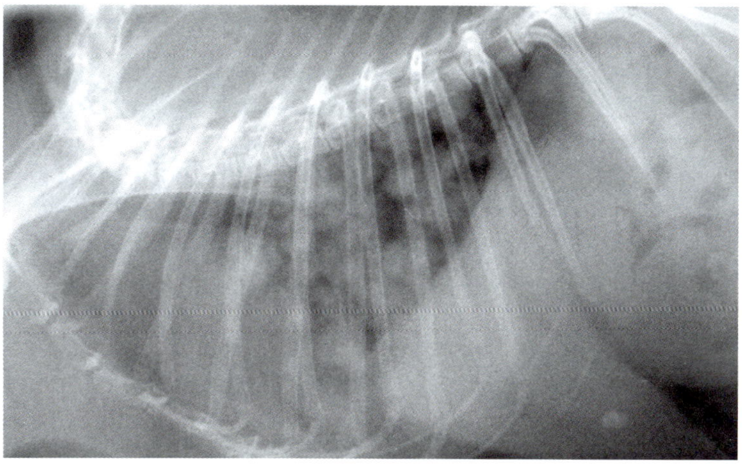

Fig. 20.23 Lung metastases secondary to uterine adenocarcinoma in a rabbit (same patient as Fig. 20.34). Multiple round soft-tissue opacity nodules are recognized throughout the lung fields. Additional findings include hepatomegaly and focal mineralization of the hepatic parenchyma.

20.6 Disorders of the abdomen

20.6.1 Diseases of the gastrointestinal tract

Foreign bodies

Gastrointestinal foreign bodies are commonly seen in ferrets, which have a tendency to chew on inappropriate material due to their playful and inquisitive nature. Young ferrets appear to have a preference for rubber and foam substances. Animals present with inappetence, anorexia, lethargy, diarrhoea and occasionally vomiting and hypersalivation.

RADIOGRAPHIC FINDINGS The actual foreign body is often not visible, but affected animals often show signs of obstructive ileus or impaired gastric emptying.

Gastric dilatation

An overly distended stomach in guinea pigs may be seen secondary to inappetence (dental diseases), malnutrition, parasite infestation or infections. Gastric dilatation and volvulus is an important differential diagnosis and should be ruled out.

RADIOGRAPHIC FINDINGS A severely dilated stomach can occupy half the abdomen (meteorism). Even without obvious compartmentalization and an opaque soft-tissue band subdividing the stomach, a severely gas-distended stomach in guinea pigs raises concern for gastric dilatation and volvulus.

Gastrointestinal hypomotility (stasis)

This is common in rabbits and results in markedly gas-distended gastrointestinal segments (meteorism), with dehydrated ingesta in the stomach and caecum (Fig. 20.24). Possible causes include inappetence (e.g. secondary to dental diseases), pain, dysbiosis, coccidiosis, administration of inappropriate antibiotics and sudden dietary changes.

Bezoars

These are fairly common in rabbits (in stomach, duodenum and cranial jejunum), guinea pigs (especially in the stomach of long-haired breeds) and rats (in the stomach) and may result in gastrointestinal obstruction. Secondary **gastric rupture** is a possible complication in rabbits. Older ferrets may also develop (tricho)bezoars.

RADIOGRAPHIC FINDINGS Bezoars and inspissated ingesta are not always visible on survey radiographs. A crescent-shaped gas deposit adjacent to an intraluminal structure is characteristic of this condition (Fig. 20.25) but is not always present.

Following oral administration of positive **contrast medium** (3–6 ml of barium sulphate suspension), contrast medium surrounds the intraluminal structure and shows a filling defect. Due to the complex nature of bezoars, they often only show incomplete and delayed (often by several hours) uptake of contrast medium (Fig. 20.26).

A dilated and predominantly fluid-filled stomach with a central gas accumulation is occasionally seen (Fig. 20.27) and suggests a partial obstruction in the region of the pylorus or cranial duodenum which is commonly caused by a bezoar.

Caecal tympany

This condition results in marked gas dilatation (meteorism) of the ventrally located caecum, which appears distended and notably septate (Fig. 20.28).

Obstipation

This is most commonly seen in chinchillas and less commonly in guinea pigs, rabbits (usually affecting the caecum) or degus. Possible aetiologies include dental diseases, painful processes and dehydration.

20.6.2 Diseases of the liver

Hepatomegaly may be seen in lymphoma in rabbits, guinea pigs or ferrets. In the latter, concurrent splenomegaly or intestinal involvement are common. In rabbits, hepatic fibrosis due to coccidiosis and hepatic congestion due to cardiac diseases are occasional causes of hepatomegaly and are sometimes associated with ascites.

RADIOGRAPHIC FINDINGS As in other animals, hepatomegaly results in caudodorsal displacement of the stomach. Detailed assessment of the liver in rodents and rabbits may be hampered by superimposition of ingesta within gastrointestinal tract segments.

20.6.3 Diseases of the urinary tract

A noninvasive ultrasound examination is generally the modality of choice to evaluate possible diseases of the urogenital tract in small mammals. Radiographically notable renal diseases are rarely seen in chinchillas.

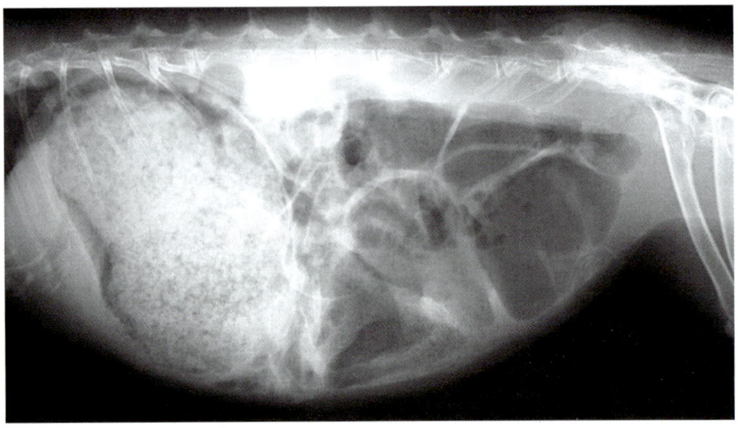

Fig. 20.24 Gastrointestinal stasis in a rabbit. The stomach is markedly distended with gas and ingesta, and the caecum is severely dilated with gas (meteorism).

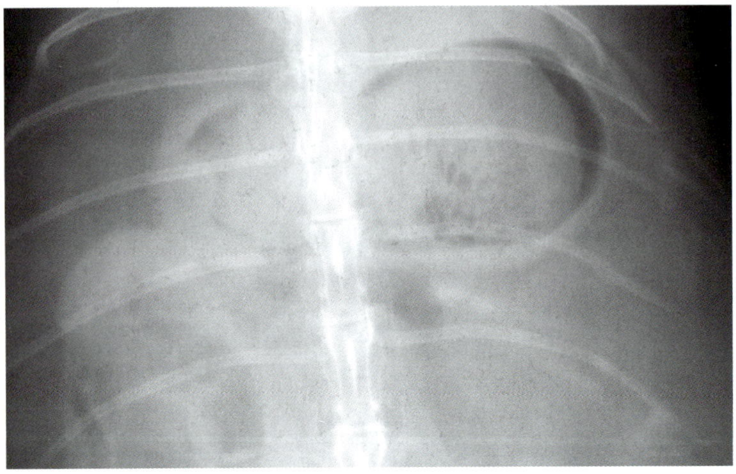

Fig. 20.25 Bezoar in a rabbit. The cropped and magnified image of a ventrodorsal abdominal radiograph shows a typical crescent-shaped gas opacity rim surrounding the bezoar within the gastric lumen.

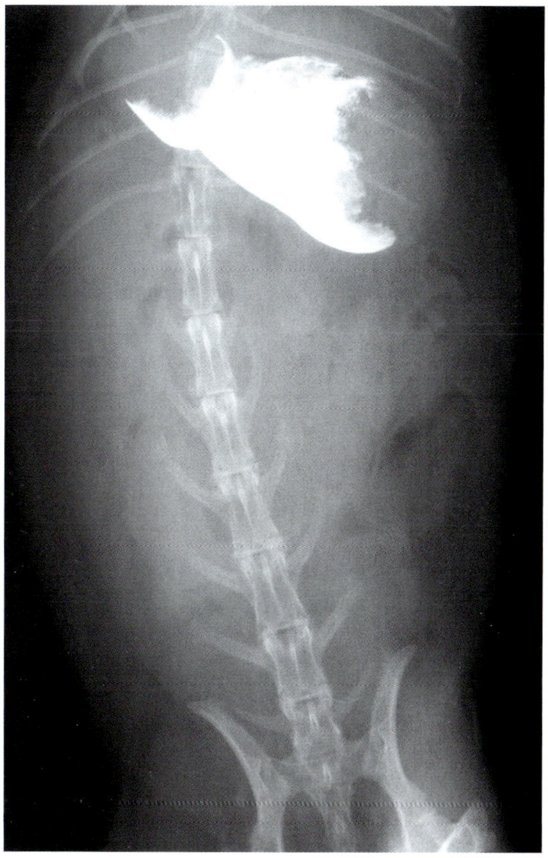

Fig. 20.26 Two bezoars associated with the stomach in a rabbit. Contrast medium has been administered for further evaluation and demonstrates large intraluminal filling defects associated with the fundus and pylorus, respectively.

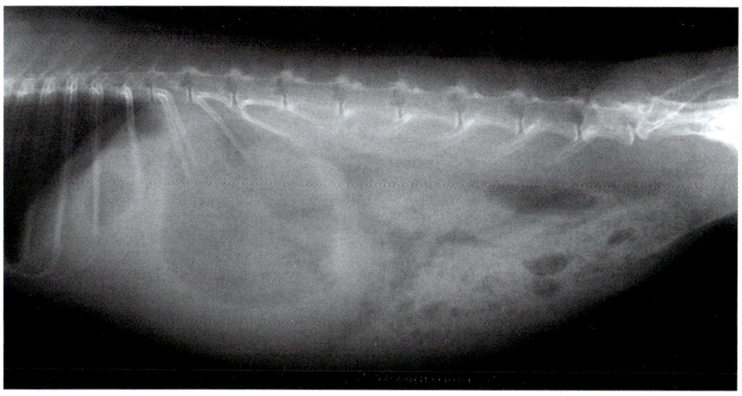

Fig. 20.27 Fluid- and gas-dilated stomach in a rabbit indicative of an obstruction at the level of the pylorus or duodenum. A bezoar was diagnosed intraoperatively.

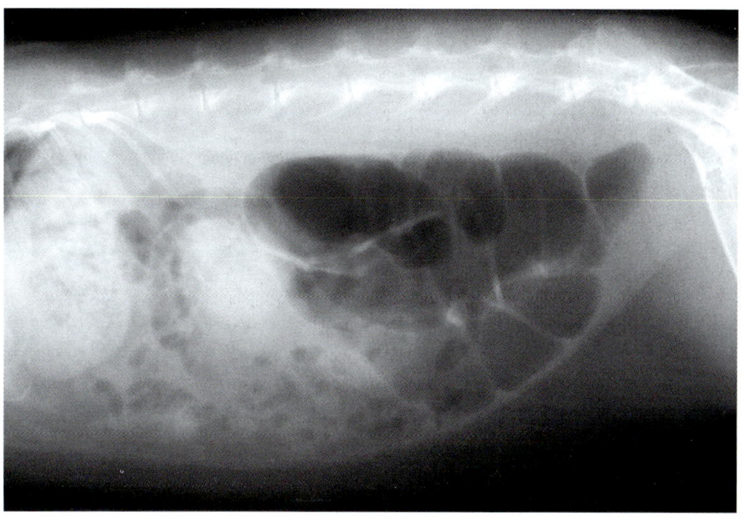

Fig. 20.28 Tympany of the caecum in a rabbit. The dilated caecum is easily recognized based on its septations.

Nephrocalcinosis and urolithiasis

Rabbits are notorious for urolithiasis, which is associated with their unusual calcium metabolism. Calcium is not only resorbed by active transport and passive resorption occurring in the gastrointestinal tract, but the kidneys (which are predominantly responsible for calcium excretion) are also able to resorb calcium. In addition, the blood calcium levels in rabbits are significantly higher than in other mammals. Thus **nephrocalcinosis**, **sediment** within the urinary bladder and **uroliths** associated with renal pelves, ureters, urinary bladder and urethra are common in this species. Cystoliths are also common in guinea pigs. Urolithiasis (struvite) is rare in ferrets.

Urethral calculi may be located very far caudally, and radiographs including the entire pelvis and perineum may be indicated for full evaluation depending on the patient's history.

Renal calculi may become displaced from the kidney into the ureter and may result in **ureteral obstruction** and secondary hydronephrosis and hydroureter.

RADIOGRAPHIC FINDINGS With nephrocalcinosis, radiating linear mineralization is visible within the renal parenchyma (Fig. 20.29). As mentioned above, the urinary bladder in rabbits may appear almost as opaque as contrast medium due to the high calcium content in urine (Fig. 20.30). A large amount of **sediment** may cause the urinary bladder to appear homogeneously mineral opaque. **Urinary bladder and urethral calculi** are usually rounded and may have a layered appearance or a rough surface (Fig. 20.31). The radiographic opacity and thus the visibility of uroliths and urinary sediment depends on their composition. Triple phosphate, calcium oxalate, calcium carbonate, ammonium urate and silicate are mineral opaque, while cystine and urate calculi are radiolucent and may be difficult or impossible to visualize on a radiograph. In addition, their visibility depends on the amount and opacity of the surrounding urine.

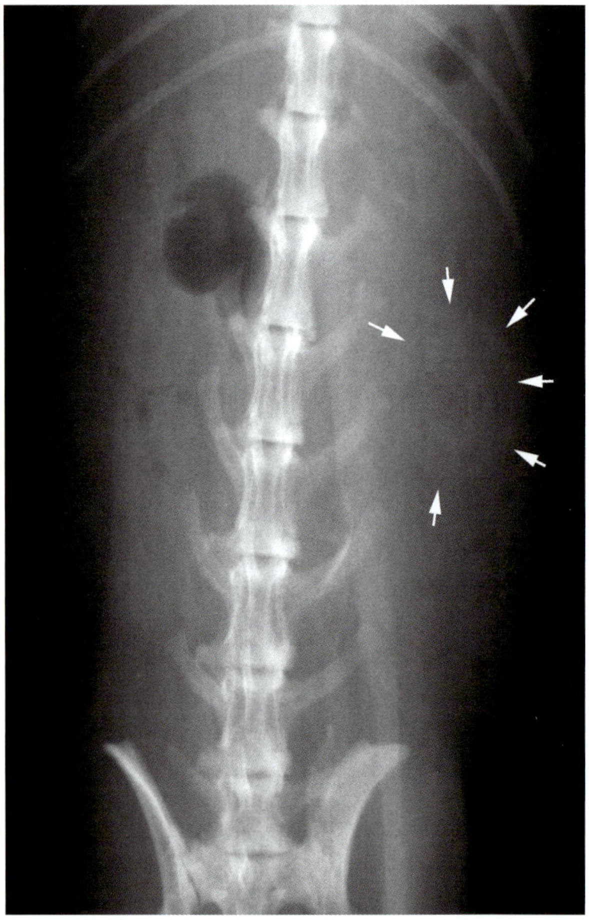

Fig. 20.29 Nephrocalcinosis in a rabbit. The left kidney is mineral opaque and easily recognized (arrows).

Cystitis

Apart from visualization of the uroliths which are commonly present, a radiographic diagnosis of cystitis is not possible.

Hydronephrosis and hydroureter

Hydronephrosis is occasionally seen as a postoperative complication following spaying in ferrets. If hydronephrosis and/or hydroureter are suspected based on survey radiographs (e.g. in the case of unilateral renomegaly), an **excretory urography** may aid in further evaluation. This involves injection of iodinated contrast medium (400 mg

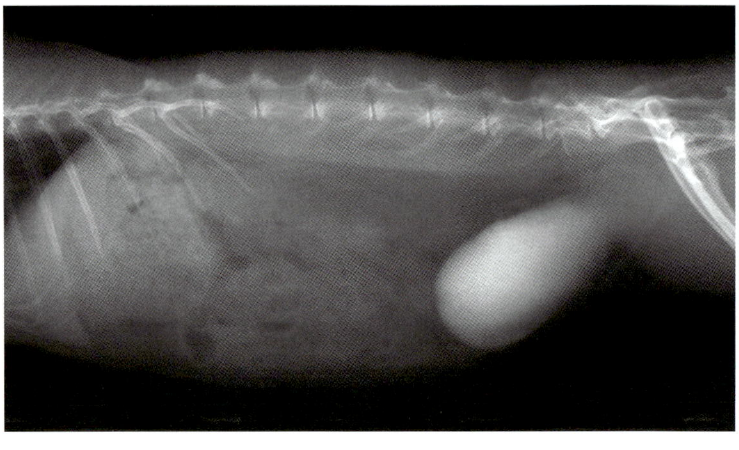

Fig. 20.30 Large amount of urinary sediment in a rabbit. The urinary bladder content is nearly as opaque as contrast medium.

I/kg), either intravenously or subcutaneously. The evaluation is principally the same as in dogs and cats (see section 14.2.1). Orthogonal radiographs are acquired immediately following contrast medium administration and after 5 and 10 minutes. In advanced renal disease, the parenchymal phase may be delayed by up to an hour (Fig. 20.32).

Renal cysts

Renal cysts are common in ferrets but are not radiographically visible.

20.6.4 Diseases of the reproductive tract

Diseases of the uterus

Uterine neoplasia is common in rabbits and guinea pigs. Rabbits usually develop adenocarcinomas with secondary mineralization, and guinea pigs develop leiomyosarcomas.

Endometrial hyperplasia, **pyometra**, **mucometra** and **hydrometra** are commonly seen in rabbits and ferrets and sometimes in hamsters.

RADIOGRAPHIC FINDINGS Severe uterine enlargement (Fig. 20.33) can result in diffuse increased soft-tissue opacity without distinct structures within the caudal abdomen. Identification of organ margins may be difficult due to the adjacent large caecum. A definitive diagnosis can be established by means of ultrasonography. Mineralization of the uterus is predominantly seen with neoplasia (Fig. 20.34).

Pathological pregnancies

These include **overly large fetuses** and **fetal death** (emphysematous fetus, mummified fetus). Pathological pregnancies are most commonly seen in guinea pigs but also occur in rabbits.

RADIOGRAPHIC FINDINGS As in dogs and cats, abnormal fetuses are recognized based on abnormally straight alignment, abnormal position of the head or extremities, resorption or abnormal mineralization of the skeleton, and occasionally endometrial or fetal gas inclusions (Fig. 20.35 and 20.36).

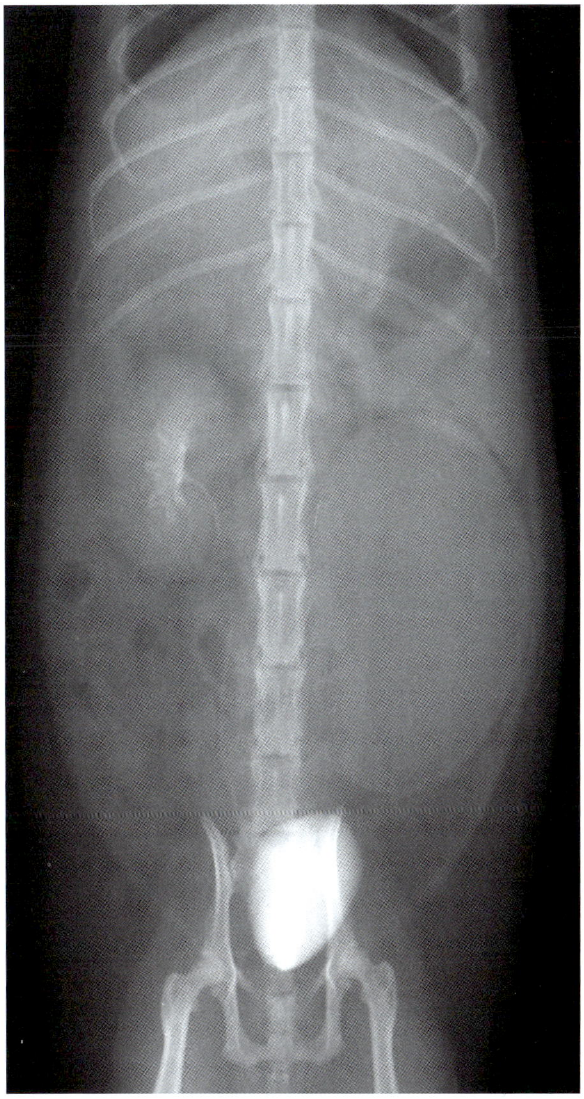

Fig. 20.32 Left-sided hydronephrosis following spaying in a ferret. Excretory urography demonstrates marked enlargement of the left renal silhouette with faint peripheral rim contrast enhancement. The left ureter is not visible. The right kidney and ureter are normal.

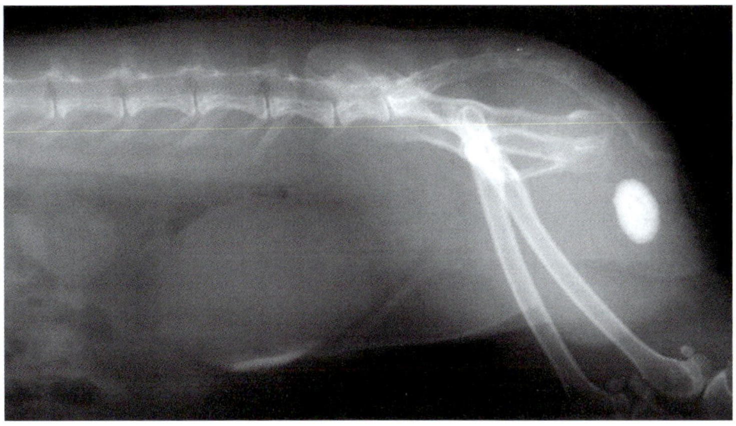

Fig. 20.31 Urolithiasis in a rabbit. A large radiating and layered calculus is noted in the caudal urethra.

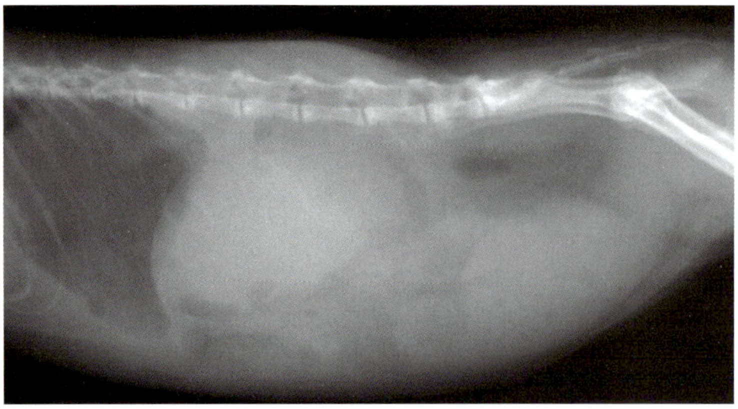

Fig. 20.33 Ovarian cysts and pyometra in a guinea pig. The enlarged ovaries are visible in the dorsal abdomen as globoid soft-tissue opacity structures. The fluid-filled uterus is recognized in the caudal abdomen as a tubular soft-tissue opaque structure.

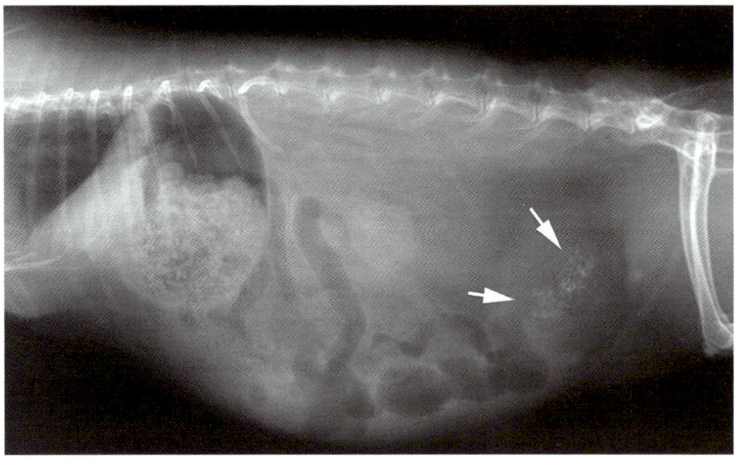

Fig. 20.34 Uterine adenocarcinoma with mineralization in a rabbit (same patient as in Fig. 20.23). A mineralized mass lesion is noted cranial to the urinary bladder (arrows).

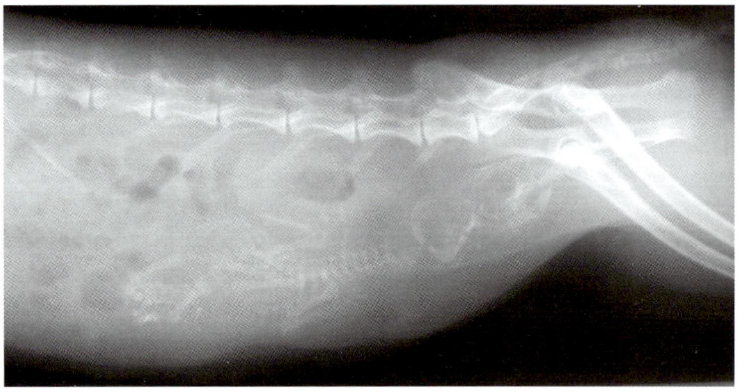

Fig. 20.35 Pathological pregnancy in a rabbit. A single fetal skeleton is located cranial to the pelvic inlet; it is abnormally stretched and has malformation of the skull.

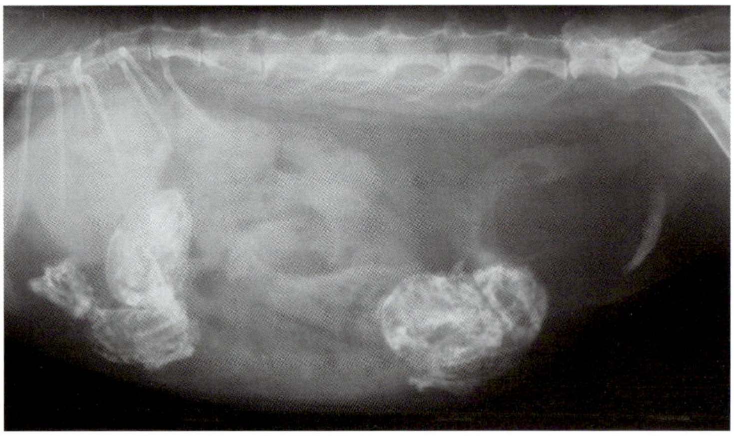

Fig. 20.36 Pathological pregnancy in a rabbit. Two mummified fetuses are noted in the cranial and mid-ventral abdomen.

Ovarian cysts

These are predominantly seen in guinea pigs and can reach considerable size.

RADIOGRAPHIC FINDINGS Ovarian cysts appear as globoid, homogeneously soft-tissue opaque, often well-circumscribed structures caudal to the kidneys. With increasing size, they may result in displacement of other abdominal organs (see Fig. 20.33).

Mammary tumours

These are common in mice and rats and often metastasize to the lungs in mice.

20.6.5 Other abdominal diseases

In rabbits, intra-abdominal **abscesses** are occasionally seen which can reach an impressive size (Fig. 20.37). The aetiology usually remains undetermined. In rare instances, gas-filled abscesses may lead to confusion with gastrointestinal tract segments.

Ascites can be seen, for example, secondary to heart disease and, depending on the amount of abdominal effusion, results in decreased visualization of abdominal organs (Fig. 20.38). With severe ascites only gas-filled intestinal segments may be visible.

Splenomegaly is most common in ferrets with lymphoma and may rarely be associated with radiographically visible lymph node enlargement (Fig. 20.39).

Enlargement and sometimes calcification of the

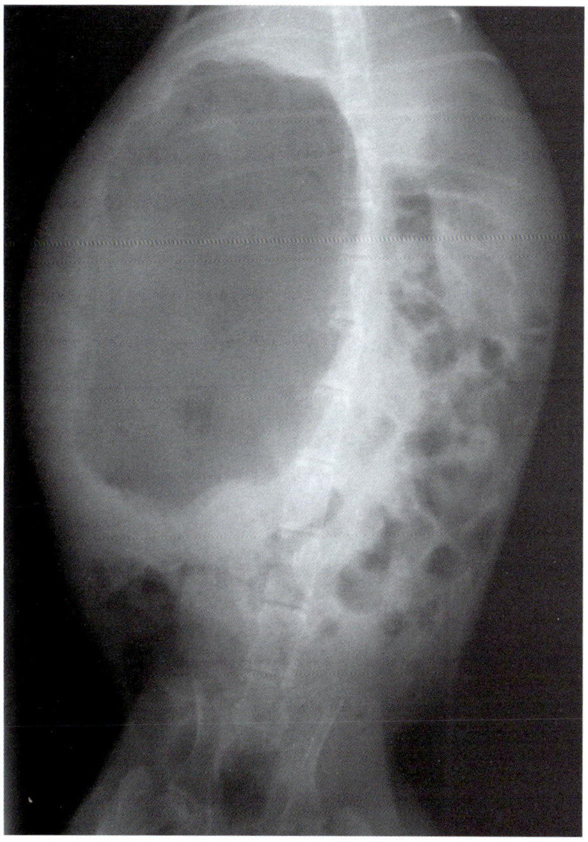

Fig. 20.37 Intra-abdominal abscess in a rabbit. On the ventrodorsal abdominal radiograph, there is a large gas-filled abscess occupying the entire right abdomen. (Courtesy of Dr Florian and Dr Margit Teufel, Vienna)

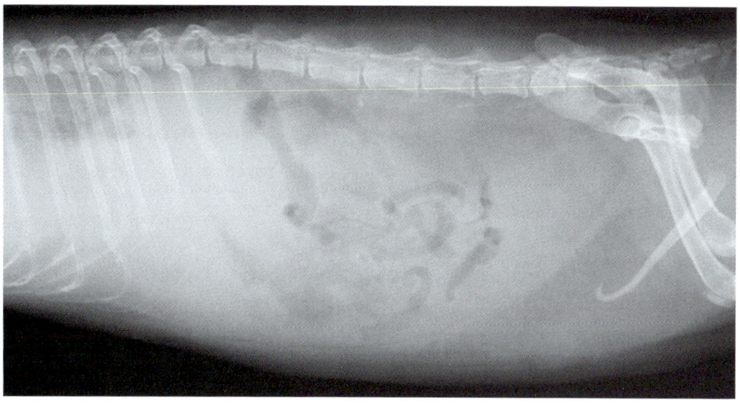

Fig. 20.38 Ascites in a ferret. There is generalized loss of abdominal serosal margin detail, and only individual gas-filled intestinal segments are visible. Concurrent pleural effusion is noted in the visible part of the thorax. Note the hook-shaped os penis.

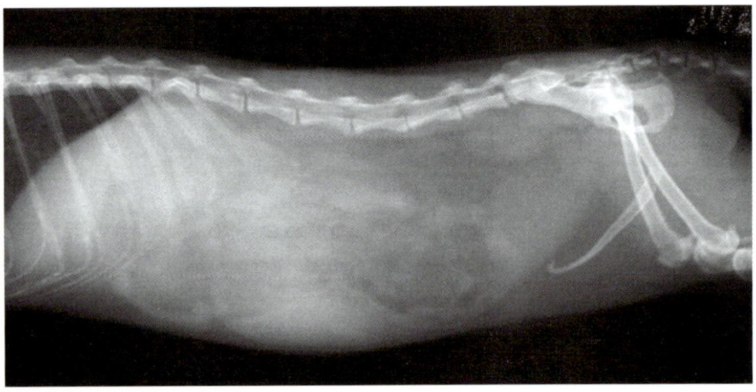

Fig. 20.39 Lymphoma in a ferret. Splenomegaly and enlargement of the sublumbar lymph nodes are noted. An incidental chronic coxofemoral joint luxation is also evident.

adrenal glands is most common in ferrets and usually diagnosed or verified by means of ultrasonography rather than radiographs.

References and further reading

Bach C. Röntgenanatomische Untersuchungen über die postnatale Entwicklung der Epi- und Apophysen der Beckengliedmaße beim Zwergkaninchen der Rasse Farbenzwerge blau (*Oryctolagus cuniculus f.domestica*). Dissertation, Hannover, 1984.

Barone R, Pavaux C, Blin CP, Cuq P. Atlas d'Anatomie du Lapin. Paris: Masson 1973.

Böhmer E. Röntgendiagnostik bei Zahn- sowie Kiefererkrankungen der Hasenartigen und Nager. Part 1: Tierartspezifische Zahn und Kieferanatomie sowie Pathologie, Indikationen für die Röntgendiagnostik. Tierärztl Prax 2001; 29: 316–27.

Böhmer E. Röntgendiagnostik bei Zahn- sowie Kiefererkrankungen der Hasenartigen und Nager. Part 2: Interpretation von Röntgenaufnahmen und tierartspezifische Fallbeispiele. Tierärztl Prax 2001; 29: 369–83.

Böhmer E, Köstlin RG. Zahnerkrankungen bzw. -anomalien bei Hasenartigen und Nagern. Diagnose, Therapie und Ergebnisse bei 83 Patienten. Prakt Tier 1988; 11: 37–51.

Crossley DA, Jackson A, Yates J, Boydell IP. Use of computed tomography to investigate cheek tooth abnormalities in chinchillas (*Chinchilla laniger*). J Small Anim Pract 1998; 39: 385–9.

Ewringmann A, Glöckner B. Leitsymptome bei Meerschweinchen, Chinchilla und Degu: diagnostischer Leitfaden und Therapie. Stuttgart: Enke 2005.

Ewringmann A, Göbel T. Heimtierkrankheiten. Stuttgart: Ulmer 2005.

Ewringmann A. Leitsymptome beim Kaninchen: diagnostischer Leitfaden und Therapie. Stuttgart: Enke 2005.

Fehr M. Diagnostische Radiologie bei Heimtieren. Kleintier Prax 1985; 30: 377–80.

Harcourt-Brown F. Textbook of Rabbit Medicine. Butterworth Heinemann 2002.

Harcourt-Brown F, Chitty J. BSAVA Manual of Rabbit Surgery, Dentistry and Imaging. BSAVA 2013.

Kattinger P, Ewringmann A, Weyland J, Skrodzki M. Kardiologische Untersuchungen beim Kaninchen. Kleintier Prax 1999; 44: 671–2.

Krautwald-Junghanns ME, Pees M, Reese S, Tully T. Diagnostic Imaging of Exotic Pets: Birds, Small Mammals, Reptiles. Hannover: Schlütersche 2011.

Künzel F, Kolm U, Böhler A, Url A. Mitralklappeninsuffizienz infolge einer Papillarmuskeldysfunktion bei einem Kaninchen. Tierärztl Prax 2005; 33: 423–30.

Lorinson D. Grundlagen und Methodik der Behandlung von Frakturen und Luxationen beim Zwergkaninchen. Habilitationsschrift, Wien 1998.

Quesenberry K, Carpenter JL. Ferrets, Rabbits and Rodents: Clinical Medicine and Surgery. Philadelphia: Saunders 2004.

Silverman S, Tell LA. Radiology of Rodents, Rabbits and Ferrets. An Atlas of Normal Anatomy and Positioning. St. Louis: Elsevier Saunders 2005.

Supakorndej P, Lewis RE, McCall JW, Dzimianski MT, Holmes RA. Radiographic and angiographic evaluation of ferrets experimentally infected with *Dirofilaria immitis*. Vet Radiol Ultrasound 1995; 36: 23–9.

Wissdorf H, Vargas L, Harder E. Röntgenbefunde am Schultergliedmaßenskelett des wachsenden Kaninchens. Kleintier Prax 1983; 28: 386–91.

Wissdorf H, Vargas L. Röntgenanatomische Darstellung der postnatalen Entwicklung von Epi- und Apophysen an Os coxae und Articulatio coxae beim Weissen Neuseeländer Kaninchen (*Oryctolagus cuniculus f.domestica*). Prak Tier 1984; 65: 594–6.

Reptiles

21

Michaela Gumpenberger, Jürgen Schumacher and Marcy Souza

Over the past two decades, **reptiles** have evolved into an important component of small animal practice. Reptile owners expect the same competence from a veterinarian as small animal clients. It is important for the veterinary practitioner to acquire a solid knowledge base not only of reptile husbandry, diseases and therapy, but also of the anatomy of different species and pathophysiology of various diseases, which often differ significantly from mammals and birds.

A radiographic examination is an important diagnostic tool that provides a good general overview of the patient (in most animals, whole body radiographs are obtained). In chelonians, which over 250 million years of evolution have developed a shell that partially or completely interferes with physical examination of the coelomic cavity, whole body radiographs serve as a routine part of a thorough clinical examination.

More than 8,000 species of reptiles are known today. This chapter can only provide an overview of the anatomy, indications for radiographic examination and most important diseases with their imaging findings in chelonians (turtles and tortoises), lizards and snakes commonly held in captivity. It is advisable to obtain and catalogue comparison radiographs of healthy partner animals, as well as rare and even deceased specimens, to allow comparison with patient radiographs if needed. Even though the body of pertinent literature is relatively large, information on every captive reptile species is not available.

The authors make no claim that the information provided regarding anatomy and diseases in this chapter is complete.

21.1 Anatomy and indications

21.1.1 Anatomy

Almost all reptiles share the common characteristic of a single body cavity (pleuroperitoneal cavity, coelom), which in contrast to mammals lacks a diaphragmatic subdivision into a thoracic and an abdominal cavity (with one exception: crocodiles).

Chelonians

The most striking feature in these reptiles is their **shell**. While the upper shell (carapace) has the shape of a hemisphere in terrestrial tortoises, it is typically flatter in freshwater and marine chelonians (turtles and terrapins). Tortoises usually have five neural or vertebral scutes, four pairs (left and right) of pleural scutes and numerous marginal or rim scutes. The most cranial marginal scute is also referred to as nuchal scute. The lower shell (plastron) consists of paired intergular, gular, humeral, axillary, pectoral, abdominal, inguinal, femoral and anal scutes. The carapace and plastron are joined by connecting bridges. In aquatic and other soft shell chelonians, the number of scutes may be reduced or replaced by a leathery skin. Box turtles, hinge-back tortoises and Asian box turtles have wide gaps associated with their plastron which should not be confused with fractures. The number and shape of the bony shell components generally do not correspond to those of the overlying horny scutes. Only the bony plates and the sutures separating them are usually visible on radiographs.

The shell typically includes the **shoulder** and **pelvic girdle**. Most chelonians have eight mobile cervical **vertebrae**. The transverse processes of the thoracolumbar vertebrae (e.g. 9–10 in Hermann's tortoises) are fused to the overlying bony shell along with the ribs. A sternum is absent.

The porous sponge-like **lung** is located dorsally and, depending on the animal's nutritional status and the extent of ventrally located coelomic organs (urogenital and gastrointestinal tract), occupies approximately 50% of the coelomic cavity. The trachea begins in the oral cavity and bifurcates into two mainstem bronchi in the cranial neck. The lung in chelonians does not have alveoli or bronchioles. The **heart** is bordered by two **liver** lobes. The gallbladder is located adjacent to the right liver lobe or slightly caudal to it. The **stomach** in most chelonians is folded and located in the left cranial half of the coelomic cavity. It should always contain gas and is easily recognized. The pylorus is in a right paramedian location. The **caecum** (in the right caudal coelom) and the **colon** are prominent in herbivorous chelonians. The colon terminates in the

coprodeum. The rounded **spleen** is located dorsomedial to the stomach. The **kidneys** are located at the level of or dorsocranial to the coxofemoral joints. Macroscopically, they lack a subdivision into cortex, medulla or renal pelvis. The **urinary bladder** may be pear-shaped or multilobulated. Additional so-called accessory bladders may be present. These terminate in the urodeum. The gonads are located cranioventral to the kidneys. The uterus is bicornuate and terminates in the urodeum. A large clitoris is notable in female chelonians.

Reptiles lack organ or mesenteric fat. Coelomic organs cannot be distinguished radiographically and are of uniform homogeneous soft-tissue opacity. The presence of gas or ingesta helps with identification of gastrointestinal tract segments. Only eggs that have a mineralized shell are visible on radiographs. Schematic anatomic drawings of a chelonian can be found in Figure 21.1.

Snakes

The **skeleton** of a snake basically consists of the skull, vertebrae and ribs. The shoulder girdle and sternum are completely absent, and only vestiges of the pelvis may be present. With the exception of two cervical and the caudal vertebrae, all (precloacal) vertebrae (up to 430!) have a free-ending pair of ribs. Ribs in proximity of the cloaca may be forked.

Due to the elongated body shape of these animals, the inner organs are arranged in a linear fashion and usually oriented one after another. When subdividing a snake into quarters from the head to the cloaca, the **heart** is located at the transition zone from the first to second quarter. The **trachea** is located dorsal to the heart. The **lung** is a saccular structure located caudal to the heart and dorsal to the liver. The left lung in most snakes is reduced or absent (except in Boidae whose left and right lungs are of similar size). The caudal part of the (right) lung can function as an air sac. The **gallbladder** is located caudal to the usually undivided liver and forms a triad with the spleen and pancreas. The thin-walled **oesophagus** continues without a distinct transition into the **stomach**, which is located approximately at the mid body (halfway between head and cloaca). The caudal half of the coelom contains intestinal segments and the urogenital tract. The **small intestine** is fairly straight. Boas and pythons only have a small **caecum**. The **kidneys** are paired and resemble rolls of coins. The right kidney is located slightly cranial compared with the left. A **urinary bladder** is absent. As described for chelonians, coelomic organs in snakes are difficult to differentiate unless they contain gas or radiopaque ingesta. A schematic anatomic drawing of a normal snake can be found in Figure 21.2.

Lizards

The anatomy of the **skeleton** is similar to that of mammals. However, there are ribs associated with every vertebra (except the cervical and caudal vertebrae). The extremities usually have five digits with a variable number of phalanges.

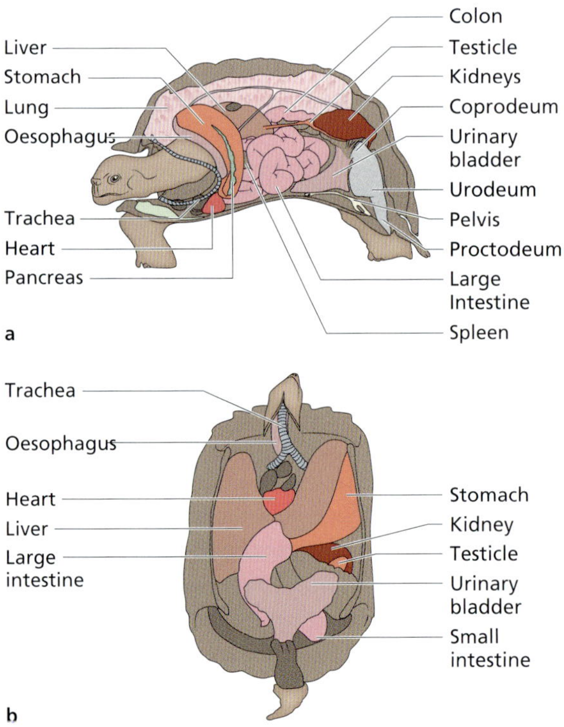

Fig. 21.1 Schematic illustration of the inner organs in a chelonian in sagittal **a** and ventral **b** views.

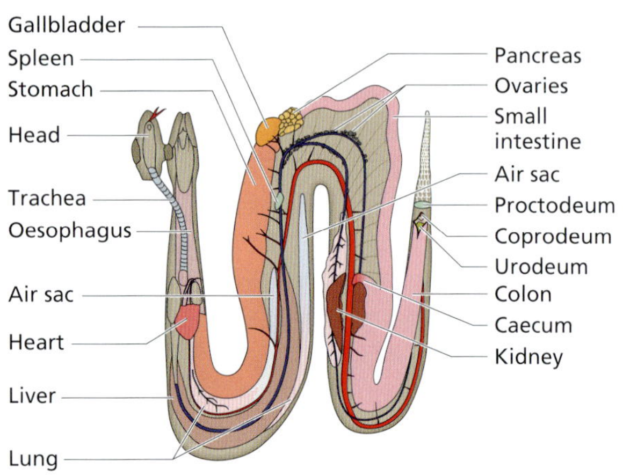

Fig. 21.2 Schematic illustration of the inner organs in a snake (ventral view).

The **lungs** occupy the cranial (craniodorsal) half of the coelomic cavity and, depending on the species, may have few or no subdivisions. Primitive 'unicameral' lungs are hollow sacs, and the respiratory epithelium is limited to the luminal surface. Traditional pulmonary patterns seen in mammals are thus not found. Even though the **heart** in lizards is located at the level of the lungs, it is often not visible because it is located in the cranial thoracic aperture and surrounded by the shoulder girdle. Like chelonians, herbivorous lizards have a prominent large intestine which may interfere with visualization of other organs. The **kidneys** in lizards are located in the caudodorsal coelom in intimate association with the vertebral column. In normal animals, they barely extend beyond the cranial margin of the osseous pelvis and thus are not radiographically visible. A paired **fat pad** serves as a storage organ and is located ventrally in the mid to caudal coelomic cavity.

As in other reptiles, a contrast study is often necessary for localization and examination of the gastrointestinal tract.

21.1.2 Indications

Reptiles are often presented with nonspecific symptoms such as anorexia or lethargy. Particularly in chelonians, radiographs are an important diagnostic aid complementing a thorough history and clinical examination. Due to the poor or absent distinction between coelomic organs on radiographs, the use of additional imaging modalities such as ultrasound or computed tomography (CT) is often necessary.

Chelonians

The most common reasons for presentation include egg binding, pneumonia, renal diseases (commonly gout) and metabolic bone diseases. Other indications include trauma (shell fractures, pulmonary haemorrhage), suspected foreign body obstruction or obstipation. The presence of urinary bladder sediment and calculi varies between geographical regions.

Snakes

Common indications for a radiographic examination include disorders of the musculoskeletal system (e.g. vertebral fractures or osteomyelitis) and of the reproductive tract (e.g. egg binding), as well as obstipation or pneumonia. Snakes are generally easy to palpate and examine by means of ultrasonography.

Lizards

A radiographic examination is most commonly performed to evaluate the musculoskeletal system (e.g. metabolic bone disease and fractures) and the reproductive tract (e.g. egg binding). Obstipation or foreign body ingestion may also occur and require evaluation.

21.2 Radiograpic technique and positioning

21.2.1 General principles

Generally, all radiographic examinations in reptiles should include two orthogonal radiographs as in mammals. Most patients (except crocodiles, large lizards and venomous snakes) can be examined without sedation or anaesthesia. **Sedation** or **anaesthesia** may be necessary in some patients. The reader is referred to anaesthesia texts for information on suitable sedation/anaesthesia protocols for different reptilian species.

Most radiographs of chelonians and lizards are acquired as **whole body radiographs** because of the small size of the patient. Animals are placed directly on the cassette (tabletop technique). Only very large reptiles require the use of a grid during radiographic examination. For detailed examination of extremely small species and for radiographs of the extremities or head, high-detail mammography film–screen combinations can be useful.

Correct positioning is important in all patients to achieve diagnostic quality radiographs and be able to recognize pathological abnormalities (especially of the head and spine). Differences in positioning and exposure factors for different reptile species are covered below.

Chelonians

Radiographs in most chelonians can be obtained without sedation. However, aquatic turtles can be aggressive, and all chelonians can move unexpectedly fast. If possible, the head and extremities should be positioned outside the shell to minimize superimposition artefacts.

Baseline radiographs in chelonians consist of a dorsoventral (DV) and a lateral view. For complete evaluation of the lungs, an additional craniocaudal (CrCd) view is necessary.

The DV view is acquired with a tabletop technique and a vertical beam path. The central beam is aimed at the third/middle vertebral scute.

Lateral and CrCd radiographs are best acquired using a horizontal beam because this positioning is better tolerated by the patients and allows ventrally located coelomic organs to remain in their physiological positions and not interfere with evaluation of the lung field (Fig. 21.3). Patients are positioned on wooden blocks or boxes, and the X-ray cassette is positioned vertically behind the animal using positioning aids (e.g. wooden angles). If the X-ray tube cannot be turned into a horizontal position, animals can be affixed to a wooden block by means of adhesive tape and turned on their side, which assures fairly symmetric lateral positioning. However, some coelomic organ displacement is likely to occur with this positioning. On a lateral view, the central beam is aimed at the boundary between the marginal and costal scutes. On a CrCd view, the beam is aimed at the nuchal scute, and the examiner should take care that the patient's head is not superimposed with the lungs.

Exposure parameters for DV views are similar to those used for radiographs of a similarly large dog's head. Depending on the system, exposure is increased by 5–10 kV for lateral and CrCd views. If using conventional film, several exposures with variable exposure parameters can be exposed on the same film in very small patients.

The **DV view** is especially useful in the assessment of the shell, gastrointestinal tract and shelled calcified eggs. A unilateral increase in opacity within the coelomic cavity due to lung disease is only seen in severe cases.

Lateral views allow evaluation of the respiratory tract, renal size, gastrointestinal tract, shell and skeleton (complementary to other views), as well as urinary bladder content and shelled eggs.

CrCd views almost exclusively aid in evaluation of the lungs but can yield complementary information in the assessment of the shell and skeleton (Fig. 21.4).

For radiographs of individual extremities, it is advisable to extend them outside the shell using tape, and to decrease the exposure parameters accordingly.

Radiographic evaluation is performed using a systematic approach. The following is one possible order in which to assess structures: (1) shell/skeleton, (2) gastrointestinal tract, (3) urinary tract, (4) reproductive tract, (5) respiratory tract and (6) other changes. For localization and description of abnormalities, the coelom can be mentally divided into four parts on the DV view (right cranial, left cranial, right caudal and left caudal coelomic quadrants). For example, the stomach is always located within the left cranial quadrant, while the pylorus is located immediately right paramedian in the mid-coelomic cavity.

Snakes

For some indications (such as exclusion of a radiopaque foreign body), or when dealing with an aggressive patient, an initial DV whole body radiograph may be acquired as a general overview. In select cases, the snake may even remain in its container (Fig. 21.5). Appropriate DV and lateral views with a vertical beam path can either be acquired using manual fixation or after placement of the patient in a plastic tube. This is achieved by allowing the patient to crawl into the tube on its own. Tubular structures can be used for positioning, including old exposed radiographic film that has been rolled up. This approach allows minimization of motion artefacts and optimizes an extended position. For many snakes, multiple successive radiographs are necessary to cover the entire length of the body. Individual body segments should be marked with lead or other metallic markers (e.g. paper clips) taped to the patient. If using conventional radiographic film, several collimated views of different sections of the patient can be exposed on the same radiograph. Exposure parameters are similar to those used for the paws of rabbits, cats or dogs of a similar diameter. Generally, a mAs/kVp combination resulting in a wide range of grey shades (i.e. relatively low in contrast) is preferable.

Lizards

Most small lizards and iguanas, especially patients that are handled frequently, can be placed directly on the cassette or in a thin-walled plastic box (e.g. Tupperware) for DV views. Lateral views are acquired as for chelonians with the animal positioned on a wooden block or cardboard box and using a horizontal beam view. Larger lizards are handled in a similar way to small animals. For chameleons, a small branch can be offered as a perch (see Fig. 21.8), so manipulation of animals for lateral views can typically be avoided.

Exposure parameters for larger lizards are similar to those used for dogs and cats; exposure parameters for smaller reptiles are similar to those used for guinea pigs or mice.

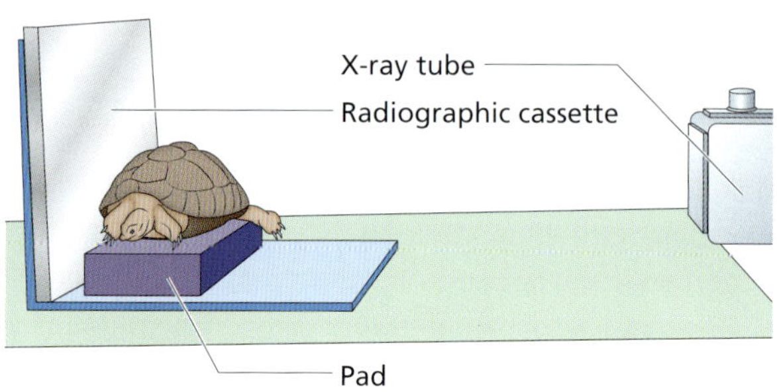

Fig. 21.3 Positioning of a chelonian for a lateral horizontal beam radiograph. The X-ray tube and thus the primary beam are parallel to the ground. The radiographic cassette is positioned perpendicularly behind the animal. The patient is positioned on a radiolucent pad (e.g. foam or cardboard) to allow imaging of the entire ventral coelom and shell. Lateral radiographs in a (calm) lizard can be acquired in the same fashion. For a craniocaudal (CrCd) view, the X-ray tube and cassette are left unchanged in position and the patient is rotated 90° to face the tube. On a lateral view, the central beam is aimed at the border between the marginal and costal scutes. On a CrCd view, the beam is aimed at the nuchal scute. The extremities and head should be extended outside the shell if possible.

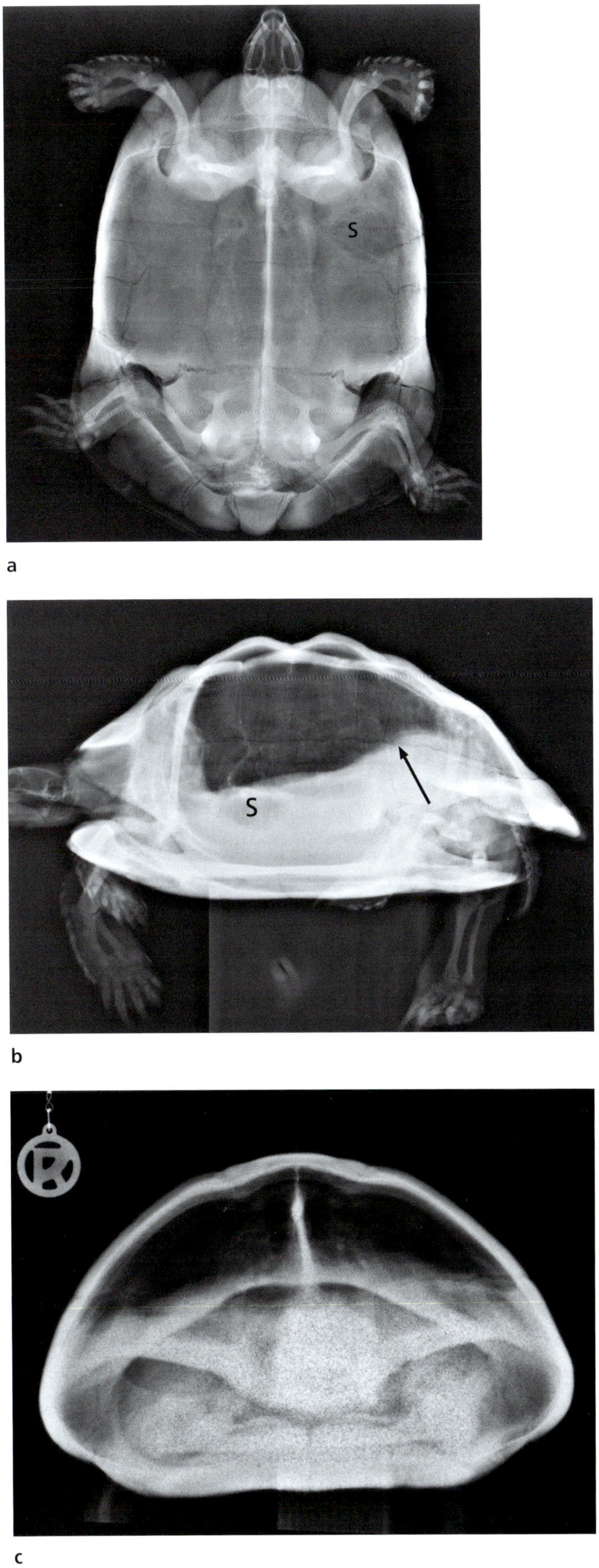

Fig. 21.4 Radiographs of a clinically healthy Hermann's tortoise in a DV a, lateral b and CrCd c beam direction.

a The DV view allows evaluation of the homogeneous mineralized shell. The sutures between individual bone plates are visible as sharply marginated, mildly serrated lucent lines. The margin between the abdominal and femoral plates of the plastron is prominent. The stomach (S) is located in the left cranial quadrant and contains only a small amount of gas. The pylorus is mostly soft-tissue opaque and cannot be distinguished.

b, c The lateral b and CrCd c views are acquired with a horizontal beam view. It is important to take care that positioning aids such as the wooden block used in b are non-opaque and do not interfere with interpretation. These views are especially useful in the evaluation of the dorsally located radiolucent lung. It is important to recognize shell structures superimposed with the lung fields and not misinterpret them as a pathological lung pattern. (This is particularly common in metabolic disorders resulting in a honeycomb appearance of the shell. Inexperienced investigators tend to misinterpret this finding as a 'bronchial lung pattern'). Ventrally located coelomic organs cannot usually be differentiated, with the exception of the gas-filled stomach (S). A horizontal lucent line (arrow) located at the mid-level of the coelomic cavity on the lateral view b represents a suture between the pleural and marginal scutes and is only visible with a perfectly horizontal beam angle. An additional possible artefact in side-necked turtles is related to the S shape of the cervical spine located on the midline within the shell when the head is withdrawn. On the CrCd view c, numerous pinpoint dark dots are superimposed with the coelomic soft tissues: This is a typical artefact on underexposed (low mAs) digital radiographs (so-called quantum mottle) (R = right).

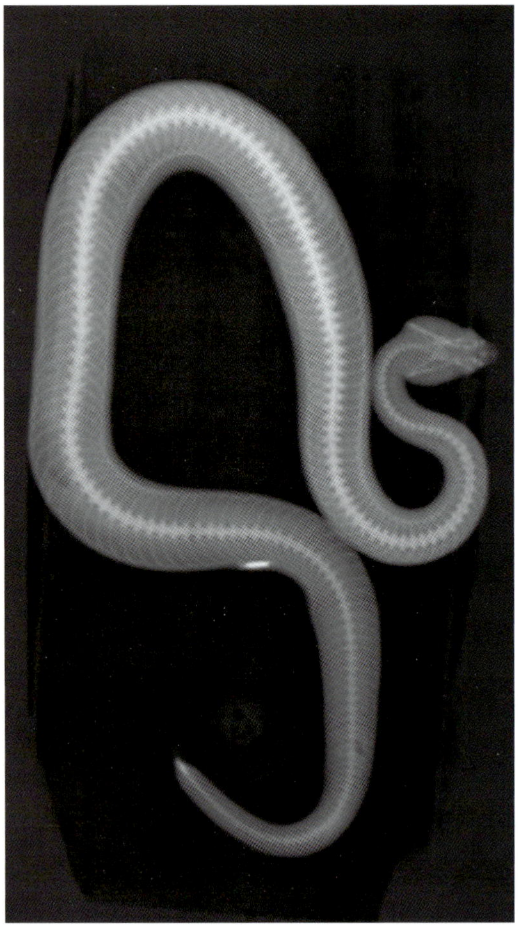

Fig. 21.5 Whole body DV view of a normal snake in a box used for patient transport. The radiograph is of limited diagnostic quality due to inadequate positioning and lack of an orthogonal projection, but allows the investigator to evaluate osseous structures, determine whether the animal is gravid and rule out the presence of radiopaque foreign bodies. One advantage of this limited technique is that the snake does not need to be fixated or manipulated, and aggressive animals can stay within their container. Radiographs of animals that are curled up within a sac are usually insufficient even as survey films.

21.2.2 Contrast procedures

Contrast examination of the gastrointestinal tract

An upper gastrointestinal (GI) contrast study is useful to evaluate the morphology and function of the gastrointestinal tract and identify non-radiopaque foreign bodies or infiltrative diseases (granulomas or neoplastic lesions) which are less common. As reptiles are poikilothermic animals, contrast medium transit time depends on the ambient temperature. Species, health status, season and diet also affect the motility of the gastrointestinal tract. Before administration of contrast medium, it is imperative to keep the patient in a temperature range (usually approximately 28–35°C) that is optimal for the respective species. This can be accomplished by use of a hot lamp in a small terrarium or box. Overheating must be avoided. Adequate hydration of the patient is also important.

The **contrast medium** (barium sulphate suspension, 10–15 ml/kg) is administered by means of a tube. DV and lateral **radiographs** are acquired immediately after contrast medium administration and repeated approximately every hour until contrast medium has reached the caecum (usually after 12–24 hours). Contrast medium remains visible within the caecum and colon for up to approximately 4 weeks. The patient temperature must be kept at physiological levels during the entire duration of the study. As in mammals, **evaluation** includes the position of gastrointestinal segments, gastrointestinal transit time, luminal diameter and margin of the contrast column. Ionic iodinated contrast media are hyperosmolar and should not be used in dehydrated reptiles.

Excretory urography

To evaluate the kidneys and ureters, iodinated nonionic contrast medium (800–1,000 mg I/kg) is administered intravenously into the jugular or dorsal tail vein. Serial DV and lateral radiographs are obtained immediately, after 30 seconds and 2, 5, 15, 30 and 60 minutes. In chelonians, ultrasonographic or CT examination may allow easier evaluation of the urinary tract than a contrast study.

Cystography

In chelonians, contrast medium can be instilled directly into the urinary bladder to facilitate diagnosis of mural or intraluminal filling defects.

21.3 Disorders of the musculoskeletal system

As in other animals, radiographic examination in reptiles is well suited to diagnosing abnormalities of the osseous skeleton. The most common disorders in chelonians and lizards include imbalances in mineral metabolism and traumatic fractures, while traumatic lesions secondary to inappropriate husbandry and infectious processes (such as osteomyelitis of the spine and ribs) predominate in snakes.

21.3.1 Metabolic bone diseases

The most common metabolic bone disease in chelonians and lizards is secondary hyperparathyroidism, which is usually nutritional in cause or may be caused by renal disease. Even though the pathogenesis is different, fibrous osteodystrophy, osteoporosis, osteomalacia and rickets are also included in this category. Disorders of mineral metabolism in reptiles are usually caused by inappropriate husbandry.

RADIOGRAPHIC FINDINGS In affected chelonians, the shell is characterized by heterogeneous bone plates of decreased opacity and with a honeycomb appearance, bumps on the individual neural plates and flattening of the carapace (depending on the time of onset and severity of disease; Fig. 21.6 and 21.7). In lizards, a generalized decrease in bone opacity accompanied by a notably thin cortex of the long bones and loss of the normal trabecular pattern is noted (Fig. 21.8). Multifocal pathological fractures (often greenstick fractures) are common and result in abnormal angulation of one or multiple bones, especially the long bones (Fig. 21.9 and 21.10). These fractures remain visible on radiographs even after correction of the underlying problem.

21.3.2 Osteomyelitis and septic arthritis

Inflammatory skeletal diseases are commonly seen affecting the extremities of lizards, as well as the spines of snakes. Lytic changes in affected bones predominate (Fig. 21.11), while new bone proliferation is uncommon. Adjacent soft tissues are often notably swollen. Gas inclusions are rarely observed.

Shell necrosis predominantly affects the plastron and appears as round lytic foci. These foci of necrosis can give rise to larger abscesses within the coelomic cavity (Fig. 21.12). Sequestration of the bone plates can occur following coeliotomies.

21.3.3 Fractures and luxations

Trauma can result in fractures and luxations in reptiles as in mammals. While fractures of the extremities are common in lizards, shell fractures predominate in chelonians (Fig. 21.13).

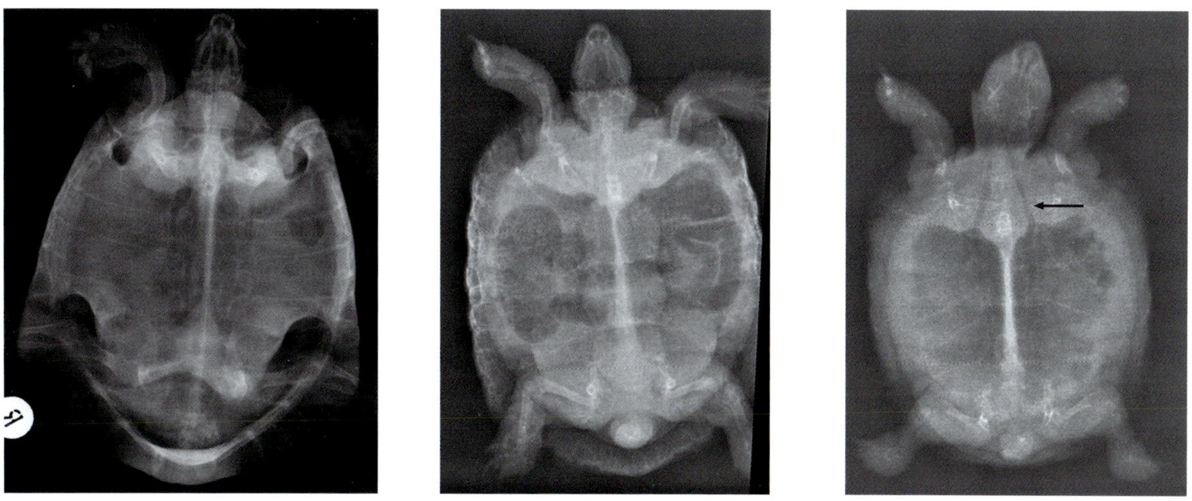

a b c

Fig. 21.6 Comparison DV radiographs of three Hermann's tortoises with disorders of mineral metabolism and secondary hyperparathyroidism of differing levels of severity.

a Male animal with an early or mild disorder of mineral metabolism. The margins of the bony plates show increased sclerosis and the shell is mildly heterogeneous (R = right).

b Female animal with evidence of extensive loss of mineralization and a marked honeycomb appearance of the shell. The compacta of individual bone plates is multifocally disrupted, and the remaining bony parts of the shell appear mesh-like. Marked gas distension of the intestinal tract is also evident.

c Young animal with severe changes. Normal osseous mineralization is mostly absent. The entire animal is soft-tissue opaque, with focal areas of increased opacity in the regions of the shoulder and pelvic girdle. Concurrent findings include visible bronchi (arrow) and decreased size of the lung fields due to concurrent moderate ascites. Inadequate husbandry and nutrition also resulted in disproportionate growth; the extremities are small in relation to the size of the shell.

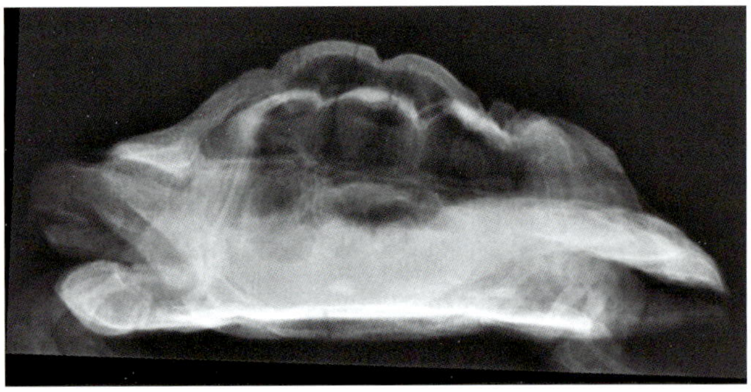

a

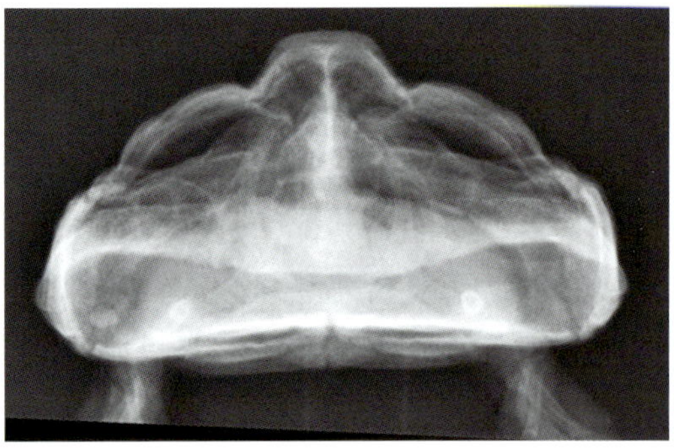

b

Fig. 21.7 Lateral a and CrCd b radiographs of an approximately 6-year-old Hermann's tortoise with disturbances in mineral metabolism. The shell not only has a honeycomb appearance, but the carapace is sunken in with pyramid-like protrusions of individual bone plates (especially neural plates). Abnormalities superimpose with the lung fields, which hampers evaluation for possible lung abnormalities.

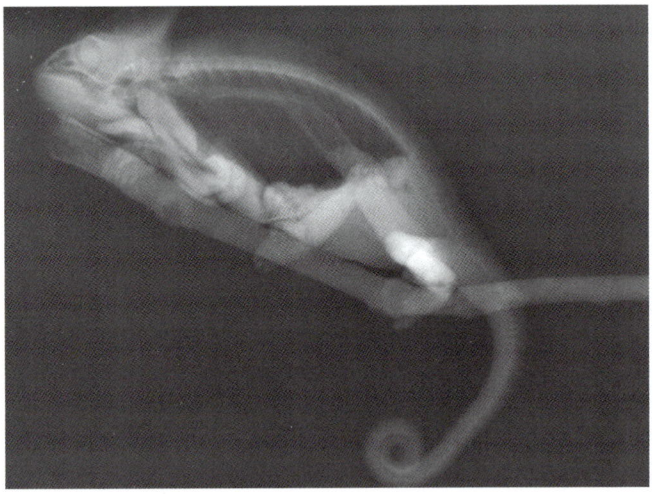

a

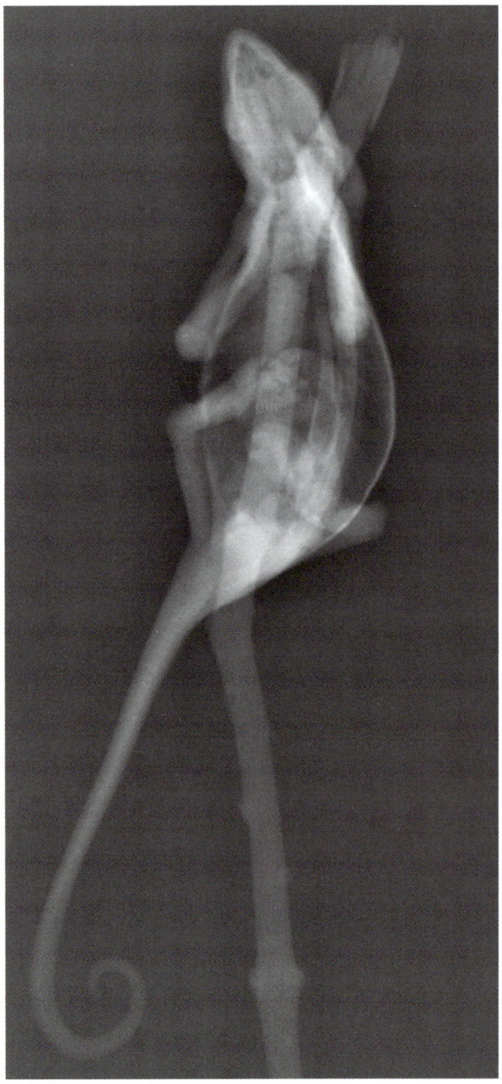

b

Fig. 21.8 Lateral a and DV b radiographs in an adult veiled chameleon. The entire skeleton is characterized by decreased radiographic opacity, thin cortices and a decreased trabecular pattern. The long bones are barely visible. The small wooden branch used for positioning appears more opaque than any part of the skeleton.

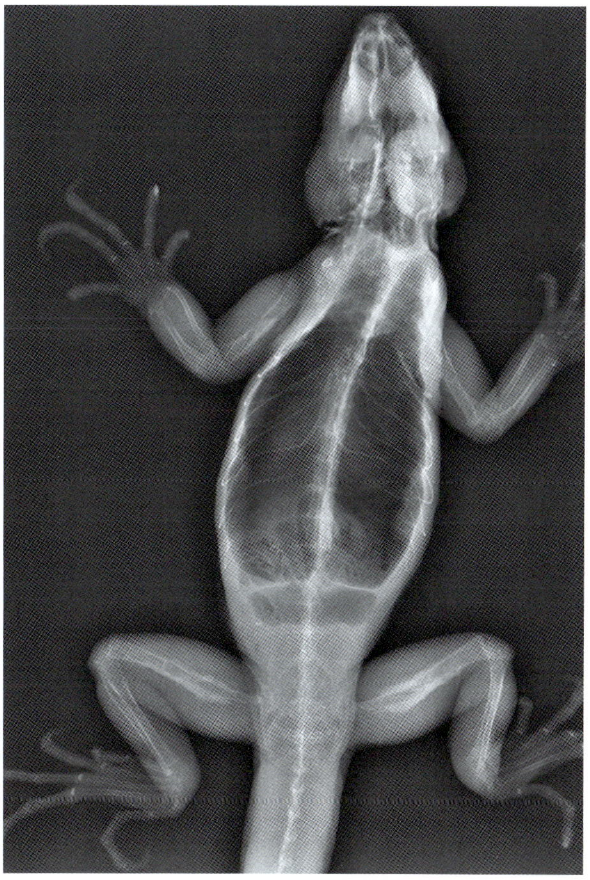

Fig. 21.9 DV radiograph of a green iguana with secondary hyperparathyroidism. Chronic fractures are noted associated with both femora, and there is an acute oblique or spiral fracture of the right humerus. There is a generalized decrease in bone opacity, and the cortices of the long bones are thin. The animal was previously treated for obstipation. Residual inspissated ingesta are still noted within the intestinal tract. The lung fields are large and extend far into the caudal half of the coelom.

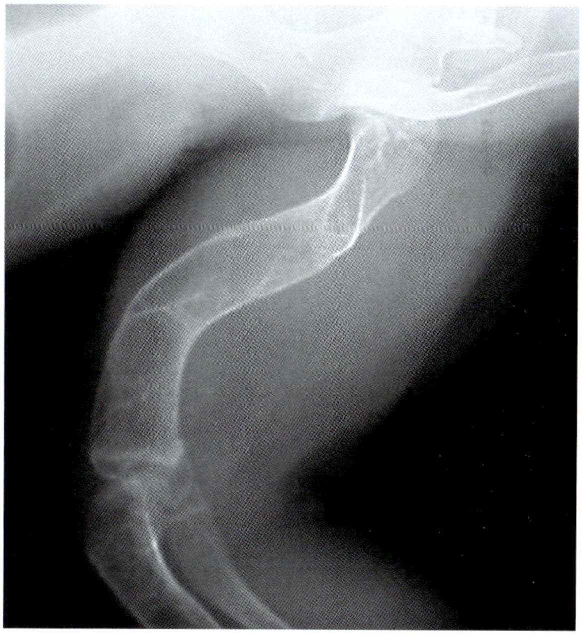

Fig. 21.10 Lateral radiograph of the proximal hind limb in a lizard. There is evidence of metabolic bone disease with a pathological fracture and resulting abnormal angulation of the long bone.

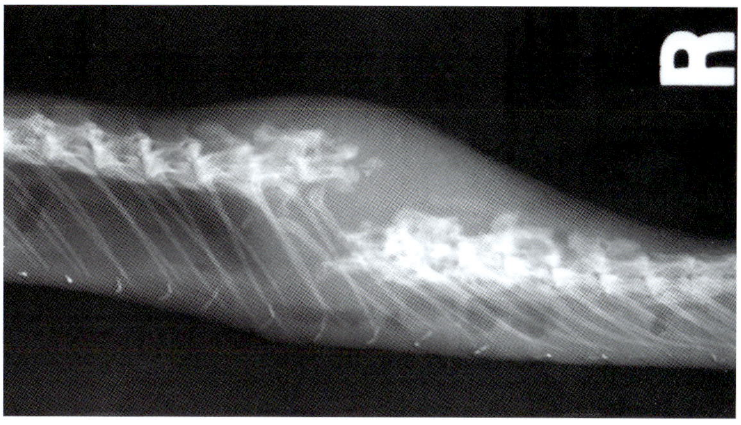

Fig. 21.11 Severe osteomyelitis in a snake. There is marked soft-tissue swelling and luxation associated with the spine. Multiple vertebrae show mostly lytic and to a lesser degree osteoproliferative changes (R = right).

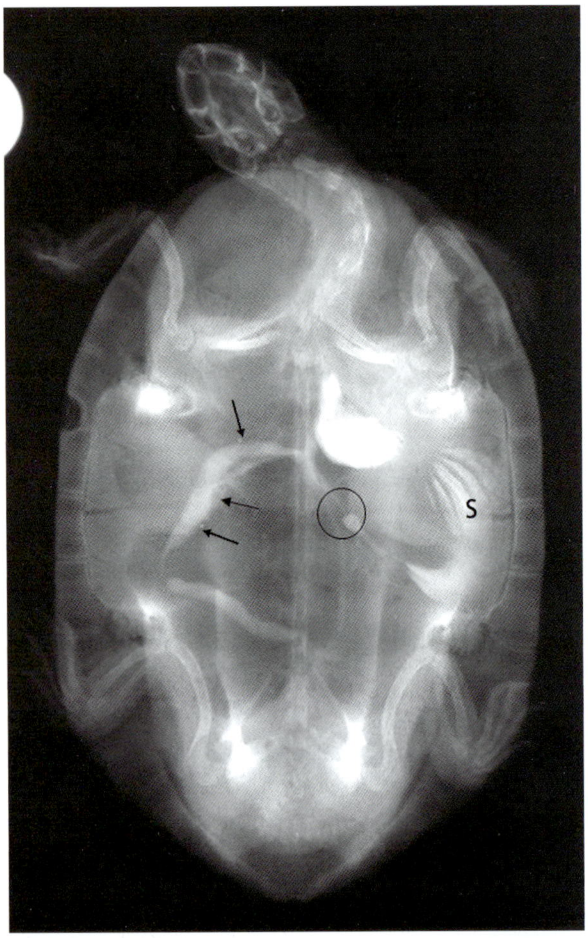

Fig. 21.12 DV radiograph obtained during an upper GI contrast study in an aquatic turtle. Caudal displacement of the stomach was already noted on survey radiographs. The contrast study not only shows caudal displacement of the stomach (S; note distinct peristalsis and prominent folds) but also leftward and caudal displacement of the pylorus (always recognized as a focal filling defect; indicated by a circle) and leftward displacement of the duodenum (arrows). Intestinal segments are displaced by round soft-tissue opacity masses. Regions of necrosis are recognized as focal lucent defects within the shell. A necropsy confirmed that these necrotic regions served as a pathway for disease spreading into the coelomic cavity with abscess formation, which ultimately resulted in displacement of the intestinal tract and adhesions with the duodenum.

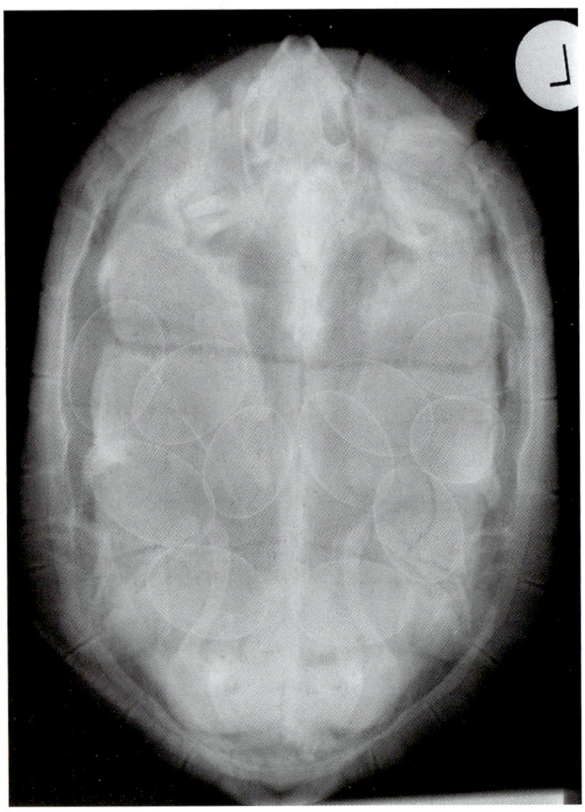

a

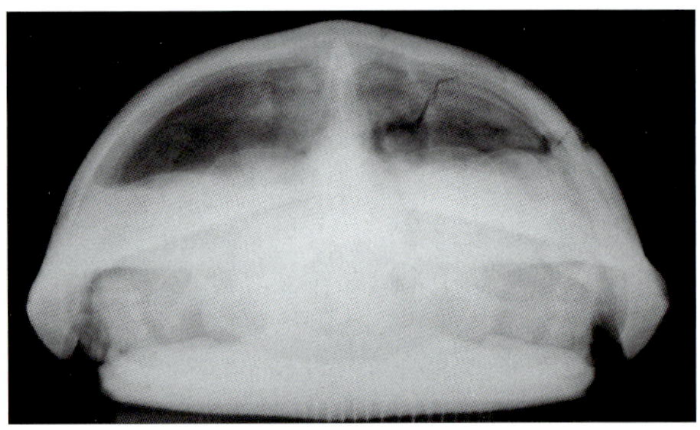

b

Fig. 21.13 DV a and CrCd b radiographs of a European pond turtle that was hit by an automobile. Several fractures are associated with the left half of the shell, especially cranially. On the CrCd view, regions of heterogeneous increased opacity are associated with the lung adjacent to the fracture lines, consistent with pulmonary haemorrhage. Additionally, late-term development of 11 eggs is noted (L = left).

Fracture healing initially occurs by means of a fibrous callus, which is not visible radiographically. Bony healing takes significantly longer than in mammals (6–18 months for the chelonian shell). Extremity fractures in chelonians are rare due to the protective mechanism of the shell and should prompt an evaluation, for example using CT to rule out abscesses in the surrounding soft tissues which would raise concern for a pathological fracture (Fig. 21.14).

Dog bites to chelonians can result in the loss of larger parts of the shell and lead to punctures into the coelomic cavity.

21.3.4 Other diseases

These are comparatively rare in reptiles. Nutritional hypervitaminosis D can result in exuberant new bone formation (especially around vertebrae and ribs) and mineralization of soft tissues (especially the great vessels) and is most commonly seen in lizards (Fig. 21.15).

21.4 Disorders of the head

Radiographs of the head in reptiles are usually indicated to evaluate soft-tissue and bone changes of the upper and lower jaw related to trauma or infection, and possibly to assess the auricular system (otitis media; Fig. 21.16). Due to the marked variation between species and for a confident diagnosis of an abnormal finding, detailed knowledge of the normal anatomy in the respective reptilian species is imperative. Patient positioning follows the same principles as in small animals. Sedation is often necessary for adequate positioning. The investigator should not be tempted to position his/her hands in the primary beam to manually position the animal!

21.5 Disorders of the cardiovascular system

Common cardiovascular abnormalities diagnosed on radiographs in reptilian species are cardiac insufficiency with resulting pulmonary oedema, and mineralization of vascular walls.

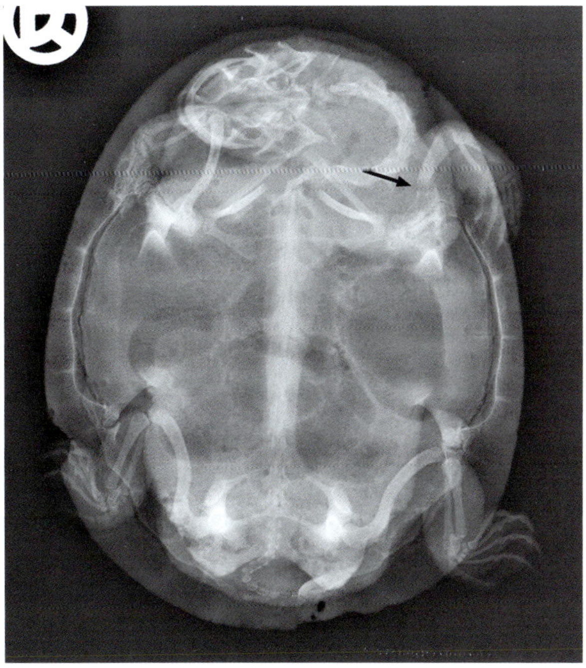

Fig. 21.14 Aquatic turtle with multiple regions of shell necrosis (indicated by round lytic lesions associated with the shell) and a fracture of the left humerus (arrow) with focal soft-tissue swelling. Fractures of the humerus and femur in chelonians usually indicate a pre-existing bone lesion as the extremities are well protected from trauma by the overlying shell. A CT examination performed in this case confirmed an extensive abscess which had caused lysis and osteomyelitis of the cranial margin of the left shell bridge. This fracture is thus considered pathological in nature. The multiple regions of shell necrosis in this patient likely served as pathway for infection. Note the horizontal S-shaped curvature of the cervical spine allowing withdrawal and protection of the head in the cranial shell in this side-necked turtle (R = right).

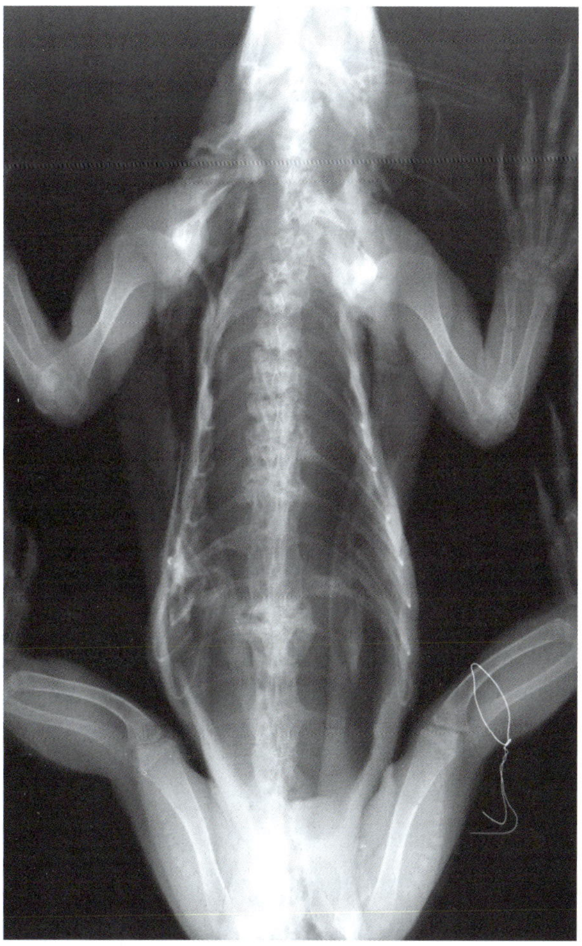

Fig. 21.15 Post mortem DV view (following removal of coelomic organs) in an adult male green iguana which received a teaspoon of vitamin/mineral supplement on a daily basis. This overdose resulted in severe hypercalcaemia which manifested as new bone proliferation along the entire spine and several ribs, as well as vascular mineralization.

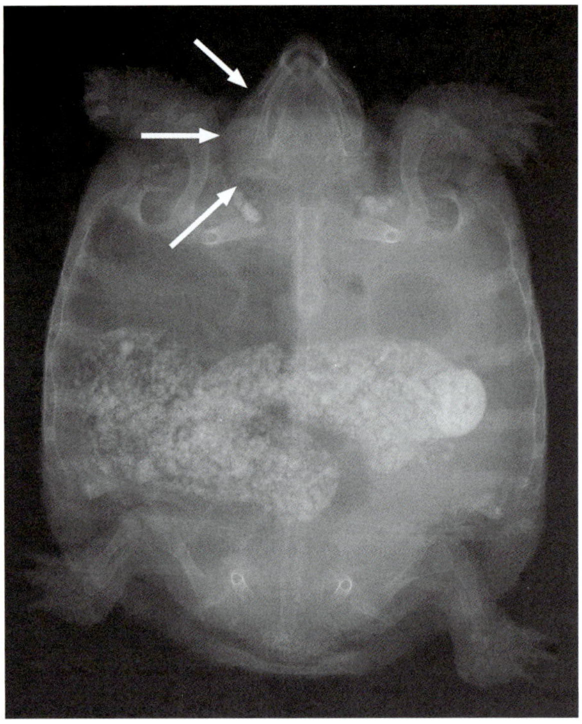

Fig. 21.16 DV radiograph of a juvenile moribund Hermann's tortoise with obstipation, left-sided pneumonia and right-sided otitis media. Otitis was considered an incidental finding in this case, but resulted in swelling at the level of the tympanic shield (arrows). Extension of the head would have been required for better radiographs.

Chelonians

Diseases of the heart and vessels cannot usually be diagnosed radiographically, because these structures are masked by surrounding organs and the shell. To evaluate the heart for pathological changes, advanced procedures such as ultrasound or CT are indicated. Changes in the large vessels are occasionally noted on craniocaudal and lateral views, especially in the case of mineralization of the vessel walls.

Snakes

Radiographic diagnosis of heart and vascular diseases is easier in snakes than in other types of reptiles. Radiographs in two planes are necessary to assess the extent of abnormalities. With generalized enlargement of the cardiac silhouette, pericardial effusion should be considered as a possible differential diagnosis for cardiac insufficiency. Echocardiography is routinely performed in snakes for further evaluation.

Lizards

The heart is difficult to evaluate radiographically because it is located far cranially in the coelomic cavity and contained within the shoulder girdle; this is especially true in iguanas and geckos. The heart and large vessels in monitor lizards are located further caudally and can be better evaluated radiographically using a lateral view.

21.6 Disorders of the respiratory tract

The lung is best evaluated on a lateral view (all reptiles) and on a craniocaudal view (chelonians). When evaluating the lung, the investigator must consider that the appearance and size of the lung fields are affected by adjacent structures. Cachexia results in enlargement and the impression of decreased opacity in the lung fields (Fig. 21.17). Conversely, space-occupying processes in the coelomic cavity or fluid accumulations can compromise the lung field (Fig. 21.18).

Pneumonia is the most common respiratory disease in reptiles. It is usually caused by bacterial organisms, but viral, fungal and parasitic infections are also possible. Pulmonary compression in chelonians often results in clinical symptoms resembling pneumonia. Radiographs can help avoid inappropriate treatment (Fig. 21.19).

> The clinical examination of a chelonian should ALWAYS include radiographs!

RADIOGRAPHIC FINDINGS Depending on the type of pneumonia (productive/'moist' or 'interstitial'), affected **chelonians** show extensive gravity-dependent regions of increased pulmonary opacity, often forming the shape of a sail, or focal reticular regions of increased opacity within the lung fields (Fig. 21.16 and 21.20). Abscesses or granulomas typically result in generalized, or rarely nodular, opacities within the lung fields (Fig. 21.21). Alveolar or bronchial patterns as seen in mammals are not recognized in reptiles. With unilateral pneumonia, emphysema of the contralateral lung is common, which is best seen on craniocaudal views.

Pneumonia in **snakes** usually results in increased density of the peripheral respiratory epithelium, which may

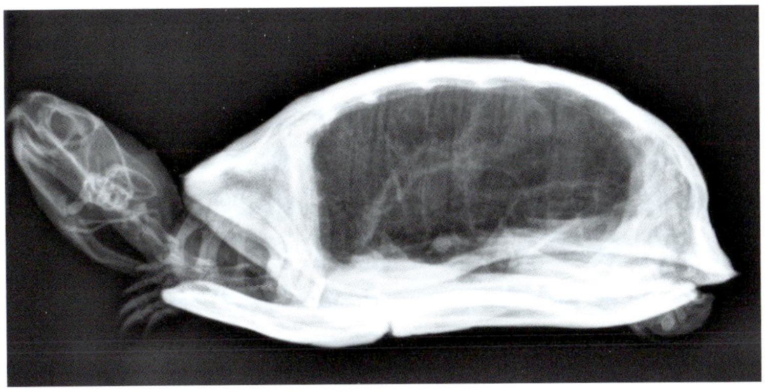

Fig. 21.17 Enlargement of the lung fields and associated decreased radiopacity of the lung secondary to severe cachexia in a chelonian.

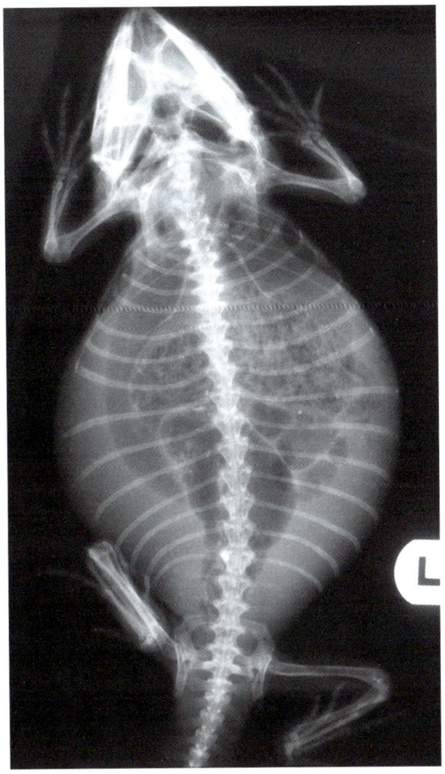

a

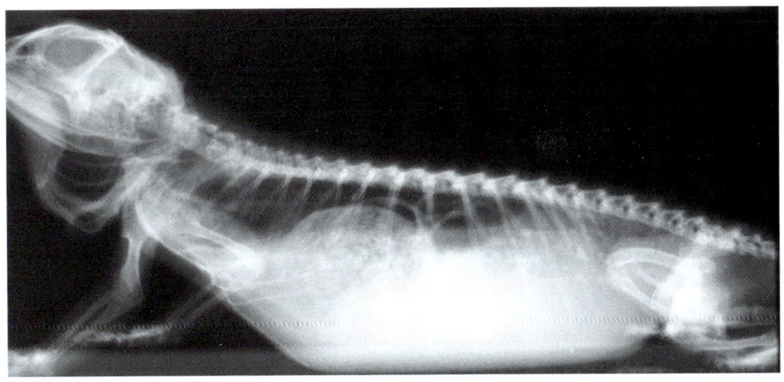

b

Fig. 21.18 Decreased size of the lung field due to severe coelomic effusion in a bearded dragon lizard.
a Abdominal distension seen on the DV view initially gives the impression of a well-nourished animal (L = left).
b The horizontal beam lateral view demonstrates a distinct fluid interface. Extensive gas accumulation within the intestinal tract is also pathological.

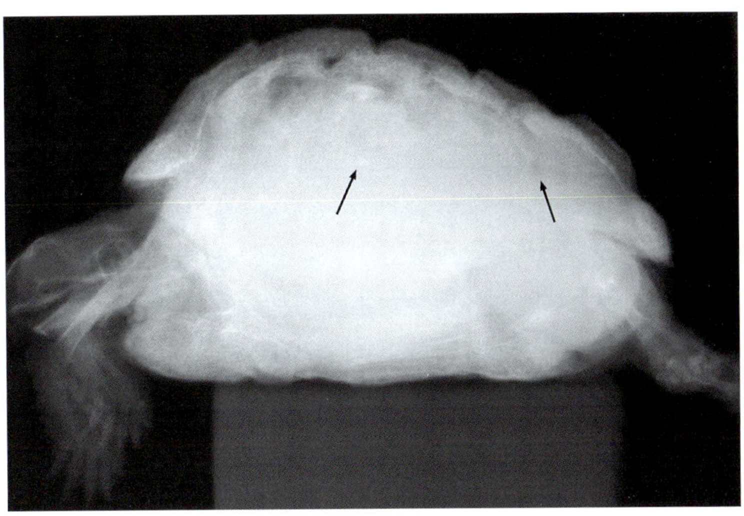

Fig. 21.19 Severely decreased size of the lung field in a juvenile Hermann's tortoise presented with dyspnoea following unsuccessful empirical treatment for pneumonia. The lung field is reduced to a small gas opacity region within the craniodorsal aspect of the shell. The intestinal tract (indistinct gas- and ingesta-filled intestinal segments indicated by arrows) is elevated dorsally. Urine retention was suspected and confirmed by means of ultrasonography. Note the open mouth (mouth breathing due to dyspnoea). The honeycomb appearance of the shell indicates poor husbandry.

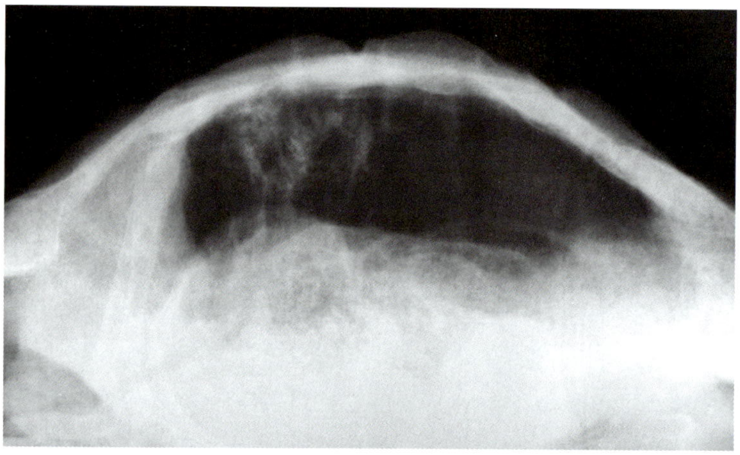

Fig. 21.20 Focal regions of increased opacity with a reticular pattern in the lung of an adult Hermann's tortoise. These were residual changes from an extensive 'interstitial' pneumonia.

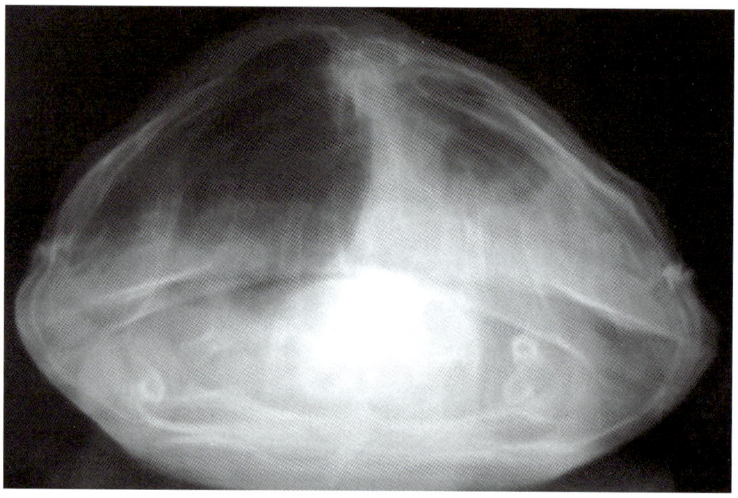

Fig. 21.21 Extensive sail-like infiltrates associated with the left lung in a red-eared slider. The right lung is emphysematous. Subsequent CT examination and necropsy identified numerous small abscesses throughout the entire coelomic cavity. This complex disease process cannot be visualized on the radiograph, which only shows an apparently 'simple' pneumonia.

result in patchy regions of increased opacity. With fluid accumulation in the central lumen, soft-tissue opacity within the lung fields increases.

In **lizards**, lung fields that are relatively small in size and patchy regions of increased opacity are the predominant findings. It is important to recognize that the overlying scales vary in shape depending on the species and may result in artefacts when superimposed over the lung fields, which may be confused with abnormal pulmonary patterns.

As in mammals, CT examination of the lung(s) in reptiles is highly rewarding.

Pulmonary haemorrhage is most commonly seen in chelonians with shell fractures and appears as a region of increased opacity (see Fig. 21.13).

Other respiratory diseases (e.g. neoplasia, anthracosis and foreign body inhalation) have been documented in individual cases but are less common than inflammatory processes.

21.7 Disorders of the gastrointestinal tract

The most common diseases of the gastrointestinal tract in reptiles include gastroenteritis caused by various infectious agents (viruses, bacteria, fungal organisms and parasites), foreign bodies, obstipation and mechanical or paralytic ileus. Neoplastic lesions are rare.

Radiographic findings It is important to note that the stomach of chelonians and most other reptiles physiologically contains a certain amount of gas. The small intestine typically only contains fluid. The large intestine may contain variably small gas accumulations in addition to faecal matter.

Survey radiographs are often unrewarding in **gastroenteritis**, but may on occasion demonstrate unusual gas accumulations within the gastrointestinal tract. An upper GI contrast study may show infiltrative abnormalities of the intestinal wall (Fig. 21.22) or changes in gastrointestinal transit time. However, a diagnosis is usually achieved by other means (endoscopy or parasitic, neurological or cytological examination).

The radiographic diagnosis of a metal or bone opaque **foreign body** within the gastrointestinal tract of a reptile is straightforward (Fig. 21.23). Non-opaque foreign bodies are a challenge and are usually diagnosed by means of advanced imaging (ultrasound, upper GI contrast study) as in dogs and cats.

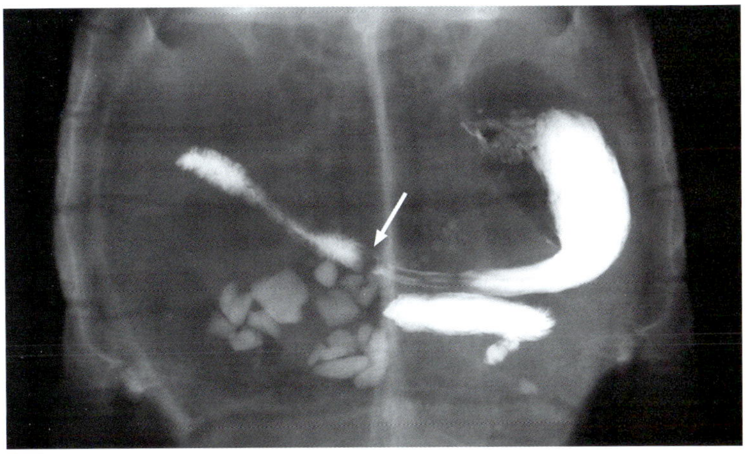

Fig. 21.22 Magnified partial DV view of a Hermann's tortoise during an upper GI barium sulphate contrast study. The pylorus (arrow) appears as a focal filling defect immediately to the right of midline. The duodenum and most cranial aspect of the jejunum contain contrast medium and have an irregular frayed contour. The diagnosis was duodenitis. Several small stones are noted associated with the caecum.

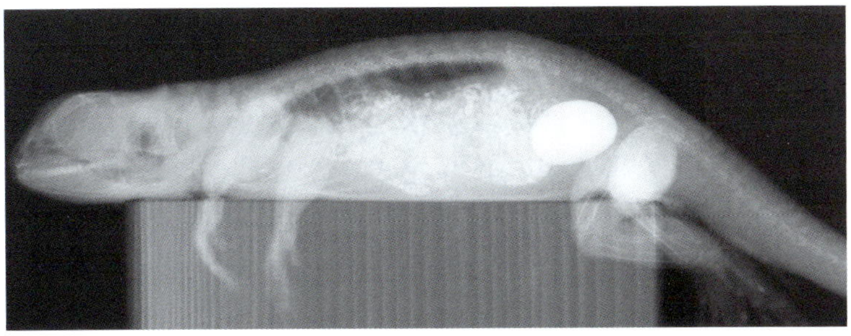

Fig. 21.23 Bearded dragon lizard that had swallowed a glass gem unable to pass through the osseous pelvis. Inspissated faecal matter has accumulated cranial to the foreign body.

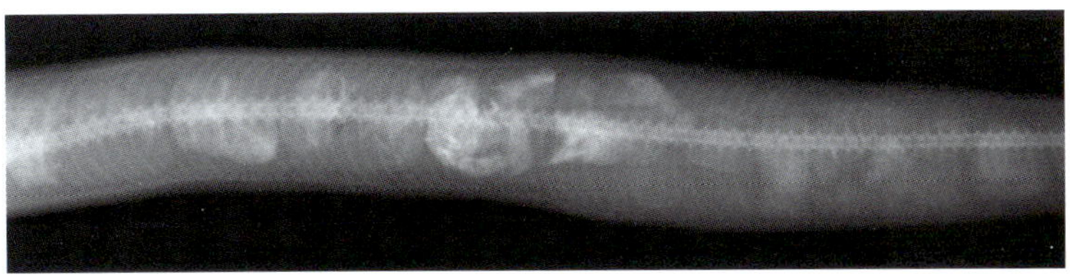

a

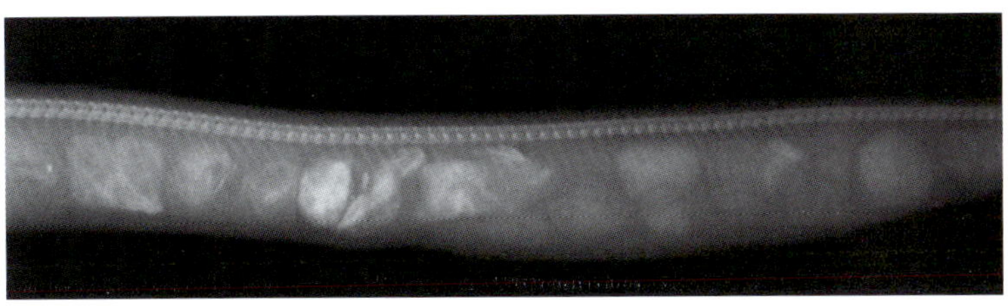

b

Fig. 21.24 DV a and lateral b radiographs of a python with numerous soft-tissue to mineral opaque rounded structures within the intestinal tract, consistent with obstipation due to so-called coproliths. It is interesting that despite obstipation (and severe clinical signs) no gas accumulation is noted.

Obstipation is a fairly common problem in chelonians and small lizards. Affected animals often present with extensive accumulation of inspissated radiopaque material within the intestinal tract (Fig. 21.16 and 21.23). Inspissated ingesta, foreign material or mass lesions may result in **mechanical ileus**, which is characterized by gas dilatation of the intestinal tract proximal to the obstructive lesion (Fig. 21.24). An upper GI contrast study can be helpful for further evaluation in select cases.

Radiographs in animals with **paralytic ileus** are typically unrewarding but may show dilatation of intestinal segments or accumulations of radiopaque ingesta ('gravel sign') (Fig. 21.25).

Gastrointestinal tract **neoplasia** is rare but mass lesions may appear on survey radiographs, depending on their size. Determination of organ association and extent of the lesion requires advanced procedures such as an upper GI contrast study, endoscopy, ultrasound or CT in most cases.

Hepatomegaly (especially secondary to lipidosis) can sometimes be suspected based on caudodorsal displacement of the stomach, but must be confirmed by means of ultrasonography or CT.

21.8 Disorders of the urinary tract

Urinary tract disorders are a common problem in reptiles. Radiographic examination plays an important role in the diagnosis of renomegaly (secondary to renal gout, purulent nephritis possibly with abscessation, or rarely neoplasia) and radiopaque uroliths. For a more detailed assessment of renal disease (specifically renal gout and glomerulonephropathy), advanced diagnostic tests and ultrasound are necessary. Ultrasound-guided biopsies of abnormal tissues are feasible, especially in snakes and lizards.

Chelonians

Marked renal enlargement is characterized by a hemispherical focal soft-tissue protrusion into the caudodorsal lung fields on lateral views (Fig. 21.26). Renal mineralization appears as plaque-like to extensive regions of increased opacity which border the caudal margin of the lung fields on the lateral view and are projected cranially to the coxofemoral joints on a DV view (Fig. 21.27). These should not be confused with intestinal contents.

Radiopaque urinary bladder calculi are also easily diagnosed on survey radiographs and may lead to confusion with pathological mineralized eggs in female animals (Fig. 21.28).

Excessive overdistention of the urinary bladder (urinary obstruction) leads to displacement of intestinal segments in a craniodorsal direction and compression of the lung fields. This should not be misinterpreted as pneumonia (see Fig. 21.19).

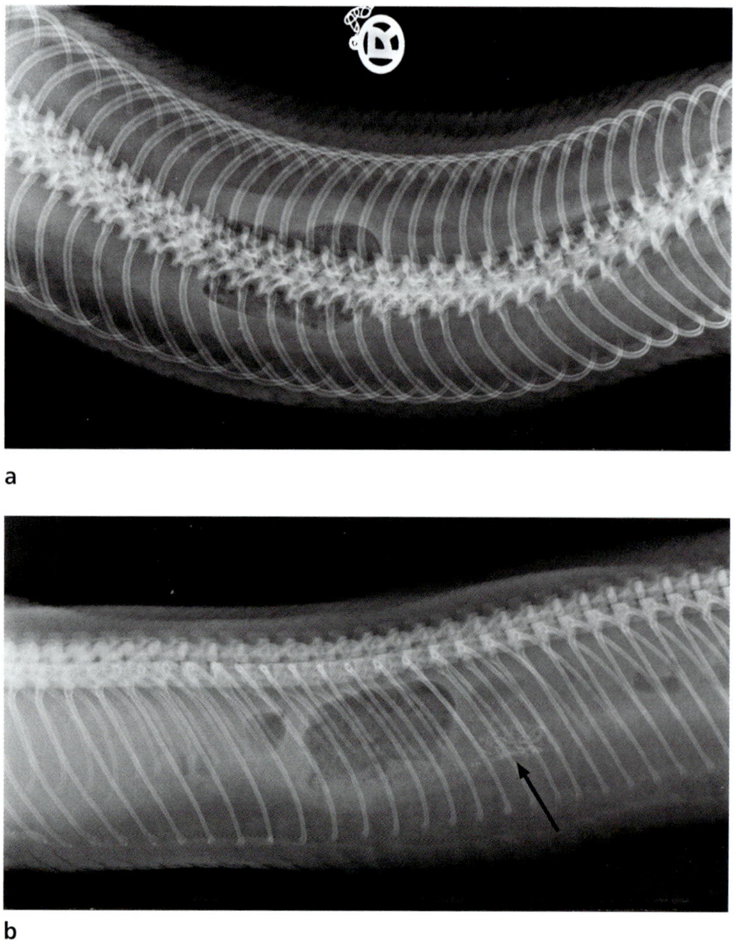

Fig. 21.25 DV a and lateral b radiographs of a tiger python showing only 10% of the body, approximately 30 cm cranial to the cloaca. There is a focal gas-dilated intestinal segment. The adjacent accumulation of small mineral opaque particles in a ventrally located intestinal segment resembles a 'gravel sign' (arrow). An intestinal abscess was diagnosed intraoperatively, which had resulted in a partial mechanical ileus. (Courtesy of Reptile Clinic, Vetmeduni Vienna, Prof Dr Zednek Knotek)

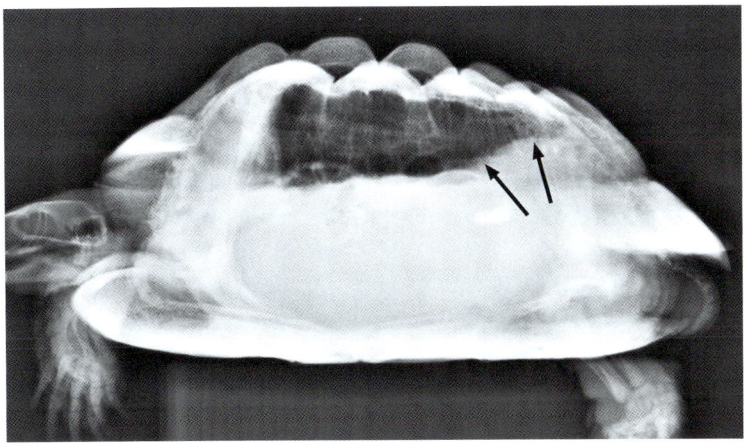

a

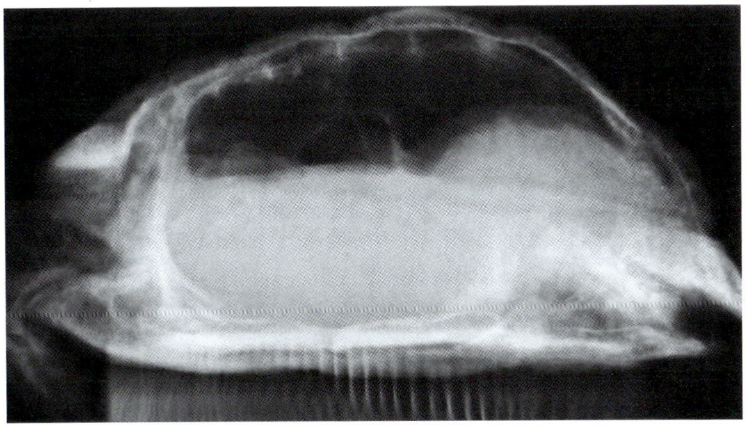

b

Fig. 21.26
a Hermann's tortoise with focal bulging of a soft-tissue opacity into the caudal lung field (arrows), which is consistent with a mild to moderate renomegaly. Renal gout was diagnosed by means of ultrasonography. Note the lumpy carapace which is indicative of inappropriate husbandry.
b Marginated tortoise with severe renomegaly due to hexamitiasis.

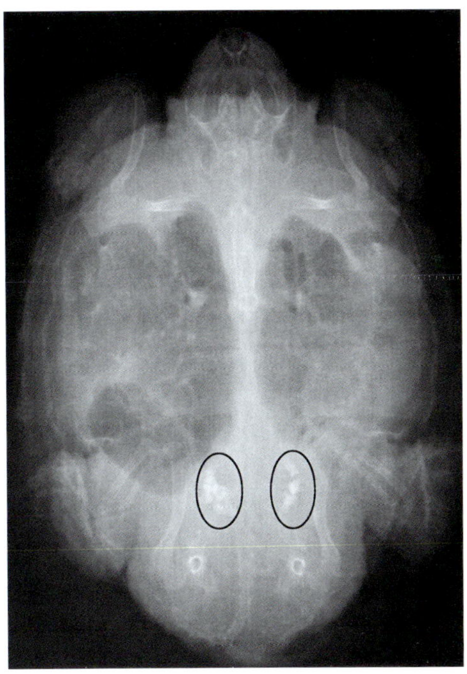

a

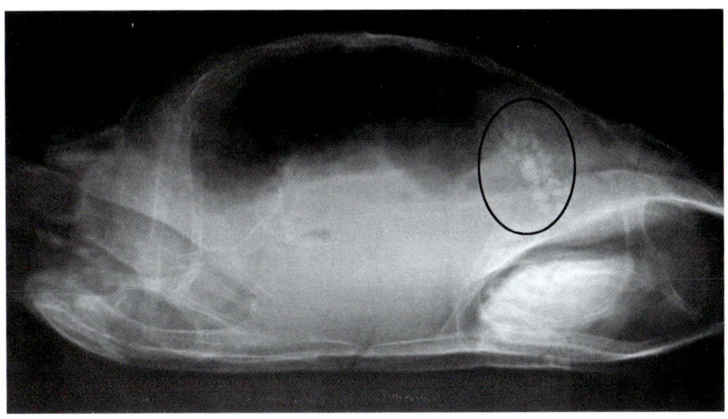

b

Fig. 21.27 DV a and lateral b radiographs of a red-eared slider with renal mineralization (circles). These should not be confused with faecal matter.

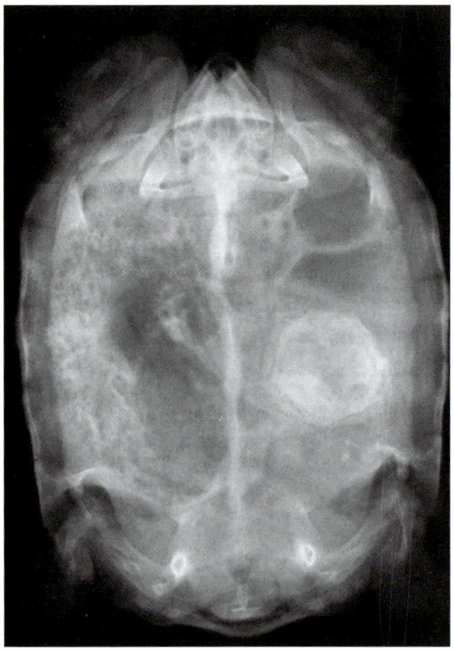

a

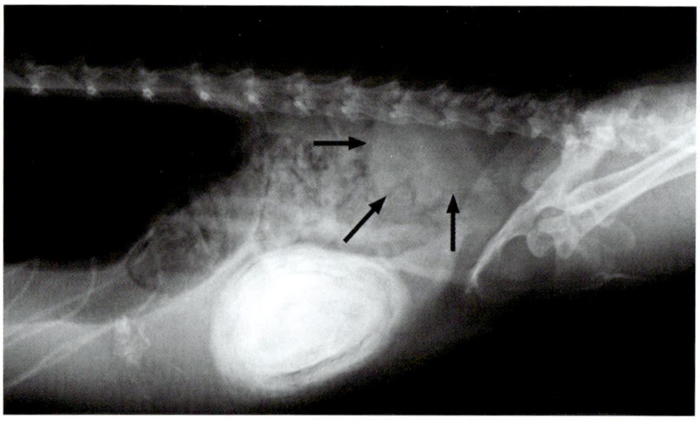

b

Fig. 21.28

a Leopard tortoise with a large layered urinary bladder calculus in the left coelomic cavity. In a female animal, this structure may lead to confusion with an egg.

b Caudal half of the body of a green iguana in a lateral view. A large urinary bladder calculus is located cranial to the pelvis. There is also evidence of renomegaly characterized by a bulging soft-tissue opacity (arrows) extending cranially to the pelvis from dorsal and resulting in secondary displacement of the intestinal tract.

Snakes

Renomegaly may appear radiographically as a focal mass lesion within the coelomic cavity. Because there is no urinary bladder, development of cystoliths is impossible, and coproliths should not be misinterpreted as such.

Lizards

The kidneys in most lizards can only be visualized if they are markedly enlarged (usually due to granulomatous or neoplastic disease) and extend cranially beyond the pelvis (Fig. 21.28b). Well-aerated lungs and air sacs in chameleons may facilitate visualization of the kidneys on a lateral view. Renomegaly may result in secondary obstipation or egg binding. Radiopaque bladder calculi are easily diagnosed on survey films.

21.9 Disorders of the reproductive tract

The most common indications for evaluation of the reproductive tract are to determine if a female is gravid, and to evaluate for egg binding. Neoplastic lesions originating from reproductive organs are rare and result in mass lesions within the coelomic cavity. The organ of origin cannot usually be determined on survey radiographs.

21.9.1 Sexing

A radiographic examination has some limited value in animal sexing by allowing identification of mineralized eggs or, less commonly, vitellogenic follicles, testicles and mineralized structures of hemipenes.

21.9.2 Diagnosis of a gravid reptile

A variable number of shelled or unshelled eggs, which may contain skeletal structures in viviparous species, is found in gravid animals (Fig. 21.29). An ultrasound examination can aid in differentiating follicles (normal versus atrophied/necrotic) and assessing viability of the young.

21.9.3 Egg binding

Egg binding can be related to various exogenous and endogenous causes. A **definitive diagnosis** can only be made if the results of the clinical examination and supporting clinical symptoms are taken into consideration and support the suspicion (Fig. 21.29b). Deformed eggs may be seen in chelonians and do not necessarily result in egg binding. Only definitively enlarged eggs or excessive mineralization of eggshells are consistent with a radiographic diagnosis of egg binding (Fig. 21.30).

Radiographic **assessment** includes the number, size, shape, density and surface smoothness of the eggs, as well as the integrity of the surface and whether the eggs are uniform in appearance. Each of these parameters varies between different reptile species. For example, Hermann's and common tortoises typically lay six to ten eggs, while spider tortoises and leopard geckos only develop two eggs which reach a considerable size compared to the parent animal. It is important to note that red-eared sliders and other (semi)aquatic turtles produce less opaque and often mildly deformed eggs compared to terrestrial species. Soft shell and marine chelonians

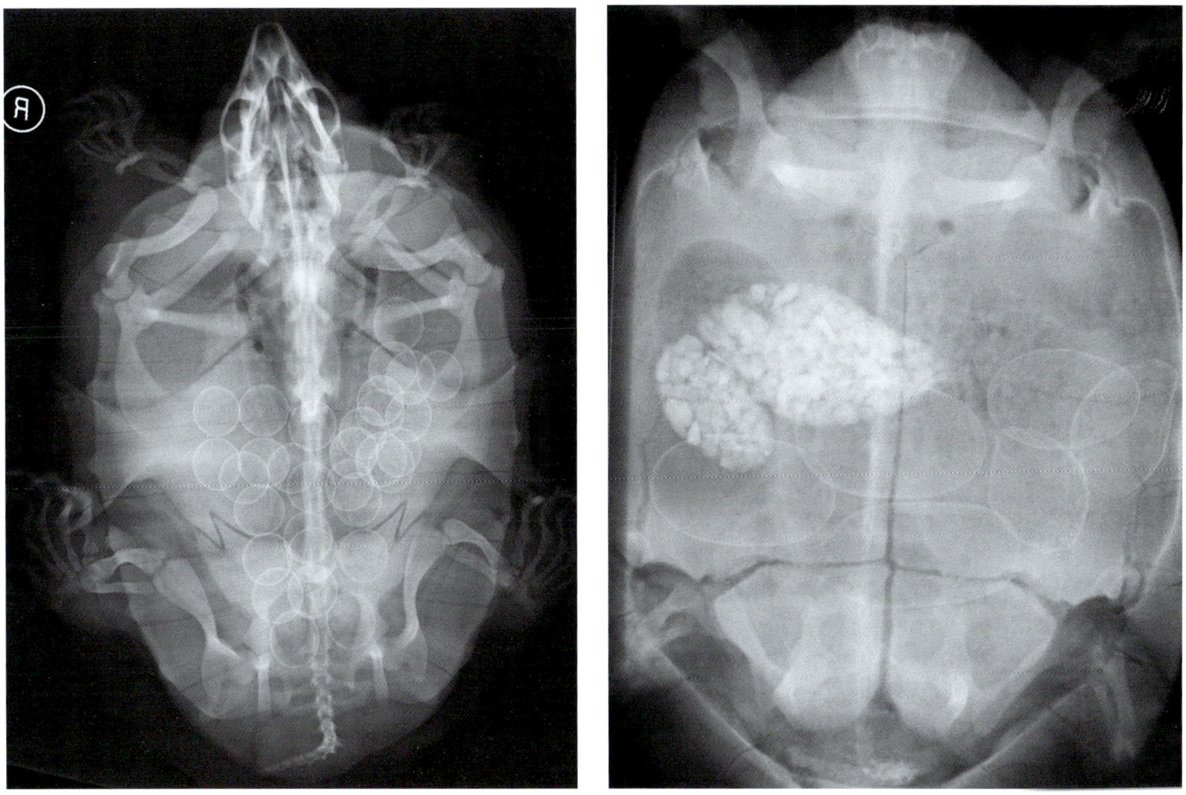

a b

Fig. 21.29a Soft shell turtle with numerous mineralized eggs. Note the unusual shape of the bone plates of the shell, which are reduced in this aquatic species. The horny scutes are replaced by a leathery skin (R = right). b Spur-thighed tortoise with partially mineralized immature eggs. Note the abnormal shape of several eggs: lemon shape, long oval with an open pole, and at least one with a distinct indentation. Despite these obvious abnormalities, a radiographic diagnosis of egg binding cannot be made in this patient. The animal was clinically normal and, although some were broken, all eggs were successfully laid one week later. Recheck radiographs following egg laying are recommended to rule out residual eggshell pieces within the coelomic cavity. The accumulation of small stones within the caecum is an incidental finding. This apparent obstipation spontaneously resolves following egg laying.

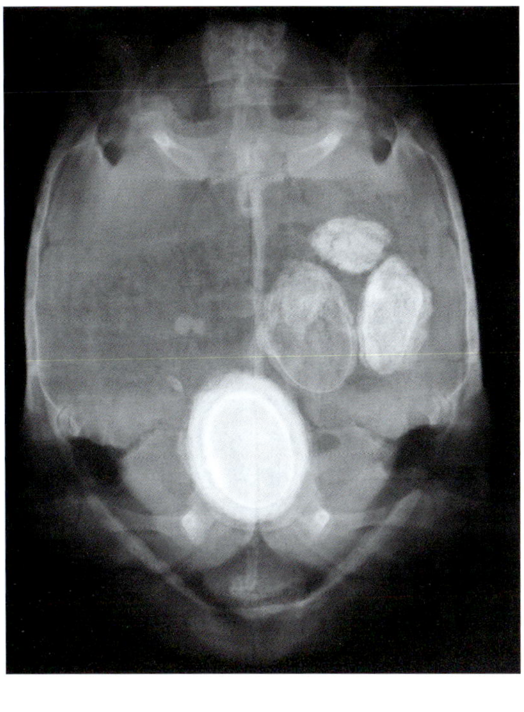

Fig. 21.30 Hermann's tortoise with a markedly oversized egg stuck in the pelvis. The marked peripheral proliferation indicates a chronic process. These findings allow a confident radiographic diagnosis of egg binding. (From Gumpenberger and Filip 2001, with permission from ÖGT)

have a large number of small and often perfectly spherical eggs. Calcified eggshells in most lizards are only recognized as a very faint rim, and notable mineralization is a pathological finding. The eggs in most snakes and lizards appear as numerous soft-tissue opaque ovoid to spherical structures within the coelomic cavity which result in pulmonary compression (Fig. 21.31 to 21.34). In Mediterranean tortoises, an accumulation of stones within the caecum is commonly observed during egg production and should not be misinterpreted as a pathological finding. Malposition of an egg within the urinary bladder is a rare finding (Fig. 21.35). A diagnosis is made by means of a retrograde cystogram or ultrasound. These eggs barely change position on recheck radiographs.

Pre-ovulatory egg binding is a special form of egg binding, during which follicles do not mature into eggs, but persist and may become necrotic. This results in a 'lumpy mass' on radiographs, which can be further evaluated by means of ultrasound or CT.

Broken eggs and leakage of contents into the coelomic cavity leads to coelomitis, which is radiographically characterized by complete loss of intracoelomic detail and decreased size of the lung fields.

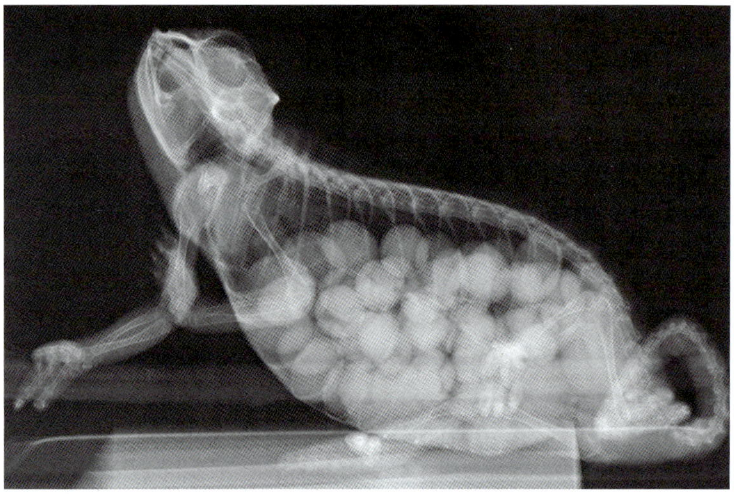

Fig. 21.31 Chameleon with a normal albeit large clutch. Note that these eggs physiologically do not have calcified shells. To minimize stress for the animal, the owner's transport box and associated wooden branch were used for positioning. The resultant asymmetric appearance of the patient is acceptable, as confirmation of a clutch was the only purpose of this radiograph.

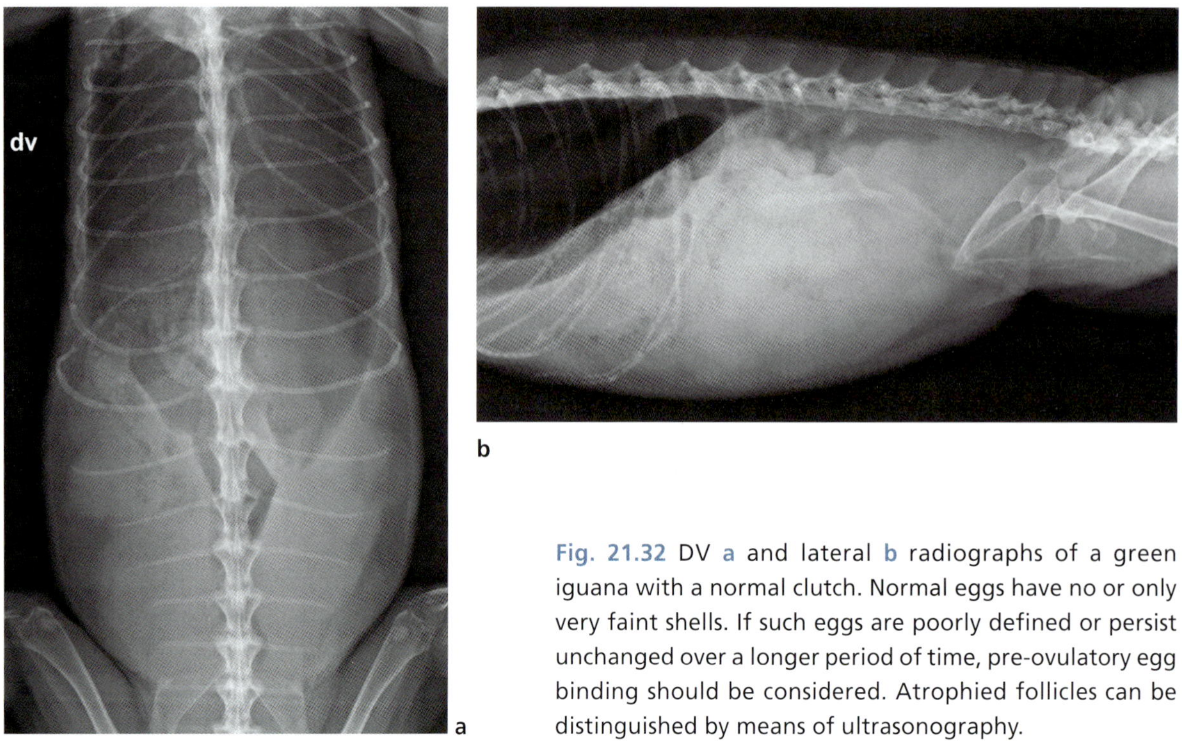

Fig. 21.32 DV a and lateral b radiographs of a green iguana with a normal clutch. Normal eggs have no or only very faint shells. If such eggs are poorly defined or persist unchanged over a longer period of time, pre-ovulatory egg binding should be considered. Atrophied follicles can be distinguished by means of ultrasonography.

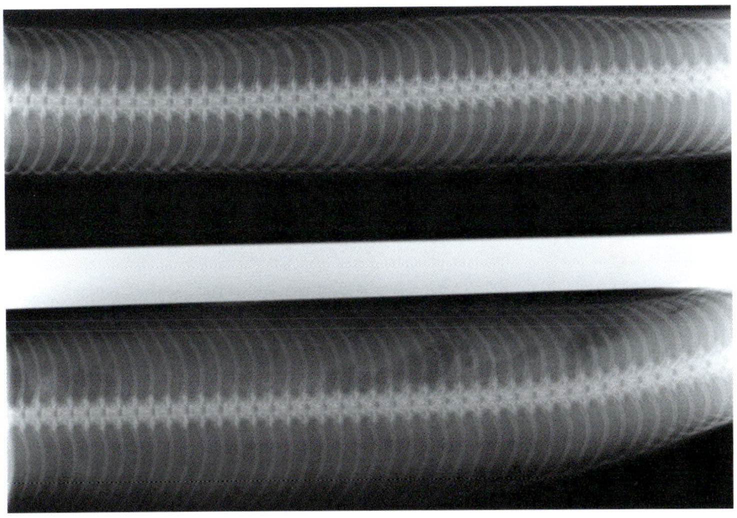

Fig. 21.33 Boa with symmetric and homogeneously soft-tissue opaque structures in the caudal half of the coelomic cavity (clutch). Vitality of the young in this viviparous species can be evaluated by means of ultrasonography.

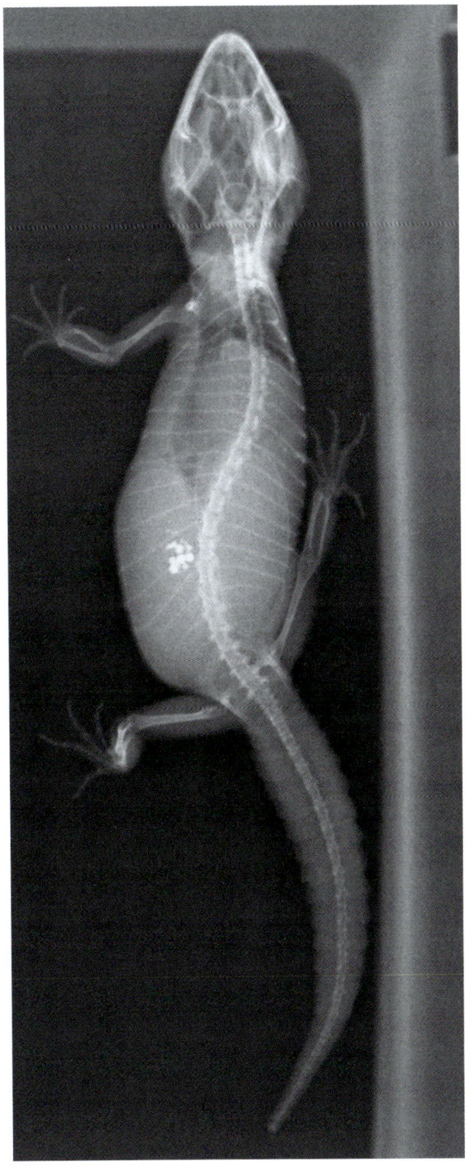

a

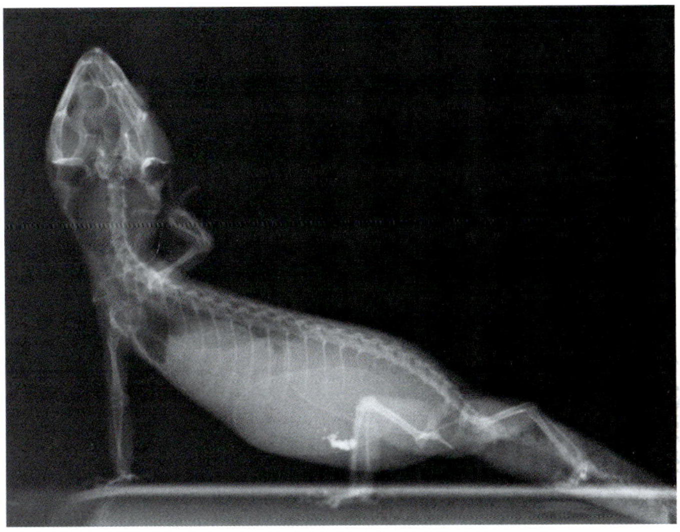

b

Fig. 21.34 DV a and lateral b radiographs of a leopard gecko with egg binding. These iguanas normally lay two eggs (as seen here), which are very large in relation to the parent animal and have an oblong shape. These eggs have soft shells (leathery when laid) to allow passage through the pelvis. The eggshells on these radiographs are notably opaque and thus too mineralized. The animal showed typical clinical signs of egg binding. Note compression of the lungs by the eggs. The patient was positioned in a thin plastic box, and on the lateral view, the animal attempted to climb up the wall, which did not interfere with diagnosis.

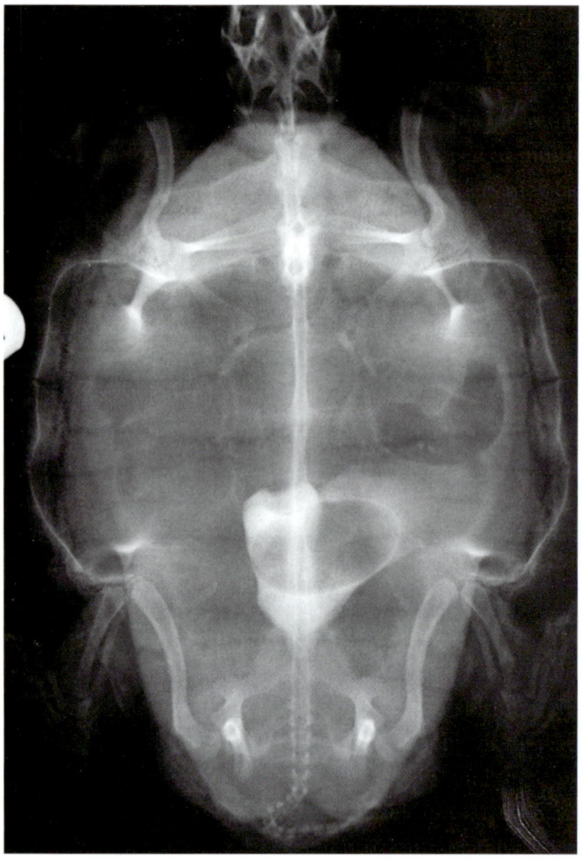

Fig. 21.35 Red-eared slider with an egg displaced into the urinary bladder. Attempts to stimulate egg laying using conservative means was unsuccessful, and a malposition was suspected. A retrograde contrast study of the urinary bladder confirms the suspicion.

21.10 Neoplastic disorders

Depending on their organ association, size and type, neoplastic lesions may be visible on routine survey radiographs. Skeletal neoplasia is rare and results in radiographic abnormalities similar to those seen in mammals (Fig. 21.36). The authors have seen one case of a vertebral metastasis secondary to renal adenocarcinoma (Fig. 21.37).

A diagnosis in chelonians is difficult as most inner organs, with the exception of the lungs, are radiographically difficult to distinguish. For a definitive diagnosis and to determine the organ association of a neoplastic process, a CT examination is usually necessary. Neoplastic diseases resulting in organomegaly are more readily diagnosed in snakes and lizards (Fig. 21.38) and may potentially be further evaluated by means of contrast studies or ultrasound.

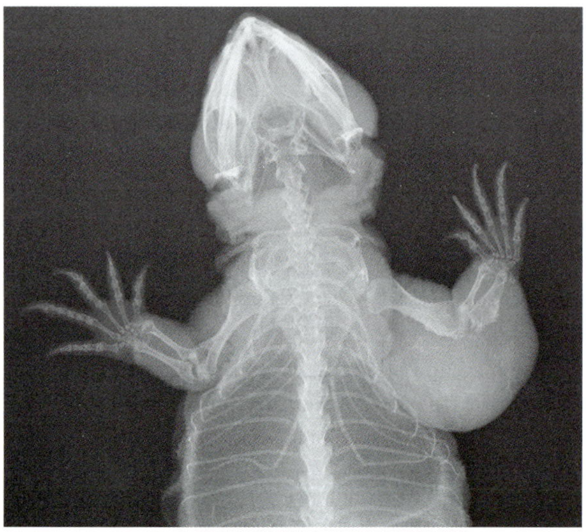

Fig. 21.36 DV view of the cranial half of a Spiny-tailed lizard. There is severe soft-tissue swelling of the left humerus with faint cloudy mineralization as well as severe periosteal reaction associated with the humerus and radius/ulna. The ultimate diagnosis was osteosarcoma.

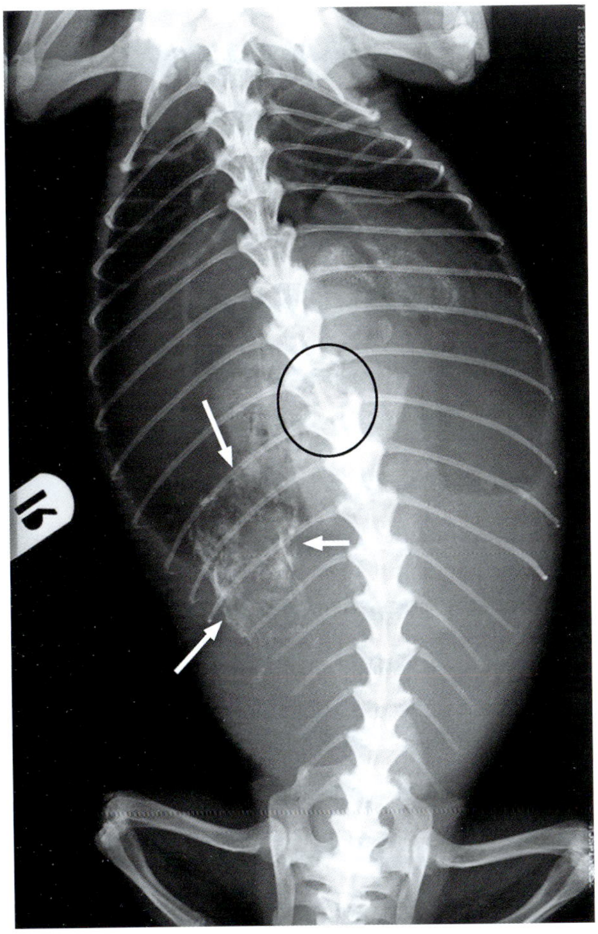

Fig. 21.37 Savannah monitor with a vertebral metastasis (circle). Heterogeneous mineral opaque material (arrows) initially resembling intestinal contents is associated with the right half of the coelomic cavity. However, these mineral opacities are located outside the intestinal tract. CT examination and subsequent necropsy identified mineralized renal neoplasia (adenocarcinoma) which was adherent to adjacent ribs. The lungs are displaced cranially and compressed by this mass lesion (R = right).

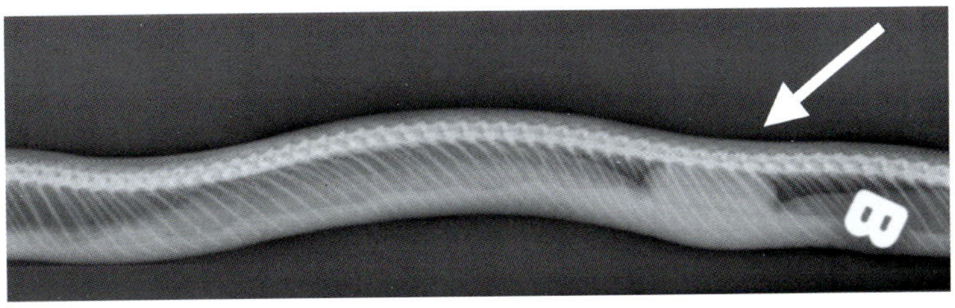

Fig. 21.38 Hepatic adenocarcinoma in a snake. The lateral view shows an ovoid mass lesion in the cranial third of the body (arrow). The diagnosis was established by means of ultrasound-guided fine-needle aspiration. Note the metallic marker ('B') used for orientation on this radiograph.

Suggested reading

Banzato T, Hellebuyck T, Vam Caelenberg A, Saunders JH, Zotti A. A review of diagnostic imaging of snakes and lizards. Vet Rec 2013; 173: 43–9.

Baur M. Untersuchungen zur vergleichenden Morphologie des Gastrointestinaltraktes der Schildkröten. Frankfurter Beiträge zur Naturkunde, Vol. 17. Frankfurt am Main: Edition Chimaira 2003; 373.

De la Navarre BJ. Common procedures in reptiles and amphibians. Vet Clin North Am Exot Anim Pract 2006; 9: 237–67.

DeShaw B, Schoenfeld A, Cook RA, Haramati N. Imaging of reptiles: A comparison study of various radiographic techniques. J Zoo Wildl Med 1996; 27: 364–70.

Filip T. Darstellung der Nieren griechischer Landschildkröten mittels Computertomographie nach intravenöser Kontrastmittelapplikation. Dissertation Vet Med, Univ Wien 2009; 95.

Garner MM, Hernandez-Divers SM, Raymond JT. Reptile neoplasia: a retrospective study of case submissions to a specialty diagnostic service. Vet Clin North Am Exot Anim Pract 2004; 7: 653–71.

Gumpenberger M. Untersuchungen am Harntrakt und weiblichen Genitaltrakt von Schildkröten mit Hilfe bildgebender Diagnostik. Dissertation Vet Med, Univ Wien 1996.

Gumpenberger M. Diagnostic imaging of dyspnoic chelonians. In: Seybold J, Mutschmann F (eds). Proceedings of the 7th International Symposium of Pathology and Medicine of Reptiles and Amphibians (Berlin 2004). Edition Chimaira 2007; 217–22.

Gumpenberger M. Diagnostic imaging of reproductive tract disorders in reptiles. Vet Clin North Am Exot Anim Pract 2017; 20: 327–43.

Gumpenberger M., Filip T. Bildgebende Diagnostik verschiedener Formen von Legenot bei Schildkröten und deren Therapie: Fallbeispiele. Wien Tierärztl Monat 2001; 88(3): 70–8.

Gumpenberger M, Hittmair K. Möglichkeiten der bildgebenden Diagnostik beim Urogenitaltrakt von Schildkröten. Erkrankungen der Zoo- und Wildtiere 1997; 38: 77–85.

Innis CJ, Boyer TH. Chelonian reproductive disorders. Vet Clin North Am Exot Anim Pract 2002; 5: 555–78.

Karlo, H. Röntgenologische Normalanatomie und gastrointestinale Kontrastmittelstudien bei Bartagamen (*Pogona vitticeps*). Dissertation Vet Med, Univ Wien 2009; 103.

Meyer J. Gastrografin as a gastrointestinal contrast agent in the Greek tortoise *(Testudo hermanni)*. J Zoo Wildl Med 1998; 29: 183–9.

Mitchell MA, Diaz-Figueroa O. Clinical reptile gastroenterology. Vet Clin North Am Exot Anim Pract 2005; 8: 277–98.

Rübel GA, Isenbügel E, Wolvekamp P. Atlas der Röntgendiagnostik bei Heimtieren. Hannover: Schlütersche 1991.

Schildger BJ. Endoskopie bei Reptilien. Dissertation Vet Med Habil, Justus-Liebig-Universität Giessen 1999.

Schumacher J, Toal RL. Advanced radiography and ultrasonography in reptiles. Sem Avian Exot Pet Med 2001; 10: 162–8.

Schumacher J. Reptile respiratory medicine. Vet Clin North Am Exot Anim Pract 2003; 6: 213–31.

Selleri P, Hernandez-Divers SJ. Renal diseases of reptiles. Vet Clin North Am Exot Anim Pract. 2006; 9: 161–74.

Silverman S. Diagnostic imaging. In: Mader DR (ed.). Reptile Medicine and Surgery. St. Louis: Saunders-Elsevier 2006; 471–89.

Sinn AD. Pathologie der Reptilien. Eine retrospektive Studie. Dissertation Vet Med, Ludwig-Maximilians-Universität München 2004.

Taylor SK, Citino SB, Zdziarski JM, Bush RM. Radiographic anatomy and barium sulfate transit time of the gastrointestinal tract of the leopard tortoise *(Testudo pardalis)*. J Zoo Wildl Med 1996; 27: 180–6.

Williams J. Orthopedic radiography in exotic animal practice. Vet Clin North Am Exot Anim Pract 2002; 5: 1–22.

Index

The suffixes *f* and *t* indicate a figure or table on that page, respectively